W9-CDB-389

2-cc

(UPP)

TCH CARDIOLOGY

Cardiovascular
Flow Dynamics
and
Measurements

CARDIOVASCULAR FLOW DYNAMICS AND MEASUREMENTS

Edited by
Ned H. C. Hwang, Ph.D.
Cardiovascular Flow Dynamics Laboratory
Department of Civil Engineering
University of Houston

and
Nils A. Normann, M.D.
Cardiovascular Engineering Laboratories
Department of Surgery
Baylor College of Medicine

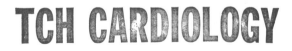

University Park Press
Baltimore · London · Tokyo

UNIVERSITY PARK PRESS
International Publishers in Science and Medicine
Chamber of Commerce Building
Baltimore, Maryland 21202

Copyright © 1977 by University Park Press

Typeset by The Composing Room of Michigan, Inc.
Manufactured in the United States of America by Universal Lithographers,
Inc., and The Optic Bindery Incorporated

Library of Congress Cataloging in Publication Data

Nato Advanced Study Institute on Cardiovascular Flow
Dynamics, Houston, Tex., 1975.
Cardiovascular flow dynamics and measurements.
Includes index.
1. Blood flow—Measurement—Congresses.
2. Hemodynamics—Congresses. 3. Cardiovascular
system—Diseases—Congresses. 4. Heart, Artificial
—Congresses. I. Hwang, Ned H. C. II. Normann,
Nils A. III. North Atlantic Treaty Organization.
Division of Scientific Affairs. IV. United States.
National Science Foundation. V. Title. [DNLM:
1. Hemodynamics—Congresses. 2. Flowmeters—
Congresses. 3. Heart, Artificial—Congresses.
WG106 N111c 1975]
RC691.6.B55N37 1975 616.1'3'0754 76-56204
ISBN 0-8391-0972-5

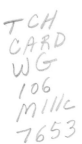

TCH CARDIOLOGY

CONTENTS

CONTRIBUTORS

Tetsuzo Akutsu, M.D., Cardiovascular Surgical Research Laboratories, Texas Heart Institute, St. Luke's Episcopal Hospital and Texas Children's Hospital, Houston, Texas 77025

Max Anliker, Ph.D., Institut für Biomedizinische Technik der Universität Zürich und der Eidgenössischen Technischen Hockschule Zürich, CH-8044 Zürich, Switzerland

Donald W. Baker, B.S.E.E., Center for Bioengineering, University of Washington, Seattle, Washington 98195

Clarence H. Brown, III, M.D., Department of Medicine, Baylor College of Medicine, Houston, Texas 77030

G. C. van den Bos, M.D., Laboratory for Physiology, Free University, Amsterdam, The Netherlands

E. S. Bücherl, M.D., Department of Surgery, Free University Berlin, Berlin, West Germany

Joseph P. Buckley, Ph.D., Director of Cardiovascular Research, College of Pharmacy, University of Houston, Houston, Texas 77004

Colin G. Caro, M.D., F.R.C.P.E., Physiological Flow Studies Unit, Imperial College of Science and Technology, London SW7 2AZ, England

Corrado Casci, D. Eng., Instituto di Macchine, Politecnico de Milano, Milano, Italy

Max Casty, Ph.D., Institut für Biomedizinische Technik der Universität Zürich und der Eidgenössischen Technischen Hochschule Zürich, CH-8004 Zürich, Switzerland

Shu Chien, M.D., Ph.D., Laboratory of Hemorheology, Department of Physiology, Columbia University College of Physicians and Surgeons, New York, New York 10032

Ruben Cronestrand, M.D., Department of Surgery, Vascular Unit, Royal Caroline Institute, Huddinge Hospital, Huddinge S-141 86, Sweden

Ronald E. Daigle, Ph.D., Center for Bioengineering, University of Washington, Seattle, Washington 98195

G. Elzinga, Ph.D., Laboratory for Physiology, Free University, Amsterdam, The Netherlands

Paul Friedli, Ph.D., Institut für Biomedizinische Technik der Universität Zürich und der Eidgenössischen Technischen Hochschule Zürich, CH-8044 Zürich, Switzerland

Roberto Fumero, D. Eng., Instituto di Macchine, Politecnico di Milano, Milano, Italy

Yuan-Cheng B. Fung, M.D., Department of Applied Mechanics and Engineering Science/Bioengineering, University of California, San Diego; La Jolla, California 92093

J. David Hellums, Ph.D., Rice University, Houston, Texas 77001

G. Wyckliffe Hoffler, M.D., NASA-Johnson Space Center, Houston, Texas 77058

A. K. M. Fazle Hussain, Ph.D., Department of Mechanical Engineering, University of Houston, Houston, Texas 77004

Ned H. C. Hwang, Ph.D., Cardiovascular Flow Dynamics Laboratory, Department of Civil Engineering, University of Houston, Houston, Texas 77044

Bhagavan S. Jandhyala, Ph.D., Department of Pharmacology, College of Pharmacy, University of Houston, Houston, Texas 77004

Carl E. Jones, Ph.D., Texas A & M University, Office of Medical Careers, Olin E. Teague Research Center, College Station, Texas 77843

Herbert Keller, Ph.D., Neurologische Klinik der Universität Zürich, CH-8006 Zürich, Switzerland

Rudolf Kubli, M.S.E. E., Institut für Biomedizinische Technik der Universität Zürich und der Eidgenössischen Technischen Hochschule Zürich, CH-8044 Zürich, Switzerland

Niels A. Lassen, M.D., Department of Clinical Physiology, Bispebjerg Hospital, DK-2400 Copenhagen NV, Denmark

John H. Lawson, Ph.D., Division of Artificial Organs, University of Utah, Salt Lake City, Utah 84112

Mustafa Lokhandwala, Ph.D., Department of Pharmacology, College of Pharmacy, University of Houston, Houston, Texas 77004

Rainer Mohnhaupt, Dipl. Ing., Chirurgische Universitätsklinik der Freien Universität Berlin, Berlin, West Germany

Franco Montevecchi, D. Eng., Instituto di Macchine, Politecnico di Milano, Milano, Italy

Robert M. Nerem, Ph.D., Physiological Fluid Mechanics Group, The Ohio State University Bio-Medical Engineering Center, Columbus, Ohio 43210

George P. Noon, M.D., Department of Surgery, Baylor College of Medicine, Houston, Texas 77030

Nils A. Normann, M.D., Cardiovascular Engineering Laboratories, Department of Surgery, Baylor College of Medicine, Houston, Texas 77030

Kim A. Parker, Ph.D., Physiological Flow Studies Unit, Imperial College of Science and Technology, London SW7 2AZ, England

Dali J. Patel, M.D., Ph.D., Vascular Physiology Section, Laboratory of Experimental Atherosclerosis, National Heart and Lung Institute, National Institutes of Health, Bethesda, Maryland 20014

Margot R. Roach, M.D., Ph.D., Departments of Biophysics and Medicine, University of Western Ontario, London N6A 5C1, Canada

P. Sipkema, Ph.D., Laboratory for Physiology, Free University, Amsterdam, The Netherlands

Sidney S. Sobin, M.D., Los Angeles County Heart Association, University of Southern California Cardiovascular Research Laboratory, University of Southern California Medical Center, Los Angeles, California 90033

D. Eugene Strandness, Jr., M.D., Department of Surgery, University of Washington School of Medicine, Seattle, Washington 98195

Volker Unger, Dipl. Ing., Chirurgische Universitätsklinik der Freien Universität Berlin, Berlin, West Germany

Ramesh N. Vaishnav, Ph.D., Department of Civil Engineering, The Catholic University of America, Washington, D.C. 20064

Regis R. Vollmer, Ph.D., Department of Pharmacology, College of Pharmacy, University of Houston, Houston, Texas 77004

N. Westerhof, Ph.D., Laboratory for Physiology, Free University, Amsterdam, The Netherlands

Derek G. Wyatt, Ph.D., Nuffield Institute for Medical Research, Oxford OX3 9DS, England

PREFACE

This volume contains the lectures presented at the 1975 NATO Advanced Study Institute on Cardiovascular Flow Dynamics, jointly sponsored by the NATO Scientific Affairs Division and the U.S. National Science Foundation. The Institute, held in Houston, Texas, October 6–17, was composed of twenty-seven invited lecturers and one hundred selected participants from eighteen countries.

The stated purpose of the NATO Advanced Study Institute Program is "the dissemination of advanced knowledge and the formation of contacts among scientists of different countries." The NATO Study Institutes differ from most international conferences and symposia by their tutorial character, the limited number of participants, and the availability of fellowships.

During the five years since the NATO-AGARD conference on "Biofluid Dynamics" in Naples in 1970, technological advances have produced new tools both for research and for clinical applications, resulting in new insights into hemodynamic mechanisms operative under normal and abnormal cardiovascular conditions. At the core of these developments is the productive interaction between individuals from engineering, physical sciences, and life sciences; the overall aim of this Institute has been to further such interactions. Thus, the program was structured to provide interdisciplinary, high level teaching, permitting in-depth treatment of each selected subject matter.

The present Institute was initiated by N. H. C. Hwang; members of the Organizing Committee were M. Anliker, N. H. C. Hwang (Director), T. Kester (NATO-SAD), N. A. Normann (Secretary), and N. Westerhof. Academic sponsors were the University of Houston and Baylor College of Medicine; the Continuing Education Center on the University of Houston campus provided ample facilities.

Based on the 1975 NATO Advanced Study Institute on Cardiovascular Flow Dynamics, jointly sponsored by the NATO Scientific Affairs Division and the U.S. National Science Foundation; held in Houston, October 6–17, 1975.

ACKNOWLEDGMENTS

On behalf of all participants, we herewith express our gratitude to NATO-Scientific Affairs Division and the U.S. National Science Foundation for making this two-week Study Institute possible. We very much appreciate the additional budgetary support received from the Fondren Foundation and the University of Houston, support made available through the efforts of Patrick J. Nicholson, Vice President of University Development; Charles V. Kirkpatrick, Dean of Cullen College of Engineering; and Francis B. Smith, Director, Office of Research and Sponsored Activities.

We thank our colleagues Ardis H. White and George Pincus for generously contributing their time, coming to our rescue in unexpected, problematic situations. We further acknowledge the excellent performance of the staffs of the Continuing Education and the Engineering Media Centers. We are especially indebted to Judy Barnett for her untiring and proficient editorial assistance. Our wives Maria and Stephanie deserve credit and thanks for their valuable suggestions and enthusiastic support.

Frequently, the note on which a meeting starts and the note on which it ends contribute framework and perspective. We were very fortunate to have the opening lecture given by Michael E. DeBakey and the closing address delivered by Arthur C. Guyton. Their active participation contributed not only luster to the Institute, but also strong moral support in our endeavor to promote international and interdisciplinary communication and collaboration.

N. H. C. Hwang
N. A. Normann

Cardiovascular
Flow Dynamics
and
Measurements

introduction

AN ENGINEERING SURVEY OF PROBLEMS IN CARDIOVASCULAR FLOW DYNAMICS

Ned H. C. Hwang

> ... I have only one excuse, but I believe it is sound: the duty, today more imperative than ever, which is incumbent on scientists to consider their discipline within the larger framework of modern culture, with a view to enriching the latter not only with technically important findings, but also with what they may feel to be humanly significant ideas arising from their area of special concern. The very ingenuousness of a fresh look at things (and science possesses an ever-youthful eye) may sometimes shed a new light upon old problems.
> ~Jacques Monod, *Chance and Necessity*~

Over the past 10 years, research in cardiovascular dynamics has not only grown considerably in size, but also in depth in some areas. Intensive efforts made by both medical and physical scientists, under the constant encouragement and support of governments and industries, have helped to establish many beachheads. Some substantial advances have been made to formulate new concepts and techniques that have been instrumental in discovering new causes and cures of some cardiovascular diseases. In the meantime, however, many research activities remain confused and flustering experiences. A periodic survey of our problems in the field and a

1

continuing effort to improve communication, or exchange of experience, are essential to keep this research moving in a forward direction.

In this chapter, a brief categorical survey is made on the flow dynamics problems involved in current cardiovascular research. The background materials are intended for those who are new or have an interest in the field. It is hoped that this chapter can be an introduction to the field for many, and to the comprehensive chapters in the book for others. My experiences in flow measurements are added to those who made major contributions in the various selected topics in the field. Several cardio-vascular flow dynamics models are briefly discussed to clarify certain basic conceptions of their significance, limitations, and applications.

Problems in cardiovascular flow dynamics may generally be classified into three categories. They are (a) problems in predictions—largely of physiologic concerns: (b) problems in applications—largely of clinical concerns; and (c) problems in measurement—both physiologic and clinical. To make an introductory survey of these categories, it is probably best to begin with a brief review of the physical properties of the cardiovascular system and the role of flow dynamics.

PHYSICAL PROPERTIES OF THE CARDIOVASCULAR SYSTEM

From an engineer's point of view, the cardiovascular system provides a field rich with flow dynamics problems. Fluid engineers have been attracted to the field from several fronts. First of all, the fact that blood flow in the cardiovascular system is basically pulsatile suggested many fluid dynamics problems that may never have been tackled during all the vast accumulation of knowledge in conventional fluid dynamics (Lighthill, 1972). Second, that the complex vascular network contains a living fluid flowing at a wide range of velocities offers great challenge in measurement. The cardiovascular system also poses a unique challenge in the design and development of circulatory prostheses and blood-contacting instrumentation. As a living fluid, blood is quite different from all other engineering fluids in many ways.

With respect to flow dynamics, description of the cardiovascular system may begin at the heart. The heart is a pair of pulsatile pumps synchronized to act simultaneously through periodic contraction of the heart muscles. Each of the pumps has two chambers. The collecting chamber is known as the atrium, and the pumping chamber is known as the ventricle. Although the two pumps are part of one organ, the architecture of the two pumps is quite different, as are their flow dynamics properties. The two pumps are arranged in series such that the outputs from the ventricles are approximately equal in quantity. The right heart forces blood through the pulmonary arteries to the lungs, where carbon dioxide is exchanged for oxygen (pulmonary circulation). The oxygenated blood is carried from the lungs through pulmonary veins to the left heart. Contraction of the left heart forces the oxygenated blood into the aorta, by which the blood is distributed to the various tissues of the body (systemic circulation).

Unidirectional flow of blood through each side of the heart is made possible by a set of two unidirectional valves in the heart. In the left heart the mitral valve is located between the left atrium and the left ventricle and the aortic valve is located between the left ventricle and the aorta. The valves in the right heart are the tricuspid valve, which is located between the right atrium and the right ventricle, and the pulmonary valve, located between the right ventricle and the pulmonary trunk. When ventricular pressure falls below atrial pressure, blood flow through the atrioventricular valves commences to fill the ventricles. During heart contraction, ventricular pressure rises above atrial pressure and the valves close to prevent retrograde flow into the atria. In the meantime, both the aortic valve and the pulmonary valve open to let the total cardiac output flow through. They close during diastole. Heart valves are thin, leaflet-type, membrane structures dynamically sensitive to the directions of the phasically changing local pressure gradients.

A normal adult heart beats at a rate of approximately 80 beats/min, at rest, with a cardiac output close to 7 liters/min. The heart rate and cardiac output may both increase according to physiologic demands. During vigorous exercise, a normal heart may deliver up to 35 liters of blood in 1 min at a heart rate of 180 beats/min.

An adult aorta has a diameter of approximately 25 mm near the aortic arch, where the wall thickness is approximately 2 mm. The aortic wall is quite elastic and stores a large portion of the cardiac energy during the ventricular ejaculation. This stored elastic energy is returned to the blood stream during diastole to drive the blood continuously downstream. The aortic diameter decreases gradually as the major arteries branch from the aortic trunk. The major arteries branch into numerous small arteries, which again branch into smaller arterioles. The arterioles feed into the capillary beds, where active diffusion and exchange of substances take place.

The venules collect blood from the other end of the capillary beds and drain it to the terminal veins. Large veins transport blood from the main venous branches to the vena cava, from which the blood flows into the right heart. The systemic veins also act as a reservoir for blood volume. It is estimated that up to 75% of the total blood volume, normally 7 liters, may be stored when the body is at rest.

Pulmonary circulation begins when blood leaves the right ventricle during ventricular contraction. Under relatively low pressure, compared with that of the systemic circulation, the blood is pumped into the pulmonary artery, which has approximately the same diameter as the aorta. The main pulmonary artery trunk extends only a few centimeters before dividing into left and right main branches. Subsequent branching of the pulmonary arteries follows approximately a pattern in which each artery divides into two daughter branches of unequal cross section until the capillaries are reached. The pulmonary capillaries, connecting to the pulmonary alveoli, form a very complex network where exchange of carbon dioxide for oxygen takes place. A venous tree collects oxygenated blood at the other end of the capillary bed, converging in ways similar to the pulmonary arterial tree, but in reverse. Through the left and right pulmonary veins, the blood is drained into the left heart. Several hypotheses have been proposed on the mechanics of pulmonary circulation. But, it was not until recently that the concept of blood circulation and gas exchange has been made clear by a mathematical model suggested by Fung, who presents a comprehensive chapter on the subject in this book. A schematic representation of the systemic and pulmonary circulations is given in Netter (1969).

Basically, all blood-vessel walls are composites of four important types of tissue: (a) The blood-contacting, endothelial lining provides a smooth pavement layer for blood flow. It also offers a selective permeability to water, sugar, red cells, and other substances passing between the blood stream and the surrounding tissues. (b) The elastic fibers form a layer just behind the endothelial lining. These fibers behave very much like coil springs. They can be extended many times their unstretched length and closely follow Hooke's law of elasticity before reaching the elastic limit. The function of elastic fibers is to provide elastic tension, which stores a large portion of the cardiac energy in potential form during systole. (c) The collagen fibers have a modulus of elasticity several hundred times greater than that of the elastic fibers. The collagen fibers are slackly folded in the vessel walls so that the vessel produces a high resistance to distension

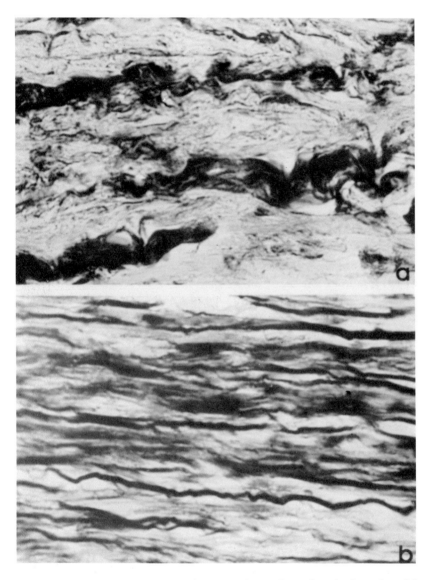

Figure 1. A: Optical micrograph of relaxed bovine aortic specimen in circumferential direction. Collagen stains are dark and elastin stains are gray (X 1500). B: Same specimen extended to λ = 1.50 (X 1500). (From Armeniades, Lake, and Missirlis, 1973.)

once the limit is approached. As an example, Figures 1A and B show the optical micrographs (1500X) of a bovine aortic specimen in relaxed and extended states, respectively. (d) The smooth vascular muscles produce active tension by contraction under physiologic controls so as to physically change the diameter of the lumen of the vessel. The greatest control of smooth muscle is in the arterioles, where it provides up to 90% of the total peripheral resistance in systemic circulation.

FLOW DYNAMIC
MEASUREMENTS IN CARDIOVASCULAR SYSTEMS

Flow dynamic measurement in the cardiovascular systems generally refers to the measurement of pressure, volumetric flow rates, or time dependent velocities in the systems. Generally speaking, measurements in cardiovascular systems are rather difficult. Not only are the measurements made on unsteady flow phenomena, but also the physical frame of reference is always moving. The heart, for example, moves in a very complex mode. To describe in precise terms the motion of the ventricular wall alone is a major task. All major blood vessels and organs move with various magnitudes that rarely can be ignored in dynamic measurements. Attempts to fix the system temporarily for dynamic measurements usually results in distortion of vessel or organ shapes, which may cause erroneous measurement results. Physiologic changes may also take place during, or because of, the measurements. With all these considerations, the reader should be forewarned that the in vivo flow dynamic measurements in cardiovascular systems are made to aid our comprehension of the system, not for exactness or meticulous precision.

Measurement of Pressure

The range of pressures in the cardiovascular system may vary from 150 mm Hg in the left ventricle to practically zero (atmospheric pressure) in the capillary beds. The periodic, pulsatile pressure waves have the same basic frequency as that of the heart.

Indirect measurements of arterial blood pressure based on Korotkoffs' sounds (Burton, 1972) are extensively used in medical practice. This is largely a clinical device, because the method provides only the systolic and diastolic pressure readings and gives no information about the pressure wave forms. Several investigators have studied the origin of the Korotkoffs' sounds; conclusions vary from laminar vortices in blood to blood turbulence, or even to vessel wall stresses. It is, however, not in the interest of this survey to review these works.

The basic requirement in cardiovascular pressure measurements is to register faithfully the *pressure variations.* This process usually involves a transducer that is in direct contact with the blood and is capable of converting the mechanical (pressure) variations into electrical signals. The signals are then amplified and recorded in a permanent or semipermanent form. In processing the signals, a certain degree of distortion from the original phenomena is expected. Precautions, therefore, must be exercised to ensure that the distortion of the pressure information is within the acceptable range and that the distortion itself is not a variable of environment or time.

For each transducer, a basic constant proportionality should be maintained between the steady level of the pressure and the recorded signal level within the measured pressure range. This proportionality can be tested and determined by a simple calibration procedure.

Faithful measurement of dynamic pressure depends, among other things, on the frequency response of the transducer. Based on Fourier (linear) theory, repeated pressure wave forms can be considered as the algebraic sum of a mean pressure value and a series of sinusoidal waves of appropriate amplitudes and phases, known as the Fourier components. For pressure waves in cardiovascular systems, the lowest frequency is the frequency of the heart and the other frequencies are integral multiples of the heart rate. It is generally believed that harmonic components higher than the tenth may not be significant to the signals. As a general rule, a transducer with a flat amplitude response of ten times that of the heart frequency, in beats per second, is adequate for most purposes. For example, for a heart rate of 120 beats/min, or 2 beats/sec, a transducer with frequency response to 20 Hz is considered sufficient.

Ideally, the pressure transducer should be placed in the field of measurement to avoid any possible transient disturbances. However, in physiologic measurements in living subjects, this is not always feasible. In many cases, catheters are used to lead the pressure signals from the field being measured to a transducer, placed a certain distance away, through liquid-filled transmission lines.

Depending on the physical properties of the transmission line and the liquid within, various transient disturbances could be introduced; these disturbances may result in great distortion of the original signals. The major concern of this type of connection is the compliance of the catheter tube. Generally speaking, the stiffer the catheter walls and the shorter the catheter length, the better the response of the system. A more rigid diaphragm in the pressure transducer also improves the fidelity of the system. Unfortunately, most of these suggested conditions are quite contradictory to those required in laboratory or clinical practices. For example, in order to bring the transducer to the field through the complicated geometry of arterial (or venous) pathways, the catheter wall must be made of rather soft and pliable materials; in cardiac catheterization of a patient, the catheter tube must be made a certain length (say, 1 meter) in order to reach the heart.

For each type of application, the catheter must be designed to meet certain requirements, while many "secondary" physical properties of the system may thus be ignored. It is, therefore, most important for the physiologist or physician who uses the catheter in the laboratory to have an adequate knowledge of the dynamics of the system. Basic understanding of properties of hydraulic transmission lines, dynamic damping, system resonance, and frequency response of the system is necessary. This information serves not only as a basis for the selection of a suitable catheter for each particular case; it also helps in making proper interpolations from the measured data.

Pressure measurements in smaller, terminal blood vessels are usually rather difficult tasks. The techniques, largely of interest in research, are limited to a few laboratories at the present time. Block (1966) reported measurements of fluctuation pressure in blood vessels down to 35 μ with a capacitance tranducer (full-scale range, 4–400 mm Hg). In his experiment, a microbore Pyrex tubing was used to connect the blood vessel and the transducer with a short cannula. Frequency response of 30–50 Hz was reported although in situ calibration procedure was not mentioned. Wiederhelm (1966) reported the use of an electrolyte-filled micropipet with a tip diameter of 0.5–5 μ. Since the electrolyte within the micropipet had a much higher electric conductivity than that of the body fluids, the fluctuation of the electrical resistance between the pipet and the external fluid was measured as the blood forced the electrolyte back into the pipet when its tip penetrated the lumen of a small blood vessel. A frequency response of 50 Hz was reported with this technique and the full-scale linearity was reported to be within 3%.

Implantable pressure transducers are used in chronic animal experiments. Most of the implantable transducers currently used in physiologic studies are the bonded strain-gauge type. The transducers are usually implanted directly in the field to be measured. The transducer surface, which is exposed to the blood stream, is coated with a thin layer of silicone film to inhibit blood clot formation. Most commercially manufactured implantable transducers have very good frequency response (up to 1 kHz), which is adequate for measurement of the wide frequency range that can be obtained in animal experiments. Because there is no connecting tubing needed between the field and the transducers, damping problems do not exist in this type of measuring system. The transducer body can be rather small (typically, 5 mm in diameter). With proper precaution, very accurate measurements of pressure or pressure differential can be obtained in situ if the transducer can be properly calibrated.

Unfortunately, in situ calibration has always been a major problem in using the implanted pressure transducer, because the strain-gauge type transducers are generally sensitive to environmental temperature changes. A strain-gauge transducer may be affected by the environmental temperature in two ways: the strain-gauge output per unit change of pressure may vary, and the baseline zero reading may be shifted. The latter usually shows a more marked change (zero shift) and may cause considerable difficulties even when rather sophisticated temperature-compensation techniques are employed.

Measurement of Flows

Measurement of blood flow in the cardiovascular system is usually carried out to determine (a) volumetric flow rate through a particular vessel (say, in liters per minute), or (b) the velocity of the blood stream at a particular point in the vessel, or (c) the fluctuations of blood velocity (both in magnitude and direction) at a certain point in the flowing blood. The high-frequency fluctuations are sometimes loosely called "turbulence" in blood flow.

In most of the relevant experiments, special instruments are designed for each of these measurements. The techniques involved in each measurement may also be different. For this reason, simultaneous measurements of two or more of the above are rarely made in an experiment at the present time. Ideally, the volumetric flow rate (a) is measured by a device, known as the flowmeter, whose output is proportional to the total volume of fluid that flows through the vessel in a given time. Categories (b) and (c) are measured by a velocity probe (commonly known as anemometer or velometer) whose output is proportional to the speed of the fluid passing the probe; it gives no account of the environment.

Determination of volumetric flow rate in a particular blood vessel has long been a clinical concern. Many clinical methods had been developed before the more sophisticated, modern instruments were commercially available. Plethysmography, as originally described by Brodie and Russell in 1905, has been used to measure total blood flow in a limb by briefly occluding the venous flow. Complete stoppage of venous return from the limb was achieved for a few seconds with a pressurized occluding cuff surrounding the limb. Then measurements were made to determine the volume change of the limb tissue distal to the cuff during the period of occlusion. It has been shown that the initial rate of volume change during the venous occlusion is equal to that of the arterial inflow. Since the venous pressure is normally much lower than the arterial pressure, it was assumed that the arterial inflow to the limb remains relatively constant and is unaffected by the cuff operation. In practice, a number of pressure levels are usually tested before the most suitable collapsive pressure is selected (Strandness, 1969). Several different types of plethysmographic equipment have been employed to measure the limb volume change. Air-filled and water-filled plethysomographs directly measure the volume change by recording the fluid displacement. The mercury strain-gauge type measures the change in limb girth, which is presumed to be linearly proportional to the volume change. The plethysmograph method, although considered a very useful and reliable method for clinical measurement of limb perfusion rate (Terry et al., 1974), provides no information as to the distribution of blood flow in any particular vessel.

The indicator-dilution method, first suggested by Fick in 1870, has become a very popular method in both laboratories and clinical practice. The method has been used clinically to determine cardiac output in patients for routine screening. It has also been used during surgery to monitor cardiac performance. With the addition of a small, built-in analog computer currently available in a commercial unit, the measurement has become very reliable. The indicator-dilution method requires a sudden injection of a certain type of indicator, such as a dye (tricarbocyanine), a thermal substance (chilled saline), or a radioactive substance, into the circulatory system. The indicator continuously mixes with the blood-stream that is passing through the vessel segment, resulting in a gradual dilution of the concentration of the indicator. The concentration is continuously monitored at a downstream station for some time after the injection.

Assuming that perfect mixing takes place instantly inside the vessel segment, a rapid rise of indicator concentration can be expected at a downstream observation site immediately after the beginning of the injection (allowing a short time lag to transport the substance from the injection site to the observation site). Thereafter, the observed concentration should gradually decay to half of its peak value at the end of the first period. The time period needed to reach the *half-value* is inversely related to the flow rate. Another equal period is needed again for the concentration to decay to half the value at the end of the first period, and so on. As a result, an exponential curve can be expected on a constant-speed recording strip when the indicator concentration is plotted against time after the injection. This curve is commonly known as the indicator-dilution curve. Based on this curve, the flow rate in the vessel can be calculated because it is inversely proportional to the area under the curve (Clark, 1967; Ganz and Swan, 1972).

The dilution technique has been used largely to determine cardiac output by passing the indicator through the heart chamber, which has been proven to be a very effective mixing pool. When the technique is applied to the measurement of blood flow rate in peripheral vessels, incomplete mixing of blood and indicator in the vessel may invalidate the method. Early theories attempted to relate the incomplete mixing to the Reynolds number of the blood vessel (defined as a ratio of the product of the mean velocity and vessel diameter to the kinematic viscosity of blood). However, in a series of experiments, our results indicate that the mixing pattern is also closely associated with the Reynolds number of the injecting jetstream (based on the jetstream velocity, jet diameter, and the kinematic viscosity of the indicator fluid). The observation was made in a series of in vitro experiments of pulsatile flow in straight plexiglas tubings (diameters varied from 3 to 20 mm).

Several operational variables are usually involved in the indicator dilution technique, such as the injectate volume, injectate solution concentration, and the catheter configuration, variations of which may alter the accuracy of the final results. On the other hand, if the injection time is kept relatively short, the final result of a dilution measurement is not affected by either the time or the mode of injection. A comprehensive review of the indicator dilution technique was given by Guyton (1963) and Guyton, Jones, and Coleman (1973). The effects of each parameter and variable involved are discussed in detail.

Cardiac output may also be measured by means of an electrical impedance method. The method is based upon the assumption that the thorax may be treated as though electrically equivalent to a homogeneous cylinder of blood; the electric resistance of the cylinder is proportional to the resistivity and the distance between the two metal band electrodes enclosing the thorax, and inversely proportional to the equivalent cross-sectional area of the cylinder. Because there is no run-off of blood from the thorax, the entire quantity of blood ejected changes the impedance of the cylinder as the "diameter" of the cylinder is assumed to increase uniformly with the ejection of blood from the heart. A small sinusoidal electric current in the frequency range 20–100 KHz is applied to two outer electrodes, of which one encircles the neck and the other encircles the abdomen. The impedance is measured from the two inner bands, which are placed at L distance apart. The impedance method provides a harmless, noninvasive method of continuously monitoring the stroke volume and cardiac output in a patient. The experimental results indicated overestimation of both stroke volume and cardiac output by the method. However, the magnitudes of changes in quantities are comparable with the other methods of measurements (Baker and Denniston, 1974; Geddes and Baker, 1975).

The electromagnetic flow meter is designed and operated on the principle of electromagnetic induction, discovered by the English physicist Michael Faraday in 1831; the principle states that when an electrical conductor moves across a magnetic field, an electric potential is created in the conductor. Since blood is an electric conductor, its flow in a vessel may be measured by first creating an electromagnetic field across the blood vessel, and then measuring the induced electric potential. It has been shown that if the dimension of the magnetic field and the physical properties of the conductor are kept constant, the generated electric potential varies linearly with the average velocity of the blood flow in the field.

Most of the commercially available electromagnetic flowmeter probes are the cuff (perivascular) type, designed to fit onto the outside diameter of the blood vessel. A tight fit between the vessel adventitia and the inner wall of the probe is essential. Intravascular catheter-tip mounted electromagnetic flowmeter probes have also been developed. The probe can be inserted into a blood vessel and placed at the site where the measurement is to take place.

Two electrodes are built into each probe to pick up the generated electric potential. Normally, the voltage induced between the two electrodes is very small; for example, for large vessels such as the aorta, the maximum induced potential should not exceed 200 μV. In smaller vessels, this value should be proportionally smaller. For measurement of venous flow near the heart, caution must be exercised because interference from the millivolt-level electrophysiologic signals may cause severe problems of cardiac arrhythmia.

Because the electromagnetic flowmeter probe is sensitive to the physical properties of the conductor on which measurements are performed, calibration of the probes should only be carried out in situ. Ex vivo calibration has little value unless it is carried out in an excised blood vessel with blood from the same subject. This is, of course, rather difficult to carry out in most experiments.

Since the electromagnetic flowmeter probes are usually used in direct contact with the blood vessel, their utilization has been mostly limited to patients in surgery or to acute animal experiments. One must also be aware that measurements of physiologic conditions carried out in the operating room may be different from those performed on patients who are awake. A few chronic measurements have been carried out in animals and in human patients. Cronestrand (Chapter 7) reports clinical experiences of applying the electromagnetic flowmeter to both acute (open wound) and chronic (implanted) measurements in vascular surgery, in patients. A comprehensive review of the basic theory, applications, and the current advances in the electromagnetic blood flowmeter is presented by Wyatt (Chapter 2).

Sounds with ultra high frequencies, say, 1 MHz and above, have very strong penetrating power. The emitted ultrasounds scatter with different patterns in different media. The pattern is also altered if the medium is in motion with a certain velocity with respect to emitted ultrasound beam. An ultrasound flowmeter is an instrument designed to measure fluid flows utilizing this basic phenomenon. Application of the ultrasound flowmeter in clinical practice or animal experimentation has the particular advantage that the technique is basically noninvasive. The need for a quantitative transcutaneous ultrasound blood flowmeter is apparent. A basic ultrasound flowmeter probe consists of two barium titanate-type crystals. An oscillator energizes one of the crystals, which transmits ultrasound waves into the medium while the second crystal receives the back-scattered sound signals. Early ultrasound flowmeters were mostly continuous-wave types. Although many of these have been built and marketed for clinical use, the devices are mostly used as flow detectors rather than flowmeters, because of their many inherent limitations.

One of the basic limitations to a continuous-wave ultrasound flowmeter is its sensitivity to all motions in the path of the second beam. If both crystals are energized, the region of sensitivity can be determined by the beam interception. A moving scatter could be localized by the intercepting region of high sensitivity. However, since the focal point is generally fixed in space, it is difficult to apply this technique to a living subject. Difficulty may also rise when more than one blood vessel passes through the region of sensitivity at the same time. All the flow signals in the beam are combined into one composite signal that cannot be separated into its elemental components.

Most of these problems are overcome by the pulse Doppler ultrasound system, which transmits bursts of ultrasound signals through the medium instead of the continuous waves. The Doppler shift of the returning echo is recorded. The distance (depth) into which the Doppler signal is sensed within a medium may be determined by the delay interval between the transmitted burst and its return to the sample gate. A range delay potentiometer may be calibrated in millimeters of tissue depth to measure the sound path length that intercepts a blood vessel. The vessel boundary can be determined by noting the depth at which the flow signals commence and the depth at which they disappear. If the angle between the sound beam and the blood vessel is known, the vessel diameter is then determined. Because the sound bursts are transmitted at very short intervals and durations, a small volume of the medium space is sampled. Through the range-gauged sampler, the detected Doppler shift frequency corresponds to the mean velocity averaged over the sampled volume. These discrete velocity measurements may be carried out across the diameter of the blood vessel lumen to map the velocity profiles within the vessel.

The size of the sample volume is apparently limited by the pulse repetition frequency (PRF) and the basic frequency of the ultrasound transmitted. For most of the commercial units presently available, the sample size is usually on the order of magnitude of 1 mm or larger. The finite size of the sample not only affects the precision of velocity measurements in smaller vessels, but also shows the measured vessel diameter to be larger than the actual one. Baker (Chapter 3) discusses the basic techniques of ultrasound blood flowmeter, while Anliker et al. (Chapter 1) discuss the clinical applications of ultrasound along with other noninvasive techniques.

Several investigators, in Europe and in the United States, have been engaged extensively in the research and development of ultrasound pulse Doppler flowmeters for measuring blood flow in smaller vessels. Hartley and Cole (1974) reported a 20-MHz directional pulse Doppler system that transmits ultrasound bursts at PRF of 62.5 kHz. The system uses a single crystal cuff probe made of a short plastic or nylon tubing. A slot cut in one side of the cylindrical cuff allows it to slip around the vessel. The system has been used to measure flow in the coronary arteries in open-chested dogs, and also has been used in chronic animal experiments by direct implantation of the probe over the coronary arteries.

A rather sophisticated transcutaneous pulse Doppler system has been developed by Anliker et al. in Switzerland for measuring flow in peripheral arteries. Current development of the noninvasive blood flow measurement systems has undoubtedly opened up a new domain in clinical diagnosis and laboratory application. Anliker et al. discuss several of these methods in Chapter 1.

Recent advances in hot-film anemometry allow detailed measurements of dynamic properties of cardiovascular flow. The instrument consists basically of a heat-velocity transducer and the supporting electronics. The transducer is a microscopic sensor strip that is made of a metal (i.e., Ni, Pt, or W) with a high thermal resistivity coefficient. The metal strip is maintained at a preset constant temperature above that of the ambient environment by passing an electrical current through the sensor film. Any fluid motion in the immediate vicinity of the film increases the heat flux from the film by forced convection. The heating current varies with the flux to maintain a constant temperature (thus constant electric resistivity) in the sensor. The product of the sensor resistivity and fluctuating heating current produces a fluctuating voltage that is calibrated against the fluid flow velocity in practical applications.

The hot-film anemometer has been utilized effectively in various engineering fluid dynamics applications for more than a decade. The device has recently been applied to cardiovascular measurements for several obvious reasons. It offers (1) fast dynamic response to the high-frequency velocity fluctuations in the disturbed flows (frequencies from DC to 5000 Hz can be easily registered by the sensor), (2) miniature size, (3) insensitivity to hydrodynamic stresses, (4) high signal-to-noise ratio, and (5) specially designed probes that allow signals to be separated into velocity components in axial and radial directions.

Ling et al. (1968a) reported their early success in measuring the detailed velocity profiles of oscillating flow in a rigid tube. The measurements were carried out in glycerin–water solution, glycerin, and dog blood. Later, the same experiment was carried out in nonlinear distensible tubes and in experimental animals. Nerem and his colleagues (1972, 1974) applied hot-film anemometry to measure blood turbulence in horse aorta and coronary arteries. The techniques of applying a hot-film anemometer for in vivo blood flow measurement are reviewed in Chapter 4 by Nerem. Our laboratory used a pair of orthogonally oriented cylindrical hot films to measure the turbulent characteristics in the near field immediately downstream from a natural human mitral valve and downstream from a natural human aortic valve. The instantaneous velocity profiles for both the axial velocity component (U), radial velocity component (V), their respective fluctuations (u') and (v'), and the corresponding Reynolds stress $(\rho \overline{u'v'})$ are measured. Our experience in measuring the transient turbulent characteristics is discussed in Chapter 21.

Measurement of cerebral blood flow presents certain unique problems. Because the four large arteries that supply blood to the brain are anastomosed in the circle of Willis at the base of the brain, one may find in many cases that more than one of these arteries are totally occluded, and yet the cerebral blood flow remains at its normal, or near normal, level (Chao and Hwang, 1972). A direct flow measurement on a single cerebral artery, therefore, does not permit conclusive information about blood flow to any part of the brain tissue. Lassen presents a comprehensive review on methods for measurement of cerebral blood flow in Chapter 5.

PROBLEMS IN PREDICTIONS

Since the early seventeenth century, knowledge of flow dynamics has been applied in clinical diagnoses of cardiovascular problems and to predict circulatory phenomena. The auscultation of abnormal heart sounds related to the abnormal flow patterns generated by lesions in the cardiovascular system and the current theories in predicting atherogenesis and thrombogenesis are two examples of the applications in modern medicine. The onset of cardiovascular surgery in the 1950s opened up a new domain of interests in flow dynamics. The diagnosis and evaluation of peripheral diseases, surgical treatment, postoperative follow-up, and pathologic examination of recovered circulatory prostheses may each be related to the dynamics of blood flow.

Description of pulsatile flow in a blood vessel inevitably involves the motion of the vessel walls. Knowledge of the mechanical properties of blood vessels in relation to pressure and flow variations has long been recognized as an important aspect in understanding the system. A great number of experimental works have been carried out in this area since the 1960s. They can be generally grouped into three major categories. The first type of work that concerns the mechanical properties of vessel wall material includes Carew, Vaishnav, and Patel (1968), who established that the arterial wall is basically incompressible, and Patel and Fry (1969), who discovered the curvilinear orthotopic nature of the aorta. The second type of work studied the tethering of blood vessel to the surrounding tissue, which restrains the motion of the blood vessel wall in the longitudinal as well as the lateral direction. The third type of work deals with the incremental properties of the vessel walls within the range of linearity corresponding to certain physiological state of deformation. For example, Patel, Janicki, and Carew (1969) studied the anisotropic nature of the aortic wall. The nonlinear behavior of blood vessel wall has also been investigated both experimentally and analytically. Patel and Vaishnav provided an up-dated review on the subject in Chapter 12.

The viscous property of blood, as a fluid, has been studied by many investigators. Although experimental results conclusively indicate that blood is Newtonian at high flow rates, it becomes quite non-Newtonian as its flow rate decreases and approaches zero. One of the peculiar characteristics of blood is that the resistance force to flow decreases, not to zero, but to a finite value as the flow rate becomes zero. This residual force of resistance is the consequence of a reversible aggregation of red cells promoted by the nonactivated fibrinogen. The non-Newtonian characteristics may impose severe restrictions on certain conventional methods of measuring the viscous properties of blood. Generally speaking, the rotational type viscometer is useful for measurement in low shear rates (shear stress up to 1 dyne/cm^2), whereas the capillary type viscometer is useful to expand the measurement toward higher values of shear rates. An extensive discussion on this subject was presented by Merrill and Pelletier (1967).

In biological and physical sciences, predictions or interpretations of prototype behavior are frequently made from observations of models. One classical example often cited is William Harvey's demonstration in 1628, in which a horse was used as the model to postulate the physiologic phenomenon of blood circulation. Cardiovascular models can generally be classified into three categories: (1) mathematical and computer models, (2) physical models, and (3) animal models. A combination of two or more of the above has also been used. The current status and the limitations of each type of cardiovasclar model are categorically discussed here.

The first question one should address in considering a model study is the *adequacy* of the model. Only then need the problem of *accuracy* of the model be considered.

A sophisticated model may take many detailed factors (parameters) into consideration. Nevertheless, such a model is also likely to introduce certain *side effects* that can cause unnecessary confusion and detract from the more basic issues. A clear conception and understanding of the limitations and functions of a particular model are essential in the selection and design of a model. Therefore, it is a good practice to begin with a simple model, as a general rule.

The simple fact that "a model is a model" indicates that no model can be made to reproduce exactly every function of the prototype. In the selection of a model, one therefore must first decide what type of information is desired and what type of information may be ignored. A model can then be selected to suit one's particular purposes.

Both qualitative observations and quantitative measurements can be carried out in one model. The qualitative observation identifies the characteristics of the system, while the quantitative measurements involve dimensions and standards of comparison. One of the particular advantages in using a model is that these observations may be repeated with controlled accuracy. Proper interpretation of a set of observations or measured data from a model requires overall comprehension and careful examination of all the factors that may cause variations in the observations or measured data. These variations may indicate either a general law that governs the behavior of the system studied, or merely indicate errors in observations.

Mathematical Models

A set of mathematical equations written to describe a certain physical phenomenon constitutes a basic mathematical model. The solution of the set of equations under given conditions predicts the behavior (or the phenomenon) in the prototype under those conditions. A simple mathematical model can usually be solved manually to provide a closed-form solution. A good example is the well-known Hagen–Poisueille equation.

Written to describe the steady laminar flow of an incompressible Newtonian fluid in a straight uniform circular tube, the Hagen–Poisueille equation states the balance of momentum in the flow field. Assuming that the pressure at a cross section does not vary with its radial position, the equation is simple enough to provide a closed-form solution by manual integration. The solution predicts a parabolic (paraboloid of revolution) velocity profile at any cross section in the tube. Furthermore, integration of the velocity profile over the cross-sectional area yields the flow rate, which is proportional to the pressure gradient and the fourth power of the tube diameter.

Although the Hagen–Poisueille model was frequently quoted in the early medical literature, it has unfortunately been misused frequently in many cardiovascular applications, most of which were made because certain conditions under which the basic model had been set up were arbitrarily ignored. For example, the limited length between major branchings and the pulsatile flow conditions that prevail in most of the larger vessels hardly allow fully developed laminar flow to occur in cardiovascular systems, although several investigators suggested that the "entrance length" may well be shorter for pulsatile flow. Among other locations, the required parabolic profile was found to exist in the femoral artery during a short phase (end systole) of a pulse cycle. Estimation of the flow rate based on a parabolic profile under the measured mean pressure gradient can be shown to overestimate by several times the actual value.

The first cardiovascular model that considered pulsatile flow was suggested by Otto Frank in 1899. Frank introduced the concept that the arterial tree functions as a compression chamber in a fire pump. Its mathematical and physical development is commonly known as the Windkessel model. This model, although very popularly accepted during the first half of the century, was developed at a time when little knowledge was available on cardiovascular dynamics, and has never concerned itself with the pressure-flow relationship in the arterial tree. Many of the unknown parameters were lumped together in the model without sound physical basis. In addition, some of the primary assumptions made on the model were so restrictive as to make the model totally irreconcilable with some of our current knowledge. A critical review of the assumptions involved in the Windkessel theory has been provided by McDonald and Taylor (1959).

A steady-state oscillation model, introduced by Womersley in 1958, was designed to predict both the pulsatile pressure and the associated pulsatile flow in an elastic arterial system by decomposing the pulsatile waves into Fourier components. The characteristic assumption involved in this model is that the heart beats are regular and repeatable over a relatively long period of time compared with those of an individual pulse. Other assumptions required in this model include (1) blood flow in vessels is laminar, (2) blood behaves as a homogeneous, Newtonian fluid, (3) blood flows through cylindrical tubes that do not alter their diameters until branching, (4) the vessel walls are elastic, (5) the "no-slip" condition exists at the wall, and (6) the vessel tube is long compared with the region studied.

The fundamental formula can be derived from the Navies–Stokes equation for incompressible flow in cylindrical coordinates. A nondimensional quantity, $\alpha = R\sqrt{\omega/\nu}$ (commonly known as the Womersley parameter or frequency parameter; where R is the tube radius, ω is the oscillatory angular velocity, and ν is the kinematic viscosity of blood) is introduced into the equation to transform it into a form of Bessel's equation. The solution (the phasic velocity profile) can thus be obtained as the Bessel function of the first kind and of zero order.

The nondimensional quantity α and the pipe-flow Reynolds number, R_e, are found to be the governing parameters in steady-state oscillatory pipe flows. Physically, α may be viewed as a ratio of the oscillatory inertial force (angular velocity) to viscous force, similar to that of the Reynolds number for steady pipe flow.

Conventionally, the Reynolds number has been used as the criterion to determine the transition from laminar flow to turbulent flow under steady flow conditions. When the inertial force predominates in a flow field, the Reynolds number is high and the flow is likely to be turbulent. Conversely, when the viscous force predominates, the Reynolds number is low, and the flow is likely to be laminar. Two flow fields with the same Reynolds number value are said to be "dynamically similar" flows if no other conditions are involved. The Reynolds number of 2,000 is generally quoted as the critical value. However, this experimentally determined value may vary greatly depending on many conditions of the experiment. For example, with a carefully rounded entrance leading flow from an undisturbed reservoir into a straight uniform tube, Osborne Reynolds himself was able to maintain the flow in laminar state up to $R_e \simeq 12,000$. Much higher values have been obtained by other investigators. On the other hand, the transitional value was found to be 200 in cardiovascular systems by several investigators. Therefore, it is clear that the Reynolds number is only a tool to describe the status of a flow field and it should not be used as the only reference. A model arbitrarily formulated only on the basis of a certain Reynolds number value may not have any physical significance in cardiovascular flow system.

The Navier–Stokes equations have been used as a basis for many flow dynamics problems in the cardiovascular system. Depending on the conditions given and the assumptions involved in the problem simulated, the form of the resulting mathematical equations (models) may vary from one case to another. Solution of the equations may be attained readily by direct integration in simple cases, while in the more complex forms direct solution may be very difficult to obtain, if not impossible. Numerous numerical and experimental methods have been developed to approach the latter, for which only approximate solutions can be attained despite laborious efforts. A large number of computations are usually involved, most of which require the assistance of the modern electronic computers.

Some examples of the numerical methods are the "difference differential equation" technique developed by Rideout and Dick (1967) to solve the problems of laminar pulsatile flow in peripheral arteries; the technique was used by Chao and Hwang (1972) to simulate blood flow and pressure distributions in the circle of Willis, and by Snyder, Rideout, and Hillstad (1968) to simulate the human systemic arterial tree; the finite difference method used by Hung to simulate the flow conditions in the vicinity of a prosthetic heart valve (Hung and Schuessler, 1972) and the vortex formation in a sudden geometric change of a vessel lumen (Hung, 1970) and other biological fluid problems (Hung, 1975).

Analogous to the electric power transmission line theory, a set of "hydraulic transmission line" equations was derived by replacing electric current with flow rate, electric potential with pressure, power line impedance with fluid line impedance, capacitance with compliance, and electric inductance with fluid inductance. Similar to the Womersley model, the hydraulic transmission line model also takes into consideration a homogeneous, incompressible viscous fluid flowing in distensible vessel system. The advantages of this model are that (1) it can take on any kind of wave form as input; it is not necessary for a "steady state" to exist as required by the Womersley model. For this reason, simulation can be made more physiologic, since the natural heart waves are not exactly repeatable from beat to beat. Transient-state physiologic conditions, as well as pathologic heart waves, may also be simulated. (2) The viscoelastic properties of the vessel walls can be modeled by expressing the model in complex terms, in which the real part represents the elastic properties of the wall, while the imaginary part represents the viscous properties. (3) There is no requirement of an "entrance length" on any vessel segment considered. The hydraulic transmission line model is apparently more suitable when applied to the cardiovascular system, which is known to have short sections before branching and generally complex and nonuniform geometry.

In the application of the hydraulic transmission line model, the simulated vascular system is subdivided into any number of connected, short cylindrical segments. With a given set of pressure and flow waves as the input to the system, the corresponding pressure and flow rate at any point in the system can be calculated as functions of time. This model does not provide information on velocity profiles.

A comprehensive review of basic hydraulic transmission line theory was provided by Hardung in 1963. Hwang and Chao (1974) discussed the possibility of including certain slowly varying physiologic controls and drug actions into the model. The practical problems in simulating the viscoelastic properties of the vessel walls by digital computer and hybrid computer were also discussed.

Compared with the arterial systems, the mathematical modeling of the venous system is usually far more difficult. The complexity is caused by the low transmural pressure in the venous system. Under certain conditions, some of the veins may collapse because of excessive external pressure. The mathematical relationship between the pressure and the flow in a collapsed vessel system has not been defined. Many of the recent studies indicate that the flow through a collapsing tube depends solely on the input (upstream) pressure and the pressure outside the tube, while the pressure at the downstream end does not influence the flow. This is a case hydraulically similar to that of a waterfall, in which the water elevation below the fall does not influence the flow of the fall. The term "vascular water fall" is therefore adopted for this analogy. A rigorous treatment of the subject is given by Noordergraaf and Kresch (1968).

Several attempts have been made to simulate the ventricular behavior by mathematical models. Beneken (1965) approximated the left ventricle by a thick-walled spherical shell and the right ventricle by a thinner-walled spherical shell that wraps around part of the outer surface of the left ventricular wall. The model takes into account the interaction between the left and right ventricles. Streeter et al. (1969) collected quantitative information about myocardium fiber orientation in the left ventricular wall during systole and diastole. Sallin (1969) showed, by computation, that a helical arrangement of left ventricular fiber around an ellipsoid body of revolution allows an ejection fraction of 61.2% of the maximum ventricular volume for 20% fiber shortening, which is very close to the generally accepted left ventricular ejection fraction, 60%, in a normal heart. A general mathematical formulation of the mechanical properties of the heart muscle was presented by Fung (1970).

Mathematical modeling of blood flow in capillary tubes has been investigated by many research groups (Lew and Fung, 1969; Wang and Skalak, 1969; Bugliarello and Hsaio, 1970; Skalak, Chen, and Chien, 1972).

Because of the size of the red cells (about 8 μ in diameter) relative to that of the capillary tubes (15 μ in diameter or less), blood flow in capillary tubes can no longer be assumed homogeneous. The mathematical models generally consider the red cell as a biconcave shaped disk, in which an incompressible liquid medium is contained in a very thin, flexible, slightly elastic membrane. The plasma fills the spaces between the cells and seeps around the cells to lubricate the cells as they move through the capillary tubes. A model describing the pressure-flow relationship in the plasma is known as the "bolus flow" model (Fitz-Gerald, 1972). It is generally assumed that a stream function exists, based on which the velocity components in the flow field are defined. Combined with the low-Reynolds-number Navier–Stokes equations, pressure gradients in the flow field can be compared. Recently, Perlin and Hung (in press) solved the Navier–Stokes equations for a train of particles moving through a capillary tube.

Although many sophisticated numerical techniques have been developed to attain solutions from these models under various presumed conditions, the model studies can provide little more than qualitative information at the present time, because of the lack of basic understanding about the red cell membrane and the mechanical properties of the capillary walls.

Problems of pulmonary hemodynamics become particularly interesting when the vascular beds are approached. Many models have been proposed for study of pulmonary flow dynamics in the past (e.g., Weiner et al., 1965; Pollack, Reddy, and Noordergraaf, 1968; Milnor et al., 1969). The system has never been properly expressed until recently. A comprehensive model of the sheet flow in alveolar septa, in the presence of the relatively large, flexible red cells, was first presented by Fung and Sobin in 1969. The readers are referred to Chapter 17 of the present book for the recent development of the model.

Attempts have also been made mathematically to model the diffusive exchange of drugs between capillary plasma, intracellular and extracellular spaces (Jacquex, Bellman, and Kalaba, 1960), and the uptake and distribution of anesthetics (Eger, 1963*a, b*). Various statistical models have also been developed that are not included here.

PHYSICAL MODELS

One of the most frequently used models in biologic studies is the ex vivo physical model. Physical models are usually constructed with nonbiologic materials to simulate a certain biologic phenomenon. Compared with the mathematical model described above, physical model simulation is a rather simple and direct process that permits repeated studies to be carried out under predetermined test conditions over arbitrarily long periods of time. An added advantage of the physical model is the easy accessibility for carrying out measurements under most circumstances. However, the main disadvantage of the model is its limited versatility, particularly the limitations on the number of parameters that may be included.

Observations made directly from the physical model may not always represent the true phenomenon in a quantitative sense. Total comprehension of the assumptions involved in designing of the model and its limitations is necessary before meaningful interpretation on the obtained data can be made.

Physical models may be generally classified into three categories, based on the forms of the models:

1. Geometric models are scaled reproductions (reduced, enlarged, or full sized) of the prototype. Close geometric similarity between the model and the prototype is emphasized in this type of model.

2. Distorted models are built to maintain a certain dynamic similarity (forces, velocities, accelerations, etc.) between the model and the prototype. Since the dynamic conditions in an enlarged (or reduced) model may not be the same as those existing in the prototype system, distortion of proportionality in the model may be necessary in one or more dimensions to achieve the desired dynamic similarity. As a result, the model and the prototype may share only limited resemblance in geometric shapes.

3. Dissimilar models bear no geometric resemblance to the prototype. Only analogous physical principles that exist between the two make it possible to study a certain phenomenon in the prototype by means of the model. For example, the dynamic distribution of blood flow and pressure in an arterial tree may be predicted by measurements obtained from an electric circuit analog.

To simulate a cardiovascular system with an ex vivo physical model should not be taken as a simple task. The most difficult part in designing a physical model is to select the primary parameters that must be included in the model. Other parameters that are judged to have only secondary importance in the phenomenon must be omitted from the design. This is the result of the severe restriction of any physical model in which only a limited number of parameters may be included. More important, however, is the concern that the effect of any secondary parameters may sometimes seriously distort the data in the less versatile model (compared with the prototype). Unless a well-comprehended design procedure is incorporated, the model may be no more useful than a demonstration device.

A few of the important physical properties of the cardiovascular system frequently considered in physical models are (1) viscosity of blood as a fluid, (2) pulsatile pressure and flow waves, (3) distensible vessel walls, (4) peripheral resistance and vascular input impedance, and (4) system compliance. Other conditions that may also be considered in certain special cases include the vascular control mechanisms and the boundary motion of a particular region in the system.

As mentioned before, it is generally agreed that, in a great portion of the cardiovascular system, blood may be treated as a homogeneous, Newtonian fluid. The absolute viscosity of whole blood (40–50% hematocrit at 37°C) is approximately 0.04 poise. Among other physical properties mentioned above, blood viscosity is found to be the easiest to simulate. Although several testing fluids have been suggested to match blood's viscosity, most investigators have found that a simple glycerine–water solution is quite satisfactory for most purposes. 36.7% (by weight) glycerine solution in water has been used as blood analog fluid in our laboratory for study of flow characteristics of natural and prosthetic heart valves. Hot-film measurements of the mean velocity profiles, turbulent intensities, and Reynolds stresses in the flow field showed no significant difference between results from the analog fluid and those of canine blood within the frequency range measured. Recently, Blick, Sabbah, and Stein (1975) reported the effect of hematocrit on the turbulent characteristics. The effect becomes more important when high-frequency fluctuations are considered. The authors postulated that the wakes of red blood cells may be the cause in their findings. This explanation is, however, questionable, considering the magnitude of the wakes that might be produced by the cells and the size of the eddies that can be measured by the film sensor they used in the experiment.

Pulsatile pressure and flow waves may also be simulated with reasonable accuracy with relatively simple equipment in a mock-up flow loop. Although several mechanisms have been suggested by different investigators, most of the systems are either of two basic types: the fluid in the system is either propelled by a positive-displacement pump or by a pressure-controled pump. The former usually incorporates a cam-driven piston pump with a preset stroke volume, while the latter involves a variable-pressure reservoir in which periodically pressurized fluid pulses through the system. With a properly designed control mechanism, both systems are capable of varying stroke volume, pulse rate, and systolic or diastolic periods. Both mechanisms have been used in our laboratory in flow loops designed for the testing of heart valve prostheses. In our experience, the control-pressure type is easier to adjust and reproduces pressure and flow waves more closely resembling those of physiologic wave forms.

Flexible tubings made of various types of materials are used in models to simulate vessel walls. The most frequently mentioned materials are tygone, rubber, or other types of polymer products. Directional reinforcements have also been used in combination with these materials to simulate the anisotropy of the vessel wall systems.

The mechanical properties of the vascular walls are rather complex in nature, as previously discussed. The natural vessel wall material consists of at least three basic types of tissue fiber: elastin, collagen, and muscle cells. The proportion of fiber types varies from largely elastin in the aorta to mostly smooth muscle cells in the arterioles, where the vascular walls become almost pure viscous in behavior. Exact simulation of these properties by a man-made material is apparently impractical. Quantitative information may be attained from physical models with limited inclusion of premeasured wall properties, such as the bulk elasticity.

Normally, a rigid wall model may provide a satisfactory solution to many cardiovascular problems investigated. Unless a well-designed distensible model is available, many investigators have found that an arbitrarily selected distensible tubing can produce certain misleading information that may further confuse the basic issue searched by the model study. The hydrodynamic effect in rigid tube was investigated by Scarton and Rouleau (1973).

The ability to reproduce the physiologic pressure and flow wave forms in the model system depends on the system's compliance and impedance. Early experiments carried out in our laboratory incorporated a simple resistance clamp and a 6-in.-diameter, drum-shaped compliance box in our mock-up flow loop. The box consists of a flexible silastic bag sealed in the plastic drum, into which pressurized air is applied to vary the system capacitance. With a pneumatically driven diaphragm pump as the power source that circulates the fluid, the resulting pressure and flow waves were shown to be similar to the physiologic wave forms (Wieting, Hwang, and Kennedy, 1972).

Although the system was found to be satisfactory for most of the projects carried out, it has come to our attention that the pressure waves need to be refined for detailed flow studies on heart valves. A linear resistance series was installed along with an air-chamber-type capacitance to match more closely the transient characteristics of the cardiovascular system.

Simulation of the cardiovascular system compliance and impedance by a physical model has been investigated by many investigators (Taylor, 1966a, b, c, 1969; Westerhof, Elzinga, and Sipkema, 1971).

Physical simulation of the boundary motions in a cardiovascular system has been a rather controversial subject. Bellhouse and Bellhouse (1969) constructed a bag model to simulate the left ventricle. In their model, the external surface of the bag was sealed in a pressurized box. By varying the pressure in the box, motion of the bag was instituted. Reul et al. (1974) fabricated a model aorta including all its major branches and the left heart with a flexible material. Two interconnected inner bags were used to represent the endothelium surfaces of the left atrium and the left ventricle. The entire system was suspended in a rigid, water-filled Perspex box in order to compensate for the hydrostatic pressure gradient. With the displacement of a piston, pressure is transmitted to the ventricle membrane by a connecting tube. The membrane motion is thus in accordance with the given shape of a cam that drives the piston.

From a dynamic point of view, any motion could normally be described in three terms. They are (1) displacement, which is the distance traveled by an element during a particular event; (2) speed, the time rate of change of the displacement; and (3) acceleration, the time rate of change of speed. The dynamic simulation of a boundary in motion, therefore, must include all three terms of all elements of the entire boundary in consideration. The models currently reported in literature may, at their best, reproduce the boundary displacement during a cardiac cycle. In detailed study of the flow patterns within the boundary, the validity of such a unilateral simulation becomes highly questionable.

With proper understanding of these limitations, judicious use of physical models for study of certain cardiovascular flow phenomena could be most profitable. A number of successful applications are discussed by Roach (Chapter 14), whose experience in effectively utilizing physical models in cardiovascular flow dynamics research becomes highly quotable.

ANIMAL MODELS

It is well known that certain anatomic and physiologic similarities exist between human and many animal species. Experimental results obtained in animals are often extrapolated to predict certain physiologic or pathologic phenomena in humans. Strictly speaking, not all animal experiments should be referred to as "models." Many of the experiments represent merely a qualitative analog between the species. Animal experiments carried out in cardiovascular research usually bear rather strict restrictions on certain similarity criteria or experimental parameters. They must be carefully examined and evaluated before any quantitative interpretation may be drawn from the experimental data.

One example of this situation is the dog model used by Fry (1968) to investigate the mechanisms of atherogenesis. Based on his initial observation made on the animal model, Fry claimed that the development of atherosclerotic lesions in the arterial system is associated with high local wall shear stress conditions. For normally occurring atheroma in humans, Caro, Fitz-Gerald, and Schroter (1971), however, discussed the possible reasons for the appearance of fatty streaks and early atheroma in regions of relatively low wall shear. Convincing results were also produced through a theoretic model proposed by the same group. The predictions from the two models of atherosclerotic development, both based on local wall shear conditions, seem contradictory. Caro et al. suggested that a distinction must be made between the atherogenetic patterns occurring in (high cholesterol fed) experimental animals and those spontaneously developed in humans. A common, complementary ground had not been achieved until more carefully conducted experiments were carried out recently (Caro, 1974; Fry, 1974). Caro discusses the mechanical factors in atherogenesis, the experimental procedure, and data interpretations in Chapter 13.

The apparent advantage in using an animal model is the anatomic and physiologic similarities that exist between the species. Most of the problems in model fabrications, as discussed previously, are no longer present. On the other hand, an animal model is rarely allowed the freedom of selectively adding (or omitting) any experimental parameter to (or from) the model. Furthermore, the reaction of different organisms to the control of certain parameter(s) may be different in the different species. To isolate some of the influences and to eliminate the different reactions to external stimuli may also be very difficult.

From a purely flow dynamics point of view, the two basic parameters to be considered in selecting an animal model are the Reynolds number, $R_e = \rho VD/\mu$, and the frequency parameter $\alpha = R \sqrt{\omega/\nu}$. The former correlates the vessel diameter and mean velocity of blood flow in the vessel. The latter correlates the vessel diameter and the basic heart frequency.

The mean values of the frequency parameter α, evaluated at the aortic root, in several different mammalian species, were computed by McDonald as shown in Table 1.

Klimes (1974) drew data from several investigators and showed that logarithmic relationships existed between (a) the weight and the radius of the aortic root; (b) the weight and the heart rate frequency; and (c) the weight and the frequency parameter, in most of the mammalian species.

Other parameters that may be considered in using an animal model include: the systolic and diastolic pressure; the change of vessel diameter in relation to pressure changes, $\Delta D/\Delta p$, which is directly proportional to the modulus of elasticity of the vascular wall; the cardiac output; the

Table 1. Some values of α in different mammalian species as evaluated at the root of aorta (from data in Clark, 1967, relating to heart rates and aortic cross-sectional area)

Species	Pulse rate/min	Radius (cm)	α (fundamental)
Mouse	600–730	0.03–0.01	1.19–1.74
Rat	360–520	0.045–0.095	1.38–3.5
Rabbit	205–220	0.17	3.92–4.07
Cat	180	0.2	4.4
Dog	72–125	0.55–0.6	8.27–10.68
Man	55–72	1.08–1.11	13.5–16.7
Ox	43	2.0	21.1
Elephant	40–50	4.47	48–51

peripheral resistance; the distribution of blood flow to the major organs; and the gross anatomy of the vascular system studies. Young and Cholvin (1966) discussed the possibilities of correlating certain of these parameters (with or without dimensions) that might elucidate the relationships for different individuals of the same or different species.

Selective combination of any two or more of the above models can be used in the study of a particular problem. Westerhof et al. (Chapter 11) study the dynamic relationship between the left side and the right side of the heart with an isolated cat's heart and an artificial flow loop to simulate the vascular system.

PROBLEMS IN APPLICATIONS

Based on the principle of flow dynamics, many circulatory prostheses are designed to assist blood circulation in various critical pathologic cases. Flow dynamic principles are also applied in current clinical diagnoses and cardiovascular reconstruction procedures.

Several types of artificial circulatory devices have been developed for clinical uses since the onset of cardiovascular surgery in the 1950s. Those involving the principles of hemodynamics are basically three types: (1) heart valve prostheses, (2) vascular graft prostheses, and (3) mechanical circulatory assist devices. Strandness presents a broad-based overview on flow dynamics in circulatory pathophysiology from a vascular surgeon's point of view in Chapter 8, while Noon discusses several specific flow related problems in cardiovascular surgery (Chapter 6).

Heart valve prostheses are designed to replace diseased or deformed natural heart valves. Currently, heart valve prostheses have been designed and fabricated in dozens of different geometries, several hundred thousand of which have been implanted in patients in the past two decades. Although the surgical procedures involved have been well accepted in common practice, the long-term success of each type of valve replacements has remained a controversial issue. Casci presents an engineer's view on the design and testing of prosthetic heart valves in Chapter 22.

Basically, natural heart valves are unidirectional check valves. Although the anatomic structure varies somewhat among the four valves (mitral, aortic, tricuspid, and pulmonary) in a heart, they all consist of a number of leaflets that open and close freely under the periodically changed pressure gradients. The body of the leaflet consists of a layer of tough interlacing fibers of connective tissue that are covered by smooth endothelium linings. The admirable properties are naturally difficult, if not impossible, for any mechanical heart valve prosthesis to match.

Other than the biologic, material, and surgical technique problems that one must overcome in the fabrication and implantation of a mechanical heart valve prosthesis, the problems in hemodynamics have been a major concern in the design of the heart valves. To understand this problem, one should take both the macroscopic and the microscopic points of view. Macroscopically, a mechanical valve must provide the maximum degree of competency (little or no flow regurgitation during valve closing), and it must be sensitive to the change of pressure gradient. Areas of stasis in the flow field must be avoided to prevent formation of local thromboses.

From a microscopic point of view, both red blood cells and platelets are rather sensitive to mechanical stresses in the field. Inadequately designed heart valve prostheses may generate excessive stresses that could seriously damage the blood in patients. Therefore, the blood-contacting surface of a mechanical valve prosthesis must be carefully polished to "microscopic" smoothness. Regions of excessively high shear stresses or high impact forces in the field must also be carefully eliminated.

Another important factor to be considered is blood damage due to mechanical forces. Over the past 10 years, many researchers have devoted their time and effort to the subject, e.g., Blackshear (1972) and Brown et al. (1975). Hellums and Brown in Chapter 20 review their many years experience in research on blood damage by mechanical forces, particularly by viscous shear force. Chien, on the other hand, provides a more basic approach to the problem in Chapter 19, in which the ultrastructure and the biochemical and biophysical properties of red cell membrane are examined in light of the various disturbances (osmotic, mechanical, thermal, or chemical).

Better understanding of blood damage by frequency dependent mechanical stresses is yet needed (Sutera and Mehrjarki, 1975). We believe that the transient eddies in blood flow detected by recent hot-film measurements (Hwang et al., in press) may also cause more damage to blood cells than previously reported. These eddies are "submacroscopic" in size (approximately in the order of magnitude of 1 mm or smaller). They are invisible to the conventional flow visualization techniques because of their small sizes and short life span. However, the scale (size) of these eddies is apparently more comparable with that of the red blood cells. It is probably easier for the blood cells to "see" and "feel" these eddies than for human eyes to see them (visualization techniques). The intensity of the "submacroscopic" eddies generated by mechanical replacement valves, or other circulatory assist devices, is expected to be much higher than that of the natural system. The corresponding shear stresses, known as the Reynolds shear stresses, are also expected to be significantly higher.

The transient turbulent characteristics of natural human valves have been investigated in our laboratory. A pair of orthogonally oriented cylindrical hot-film anemometer probes are used to measure both the axial and radial components of transient eddy intensities and the level of Reynolds stresses in the field close to the valve. The statistical structure of these "submacroscopic" eddies and the detailed techniques involved in the measurement are discussed in Chapter 21.

Direct vascular surgery for correction of arterial lesions may present many problems of a flow dynamics nature. The entire step-by-step procedure, beginning with the physician's attempt to make the correct diagnosis, to localize and assess the state of the diseased arteries, and to determine the functional disability of the diseased arteries, and including the decision on surgery, surgical procedure, postoperative evaluation, and follow-up, all may involve various degrees of flow dynamics at each stage. This subject is comprehensively reviewed by Strandness in Chapter 8.

Angiography is the principal tool in the final evaluation of most of the severe vascular lesions. The technique generally involves x-ray assessment of the vascular dimensions by injection of radiopaque dye directly into the vessel lumen at a location proximal to the lesions in question. Although the technique has been proved a very valuable procedure in clinical diagnosis, certain inherent difficulties limit its application in hemodynamic research. Questions involving the mixing patterns of the injected dye (a jet stream) with the flowing blood stream, and other matters of flow dynamics origins, make it impossible to obtain accurate measure of the time-dependent, local velocity distributions. Direct evaluation of the detailed vessel geometry by means of angiograms (superpositions, use of bi-plane projections, etc.) is also very difficult because of the limited resolution and other problems.

Failures in surgically reconstructed arteries that occur shortly after the procedure are usually related to the surgical techniques. However, the causes of late failures in reconstructed arteries have stimulated interesting discussions among flow-dynamists and surgeons. In earlier publications, Szilagyi et al. (1956, 1960) discussed the various configurations in surgically revascularized arteries. A systematic evaluation was attempted to relate the causes of late failures to the various techniques involved in arterial grafting. Experimental approach on the subject has also been reported (Imparato et al., 1972). Recently, Kennedy et al. (1974) discussed some of their preliminary finds concerning relationships between the hydraulic factors and long-term success in revasculated coronary arteries.

Over the past two decades, thousands of patients have undergone vascular reconstruction surgery. This large population could have provided invaluable information for the correlations if the patients were followed up systematically. Although only a few such follow-up systems have existed over a significant period of time, a careful examination of these findings for the roles of flow dynamics in the late failure of reconstructed arteries may prove to be very interesting.

Mechanical circulatory assist devices have been designed to partially or totally take over the function of a failing heart. Their role is to maintain the normal body functions on a temporary basis while favoring recovery of damaged myocardium. Generally, this goal may be accomplished in combination with other means, e.g., drug therapy or surgical intervention.

Presently, there are a variety of mechanical circulatory assist devices available or under development, most of which may generally be classified into the following categories:

1. External compression techniques are relatively simple to employ clinically. Periodic external compression of a certain portion of the patient's body may assist circulation of blood if the pulsatile waves are synchronized with that of the heart. Although the method is noninvasive and easy to apply, the efficiency of this method limits its applications.

2. Veno-arterial extracorporeal circulation with oxygenation, commonly known as the "heart–lung bypass," is currently accepted as a common practice in open-heart surgery. During the surgical procedure, the patient's heart is temporarily bypassed, while the cardiopulmonary bypass system takes the venous blood through an artificial oxygenator and pumps it back into the arterial system. At the present time, the general concern is the relatively high hemolysis rate, which is thought to be related to the design of the oxygenator and the pump system. Total bypass is rarely used for more than a few hours in any single application.

3. Diastolic intra-aortic counter pulsation involves a relatively simple procedure in which balloon is installed in the descending aorta. By periodically inflating and deflating the balloon, triggered by the patient's ECG, diastolic pressure is augmented to enhance circulation in the myocardium.

The method requires precise phase displacement and perfect synchronization with heart action. The method has been proved to be very successful in increasing coronary blood flow and in reducing the load on a failing left ventricle.

4. The left ventricular bypass pump is designed to partially or totally take over the function of a failing left ventricle. It consists of a pneumatically driven diaphragm pump incorporating two unidirectional check valves, one at the inlet and one at the outlet of the pump. Surgical procedure is required to connect the inlet to the left heart and the outlet to the aorta or a peripheral artery. An external pulser delivers compressed gas to the pump housing in which the diaphragm is periodically pushed (systole) and relaxed (diastole) at a controlled pulse duration and rate. The operation of a mechanical circulatory assist device is not a simple mechanical matter, because it must keep up with the physiologic conditions and demands at all times. Normann presents in Chapter 23 a discussion of the operational aspects of mechanical circulatory assist.

5. The total orthotopic cardiac pump is designed as the total replacement of the heart by means of a pair of pumps. Extensive research and development of total heart replacement have been carried out at several centers in the United States, Europe, and Japan. Basic developments and current status of the total mechanical heart are discussed in Chapter 24 by E. S. Bücherl, R. Mohnhaupt, J. H. Lawson, and T. Akutzu.

Several flow dynamics related problems, which are the common concern of all the circulatory assist devices, are briefly reviewed here in general terms.

The question of steady flow or pulsatile flow has been debated among investigators. Although a certain number of the blood pumps currently in clinical use are basically steady-flow pumps, many arguments favor the pulsatile flow as more physiologic. Wesolowski (1955) showed that the absence of pulsation favors acidosis, capillary stasis, and edema. In addition to pulsed perfusion, it is also interesting to note that pulsatile pressure waves change slope and become attenuated as they propagate downstream. The rapid rise of pressure during the systolic phase of a cardiac cycle may well have a physical or physiologic significance from a pure flow dynamics point of view. Before these questions can be answered with any scientific certainty, it is apparently advisable that circulatory assist devices should be designed to reproduce the physiologic wave forms.

The ability of a circulatory assist device to produce physiologic wave forms can be examined by testing the device on a mock-up fluid loop. The mechanical properties of the testing loop (vascular impedance, compliance, inductance, etc.) can be made to match those of the physiologic, as previously discussed.

The problem of *synchronization* of an artificial circulatory device with the natural heart arises when the device is used to partially assist a failing heart. Among the four basic types of circulatory assist devices mentioned above, in only two types (external body compression and diastolic aortic counter pulsation) do the function of the device depend on the rigorous synchronization with the heart. For the other two types of devices, current data from animal experiments seem to indicate that the synchronization may not be necessary. More information is needed to identify definitely the physiologic effects of the asynchronization. From a flow dynamics point of view, however, it has been shown by several investigators that synchronizing the circulatory assist device with the heart may facilitate the efficiency of the device.

The question of *competition with the natural heart* causes great clinical concern when the assist device is functioning simultaneously with the natural heart. Several control schemes have been proposed. Ideally, certain important pathologic parameters in the patient should be fed into the control system that governs the performance of the assist device. In conjunction with the left ventricular bypass pump developed in the Baylor laboratories, Normann et al. have introduced a new and efficient method for monitoring and closed loop control of pneumatically driven blood pumps; the method, discussed in Chapter 23, is based on the continuous measurement of electrical capacitance across the gas space within the pump.

The flow dynamics problems associated with a total heart replacement stand in a class by themselves. First of all, two pumps, functioning in series, are separated by the systemic circulation on one side and the pulmonary circulation on the other. Between the "left heart" and the "right heart," a basic level of hydrodynamic communication must be maintained at all times. During the equilibrium state, the output of the two "ventricles" must be exactly the same in order to avoid accumulation of blood volume in one portion of the circuit. Also, in the transient state, the balance of flow must be automatically adjusted to the ratio of the pulmonary and systemic impedances. A series of well-planned studies on the subject of hydrodynamic "cross talk" between the left heart and the right heart have been carried out by Elzinga and Westerhof (1974). An electrically paced cat heart was used in their study in connection with a specially designed mock-up flow loop that simulates the hydrodynamic functions of the systemic circulatory system. Westerhof et al. provide a quantitative analysis of the arterial system and the heart in light of pressure—flow relationship (Chapter 11).

FUNDAMENTALS AND ADVANCES

The last part of this book is especially directed toward the basic fundamentals and current advances in the field of cardiovascular flow dynamics. Our colleague, A.K.M.F. Hussain, contributes Chapter 15 on the basic principles of fluid mechanics of relevance to the cardiovascular system. Parker discusses in Chapter 16 the instability problem of blood flow in a circular tube; some of the flow dynamics techniques that he specifies are both interesting and stimulative.

In Chapter 10 Jones presents a broad review of the physiologic control mechanisms on both the heart and the peripheral circulation. A graphical analysis method is presented by which the effects of the various factors can be determined. In Chapter 18 Buckley discusses drug actions on cardiovascular functions. Compounds acting directly on alpha and/or beta adrenergic receptors, and hormones such as angiotensin II, that act both directly and indirectly on vascular tone and cardiac activity, are discussed in detail.

In connection with our space activities, Hoffler (Chapter 9) reports the cardiovascular studies performed on U.S. space crews. Efforts in this early investigation of physiologic alterations under zero-gravitational or multi-gravitational conditions, and the recent advances in that field, may open up a new domain of interests in cardiovascular flow dynamics.

REFERENCES

Armeniades, C. D., L. W. Lake, and Y. F. Missirlis. 1973. Histological origin of aortic tissue mechanics. Appl. Polym. Sym. 22:319–339.

Baker, L. E., and J. C. Denniston. 1974. Noninvasive measurement of intrathoracic fluids. Chest 65:(Suppl.) 35S–37S.

Bellhouse, B. J., and F. H. Bellhouse. 1969. Fluid mechanics of the mitral valve. Nature 224:615.

Beneken, J. E. W. 1965. A mathematical approach to cardiovascular function. The uncontrolled human system. Int. Rep. 2.4 5/6. Inst. of Med. Physics. TNO, Utrecht, The Netherlands.

Berguer, R., and N. H. C. Hwang. 1974. Critical arterial stenosis: A theoretical and experimental solution. Ann. Surg. 180, 1:39.

Blackshear, P. L. 1972. Mechanical hemolysis in flowing blood. *In* Y. C. Fung (ed.), Biomechanics, p. 501. Prentice-Hall, Englewood Cliffs, N.J.

Blick, E. F., H. N. Sabbah, and P. D. Stein. 1975. Red blood cells and turbulence. Proceedings of the Fourth Annual Symposium on Turbulence in Liquids. University of Missouri, Rolla, Missouri, September 22–24, 1975.

Block, E. H. 1966. Low compliance pressure gauge. *In* R. F. Rushmer (ed.), Methods in Medical Research, Vol. II. Year Book Medical Publishers, Chicago.

Brodie, T. G., and A. E. Russell. 1905. On the determination of rate of blood flow through an organ. J. Physiol. 32:47.

Brown, C. H., R. F. Lemuth, J. D. Hellums, L. B. Leverett, and C. P. Alfrey. 1975. Response of human platelets to shear stress. Trans. A.S.A.I.O., XXI: 35.

Bugliarello, G., and G. C. C. Hsaio. 1970. A mathematical model of the flow in the axial plasmatic gaps of the smaller vessels. Biorheology 7:5.

Burton, A. C. 1972. Physiology and Biophysics of the Circulation. 2nd Ed. p. 112. Year Book Medical Publishers, Chicago.

Carew, T. E., R. N. Vaishnav, and D. J. Patel. 1968. Compressibility of the arterial wall. Circ. Res. 23:61.

Caro, C. G., J. M. Fitz-Gerald, and R. C. Schroter. 1971. Atheroma and arterial wall shear: Observation, correlation, and proposal for a shear dependent mass transfer mechanism for atherogenesis. Proc. Roy. Soc. Lond. (Biol.) 117:109.

Caro, C. G. 1974. Transport of [14]C-4 cholesterol between perfusing serum and dog common carotid artery. Cardiol. Res. 8:194.

Chao, J. C., and N. H. C. Hwang. 1972. Functional dynamics of the Circle of Willis. TIT J. Life Sci. 2, 3:81.

Clark, C. 1967. A local thermodilution flowmeter for the measurement of venous blood flow in man. Med. Bio. Eng. 6:133.

Eger, E. I. 1963(a). A mathematical model of uptake and distribution. *In* E. M. Papper and R. J. Kitz (eds.), Uptake and Distribution of Anesthetic Agents. McGraw-Hill, New York.

Eger, E. I. 1963(b). Applications of a mathematical model of gas uptake. *In* E. M. Papper and R. J. Kitz (eds.), Uptake and Distribution of Anesthetic Agents. McGraw-Hill, New York.

Elzinga, G., and N. Westerhof. 1974. End diastolic volume and source impedance of the heart. *In* A. Guz (ed.), Physiological Basic of Starlings Law of the Heart, p. 241, CIBA 24.

Fitz-Gerald, J. M. 1972. The mechanics of capillary blood flow. *In* D. H. Bergel (ed.)., Cardiovascular Fluid Dynamics, Vol. 2, p. 209. Academic Press, London.

Frank, O. 1899. Die Grundform des Arteriellen Pulses. Erst Abhandlung. Abhandlung. Mathematische Analyse., Z. Biol., 37:483.

Fry, D. L. 1968. Acute vascular endothelial changes associated with increased blood velocity gradients. Circ. Res. 22:165.

Fry, D. L. 1974. Some arterial changes associated with hemodynamic events. *In* R. M. Nerem (ed.), Proceedings, Fluid Dynamic Aspects of Arterial Disease, Ohio State Univ., Sept 19–20, p. 64.

Fung, Y. C. 1970. Mathematical representation of the mechanical properties of heart muscles. J. Biomech. 3:381–404.

Fung, Y. C., and S. S. Sobin. 1969. Theory of sheet flow in the lung alveoli. J. Appl. Physiol. 26:472–488.

Ganz, W., and H. J. Swan. 1972. Measurement of blood flow by thermal-dilution. Am. J. Cardiol. 29:241.

Geddes, L. A., and L. E. Baker. 1975. Principles of applied biomedical instrumentation. *In* Detection of Physiological Events by Impedance. Chapter 10, 2nd Ed. John Wiley & Sons, New York.

Guyton, A. C. 1963. Circulatory Physiology. W. B. Saunders, Philadelphia.

Guyton, A. C., C. E. Jones, and T. G. Coleman. 1973. Circulatory Physiology, Cardiac Output and Its Regulation. W. B. Saunders, Philadelphia.

Hardung, V. 1963. Propagation of pulse waves in visco-elastic tubings. Handbook of Physiology, Vol. 1, p. 107. Section on Neurophysiology. American Physiology Society, Washington, D.C.

Hartley, C. J., and J. S. Cole. 1974. An ultrasonic pulsed Doppler system for measuring blood flow in small vessels. J. Appl. Phys. 37,4:626–629.

Hung, T. K. 1970. Vortex in pulsatile flow. Proceedings of the Fifth International Congress on Rheology, Vol. II. University of Tokyo Press, Tokyo.

Hung, T. K. 1975. Development of computational method for biofluid dynamics. Preprint No. 2744, ASCE, Structural Engr. Conf., New Orleans, La.

Hung, T. K., and G. B. Schuessler. 1972. Computational analysis as an aid to the design of heart valves. Advances in Bioengineering, Chemical Engineering Progress, Symposium Series, Vol. 67, p. 8.

Hwang, N. H. C., and C. Chao. 1974. Applications of the hydraulic transmission line equations in model analogy of the circulatory system. *In* D. Gisheta (ed.), Prospectives of Biomedical Engineering II. Madras, India.

Hwang, N. H. C., A. K. M. F. Hussain, P. W. Hui, and T. Stripling. Turbulent flow through a natural human neutral valve. J. Biomech. In press.

Imparato, A. M., A. Bracco, G. E. Kim, and R. Zeff. 1972. Intimal and neointimal fibrous proliferation causing failure of arterial constructions. Surgery 72, 6:1007.

Jacquez, J. A., R. Bellman, and R. Kalaba. 1960. Some mathematical aspects of chemotherapy–II: The distribution of drug in body. Bull. Math. Biophys. 22:309.

Kennedy, J. H., D. W. Wieting, N. H. C. Hwang, M. S. Anderson, R. J. Bayardo, J. F. Howell, and M. E. DeBakey. 1974. Hydraulic and morphologic study of fibrous intimal hyperplasia in autogenous saphenous vein bypass grafts. J. Thorac. Cardiovasc. Surg. 67, 5: 805.

Klimes, F. 1974. Research into flow on a model of the aorta and on mechanical systems for the assistance of the heart. Rev. Czech. Med. 20, 4: 210–221.

Kresch, E., and A. Noordergraaf. 1969. A mathematical model for the pressure-flow relationship in a segment of vein. IEEE Trans. Bio-Med. Eng. BME-16: 296–307.

Lew, H. S., and Y. C. Fung. 1969. The motion of the plasma between the red cells in the bolus flow. Biorheology G: 109.

Lighthill, J. M. 1972. Physiological fluid dynamics: A survey. J. Fluid Mech. 52,3: 475–497.

Ling, S. C., H. Atabek, D. L. Fry, D. J. Patel, and S. Janicki. 1968(a). Application of heated-film velocity and shear probes to hemodynamic studies. Circ. Res. 23:789.

Ling, S. C., H. B. Atabek, and J. J. Carmody. 1968(b). Pulsatile flow in arteries. Proceedings Internat., Congress of Applied Mechanics, Stanford University, Stanford, Calif., p. 277.

McDonald, D. A., and M. G. Taylor. 1959. The hydrodynamics of arterial circulation. In Progress in Biophysics, Vol. 9, p. 107. Pergamon, London.

Merrill, E. W., and A. Pelletier. 1967. Viscosity of human blood: Transition from Newtonian to non-Newtonian. J. Appl. Phys. 23,2: 178.

Nerem, R. M., W. A. Seed, and N. B. Wood. 1972. An experimental study of the velocity distribution and transition to turbulence in the aorta. J. Fluid Mech. 52, 1:137.

Nerem, R. M., J. A. Rumberger, D. R. Gross, R. L. Hamlin, and G. L. Geiger. 1974. Hot-film anemometer velocity measurements in arterial blood flow in horses. Circ. Res. 34:193.

Netter, F. H. 1969. Heart. CIBA Collection of Med. Illustration, Vol. 5:40.

Noordergraaf, A., and E. Kresch (eds.). 1968. The Venous System: Characteristics and Function. A Biomedical Engineering Approach. IEEE Trans. Bio-Med. Eng. BME-16:233.

Normann, N. A., M. E. DeBakey, G. P. Noon, and J. N. Ross. 1973. Monitoring and closed-loop control of pneumatic blood pumps. Cardiovasc. Res. Center Bulletin 12: 3–12.

Normann, N. A., G. P. Noon, M. E. DeBakey, and J. N. Ross. 1974. Automatic control of pneumatic blood pumps. Trans. Amer. Soc. Artif. Int. Organs 20:685–690.

Patel, D. J., and D. L. Fry. 1969. The elastic symmetry of arterial segments in dogs. Circ. Res. 24:1.

Patel, D. J., J. S. Janicki, and T. E. Carew. 1969. Static anisotropic elastic properties of the aorta in living dogs. Circ. Res. 25:765.

Patel, D. J., and N. Vaishnav. 1972. The rheology of large blood vessels. In D. H. Bergel (ed.), Cardiovascular Fluid Dynamics, Vol. 2, Ch. 11. Academic Press, London.

Perlin, A., and T. K. Hung. Flow development of a train of particles in capillary. J. Engr. Mech., Div. ASCE. In press.

Pollack, G. H., R. W. Reddy, and A. Noordergraaf. 1968. Input impedance wave travel, and reflections in the human pulmonary arterial tree: Studies using an electric analog. IEEE Trans. Bio-Med. Eng. BME-15:151.

Reul, H., B. Tesch, J. Schoenmackers, and S. Effert. 1974. Hydromechanical simulation of systemic circulation. Med. Bio. Eng. 431–436.

Rideout, V. C., and D. E. Dick. 1967. Difference-differential equation: for fluid flow in distensible tubes. IEEE Trans. Bio-Med. Eng. BME-14:171.

Sallin, E. A. 1969. Fibre orientation and ejection fraction in the human left ventricle. Biophys. J. 9:954.

Scarton, H. A., and W. T. Rouleau. 1973. Axisymmetric waves in compressible Newtonian liquids contained in rigid tubes: Steady periodic mode shapes and dispension by the method of eiganvalleys. J. Fluid Mech. 58,3:595.

Schultz, D. L. 1972. Pressure and flow in large arteries. In D. H. Bergel (ed.), Cardiovascular Fluid Dynamics, Vol. 1, Chap. 9. Academic Press, London.

Skalak, R., P. H. Chen, and S. Chien. 1972. Effects of hematocrit and rouleux on apparant viscosity in capillaries. Biorheology 9:67.

Snyder, M. E., V. C. Rideout, and R. J. Hillstad. 1968. Computer modeling of the human systemic arterial tree. J. Bio. Mech. 35.

Strandness, D. E., Jr. 1969. Peripheral Arterial Disease: A Physiologic Approach. Little, Brown, Boston, p. 163.

Streeter, D. D., H. M. Spotmitz, D. J. Patel, J. Ross, and E. H. Sonneblick. 1969. Fibre orientation in the canine left ventricle during diastole and systole. Circ. Res. 24:339.

Sutera, S. P., and M. N. Mehrjarki. 1975. Deformation and fragmentation of human RBC in turbulent shear flow. Biophys. J. 15:1.

Szilagyi, D. E., J. G. Whitcomb, and P. Waibel. 1960. The laws of fluid flow and arterial grafting. Surgery 47.

Szilagyi, D. E., J. G. Whitcomb, and R. F. Smith. 1956. The causes of late failure in grafting therapy of peripheral occlusive arterial diseases. Am. Surg. 144:611.

Taylor, M. G. 1966(a). The input impedance of an assembly of randomly branching elastic tubes. Biophys. J. 6:29.

Taylor, M. G. 1966(b). Wave transmission through an assembly of randomly branching elastic tubes. Biophys. J. 6:697.

Taylor, M. G. 1966(c). Use of random excitation and spectral analysis in the study of frequency-dependent parameters of the cardiovascular system. Circ. Res. 18: 585.

Taylor, M. G. 1969. Arterial impedance and distensibility. In A.P. Fishman and H. H. Hecht (eds.), The Pulmonary Circulation and Interstitial Space, p. 341. University of Chicago Press, Chicago.

Terry, E. N., R. H. Clauss, L. R. Rouen, and W. Ridsch. 1974. Blood flow and perfusion, their true meaning. IX International Congress of Angiology, Florence, Italy, April 3–7.

Wang, H., and R. Skalak. 1969. Viscous flow in a cylindrical tube containing a row of spherical particles. J. Fluid Mech. 38:75.

Weiner, F., E. Morkin, R. Skalak, and A. P. Fishman. 1965. Wave propagation in the pulmonary circulation. Circ. Res. 19:834.

Westerhof, N. G. Elzinga, and P. Sipkema. 1971. An artificial arterial system for pumping hearts. J. Appl. Physiol. 31,5: 776.

Wiederhelm, C. A. 1966. Servo micropipet pressure recording technique. In R. F. Rushmer (ed.), Methods in Medical Research, Vol. 2, p. 199. Year Book Medical Publishers, Chicago.

Wieting, D. W., N. H. C. Hwang, and J. H. Kennedy. 1971. Fluid mechanics of the human mitral valve. AIAA paper No. 71-102, AIAA 9th Aerospace Sciences Meeting, New York.

Wieting, D. W., N. H. C. Hwang, and J. H. Kennedy. 1972. Testing of prosthetic heart valves. In J. H. K. Vogel (ed.), Long-term Prognosis Following Valve Replacement. S. Karger, Basel.

Womersley, J. R. 1958. The mathematical analysis of the arterial circulation in a state of oscillatory motion. Wright Air Development Center Tech. Rep. WADC-TR 56-614.

Young, D. F., and N. R. Cholvin. 1966. Application of the concept of similitude to pulsatile blood flow studies. Biomedical Fluid Mech. Symp., ASME. Denver, Colo., April 25–27, pp. 78–88.

Cardiovascular Flow Dynamics and Measurements
Edited by N. H. C. Hwang and N. A. Normann
Copyright 1977   University Park Press   Baltimore

chapter 1

NONINVASIVE MEASUREMENT OF BLOOD FLOW

Max Anliker,
Max Casty, Paul Friedli, Rudolf Kubli, and Herbert Keller

ABSTRACT

New ways of obtaining noninvasively diagnostic information on peripheral vessel disease and in some circumstances also on certain disorders of the heart are offered by recent designs of multichannel ultrasonic velocity profile meters. They yield quantitative data on flow patterns in large blood vessels near the skin in terms of the instantaneous spatial velocity profiles, their variations during the cardiac cycle, and the instantaneous volume flow rates evaluated by integrating the profiles over the cross section whose diameter is determined by echo ranging. Examples of measurements in the common carotid artery, axillary artery, and femoral artery are described.

By way of television microscopy and computer-assisted image analysis the speed of red blood cells is determined on line in human nailfold capillaries. A spatial correlation process reveals that the speed may exceed 2 mm/sec and exhibit an oscillatory pattern that is in phase with the flow pulse generated by the heart.

On-line computer thermography is described as a method of assessing changes in regional blood flow. Certain pathologic features of the temperature pattern and the surface vein distribution are characterized by parameters and evaluated within seconds after the digital recording of the thermogram. The abnormal features are displayed graphically as well as in alphanumeric form on the color-coded thermogram. The system and method developed are applied in a breast cancer detection project.

1 INTRODUCTION

The noninvasive evaluation of changes in the cardiovascular system caused by diseases, aging, unusual environments like space flight, and by normal

43

regulatory mechanisms has been given much attention during the past 15 years (Strandness et al., 1969; Baker, 1970; Anliker, 1971; Darling et al., 1972; Fronek et al., 1973; Brunner et al., 1975; Planiol and Pourcelot, 1974; Rutishauser et al., 1974; Bollinger, Brunner, and Anliker, 1974a; Peronneau, 1974; Daigle et al., 1975). A considerable number of research projects in this area have been supported by NASA because astronauts have shown cardiovascular adaption during space flight (Anliker, 1971). Most of the material presented here is the result of an interdisciplinary group effort within the Swiss Federal Institute of Technology in Zürich and the Medical School of the University of Zürich. To some extent the findings are based on earlier studies carried out at Stanford University and at the Ames Research Center of the NASA at Moffett Field in California.

Although there is still relatively little information available on the flow patterns in the various segments of the circulatory system of man, one finds a substantial amount of corresponding canine data in the literature. Theoretical studies of blood flow in man are therefore often based on the working hypothesis that the basic mechanical and physiologic behavior of the canine and human vascular trees is similar. Presupposing the admissibility of this hypothesis, one concludes from the results of mathematical model studies of the canine arterial system that pressure and flow pulses in human arteries alter their typical and vessel-dependent patterns in response to changes in cardiac function and anatomic as well as physiologic features of arterial conduits (Anliker, Rockwell, and Ogden, 1971). In other words, the flow pulses are expected to exhibit diagnostic information.

Recent theoretic investigations of the flow and pressure pulses in arteries confirm the diagnostic possibilities offered by measurements of the temporal variation of the volume flow rate in various vessels (Westerhof et al., 1969; Rockwell, Anliker, and Elsner, 1974; Raines, Jaffrin, and Shapiro, 1974; Cheng, Robertson, and Clark, 1974). Elsner (1975) used the one-dimensional method of characteristics to compute the pressure and flow in a human arterial conduit as a function of time and distance from the heart. It includes the effects of the viscosity of the blood and the viscoelasticity of the arterial wall. Moreover, it takes into account various nonlinear phenomena such as the increases of area and wave speed with pressure as well as the convective contribution of the flowing blood to the wave speed. Because no human data were available on the increase of the wave speed with pressure, the corresponding findings of canine in vivo studies were utilized (Anliker et al., 1971). A significant improvement over earlier mathematical models (Anliker et al., 1971; Rockwell et al., 1974) appeared to be the simulation of the branches in terms of a continuously distributed flow—rather than pressure-dependent seepage through the wall. The pulse patterns predicted agree reasonably well with the direct human pressure measurements reported in the literature and with the flow data determined noninvasively by means of ultrasound and described partly in Section 2 and elsewhere (Brunner et al., 1974; Bollinger et al., 1974a; Doriot et al., 1976; Anliker, 1976).

In view of the functions of the circulatory system, one is inclined to attribute particular importance to the quantification of the blood flow and transport phenomena in the capillary bed. So far very little is known about the hemodynamics in microvessels and the transcapillary mass transport in human tissues. However, with the help of television microscopy it has become possible to evaluate the speed of red blood cells (RBC) in certain capillaries of man, such as those of the nailfold (Bollinger et al., 1974b). In principle, this technique also permits a study of exchange processes that take place across the walls of microvessels.

In measuring the RBC speed in capillaries of the nailfold, three essential observations were made. First, there is a substantial variability of the resting flow rate from subject to subject. Second, the RBC speed is often too high to be quantified by videomicroscopy at conventional frame rates of 50 or 60 images per second. Third, the frame-to-frame analysis and the videodensitometric method may yield differing results when the two-slit technique is employed and the speed is determined by a temporal correlation process (Hollinger et al., 1975). The first observation implies that it may be practically impossible to differentiate normal microcirculatory behavior from a mildly pathologic one by merely quantifying resting flow rates. One may, therefore, have to resort to a physiologic maneuver like a reactive hyperemia for a sharper diagnostic evaluation of microcirculatory disorders. During such a maneuver, however, the RBC speed will very likely exceed the maximum speed that can be measured with currently used video techniques. These facts, together with the third observation, suggested the development of an alternative approach in the methodology (Anliker and Kubli, 1976). A brief description of such an alternative approach and some of the first results it yielded are described in Section 3.

To assess changes in regional blood flow, one applies different methods depending on the nature of the tissues involved. For example, the perfusion of limbs is frequently evaluated by plethysmography, that of inner organs primarily by isotope techniques, and that of body parts directly connected to the skin by thermography (Wallace and Cade, 1974). In recent years, there has been an increasing interest in the use of thermography. Its medical significance lies in its ability to identify unusual topographic variations of the skin temperature. Deviations from usual surface temperature distributions of the body are primarily caused by abnormal levels in regional blood flow. The associated heat transfer is thus predominantly effected by convection in terms of an altered flow through the surface veins.

To date, no sharply defined criteria have been established for pathologic patterns of the skin temperature. A pattern is generally considered unusual if it exhibits a certain degree of asymmetry with respect to the sagittal plane, or if it contains hot spots, i.e., areas in which the temperature exceeds the expected temperature by a certain amount, for instance, 1.5°C. In spite of the vagueness of these criteria, the studies reported in the literature indicate a variety of diagnostic possibilities of thermography, especially with regard to the following disease categories and specific illnesses (Wallace and Cade, 1974):

Neoplastic diseases, in particular, cancer of the female breast.
Circulatory disorders, for example, occlusions of extracranial vessels or
    other peripheral vascular diseases.
Musculoskeletal injuries, such as herniated lumbar disks.
Burns
Inflammatory diseases, for example, arthritis or acute appendicitis in
    children.

Nevertheless, clinical thermography has not yet established itself as a widely accepted diagnostic procedure. This may be because the results have been somewhat heterogeneous. The customary visual evaluation procedure simply leaves too much room for a subjective interpretation, especially when the symptoms are weak, and incisive diagnostic information would be particularly appreciated by the examining physician.

There are two important shortcomings of conventional thermography applications. One is the difficulty of the human eye in quantifying unusual features in the distribution of the skin temperature on the basis of a thermogram, especially when the temperature variation is displayed in terms of a gray scale. The other is the restriction to stationary temperature distributions, which may very likely yield less conclusive diagnostic information than thermograms recorded during a dynamic situation enforced, for example, by a controlled cooling or warming process. To provide a better quantitative evaluation of unusual features of the temperature distribution and to permit the identification of new diagnostic parameters, a computer-assisted digital mapping procedure and color-coding of thermograms have been implemented (Anliker and Friedli, 1976). Some of the technical aspects of this procedure and recent results are presented in Section 4.

2 QUANTITATIVE EVALUATION OF FLOW CONDITIONS IN CERTAIN LARGE HUMAN ARTERIES BY MEANS OF ULTRASOUND

The instantaneous velocity profiles in larger blood vessels near the skin can be determined noninvasively and reproducibly with the aid of a multichannel pulsed ultrasound velocity meter. Such an instrument was designed and built at the Institut für Biomedizinische Technik in Zürich on

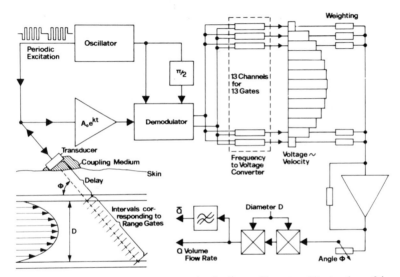

Figure 1. Multichannel pulsed ultrasound velocity profile meter. Short pulses of 4 or 8 sine waves with a frequency between 6 and 8 MHz are radiated across a vessel from a transducer placed on the skin. The pulse repetition frequency is about 20 kHz. During the intervals between successive pulses, the transducer is used as a receiver of the echo signals, which are amplified with a range-compensated gain. To allow for a spatial resolution of the Doppler frequency and hence the velocity, the echo signals emanating from within the vessel lumen are range gated, demodulated, sampled, and processed in parallel fashion by a set of 7–14 channels. Sign and magnitude of the velocity determined by the individual channel are based on the echoes received from a depth range corresponding to the times the channel begins and ends sampling the demodulated signal (Doriot et al., 1976). The velocities obtained in this manner are weighted by the areas of the associated half-annuli, added and multiplied twice by the vessel diameter after taking into account the angle ϕ. One thus arrives at the volume flow rate Q and by filtering or time averaging this quantity one obtains $\bar{Q}$.

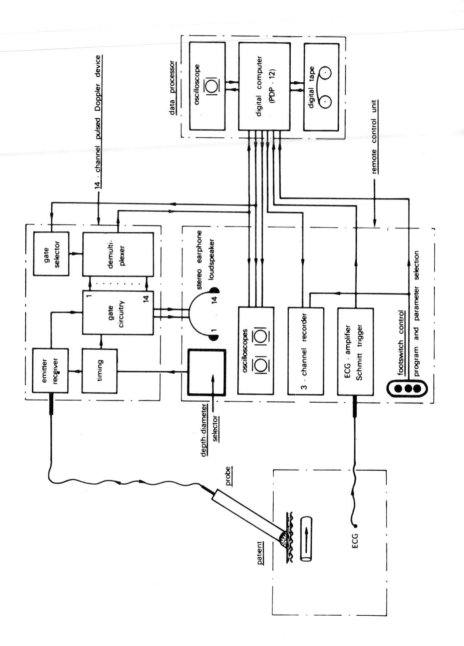

the basis of earlier work at Stanford University. Although the principle of operation of this velocity profile meter and some of its technical features have already been described elsewhere (Anliker, 1976; McLeod, 1974), a short review of the essential aspects is given here to facilitate the discussion of the limitations of the instrument and its clinical applications. Schematic diagrams of two different clinical systems currently used in the medical center of the University of Zürich are given in Figures 1 and 2. The principle of operation of the multichannel velocity meter is outlined in Figure 1.

To evaluate the phasic variations of the volume flow rate Q caused by the cardiac functions and respiration, the instantaneous velocity profiles have to be integrated over the cross section of the vessel. For the determination of the mean flow rate $\bar{Q}$, the instantaneous volume flow rate Q is integrated with respect to time. The evaluation of Q implies, however, a measurement of the vessel diameter and some indication that the cross section is circular. In addition, it must be assumed that any possible asymmetry of the velocity distribution across the vessel is in the mean equivalent to a corresponding asymmetry of the velocity profile obtained along the axis of the ultrasound beam. Within these restrictions, the volume flow rates can readily be evaluated by supplementing the velocity profile meter with a hard-wired hybrid computer (Figure 1) or connecting it to a PDP 12 computer (Figure 2). The integration procedure in determining Q is illustrated in Figure 3. Statistical fluctuations and artifacts may sometimes cause distortions of the instantaneous velocity profiles and the associated flow pulse when measurements are only carried out over a single cardiac cycle. To minimize distortions, the data are averaged digi-

---

Figure 2. Computer-assisted multichannel pulsed ultrasound velocity meter. A velocity profile meter with 14 channels has been modified for computer control. At uniform time intervals a PDP-12 computer synthesized a spatial velocity profile across the lumen by linearly interpolating the corresponding values of the 14 individual velocity–time functions generated by the set of channels. Instantaneous volume flow rate Q and the associated mean velocity v are evaluated by the computer. The ECG of the patient triggers both the PDP-12 computer and the display of Q and v on the oscilloscope. Within 500 μsec the velocity values of the frequency-to-voltage converters of the 14 channels are sampled and read into the A/D converter of the computer. By means of a foot switch, a command is given to the computer to average the velocity–time functions, the velocity profiles, and Q and v for 20 successive heart beats. The averaged data are immediately displayed on an oscilloscope and may be stored on a DEC tape for recall and comparison. With this system the total depth range of the 14 channels is usually set with the aid of the audio signals from channels 1 and 14 and by observing consecutive instantaneous velocity profiles.

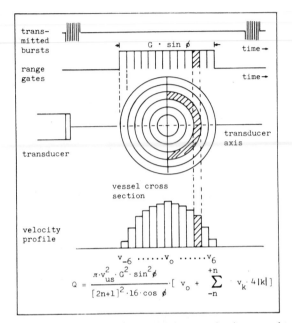

Figure 3. Integration of velocity profiles. The cross section is assumed to be circular and subdivided into annuli whose widths correspond to the depth interval of the individual channel. When the number of channels is odd, the central annulus degenerates into a circle with a diameter equal to the width of the other annuli. The velocity determined by any one of the channels is considered to be constant over the corresponding half-annulus as shown. For an odd number $(2n + 1)$ of channels the volume flow rate is given by the formula at the bottom of the figure. v_{us} is the speed of the ultrasound in blood and v'_k the velocity of channel k in the direction of the ultrasound beam.

tally for 8–20 successive heart beats. In the system shown in Figure 1, this is done by means of an iterator as schematically delineated in Figure 4.

A theoretic analysis and tests of the velocity profile meter and of the procedure involved in its application helped to identify the features and parameters that primarily limit the accuracy of the instrument (Doriot et al., 1976; Anliker, 1976). Flow studies on simulated arteries of various diameters have been carried out to document the different kinds of profile distortions caused by improper placements of the gates (see Figure 1), relatively high ratios of transducer diameter to vessel diameter, and by lengthening the ultrasound pulse (Doriot et al., 1976; Anliker, 1976). Corresponding errors in the volume flow rate determined from these profiles were evaluated with the help of flow-rate measurements, using beaker and stop watch. When the gates were properly placed, the errors

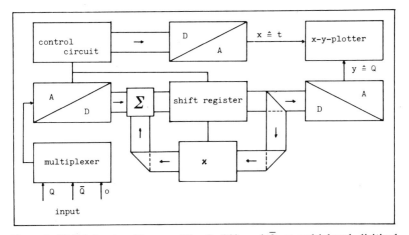

Figure 4. Digital iterator. The quantities 0, $Q(t)$, and $\overline{Q}$ are multiplexed, digitized, and stored in a shift register of 1,024 words with 10-bit resolution. Of the 1,024 words the first 8 are always set equal to zero, the next 1,008 places are used to store the values of $Q(t)$, the next 4 contain the value of $\overline{Q}$ and the last 4 are again set equal to zero. The shift register is part of a feedback loop with which seven-eighths of the previous shift register content is added to the new data. The cycle time of the loop is 1 sec. In the starting phase the control circuit sets $\kappa = 0$ for one cycle and then $\kappa = 1$ for the next 8 consecutive cycles, and after that $\kappa = \frac{7}{8}$. Upon command the control circuit stops the feedback loop, activates the $x-y$ plotter and initiates the read-out process from the shift register.

were generally within ±5% for stationary as well as pulsatile flow conditions. When transcutaneous measurements were simulated on anesthetized dogs by interposing muscle tissue between the exposed thoracic aorta and the transducer, the errors were generally within ±20%. This increase from ±5% to ±20% is mostly the result of inaccuracies in the determination of the lumen diameter and of the angle ϕ between the axis of the ultrasound beam and that of the vessel.

For clinical applications, a special transducer holder was designed that includes a goniometer. It is illustrated in Figure 5 and permits the rotation of the transducer about an axis that intersects the vessel axis at an angle of 90°. This holder enables a rather precise evaluation of the vessel diameter and a careful positioning of the gates across the lumen (Doriot et al., 1976; Casty, 1976). Following the procedure described in earlier publications, the overall accuracy of the trascutaneous volume flow determination is normally expected to be within ±20%.

When the aim of a clinical flow study is the identification of anatomic changes in the vasculature near the observation site, it may be advan-

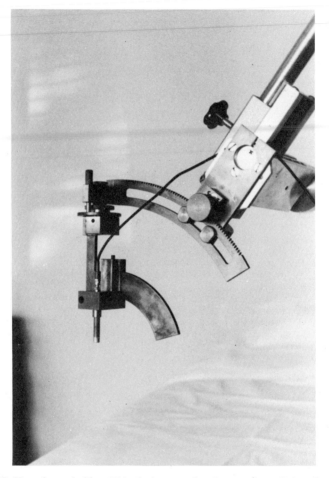

Figure 5. Transducer holder. This device permits the rotation of the ultrasound transducer about an axis that is perpendicular to the plane defined by the vessel and beam axes and that intersects the vessel axis. Accordingly, the velocity profile may be recorded at the same section where the diameter has been determined by echo ranging. A goniometer scale allows for a precise selection of the angle ϕ between the vessel axis and that of the ultrasound beam.

tageous to examine not only the flow pulse but also the variations of the instantaneous velocity profiles with the different phases of the cardiac cycle (Brunner et al., 1974; Doriot et al., 1976; Anliker, 1976). For example, the presence of plaques may give rise to asymmetries in the instantaneous velocity profiles and also to fluctuations in their form when they are monitored over several heart beats. Also, velocity profiles recorded at different points of an aneurysma, as illustrated in Figure 6, may reveal pathologic features of the arterial conduits. The profiles shown were recorded on a storage oscilloscope with the help of an ECG triggered sampling circuit. It allows for the continuous display of eight profiles

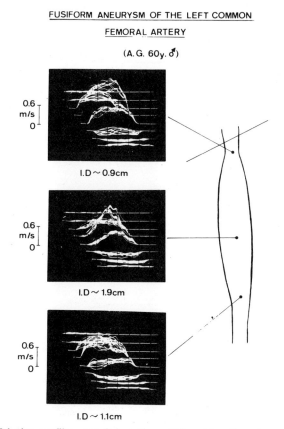

Figure 6. Velocity profiles recorded at three different locations in an aneurysma. Eight instantaneous velocity profiles are recorded at identical intervals uniformly distributed over the cardiac period beginning with the R peak of the ECG. The profiles have been superimposed for 10 successive heart beats and are displayed in a staggered formation for easier evaluation. They exhibit a more pronounced variability at the points where the blood enters and leaves the aneurysma than in its center. This variability seems to be associated with the accelerating and decelerating phases of the flow. The profiles recorded in the center of the aneurysma, where the inside diameter (I.D.) is approximately 1.9 cm, seem more closely of parabolic form during the systolic phase of the flow pulse than is the case at the entrance and exit.

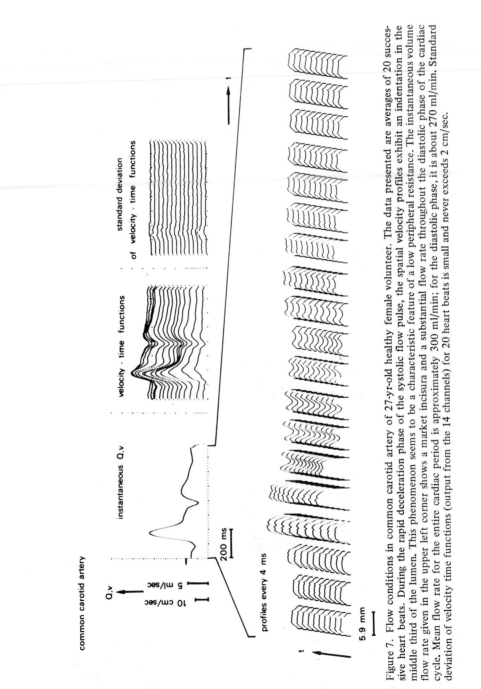

Figure 7. Flow conditions in common carotid artery of 27-yr-old healthy female volunteer. The data presented are averages of 20 successive heart beats. During the rapid deceleration phase of the systolic flow pulse, the spatial velocity profiles exhibit an indentation in the middle third of the lumen. This phenomenon seems to be a characteristic feature of a low peripheral resistance. The instantaneous volume flow rate given in the upper left corner shows a market incisura and a substantial flow rate throughout the diastolic phase of the cardiac cycle. Mean flow rate for the entire cardiac period is approximately 300 ml/min; for the diastolic phase, it is about 270 ml/min. Standard deviation of velocity time functions (output from the 14 channels) for 20 heart beats is small and never exceeds 2 cm/sec.

corresponding to eight distinct instants within each cardiac cycle and separated by a constant time interval. The superposition of these profiles for successive heart beats provides a graphic documentation of the velocity fluctuations that may be due to a variety of causes, such as instabilities in the flow induced by certain geometric features of the vessel, sinus arrhythmia, or turbulence.

More detailed information on the variation of the velocity profiles during the cardiac cycle can readily be made available when the profile meter is connected to a computer, as was done in the system outlined in Figure 2. Velocity profiles recorded every 4 msec in the common carotid artery of a 28-yr-old healthy female volunteer are illustrated in Figure 7 together with the instantaneous mean velocity and instantaneous volume flow rate plotted as a function of time. The indentation of the center of the profiles during the diminishing phase of the systolic flow pulse indicates a faster deceleration in the middle third of the vessel lumen than along the vessel wall. Such a phenomenon occurs in long circular cylindric

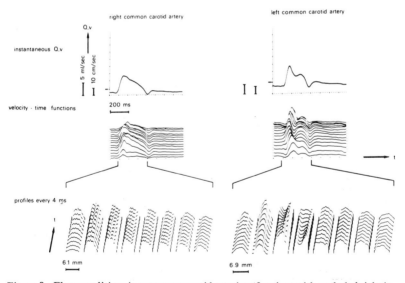

Figure 8. Flow conditions in common carotid arteries of patient with occluded right internal carotid artery. The flow pattern in the right common carotid artery of the 58-yr-old patient does not show indentation of velocity profiles during the deceleration phase. In addition, the volume flow rate during diastole is much lower than that of the healthy contralateral side. The occlusion of the right internal carotid artery appears to be responsible for a substantial increase in the peripheral resistance and a relatively low mean flow rate of 180 ml/min.

right common carotid artery before operation

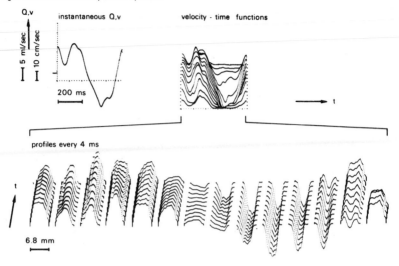

right common carotid artery 10 days after operation

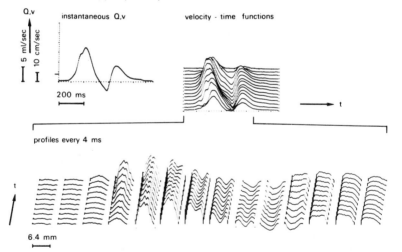

Figure 9. Flow patterns in common carotid artery of patient with aortic insufficiency before and after implantation of a Björk–Shiley valve prosthesis. Volume flow rate and velocity profiles in common carotid artery of this 28-yr-old patient clearly document a severe aortic insufficiency with a cardiac regurgitation fraction of about 75%. The back-flow fraction in common carotid artery is approximately 35%. During recovery from back flow, a reversal in the velocity direction occurs first along the vessel wall, while in the center of the lumen the velocity still indicates a flow towards the heart. This phenomenon can still be recognized after implantation of the prosthesis.

tubes under sinusoidal flow conditions. It has been predicted by Womersley (1955) and verified experimentally (Bendick, 1973) for certain values of $\alpha = R\sqrt{\omega\rho/\eta}$ where R is the radius of the lumen, ω the circular frequency of the sinusoidal flow variations, η the viscosity coefficient of the fluid, and ρ the density of the fluid. Hemodynamically, this phenomenon seems to imply a low peripheral resistance, since it has also been observed in a femoral artery proximal to a shunt (Brunner et al., 1974). Another indication for a low peripheral resistance is the relatively high mean volume flow rate Q_d during the diastolic phase of the flow pulse and by the low ratio $(Q_{max} - Q_d)/Q_d$ where Q_{max} is the systolic maximum flow rate. By contrast, as is evident from Figure 8, this ratio is substantially larger for the right common carotid artery of a patient whose right internal carotid artery is occluded; also, the indentation of the velocity profile is no longer present during the deceleration phase of the systolic flow pulse.

A particularly interesting case of a patient with aortic insufficiency is illustrated in Figure 9. The velocity profiles and flow patterns in the right common carotid artery are shown before and after implantation of a Björk–Shiley valve. Before operation, the velocity profiles do not exhibit the indentation during the late systolic phase. However, during the early systolic phase (recovery from back flow), the flow is characterized by saddle-type velocity profiles, which are also observed during sinusoidal flow in tubes for α values between approximately 4 and 9.

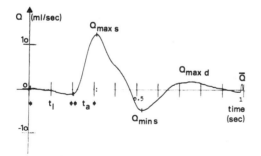

Figure 10. Instantaneous volume flow rate in the femoral of 31-yr-old healthy volunteer after period of rest. For a period of 1 sec, the instantaneous volume flow rate Q has been recorded from the shift register of the digital iterator shown in Figure 4. Also recorded are the mean flow rate $\overline{Q}$ and 0. t_1 denotes the time interval between the R peak of the ECG ($t = 0$) and the onset of the systolic flow pulse. t_a represents the rise time of the systolic peak $Q_{max\ s}$. $Q_{min\ s}$ indicates the postsystolic minimum flow rate and $Q_{max\ d}$ the diastolic maximum.

The system illustrated in Figure 1 has so far been primarily used to collect data for an atlas of normal and pathologic flow patterns in various larger arteries and veins near the skin (Casty, 1976). For example, under resting conditions, the volume flow rate Q may vary in the femoral artery of a healthy volunteer during a cardiac cycle as shown in Figure 10. This flow pattern exhibits, however, a certain degree of variability from volunteer to volunteer, as documented in Figure 11 and Table 1. This variability is also true of the axillary artery and the common carotid artery, for which sample recordings and data are given in Figures 12 and 13 and Tables 2 and 3. The variability of the resting flow patterns among healthy persons

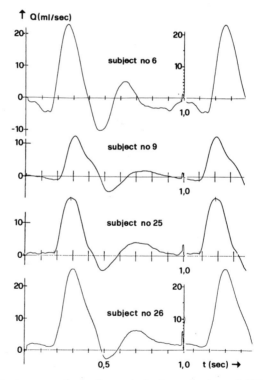

Figure 11. Instantaneous volume flow rate in femoral artery of different healthy subjects after 20-min period of rest. The curves demonstrate the variability of $Q(t)$ among different healthy subjects after resting 20 min in supine position. The corresponding values of the parameters defined in Figure 10 are given in Table 1. $t = 0$ defines the R peak of the ECG.

Table 1. Values of parameters characterizing instantaneous volume flow rate in femoral arteries of healthy volunteers under resting conditions

Volunteer no.	$\bar{Q}$ (ml/sec)	$Q_{max\ s}$ (ml/sec)	$Q_{min\ s}$ (ml/sec)	Ampl. (ml/sec)	$Q_{max\ d}$ (ml/sec)	t_1 (msec)	t_a (msec)
1	4.0	16	− 3	19	4	210	80
6	1.7	23	−10	33	5.2	160	110
7	3.3	14	− 4.5	28.5	2.3	160	95
8	1.6	10	− 3.0	13.0	1.0	200	140
9	2.2	12.5	− 4.7	17.2	1.8	200	110
17	4.4	35	−11	46	9.0	180	120
20	4.2	23	− 7.0	30	5.0	200	110
21	3.9	40	−12	52	6.3	190	90
22	6.4	40	−15	55	10.0	190	120
24	3.0	21	− 5	26	2.5	160	100
25	3.9	18	− 4.7	22.7	5.5	190	95
26	6.2	25	− 3.0	28	6.1	180	120
Mean value	3.7	23.1	− 6.9	30.9	4.9	185	107.5
S.D.	1.5	10.3	4.1	13.5	2.8	17.3	16.5

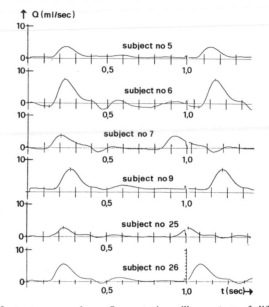

Figure 12. Instantaneous volume flow rate in axillary artery of different healthy subjects after period of rest. The curves show that the incisura cannot be precisely identified in all cases. Also, in contrast to the femoral artery, the flow does not necessarily reverse its direction in the postsystolic and diastolic phase of the cardiac cycle. $t = 0$ defines the R peak of the ECG.

may be due to a multitude of reasons. To suppress somewhat the effects of an immediate prehistory in terms of food intake, physical activity, emotional experience, etc. on the blood flow to the extremities, a physiologic maneuver is frequently imposed in the form of a reactive hyperemia. In such a maneuver all blood flow to the particular limb of interest is blocked for 3 min with the help of a pneumatic cuff. Upon release of the cuff pressure, the oxygen deficiency in the downstream part of the limb causes a distinct rise in the flow rate which, in the absence of obstructions or other impairments to flow, occurs rapidly and also decays rapidly, as illustrated in Figure 14. A representative set of data for healthy young volunteers is compiled in Tables 4 and 5. Age, weight, height, body surface area, and blood pressure of the volunteers are given in Table 6. The diagnostic significance of the parameters measured during postocclusive reactive hyperemia is demonstrated in the example that is documented in Figure 15.

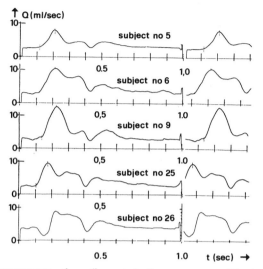

Figure 13. Instantaneous volume flow rate in the common carotid artery of different healthy subjects after period of rest. All subjects exhibit a substantial diastolic flow rate and a relatively low value for $(Q_{max\ s} - Q_d)/Q_d$ where Q_d is the mean diastolic flow rate.

3 ON-LINE MEASUREMENT OF FLOW IN HUMAN CAPILLARIES BY VIDEOMICROSCOPY AND SPATIAL CORRELATION OF IMAGES

In animal experiments the flow of blood in capillaries has so far mostly been examined with the help of the so-called double-slit technique, which allows for the on-line recording of the RBC speed in a single capillary and usually requires transillumination of the tissue (Wayland and Johnson, 1967). One of the major advantages of utilizing television microscopy and videorecorders for the study of transport phenomena in the capillary bed lies in the possibility of studying the events in a group of 6–12 capillaries rather than merely in one (Bollinger et al., 1974b; Intaglietta, Tompkins, and Richardson, 1970; Butti et al., 1975). This capability is essential, because the flow patterns in a single capillary may not be representative or typical of the microvascular bed to which it belongs. With the adaption of the double-slit technique to videomicroscopy and the development of a velocity-tracking correlator (Hollinger et al., 1975; Tompkins et al., 1974), the speed of RBCs can also be evaluated on line during recording and playback of the videotape. A schematic diagram of a system permitting such a measurement process for capillaries of the human nailfold is given

Table 2. Values of parameters characterizing instantaneous volume flow rate in axillary arteries of healthy volunteers under resting conditions

Volunteer no.	$\bar{Q}$ (ml/sec)	$Q_{\max s}$ (ml/sec)	$Q_{\min s}$ (ml/sec)	Ampl. (ml/sec)	$Q_{\max a}$ (ml/sec)	t_1 (msec)	t_a (msec)
5	1.4	4.0	0.6	3.4	1.0	150	90
6	1.0	7.5	−2.0	9.5	0.9	135	95
7	0.9	4.0	−1.5	5.5	0.5	130	95
8	0.6	4.5	−0.5	5.0	1.0	110	100
9	2.0	7.0	0.8	6.2	2.0	170	100
10	1.9	10.5	−1.0	11.5	3.2	120	100
11	1.2	7.5	−0.4	7.9	1.2	130	80
13	1.2	7.0	−0.7	7.7	1.5	120	100
14	0.8	7.0	−2.0	9.0	2.0	120	80
25	0.7	2.8	−0.3	3.1	0.6	150	80
26	1.9	5.5	−0.5	6.0	1.2	150	80
Mean value	1.24	6.1	−0.7	6.8	1.4	135	90.9
S.D.	0.5	2.2	0.9	2.6	0.8	18.0	9.2

Table 3. Values of parameters characterizing instantaneous volume flow rate in common carotid arteries of healthy volunteers under resting conditions

Volunteer no.	$\bar{Q}$ (ml/sec)	$Q_{max\ s}$ (ml/sec)	$Q_{min\ s}$ (ml/sec)	Ampl. (ml/sec)	$Q_{max\ d}$ (ml/sec)	t_1 (msec)	t_a (msec)
5	3.9	8.0	3.0	5.0	4.7	120	90
6	5.0	10.5	3.5	7.0	5.7	120	95
7	6.3	13.0	3.0	10	6.4	90	80
8	5.0	11.8	2.3	9.5	5.3	130	70
9	4.8	12.5	2.5	10	5.8	140	85
25	4.5	9.5	2.3	7.2	5.2	100	80
26	6.2	8.7	2.5	6.2	6.0	155	70
Mean value	5.1	10.6	2.7	7.8	5.6	122	81
S.D.	0.9	1.9	0.5	2.0	0.6	22	9

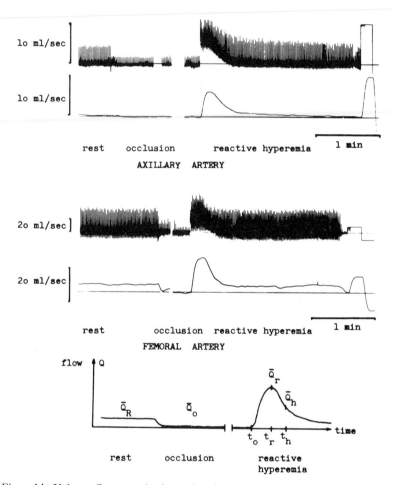

Figure 14. Volume flow rate in femoral and axillary arteries of healthy subjects during postocclusive reactive hyperemia. The recordings of instantaneous and mean volume flow rates are representative of normal peripheral circulation in the limbs of healthy subjects. Occlusion was induced by pneumatic cuff that was inflated a pressure of 300 mm Hg for 3 min. t_o denotes the time instant of release of cuff pressure, t_r that of maximum flow response. t_h defines the time at which the mean flow response decays to $\frac{1}{2}(\bar{Q}_r + \bar{Q}_s)$. The parameter values for the two recordings are listed in Tables 4 and 5.

Table 4. Results of flow measurements in femoral arteries of healthy subjects during occlusive reactive hyperemia

Volunteer no.	$\bar{Q}_R$ (ml/sec)	$Q_{max\,s}$ (ml/sec)	$Q_{min\,s}$ (ml/sec)	$Ampl._s$ (ml/sec)	$\bar{Q}_0$ (ml/sec)	$\bar{Q}_r$ (ml/sec)	t_r (sec)	t_h (sec)	$Q_{max\,r}$ (ml/sec)	$Q_{min\,r}$ (ml/sec)	$Ampl._r$ (ml/sec)
1	3.9	15	1	14	2.0	9.5	10	23	22	10	12
8	2.1	28	− 5	33	0	17.5	14	37	40	10	30
9	4.1	23	− 6	29	1.6	16.5	12.5	21	30	8	22
12	7.7	32	−13	45	1.9	31.9	11	20	50	10	40
18	6.0	28	−12	40	1.0	20.7	12	20	28	0	28
20	2.4	21	− 1	22	0.5	10.9	10	23	22	7	15
21	3.6	35	−10	45	0.5	17.0	8	37	35	7	28
22	4.9	35	−10	45	0.7	21	12	22	40	5	35
24	3.0	21	− 7	28	1.0	12.1	11	26	25	5	20
26	4.3	23	−10	33	0.1	13.1	12	18	30	0	30
Mean value	4.2	26.1	− 7.3	33.4	0.9	17.0	11.3	24.7	32.2	6.2	26.0
S.D.	1.7	6.6	4.6	10.6	0.7	6.6	1.7	6.8	9.0	3.8	8.7

Table 5. Results of flow measurements in axillary arteries of healthy subjects during occlusive reactive hyperemia

Volunteer no.	$\bar{Q}_R$ (ml/sec)	$Q_{\max s}$ (ml/sec)	$Q_{\min s}$ (ml/sec)	Ampl._s (ml/sec)	$\bar{Q}_o$ (ml/sec)	$\bar{Q}_r$ (ml/sec)	t_r (sec)	t_h (sec)	$Q_{\max r}$ (ml/sec)	$Q_{\min r}$ (ml/sec)	Ampl._r (ml/sec)
5	3.1	7.0	1.8	5.2	0	9.1	12	35	13	7	6
6	1.0	7.0	−2.0	9.0	0	8.2	10	24	15	5	9
7	1.4	6.5	−1.5	8.0	0.3	14.2	12	22	10	5	5
8	0.4	4.5	−0.5	5.0	0.1	6.9	14	22	11	5	5
9	3.0	7.5	1.5	6.0	0	12.2	12	27	15	8	7
13	1.8	6.0	0	6.0	0.3	4.9	9	21	10	2	8
23	1.3	6.0	0	6.0	0.2	6.9	13	29	12	4	8
25	1.3	3.5	0.5	3.0	0	7.0	9	22	10	6	4
Mean value	1.7	6.0	0.0	6.0	0.1	8.7	11.4	25.3	12.0	5.3	6.5
S.D.	0.9	1.4	1.3	1.8	0.14	3.1	1.9	4.8	2.1	1.8	1.8

Table 6. Physical parameters of volunteers

Volunteer no.	Age (yr)	Height (cm)	Weight (kg)	Body surface (m^2)	Blood pressure (mm Hg)
1	21	164	55	1.58	110/80
5	27	179	75	1.93	115/90
6	62	178	90	2.09	130/85
7	53	160	64	1	125/80
8	21	168	51	1.56	110/75
9	30	178	75	1.92	110/70
10	28	192	82	2.10	120/90
11	26	162	56	1.58	105/75
12	26	184	74	1.96	120/80
13	26	182	75	1.96	135/90
14	25	174	61	1.73	120/80
17	24	181	72	1.91	120/80
18	31	186	80	2.04	140/80
20	27	186	74	1.97	120/80
21	34	183	77	2.00	125/70
22	26	185	75	1.97	125/75
23	62	160	65	1.67	140/90
24	26	174	60	1.72	110/70
25	31	168	55	1.61	110/80
26	29	174	70	1.84	105/70

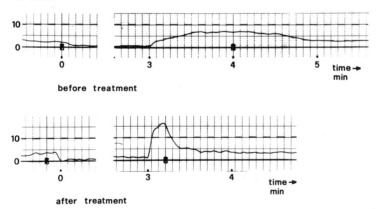

Figure 15. Postocclusive reactive hyperemia measured in the femoral artery of a 60-yr-old patient with a stenosis in the right iliac artery before and after treatment. Before recanalization of the iliac artery has been performed, the maximum of the mean flow rate is reached about 1 min after release of pressure in the cuff. The peak flow rate is approximately 7 ml/sec. A few days after treatment (recanalization) the maximum flow response is already reached 11 sec after cuff release. Besides this, the maximum mean flow rate reached is now 16 ml/sec.

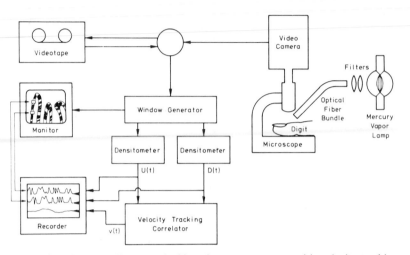

Figure 16. Schematic diagram of videomicroscopy system with velocity-tracking correlator. The nailfold of a finger or toe is positioned under a microscope (Wild M 20) and illuminated with the aid of a mercury vapor lamp. To improve the visualization of the capillary bed, the transparency of the skin is enhanced by the application of a layer of paraffin oil or clear nail polish. A segment of the capillary bed is viewed through a plan fluotar objective 6.0/0.2 and zoom by a silicon target video camera (RCA 4532). The images are displayed on a monitor and simultaneously recorded with a video tape recorder. The scale of the image is generally 2 μ per raster line. A window generator permits the placement of two separate windows of variable size at an upstream and a downstream location of the capillary in which the RBC speed is to be determined. The average density of the video signal within the two windows is evaluated by means of a dual-channel videophotometric analyzer (videodensitometer). The variation with time of the two video densities $U(t)$ and $D(t)$ is continuously recorded in graphic form. Besides this, the time delay of the downstream signal $D(t)$ is computed with the aid of a velocity-tracking correlator (Instrumentation for Physiology and Medicine, San Diego, California) and used to determine the RBC velocity.

in Figure 16. Because the video camera records 50 frames per second (60 frames/sec in the United States) the mean video signals in the two windows (slits) are sampled at intervals of 20 msec. For a determination of the speed of RBCs from their transmission time between the two windows separated by a known distance, it is necessary that the same sequence of RBCs and plasma spaces be seen at both the upstream and the downstream window. For this to be possible, the flow rate must be sufficiently small so that the plasma space or RBC seen at the upstream window is not already beyond the downstream window when the next video frame is recorded. By means of a temporal correlation of the corresponding signals $U(t)$ and

$D(t)$, the transmission time can then be determined (Hollinger et al., 1975; Tompkins et al., 1974).

Because the sequences of RBCs and plasma spaces moving through the capillaries are monitored temporally every 20 msec and spatially through the two small windows, a large portion of the motion information is discarded. Therefore, as is evident from Figure 17, the time interval between observations of signals $U(t)$ and $D(t)$, which correspond to the same plasma space and thus can be correlated, may be of the order of seconds. This implies that variations of the RBC speed that are in phase with the cardiac function are not necessarily recognized when the double-window technique is used. One way to overcome some of these difficulties and limitations inherent in the dual-window videodensitometric technique is to replace the two small windows by a single one that can be positioned over the capillary as illustrated in Figure 18. Within this window, the video signal is integrated for each line to provide a video density distribution $S(x)$ along the capillary. If the time interval between this video image and a later one can be selected such that no more than about half of the RBC plasma space sequence contained within the window has moved beyond it, then the displacement can be evaluated by a spatial correlation process as shown in Figure 19. Dividing the displacement by the corresponding time interval, one obtains a measure of the RBC speed and flow velocity.

Although the temporal correlation process utilized in the double-window technique requires an integration time of at least several seconds and thus a large number of video frames, the spatial correlation associated

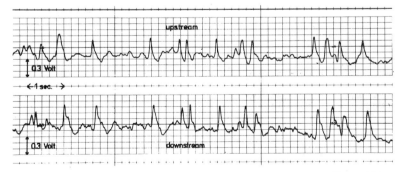

Figure 17. Recording of videodensitometer signals from nailfold capillary of 31-yr-old healthy volunteer. Large amplitude deflections are induced by longer plasma gaps. The window separation is 40 μ and the RBC speed about 0.4 mm/sec. The delay of the downstream signal $D(t)$ can be evaluated from the recording.

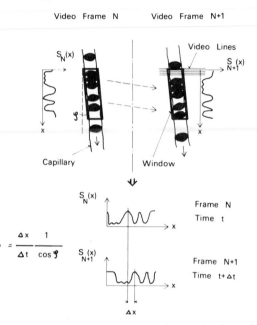

Figure 18. Graphic illustration of single-window technique for the evaluation of the RBC speed. The same capillary is schematically redrawn from video images N and $N + 1$ recorded at the times t and $t + \Delta t$. By integrating for each line the video signal within the window, one obtains a density pattern $S_N(x)$ and $S_{N+1}(x)$ along the capillary corresponding to the instantaneous distribution of the RBCs and plasma gaps. When the capillary has a sufficiently small and uniform diameter, the features of this pattern can be seen moving along the capillary as indicated in video image $N + 1$. The maximum of the spatial correlation of the density patterns $S_N(x)$ and $S_{N+1}(x)$ yields the displacement of the capillary content during the time interval Δt.

with the single-window approach requires basically only two video frames. To allow for high speeds and accordingly for very short time intervals between successive video frames to be correlated, the microscopic scene is viewed with two video cameras whose recording cycles have a precisely controlled phase difference, as schematically shown in Figure 20. Another solution would be to reduce the number of video lines per image; this, however, would lead to a reduction of the area of the capillary bed and therefore to a smaller number of capillaries that can be examined (Goodman et al., 1974). A further advantage of the system illustrated in Figure 20 is that the size, shape, and position of the window—and also the analysis of the video signal—can be chosen in a manner depending on the

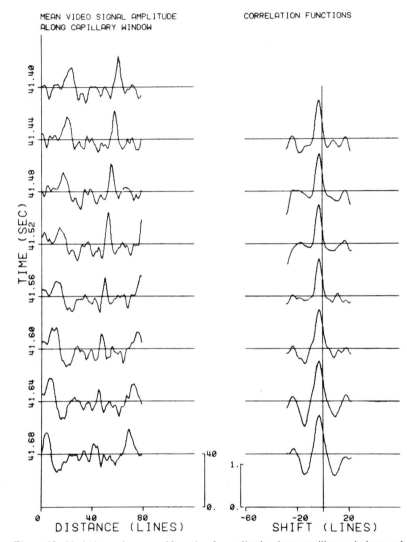

Figure 19. Variation of mean video signal amplitude along capillary window and correlation functions for successive frames. In the window data on the left-hand side a large amplitude represents a plasma gap. A comparison of these data from top to bottom reveals a displacement of the capillary content towards the left in intervals of 40 msec. The corresponding velocity is on the order of 0.15 mm/sec. The positions of the peaks of the correlation functions on the right-hand side define the displacements between successive window data plots.

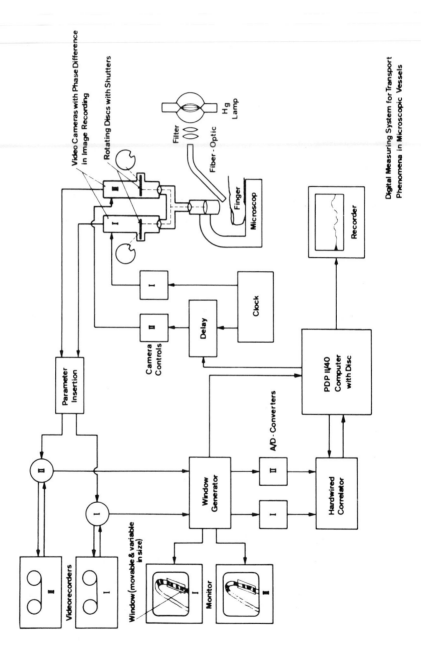

Digital Measuring System for Transport
Phenomena in Microscopic Vessels

application to be pursued. For example, for detailed studies of diameters, hematocrit, aggregation, and capillary exchange processes, the system permits the digital mapping of the video signal and the analysis of the data by the computer.

Because of the lag of the video camera utilized (RCA 4532), the video signal at any time contains, under the operating conditions considered here, between 30% and 60% of the previous image information. This causes distortions of the actual scenes (Rindfleisch et al., 1971) and accordingly impairs the velocity determination by the spatial correlation technique, especially at higher and at rapidly changing velocities. In the system illustrated in Figure 20 the variation $S(x)$ of the mean video signal amplitude along the capillary window is stored in digital form. Hence the lag effect can be reduced in a rough but computationally efficient way by continually subtracting from $S(x)$ a constant percentage of the corresponding value of the previous frame. The effect of camera lag and the reduction of the residual image are documented in Figure 21 for a simulated sequence of erythrocyte rouleaux with two plasma gaps moving with a speed of 1.2 mm/sec. It shows the computer plot of $S(x)$ before and after camera lag correction. With the lag effect largely removed, the plasma spaces and erythrocyte rouleaux are delineated much more sharply and the displacement of the capillary content, for which the correlation function assumes a maximum, can be more precisely determined. A further improvement of the velocity determination is achieved by removing the background in $S(x)$. This is done by recursive digital high-pass filtering of $S(x)$ whereby the cutoff frequency is less than 0.1 Hz and the phase response is practically zero (Goodman et al., 1974; Shanks, 1967). Measurements of RBC speeds in capillaries of the human nailfold during reactive hyperemia are in progress. Initial studies of resting flow patterns

Figure 20. Computer-assisted measuring system for transport phenomena in microscopic vessels. The capillary bed is viewed with two video cameras where recording cycles have a precisely controlled phase difference. To allow for a sharp image of the instantaneous sequence of RBCs and plasma gaps, a set of rotating shutters is exposing the cameras for a variable time interval at a preselected instant of the recording cycle. A time code generator and parameter insertion unit labels each video frame in alphanumeric and binary form so that the information can be read by the experimenter as well as the computer. The window generator enables the placement of a parallelogram whose width, length, and inclination with regard to the horizontal lines can be chosen over the capillary of interest. A/D converters permit the on-line digital mapping of the video signal at rates up to 15 MHz. To allow for an on-line RBC speed determination, a hard-wired correlator has been built that evaluates the correllelogram of the video densities along the capillary for forward and backward flow within less than 10 msec.

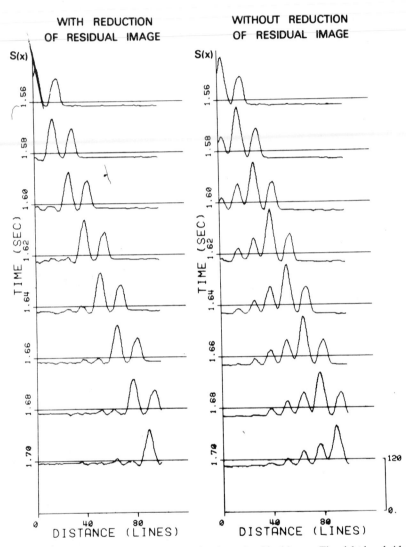

Figure 21. Effect of camera lag and reduction of residual image. The right-hand side shows the mean video signal amplitude $S(x)$ for a simulated sequence of erythrocyte rouleaux with two plasma gaps moving together with a speed of 1.2 mm/sec. The two moving bright rectangular areas that characterize the plasma gaps should appear as two peaks in $S(x)$. Because of the camera lag, a residue of the preceding image can be observed. By continually subtracting a fixed percentage (in this case 48%) of the previous $S(x)$ from the current mean video signal amplitude, the residual image is reduced as illustrated on the left-hand side.

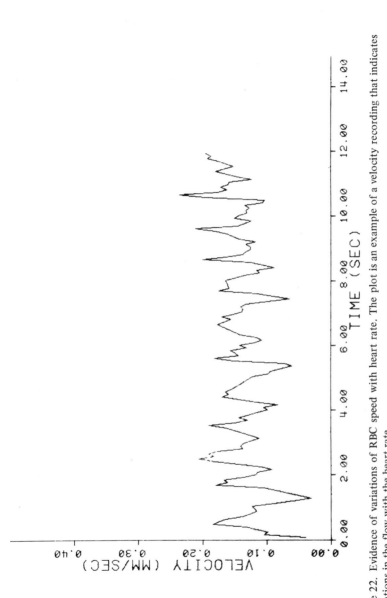
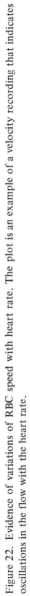

Figure 22. Evidence of variations of RBC speed with heart rate. The plot is an example of a velocity recording that indicates oscillations in the flow with the heart rate.

in such capillaries with the aid of the spatial correlation technique have shown that in some cases the RBC speed exhibits oscillations that are in phase with the heart rhythm. An example of such oscillations is given in Figure 22.

4   COMPUTER-ASSISTED THERMOGRAPHIC IDENTIFICATION OF UNUSUAL PATTERNS IN REGIONAL BLOOD FLOW

The work described here was preceded by a preliminary study of the possibilities of detecting breast cancer in female patients at the medical center of the University of Zürich. That study was carried out with a recently developed high-resolution thermograph, and the results from 650 women reconfirmed the need for a more quantitative approach in evaluating the features of the temperature distribution of the skin. The unit used is a Spectrotherm[1] Model 1000. It synthesizes an image as illustrated schematically in Figure 23. The object is scanned horizontally by a hexagonal mirror that rotates at 3,000 RPM and thus generates 300 image lines per second. Between two successive horizontal lines, a tilting mirror effects a vertical deflection of the scan level. With the help of a germanium lens, the thermal radiation of the object is focused on an infrared detector of the mercury-cadmium-telluride type that is cooled by liquid nitrogen. At the scanning speed utilized, the detector has a temperature resolution of $0.2°C$ or better. A full image consists of 525 lines with 600 points each and requires a scanning time of 1.75 sec. The storage of the thermogram in a video memory allows for a black-and-white display with a refresh cycle of 50 frames per second and thus for an immediate visual evaluation of the temperature distribution.

To permit an on-line computer analysis of the thermograms, the Spectrotherm unit was modified and interfaced with a PDP 11/40 computer. Thus, a computer-controlled thermography system was realized. Some of its principal features have been reported (Anliker and Friedli, 1976), but they are briefly reiterated here for the sake of continuity and to establish a technical basis for the description of the digital image analysis procedures developed during recent months. In this system the detector signal is not only fed into a video memory, but also digitized on line to an accuracy of 8 bits and stored by way of an asynchronous data flow

---

[1] Spectrotherm Corporation, 3040 Olcott Street, Santa Clara, California 95051.

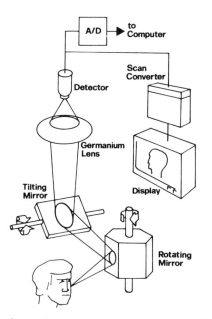

Figure 23. Principle of operation of high-resolution thermograph. The thermal radiation of a point of the object is focused on the infrared detector by means of a germanium lens. A hexagonal rotating mirror produces a horizontal scan, and a tilting mirror the vertical deflection of the scan level. To visualize the image, it is stored in a video memory and displayed on a monitor with a refresh cycle of 50 frames per second. For the on-line digital mapping of the thermogram, the infrared signal is continually digitized to 8-bit accuracy and stored on the disk cartridge of a PDP 11/40 computer. An uninterrupted data flow onto the disk is arranged through buffer memories and computer control of the tilting mirror.

of a disk cartridge of the PDP 11/40. An asynchronous data flow is required, because each horizontal line is generated by only 30% of the width of a single face of the rotating mirror. This implies that the A/D converter yields bursts of information representing individual image lines. To avoid interruptions in writing the data onto the disk, a buffer storage arrangement and a computer control of the scanning process have been designed as indicated in Figure 24. The interface between the A/D converter and the unibus contains a small hard-wired "first-in–first-out" (FIFO) buffer memory with a capacity of 384 × 8 bits. From this buffer the signal is read into a set of 12 additional FIFO memories that are split off from the core of the PDP 11/40 computer through software design. Each of these has a capacity of 512 × 8 bits. Finally, the digitized image

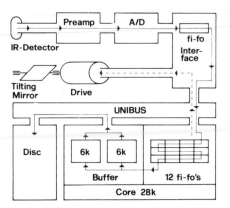

Figure 24. Buffer arrangement for on-line disk storage of thermogram. A continuous writing process for the storage of the digitized infrared image onto the disk of a PDP 11/40 computer is provided by a set of "first-in–first-out" memories and a double buffer. To prevent overflow in the 12 FIFOs of the core memory, the tilting mirror drive is controlled by the computer by way of a feed back loop.

information is double buffered in the core to increase the transfer rate onto the disk. The writing speed of the disk is not quite sufficient to accommodate the data flow dictated by the 3,000 RPM of the hexagonal mirror. Therefore, the step-wise rotation of the tilting mirror is briefly halted by the computer whenever overflow is imminent in the 12 buffer memories. By introducing a supplemental damping of the tilt drive, this intermittent stoppage does not lead to fluctuations in line positions. With this solution, the scan and digital mapping time for a thermogram can be minimized to 2.05 sec.

While the thermogram is digitally mapped onto the disk, the image information is also processed in a programmed manner by the computer and the resulting data transferred via unibus into the MOS memory of a Ramtek[2] GX 100A color display unit as shown in Figure 25. The Ramtek device permits a progressive display of the thermogram on the color monitor so that the completely processed image is available for an initial, qualitative visual assessment at the end of the scanning and digital mapping operation. A set of seven thermograms may be recorded on a single disk. To allow for a comparison of images in follow-up examinations, the digitized thermograms are transferred onto a magnetic tape.

In current medical applications of the system schematically illustrated

---

[2] Ramtek Corporation, 292 Commercial Street, Sunnyvale, California 94086.

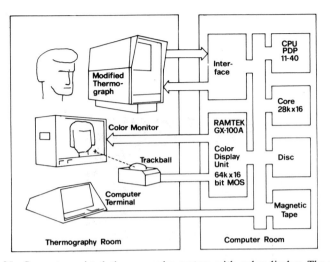

Figure 25. Computer-assisted thermography system with color display. The system consists of a modified Spectrotherm Model 1000 thermograph with a black-and-white video memory, a PDP 11/40 computer including a RKO5 disk and a Pertec T 9640 (Pertec Peripheral Equipment Division, 9600 Irondale Ave., Chatsworth, Ca. 91311) magnetic tape, a Ramtek GX 100A color display unit, a Conrac (Conrac Corporation, 600 N. Rimsdale Ave., Covina, Ca. 91722) color monitor, trackball unit, and a VTO5 computer terminal. With on-line digital mapping included, the scanning operation is completed in 2.05 sec. Simultaneous processing of the digitized infrared signal and utilization of a Ramtek graphic color display unit with a 64 k × 16 bit MOS memory permit the visualization of the thermogram as a color-coded image in terms of 512 lines, containing 512 points each, or of 256 lines with 512 points each. With these two levels of image resolution one has 4 or 8 bits available for color coding.

in Figure 25, the color-coded thermograms are usually displayed in terms of 256 lines with 512 points each. The initial color-coded temperature distribution presented at the end of the scanning operation is based on the 4 most significant bits of the infrared signal. With these 4 bits a raster of 15 colors is defined in which the colors are chosen to permit an easy distinction of the corresponding temperature intervals. The two end colors of the raster are black and white. They represent, respectively, all temperatures lower and higher than those of the neighboring colors. If a more detailed display of the temperature pattern is desired for some part of the image, the temperature interval for each of the colors can be reduced selectively from 0.5°C to 0.1°C or less as shown in Figure 26. In a color-coded thermogram the visual evaluation of the area distribution of a certain color is much more reliable than that of a certain gray level in a black-and-white infrared image. Accordingly, any asymmetries or unusual

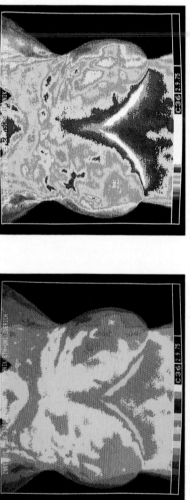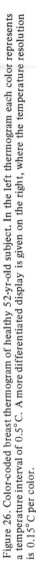

Figure 26. Color-coded breast thermogram of healthy 52-yr-old subject. In the left thermogram each color represents a temperature interval of 0.5°C. A more differentiated display is given on the right, where the temperature resolution is 0.15°C per color.

features, such as hot spots (Wallace and Cade, 1974), in the temperature pattern can be recognized more objectively by the human eye when the thermogram is displayed as a color image instead of on a gray scale basis. Of more importance, however, is the fact that the system offers a multitude of possibilities in digital image processing and establishing quantitative criteria for unusual temperature patterns. In view of its on-line capabilities, it should facilitate the extension of earlier efforts to identify a pathologic thermogram with the aid of computers (von Fournier et al., 1973; Winter and Stein, 1973; Ziskin et al., 1975).

New attempts have therefore been initiated to develop objective methods for recognizing abnormal distributions of the surface temperature of the female chest. In a first step, some features of the digitally mapped thermogram have been quantified. As illustrated in Figure 27, the geometric center and the heat center of each line of the frontal exposition are determined between the white horizontal lines at the upper end of the sternum and below the lower edges of the mammas. The distance between the two centers is normalized with respect to the width of the chest at the corresponding image line. The nondimensional value obtained in this manner is independent of the image magnification and quantifies the asymmetry of the temperature distribution on a line-by-line basis. The averages of this quantity and of its square are denoted by $\bar{\xi}$ and $\bar{\xi}^2$, called the mean of heat center deviation and the mean square of heat center deviation. $\bar{\xi}$ and $\bar{\xi}^2$ characterize the overall asymmetry of the temperature distribution with respect to the sagittal plane. Differences in the temperature patterns of the more lateral chest and mamma surfaces are not necessarily recognizable in a frontal exposition. Therefore, the corresponding asymmetries are quantified as indicated in Figure 27 from an oblique right and an oblique left view of the chest. By computing the parameter $\bar{\tau}$, defined as the difference between the mean temperatures of the corresponding marked areas (which may or may not include the axillary lymph nodes, depending on their temperature difference) of the two oblique views divided by the average of the two mean temperatures, an additional basis for a criterion is established.

A major disadvantage of color coding is that it generally obliterates the pathways of surface veins, which are to some extent recognizable when the thermogram is displayed in black and white. Because any unusual features in the temperature distribution are most likely caused by correspondingly unusual regional blood flow patterns through the surface veins, their distribution, i.e., the so-called vascularization, may reveal additional diag-

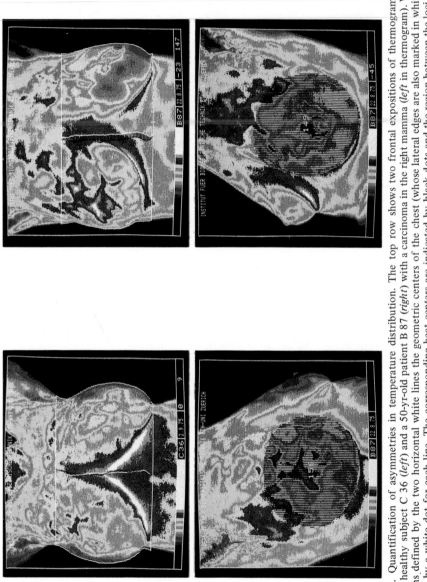

Figure 27. Quantification of asymmetries in temperature distribution. The top row shows two frontal expositions of thermograms of a 52-yr-old healthy subject C 36 (*left*) and a 50-yr-old patient B 87 (*right*) with a carcinoma in the right mamma (*left* in thermogram). Within the regions defined by the two horizontal white lines the geometric centers of the chest (whose lateral edges are also marked in white) are identified by a white dot for each line. The corresponding heat centers are indicated by black dots and the region between the loci of the two centers is shaded horizontally in black. For the healthy subject the two centers practically coincide, whereas for the patient with the cancer they are significantly separated. Accordingly, the values for ξ and ξ^2 are 0 and 9 for the left thermogram, -23 and 147 for that on the right, respectively. The bottom row shows half-right and half-left expositions of cancer patient B 87. The mamma areas are identified with the aid of the trackball unit and shaded vertically in black. For each of these areas the corresponding mean temperatures τ_l and τ_r (normalized arbitrarily) are computed with $\tau_l = 149$ and $\tau_r = 156$. One obtains $\bar{\tau} = 2(149 - 156)/(149 + 156) = 0.045$ or $-45\,^\circ/_{oo}$. For the

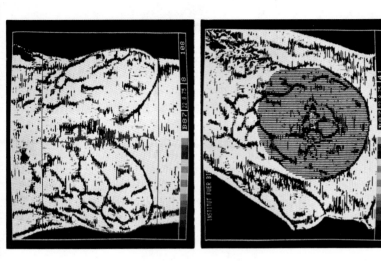

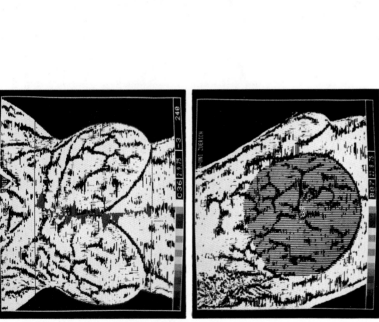

Figure 28. Identification and quantification of surface vein pattern. For the same set of thermograms shown in Figure 27 the surface veins are determined by an adaptive digital filtering process and marked in black. In the frontal expositions the asymmetry is graphically illustrated by red lines pointing towards the side that is locally less vascularized. The length of these lines is directly proportional to the asymmetry. The fluctuations of the direction seem to suggest an inadequate smoothening of η and possibly also an insufficient decisiveness of the identification algorithm. For the cancer patient B 87 one obtains $\overline{\eta} = 9$, $\overline{\eta^2} = 108$, and $\underline{\nu} = 41^0/_{00}$, while for the healthy subject C 36 the corresponding values are -3, 240, and 0, respectively.

nostic clues. By applying digital filtering techniques, it is possible to map the vasculature in terms of local maxima in the surface temperature distribution. This is demonstrated in Figure 28, which displays the distribution of the local temperature maxima without the surrounding temperature information. For the vascular pattern identified in this fashion, one can also compute corresponding asymmetry parameters $\bar{\eta}$ and $\bar{\eta}^2$, which are defined as the mean of vascular center deviation and the mean square of vascular center deviation and are computed in the same manner as are $\bar{\xi}$ and $\bar{\xi}^2$. Likewise, in analogy to $\bar{\tau}$, a parameter $\bar{\nu}$ may be defined for the vasculature contained within the marked areas of the oblique right and oblique left images as shown in Figure 28. The diagnostic significance of these parameters $\bar{\xi}, \bar{\xi}^2, \bar{\tau}, \bar{\eta}, \bar{\eta}^2$, and $\bar{\nu}$ with regard to breast tumors is now being examined by evaluating their ranges for healthy subjects and patients with proved tumors. It is hoped that they will help develop criteria for the early detection of breast cancer.

5 SUMMARY AND CONCLUSIONS

Recent designs of multichannel ultrasonic velocity profile meters offer new ways of obtaining quantitative information on the flow patterns in blood vessels near the skin. The shapes of the instantaneous spatial velocity profiles, as well as the instantaneous volume flow rates Q determined by integrating the profiles over the cross section, contain diagnostic information on peripheral vessel disease and in some circumstances also on certain disorders of the heart. Besides this, the spatial profiles and Q provide an additional basis for theoretic studies of the dynamics of the human arterial pulse. Of particular significance may be the possibility of preventing strokes by assessing the velocity profiles and the flow rates in extracranial arteries of patients with a relatively high risk of developing stenoses. Applications of the multichannel velocity meter to study the blood flow characteristics in the common carotid artery, the axillary artery, and the femoral artery are described. Some typical features of the flow patterns in these arteries are documented in sample recordings and tables for a number of healthy volunteers. Also, a quantitative analysis of the flow in the femoral and axillary arteries during occlusive reactive hyperemia is given for a group of these volunteers. Moreover, the diagnostic significance of the parameters measured is demonstrated in an example.

Television microscopy seems to be developing into an important tool for hemodynamic studies of capillaries in man. Microscopy systems involving a single video camera and utilizing the double-slit technique have a rather limited application range with regard to the speed of the red blood cells (RBC) and its temporal variations. Such systems can generally not be utilized when the RBC speed is much beyond 1 mm/sec, as may be the case in many subjects and is to be expected during a reactive hyperemia maneuver. A new system has, therefore, been developed in which a microscopic image of the capillary bed is viewed with two video cameras whose recording cycles have a precisely controlled phase difference. The cameras are modified to record all half-frames with identical line positions. The vessel of interest is surrounded by a parallelogram that forms a window within which the video signal is integrated for each line to provide a video density distribution along the vessel. A spatial correlation of the density distribution corresponding to two frames recorded within a given time interval yields a measure of the flow velocity. With the aid of a custom-made digital correlator the RBC speed can be evaluated on line (for forward or backward flow) during the videorecording process or playback. The time delay between the two frames is chosen such that the video density distributions overlap 50% at least. With a time delay of 1 msec the flow speed may be as high as 20–50 mm/sec, depending on vessel length and magnification. Also, because of the spatial correlation process, it is possible to quantify oscillatory patterns in capillary flow that are in phase with the cardiac rhythm.

Computer-assisted thermography is presented as an additional noninvasive method of assessing regional blood flow. Abnormal topographic variations of the skin temperature are, in general, primarily caused by unusual distributions in regional blood flow. By implementing an on-line digital mapping procedure for the infrared signal from a high-resolution thermograph, an immediate quantitative analysis of the temperature distribution has become possible. To facilitate the visual assessment of the features of the thermogram, it is displayed on a color monitor with the aid of a 64 k × 16-bits MOS memory and a graphic display system that provides a point raster of 512 × 512 points and 15 colors, each representing a preselected temperature interval. The time required for the scanning of an object, the processing of the infrared signal, and the visualization of the temperature pattern with a color-coding is about 2 sec. Certain pathologic features of the temperature pattern are identified by the computer within 2–5 sec and indicated graphically as well as numerically on the monitor. Moreover, by means of adaptive digital filtering techniques the surface veins can be identified on the digitally mapped thermogram and displayed for visual evaluation. Certain features of the surface vein distribution are also quantified in terms of indices in a fashion similar to the quantification of the temperature distribution. The system and methods developed are now being applied in a breast cancer detection project.

LITERATURE CITED

Anliker, M. 1971. Towards a nontraumatic study of the circulatory system. *In* Y. C. Fung, N. Perrone, and M. Anliker (eds.), Biomechanics, Its Foundations and Objectives. Prentice-Hall, Englewood Cliffs, N.J.

Anliker, M., R. L. Rockwell, and E. Ogden. 1971. Nonlinear analysis of flow pulses and shock waves in arteries. Part I: Derivation and properties of mathematical model. Part II: Parametric study related to clinical problems. J. Appl. Math. Phys. (ZAMP) 22: 217–246 (part I), 563–581 (part II).

Anliker, M. 1976. Diagnostic analysis of arterial flow pulses in man. *In* J. Baan, A. Noordergraaf, and J. Raines (eds.), Cardiovascular System Dynamics. MIT Press, Cambridge.

Anliker, M., and R. Kubli. 1976. A new on-line method of measuring high flow speeds in microscopic vessels by a dual video camera technique. Proceedings of the First World Congress for Microcirculation, Toronto, June 1975. Plenum, New York.

Anliker, M., and P. Friedli. 1976. Evaluation of high-resolution thermograms by on-line digital mapping and color-coding. Appl. Radiol. (in press).

Baker, D. W. 1970. Pulsed ultrasonic Doppler blood-flow sensing. IEEE Trans. Sonics Ultrasonics, SU-17/3: 170–185.

Bendick, Ph. 1973. A laser Doppler study of velocity profiles in oscillatory flow. Ph.D. Dissertation, Stanford University.

Bollinger, A., H. H. Brunner, and M. Anliker. 1974a. Ultraschalldiagnostik. *In* F. Loogen and K. Kredner (Hrsg.), Gefässerkrankungen, pp. 97–105. G. Witzstock, Baden-Baden/Brüssel.

Bollinger, A., P. Butti, J.-P. Barras, H. Trachsler, and W. Siegenthaler. 1974b. Red blood cell velocity in nailfold capillaries of man measured by a television microscopy technique. Microvasc. Res. 7: 61–72.

Brunner, H. H., A. Bollinger, M. Anliker, H. J. Zweifel, and W. Rutishauser. 1974. Bestimmung instantaner Strömungsprofile in der A. femoralis communis mit gepulstem Doppler-Ultraschall bei Stenosen und Verschlüssen. Deutsche Medizinische Wochenschrift 99: 3–12.

Butti, P., M. Intaglietta, H. Reimann, Ch. Holliger, A. Bollinger, and M. Anliker Capillary red blood cell velocity measurements in human nailfold by videodensitometric method. Microvasc. Res. 10 (1975) (in press).

Casty, M. 1976. Perkutane atraumatische Flussmessung in grossen haut-nahen Gefässen mit einem vielkanaligen gepulsten Ultraschall-Doppler-Gerät. Inauguraldissertation der Medizinischen Fakultät der Universität Zürich.

Cheng, L. C., J. M. Robertson, and M. E. Clark. 1974. Calculation of plane pulsatile flow past wall obstacles. Computers and Fluids 2: 363–380.

Daigle, R. E., C. W. Miller, M. B. Histand, F. D. McLeod, and D. E. Hokanson. 1975. Nontraumatic aortic blood flow sensing by use of an ultrasonic esophageal probe. J. Appl. Physiol. 38: 1153–1160.

Darling, R. C., J. K. Raines, B. J. Brener, and W. G. Austen. 1972. Quantitative segmental pulse volume recorder: a clinical tool. Surgery 72: 873–887.

Doriot, P. A., M. Casty, B. Milakara, M. Anliker, A. Bollinger, and W. Siegenthaler. 1976. Quantitative analysis of flow conditions in simulated vessels and large human arteries and veins by means of ultrasound. Excerpta Medica (in press).

Elsner, J. 1975. Mathematische Modellstudien der Druck- und Flusspulse in menschlichen Arterien. Dissertation, Eidg. Technische Hochschule Zürich.

von Fournier, D., J. Kuttig, S. Curland, and H. Poser. 1973. Auswertung von Thermogrammen mit dem Computer in der Mammakarzinom-Diagnostik. Strahlentherapie 145: 406–414.

Fronek, A., K. H. Johansen, R. B. Dilley, and E. F. Bernstein. 1973. Noninvasive physiologic tests in the diagnosis and characterization of peripheral arterial occlusive disease. Amer. J. Surg. 126: 205–214.

Goodman, A. H., A. C. Guyton, R. Drake, and J. H. Loflin. 1974. A television method for measuring capillary red cell velocities. J. Appl. Physiol. 37: 126–130.

Holliger, Ch., M. Anliker, D. Klingler, and A. Bollinger. 1975. Evaluation of an on-line videodensitometric measurement of red blood cell velocity in the capillaries of the human nailfold. Biomed. Tech. 20: 187–192.

Intaglietta, M., W. R. Tompkins, and D. R. Richardson. 1970. Velocity measurements in the microvasculature of the cat omentum by on-line method. Microvasc. Res. 2: 462–473.

McLeod, F. D. 1974. Multichannel pulse Doppler techniques. In R. S. Reuemann (ed.), Cardiovascular Applications of Ultrasound. North-Holland, Amsterdam.

Peronneau, P. A., A. Bugnon, J.-P. Bournat, M. Xhaard, and J. Hinglais. 1974. Instantaneous bi-dimensional blood velocity profiles in the major vessels measured by a pulsed ultrasonic Doppler device. In M. De Vlieger et al. (eds.), Ultrasonics in Medicine, Proceedings of the 2nd World Congress, pp. 258–268. Excerpta Medica, Amsterdam/American Elsevier, New York.

Planiol, Th., and L. Pourcelot. 1974. Doppler effect study of the carotid circulation. In M. De Vlieger, D. N. White, and V. R. McCready (eds.),

Ultrasonics in Medicine. Proceedings of the 2nd World Congress 1973. Excerpta Medica, Amsterdam/American Elsevier, New York.

Raines, J. K., M. Y. Jaffrin, and A. H. Shapiro. 1974. A computer simulation of arterial dynamics in the human leg. J. Biomech. 7: 77–91.

Rindfleisch, T. C., J. A. Dunne, H. J. Frieden, W. D. Stromberg, and R. M. Ruiz. 1971. Digital processing of the Mariner 6 and 7 pictures. J. Geophys. Res. 76: 394–417.

Rockwell, R. L., M. Anliker, and J. Elsner. 1974. Model studies of the pressure and flow pulses in a viscoelastic arterial conduit. J. Franklin Inst. 297: 405–427.

Rutishauser, W, H. H. Brunner, A. Bollinger, M. Brandestini, P. A. Doriot, and M. Anliker. 1974. Blutflussmessung in Arterien aus instantanen Strömungsprofilen mit gepulstem Doppler Ultraschall. Verh. Dtsch. Ges. Kreislaufforschg. 40: 149–153.

Shanks, J. L. 1967. Recursion filters for digital processing. Geophysics 32: 33–51.

Strandness, D. E., J. W. Kennedy, T. P. Judge, and F. D. McLeod. 1969. Transcutaneous directional flow detection: A preliminary report. Amer. Heart J. 78: 65.

Tompkins, W. R., R. Monti, and M. Intaglietta. 1974. Velocity measurement by self-tracking correlator. Rev. Sci. Instr. 45, No. 5: 647–649.

Wallace, J. D., and C. M. Cade. 1974. Clinical thermography. Crit. Rev. Bioeng. 2: 39–94.

Wayland, H., and P. C. Johnson. 1967. Erythrocyte velocity measurement in microvessels by a two-slit photometric method. J. Appl. Physiol. 22: 333–337.

Westerhof, N., F. Bosmann, C. J. De Vries, and A. Noordergraaf. 1969. Analog studies of the human systemic arterial tree. J. Biomech. 2: 121–143.

Winter, J., and M. A. Stein. 1973. Computer image processing techniques for automated breast thermogram interpretation. Computers and Biomed. Res. 6: 522–529.

Womersley, J. R. 1955. WADC Technical Report TR 56-614; Phil. Mag. 46: 199–221.

Ziskin, M. C., M. Negin, C. Piner, and M. S. Lapayowker. 1975. Computer diagnosis of breast thermograms. Radiology 115: 341–347.

Cardiovascular Flow Dynamics and Measurements
Edited by N. H. C. Hwang and N. A. Normann
Copyright 1977   University Park Press   Baltimore

chapter 2

THEORY, DESIGN, AND USE OF ELECTROMAGNETIC FLOWMETERS

Derek G. Wyatt

ABSTRACT

The theoretical basis of the electromagnetic flowmeter is described using Bevir's virtual current theory. This is applied to two-dimensional flowmeters, in which both the field and the flow are invariant in the direction of the flowmeter axis. A method of optimizing the magnetic field for least variation of sensitivity with velocity profile is given. Hemp's method of optimizing the field in three dimensions, assuming rectilinear flow, is described. An account is given of the effect of blood vessel wall, hematocrit, and surrounding tissue on flowmeter sensitivity. The uncertainties of calibration procedures are discussed. Procedures for designing flowmeter heads are mentioned, together with some practical aspects of head design. The problems of electronic design are discussed in outline, including the preamplifier, noise, detection, filters, quadrature, interference, and the properties of different magnet excitation waveforms. There are some notes on electromagnetic catheter devices, ultrasonic flowmeters, and the problems of buying an electromagnetic flowmeter.

THEORY

Bevir's Virtual Current Theory

When a conducting medium moves with velocity $\underline{v}$ in a magnetic field $\underline{B}$, a Lorentz force acts on the charge carriers, tending to separate them. This electric force acts in a direction perpendicular to the plane containing the vectors $\underline{v}$ and $\underline{B}$ and is denoted by the vector product $\underline{v} \times \underline{B}$. It results in the generation of an electric field $\underline{E}$ due to charges distributed in and

89

around the conductor; it may also result in a flow of current $\underline{j}$ in the medium. We can write

$$\underline{j} = \sigma(\underline{E} + \underline{v} \times \underline{B}). \tag{1}$$

σ is the conductivity of the medium. The electric potential U in the conductor is defined by $\underline{E} = -\text{grad}\, U$ and the difference in potential between any two points is the line integral of $\underline{E}$ between them.

Consider a conventional circular flowmeter fitted with small electrodes, between which the difference in potential, known as the signal, is measured (Figure 1). At point P let the liquid velocity be $\underline{v}$ and the magnetic field strength $\underline{B}$, resulting in an electromotive force $(\underline{v} \times \underline{B}) \cdot d\underline{l}$. Here $d\underline{l}$ is a small element of length in the direction of $\underline{v} \times \underline{B}$. In order to express the response of the flowmeter to flow throughout its sensible volume, we need to establish the proportion of $(\underline{v} \times \underline{B}) \cdot d\underline{l}$ that appears at the electrodes from every point in the liquid and sum the total. Although at first sight this appears an intractable problem, there is a remarkably simple solution of great generality and great analytic power. It depends on the fact that we can regard the liquid as a continuous network of resistances. Consider the simplest possible network shown in Figure 2.

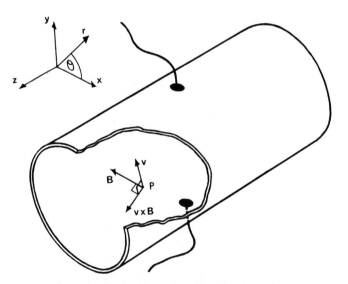

Figure 1. Circular flowmeter with point electrodes.

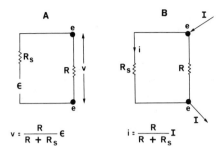

Figure 2. Voltage–current relationships in a simple network.

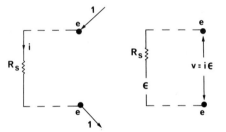

Figure 3. Current–voltage relationships in a complex network.

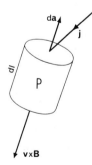

Figure 4. Cylindrical element of liquid at P.

In Figure 2A the proportion of the electromotive force ϵ that appears between the points e, e is $R/(R + R_s)$. This is also the proportion of current I from an external source that passes through R_s when ϵ is made zero (Figure 2B). If I is 1 unit, then i is the fraction of ϵ that appears between e, e. This theorem holds however complex the resistance network between R_s and e, e may be (Figure 3). It is easily proved by applying the Reciprocity Theorem for networks. Consider (Figure 4) a small cylindrical element of liquid at P, its axis coincident with the vector $\underline{v} \times \underline{B}$. The e.m.f. between the ends of the element is $(\underline{v} \times \underline{B}) \cdot d\underline{l}$. Suppose now, with the flowmeter not working, that we impose unit current between the electrodes from an external source. Let the resultant current density at P be $\underline{j}$. Then, applying our theorem, we see that the voltage between the electrodes due to $(\underline{v} \times \underline{B}) \cdot d\underline{l}$ at P when the flowmeter is operating is

$$\Delta U = (\underline{j} \cdot d\underline{a})(\underline{v} \times \underline{B} \cdot d\underline{l}) \tag{2}$$

or

$$\Delta U = \underline{j} \cdot \underline{v} \times \underline{B} \, d\tau.$$

where $d\tau$ is an element of volume. The signal between e, e due to flow everywhere within the flowmeter volume τ is

$$U = \int_\tau \underline{j} \cdot \underline{v} \times \underline{B} \, d\tau. \tag{3}$$

$\underline{j}$ has the form of a weight vector used to weight $\underline{v} \times \underline{B}$ according to its effect at the electrodes. It is more useful to obtain a weight vector that weights the local fluid *velocity* at points such as P and this is obtained by a simple vector transformation giving

$$U = \int_\tau \underline{W} \cdot \underline{v} \, d\tau. \tag{4}$$

Here $\underline{W} = \underline{B} \times \underline{j}$ and is known as the weight vector. This result is due to Bevir (1970), who gives a more rigorous proof. It must rank as the most important contribution yet to our understanding of the electromagnetic flowmeter. The current $\underline{j}$ in this equation is not to be confused with the current $\underline{j}$ that actually flows when the meter is working (Eq. 1). Here $\underline{j}$ is a compact expression that describes the geometry of the flowmeter tube and electrodes. It is applicable to tubes of any shape and to electrodes of any shape and position. The flowmeter signal U is obtained by performing the integration over the volume of the flowmeter when the magnetic field $\underline{B}$, and the current distribution $\underline{j}$ that would result by applying unit current between the electrodes, are known. j could be found experimentally by actually applying a current beteen the electrodes and measuring the current density at various points in the liquid (preferably with no magnetic field). More usually it is computed or calculated. Bevir gave the name *virtual* current to j, to emphasize that it is not actually present in a working flowmeter.

As an example of the use of virtual current, consider a flowmeter of rectangular cross section with large electrodes and a uniform magnetic field (Arnold, 1951). Liquid flows into it not necessarily parallel to its axis (Figure 5). We assume there are no edge effects at the ends of the electrodes, so the virtual current would flow in straight lines everywhere normal to the electrodes. (In fact, edge effects would not affect the properties of this flowmeter; see below.) Because $\underline{B}$ is everywhere perpendicular to j, the weight vector $\underline{W} = \underline{B} \times j$ has only one component, W_z, which has the value $Bj = B/WL$. Hence

$$U = \int_\tau \underline{W} \cdot \underline{v} \, d\tau = \frac{B}{WL} \int_\tau v_z \, d\tau = \frac{BQ}{W}. \qquad (5)$$

Q is the flow rate.

Note that since $\underline{W}$ has only the one component W_z, the product $\underline{W} \cdot \underline{v}$ has a value only for v_z, the component of $\underline{v}$ parallel to the flowmeter axis. The absence of other components of $\underline{W}$ indicates that the flowmeter is wholly insensitive to velocity components other than those parallel to the axis. This is why $U \propto Q$.

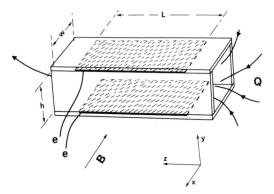

Figure 5. Rectangular flowmeter with large electrodes and uniform field.

The flowmeter is a perfect, or ideal one, since its signal is proportional to the flow rate and independent of velocity profile. Bevir showed that a necessary and sufficient condition for a flowmeter to be ideal is

$$\text{curl } \underline{W} = 0, \tag{6}$$

and from this he deduced the existence of a class of ideal flowmeters of which that just described is a special case. In this class either $\underline{B}$ or $\underline{j}$ must be uniform and the other lie in planes perpendicular to it. Figure 6 shows a more general ideal flowmeter. The sensitivity is independent of the height, which may vary along the length. The sensitivity is independent also of the electrode width in the flow direction and of electrode position. The only requirements are a uniform magnetic field, constant channel width in the direction of the field, and electrodes that are parallel to the field and invariant in shape in this direction. Figure 7 shows an experimental rectangular flowmeter of this type; it is 1 in. square in section. Provision is made for moving a jet $\frac{1}{8}$ in. diameter to different positions on a circle $\frac{3}{4}$ in. diameter centered on the flowmeter axis. The jet is situated $2\frac{1}{2}$ in. upstream from the electrodes.

Figure 8 shows the response of the flowmeter with the jet positioned either toward the electrodes or toward the side wall. The variation in response is ~2%, which, although small, is greater than might have been expected of such an accurately made flowmeter. Figure 9A shows the results of the same experiment $\frac{1}{2}$ hr after the flowmeter had been dried

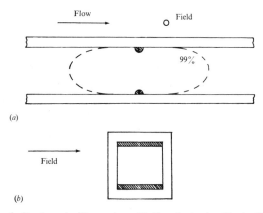

Figure 6. Rectangular flowmeter with line electrodes (Bevir, 1970).

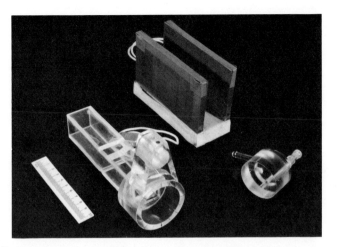

Figure 7. Experimental rectangular flowmeter, comprising 1-in.-square rectangular pipe with line electrodes, rotating jet attachment, and uniform field magnet.

and then refilled with saline. Figure 9B shows the effect of washing the flowmeter with a detergent surfactant before refilling with saline. These results reflect one disadvantage of large electrodes: any variation in surface impedance will destroy the ideal performance of the flowmeter and alter its sensitivity as well; in effect the virtual current is altered. Any deposits on the electrodes change the flowmeter characteristics, whereas flowmeters using small electrodes are not affected in this way. They merely stop working if the electrode impedance becomes high.

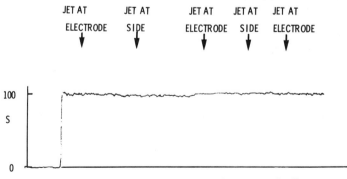

Figure 8. Result of rotating jet experiment with rectangular flowmeter.

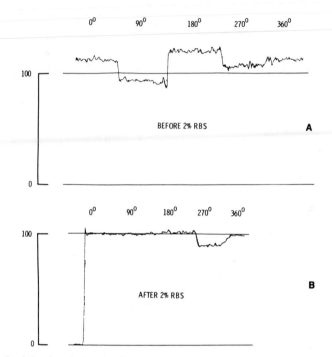

Figure 9. (A) After drying the flowmeter and refilling with saline. (B) After washing with detergent RBS25 surfactant. 0°, 180°, 360°: jet in line with electrode. 90°, 270°: jet in line with side wall.

Two-dimensional Analysis

Point-electrode flowmeters are of great importance: not only are they immune to variations in the electrode surface, but large numbers of them are in use for industrial and medical applications. The two-dimensional, circular tube point electrode flowmeter is easy to analyze and its properties are near enough to those of many practical flowmeters to be a useful guide to both principles and performance. By two-dimensional we mean here that both the velocity and the magnetic field are invariant in the direction of the pipe axis. Thus by definition both the velocity field and the magnetic field are two-dimensional. The virtual current field, however, is not two-dimensional, but it is possible to see that there is in fact an equivalent two-dimensional virtual current, and thus simplify the analysis, as follows. Since the velocity and magnetic fields are two-dimensional, no currents flow in the liquid parallel to the pipe axis. Hence all lines parallel to the pipe axis are equipotential lines and we can replace the point electrodes with line electrodes parallel to the axis without affecting the flowmeter operation. Such line electrodes give a two-dimensional virtual current and it is this that we may use (Bevir, 1971a).

The flowmeter signal is given by an integral over the cross-sectional area S of the flowmeter,

$$U = \int_S Wv \, dS. \tag{7}$$

Both W and v are functions of the position coordinates x, y (or r, θ) in the cross section and

$$W = B_x j_y - B_y j_x.$$

The virtual current is found by a two-dimensional potential calculation, yielding current lines as shown in Figure 10. We see immediately that this flowmeter will have very poor performance if used with a uniform magnetic field, at least for nonaxisymmetric flows. The virtual current density tends to infinity at the electrodes, indicating an infinite value of W here and therefore an infinite sensitivity to flow; whereas at the side walls the

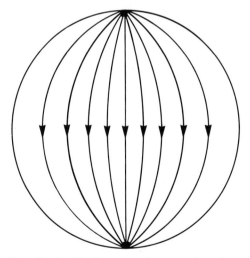

Figure 10. Two-dimensional virtual current between line electrodes in circular flowmeter.

virtual current density is lower than it is at the center, indicating a reduced sensitivity. The values of j_x, j_y are

$$j_y = \frac{2}{\pi} \sum_{m=0}^{\infty} (-1)^m r^{2m} \cos 2m\theta$$

$$j_x = \frac{2}{\pi} \sum_{m=0}^{\infty} (-1)^m r^{2m} \sin 2m\theta,$$

where r, θ are polar coordinates. r is normalized and is not greater than 1. When the field is uniform and transverse to the line joining the electrodes, $B_x = B$ (constant) and $B_y = 0$. j_y is the equivalent form of the well-known weight function for this case given by Shercliff (1962) (Figure 11). Here we see how the weight function tends to infinity at the electrodes and falls at the side walls to half its value at the center. The average value is 1. Figure 12 shows the apparatus for a jet experiment using a 1-in.-diameter circular point-electrode flowmeter with a uniform magnetic field, similar to that described using an "ideal" rectangular flowmeter. Figure 13 shows the variation in response. The large fluctuations are due to the nonideal character of this flowmeter, coupled with the turbulent flow that is

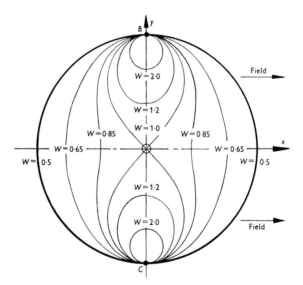

Figure 11. Weight function diagram for uniform field flowmeter with point electrodes (Shercliff, 1962; reprinted by permission).

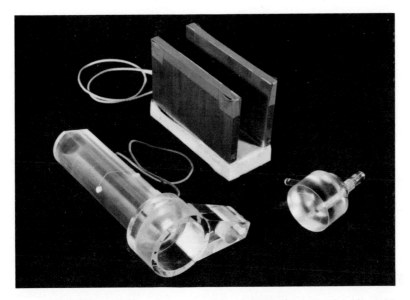

Figure 12. Experimental flowmeter, comprising 1-in.-diameter circular pipe with point electrodes, rotating jet attachment, and uniform field magnet.

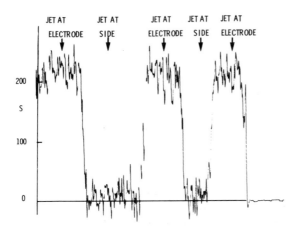

Figure 13. Result of rotating jet experiment with circular flowmeter.

occurring. Negative response is due to backflow at the electrodes when the jet is at the side walls (see also Goldman, Marple, and Scolnik, 1963).

Although the circular, point-electrode, uniform field flowmeter has this very nonuniform response to both general and rectilinear flows (rectilinear flow is flow parallel to the axis), it has an ideal response to a restricted form of rectilinear flow, namely, axisymmetric flow. The popularity of the electromagnetic flowmeter is due in large measure to this fact, even though the magnetic fields in practical flowmeters are hardly ever uniform and the flow often not axisymmetric. The axisymmetric property can be deduced by noting that since j_y is a solution to Laplace's equation, W must be a solution too. By the mean value theorem for Laplace functions it follows that the mean value of W over any circle in the pipe cross section is equal to the value at the center of the circle. If we apply this to circles coincident with the axis (Bevir, 1971a) it follows that the response of the flowmeter to axisymmetric velocity profiles is uniform.

When the magnetic field is not uniform the terms B_y, j_x have to be introduced in W. We can do this in a perfectly general way by writing B_x, B_y as series of two-dimensional field harmonics. When this is done and the terms collected up, the weight function is (Wyatt, 1972)

$$W = \sum_{m=0}^{\infty} \sum_{n=1}^{\infty} (-1)^m na_n r^{2m+\overline{n-1}} \cos(2m-\overline{n-1})\theta. \quad n \text{ (odd)} \qquad (8)$$

n is the order of harmonic and a_n the corresponding coefficient of magnetic field potential. The axisymmetric weight function, which is a function of radius only and which describes the response to axisymmetric velocity profiles, is

$$W'(r) = \frac{1}{2\pi} \int_0^{2\pi} W \, d\theta = \sum_{n=1}^{\infty} (-1)^{(n-1)/2} na_n r^{2(n-1)} \qquad (9)$$

and the signal is

$$U = 2\pi \int_0^1 W'(r)v(r)r \, dr. \qquad (10)$$

We now see explicitly that the axisymmetric weight function for the point electrode two-dimensional flowmeter is uniform (independent of radius) only when $n = 1$, that is, when the magnetic field is uniform. Any attempt to move away from a uniform field in an effort to make W more uniform and thus reduce variations in response caused by asymmetric velocity profiles will result in nonuniformity of response to axisymmetric profiles.

There is no possibility of obtaining uniform response with the two-dimensional point-electrode flowmeter, and, indeed, Bevir (1970) has proved theoretically that the point-electrode flowmeter cannot be made "ideal" even when the two-dimensional constraint on the magnetic field is removed. The most obvious way of improving the circular flowmeter is to make the virtual current more uniform by using line electrodes. Figure 14 shows a two-dimensional weight function plot for 133° line electrodes and a uniform magnetic field (Bevir, 1971a). However, there remains the problem of variable electrode impedance. A possible solution to this electrode problem is to fabricate line electrodes as indicated in Figure 15. The virtual current would be controlled by a high-resistance material rather than by variations in the relatively low-impedance electrode—electrolyte interface. It would be necessary for the resistance of the whole electrode to be low to maintain a low noise level and this implies a sufficiently large surface area. The impedance of the electrode could be continuously monitored by using a frequency that is high compared with the magnet frequency. This is an important feature of the scheme.

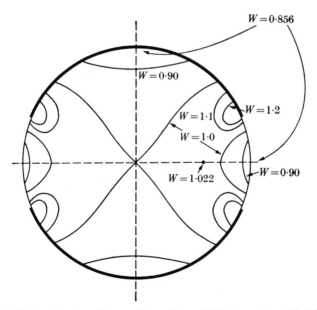

Figure 14. Weight function diagram for uniform field flowmeter with 133° line electrodes (Bevir, 1971a; reprinted by permission).

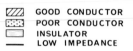

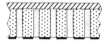

ELECTROLYTE

Figure 15. Possible method of manufacturing line electrodes.

Two-dimensional Optimization

It is possible to improve the point-electrode flowmeter by optimizing the magnetic field for least variation of weight function. The two-dimensional flowmeter field can be optimized analytically using as a criterion E, the root-mean-square deviation of weight function over the cross section

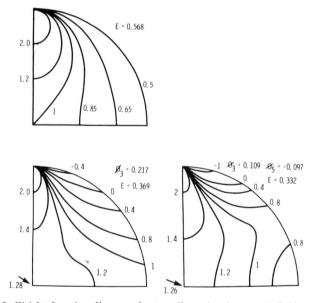

Figure 16. Weight function diagrams for two-dimensional magnetic fields. ϕ_3, ϕ_5 are the amplitudes of the third and fifth magnetic potential harmonics, $\phi_1 = 1$. The upper diagram is for a uniform field ($\phi_1 = 1$). The mean weight function is 1 in each case.

divided by the mean value $\overline{W}$ of the weight function over a circle of radius r (Wyatt, 1972):

$$E = \frac{1}{\overline{W}} \left[\frac{1}{\pi r^2} \int_0^r \int_0^{2\pi} (W - \overline{W})^2 r \, dr \, d\theta \right]^{1/2}. \tag{11}$$

The coefficients a_n of the harmonics of magnetic field potential are treated as variables and E is minimized in terms of them. Some results are shown in Figure 16. Note the reduction in size of the "bad" region near the electrodes as the number of harmonics is increased, and the corresponding reduction in E, the relative r.m.s. deviation of weight function. Figure 17 shows the axisymmetric weight functions for these fields, all

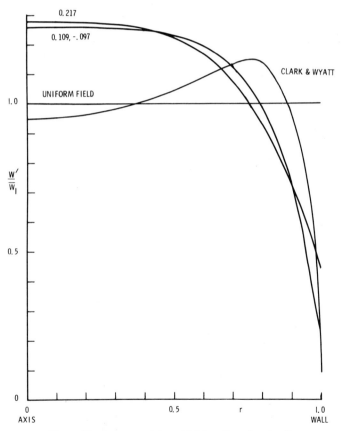

Figure 17. Axisymmetric weight functions (see text).

worse than for the uniform field as anticipated. The curve marked Clark & Wyatt is for a flowmeter currently in use in the Nuffield Institute and is referred to later.

Three-dimensional Optimization

It has been known for some years that a departure from the two-dimensional idea, by allowing the field to vary in the direction of flow as well as in the cross section, could improve the uniformity of response. Rummel and Ketelsen (1966) have described briefly an industrial flow-meter (Figure 18) in which the coils were diamond shaped. They arrived at this design by semiempirical analysis and no detailed performance figures were given. However, it is clear that coils of this kind must produce some improvement. The field and therefore $\underline{v} \times \underline{B}$ will be reduced at each side of the electrodes in the flow direction, producing a short-circuiting effect and hence a reduction in sensitivity near the electrode region where it is most needed.

The difficult problem of optimizing the magnetic field in three dimensions has been solved by Hemp (1975), again using a criterion very similar to the mean-square deviation of weight function and assuming rectilinear flow. In the three-dimensional case the optimization process cannot be

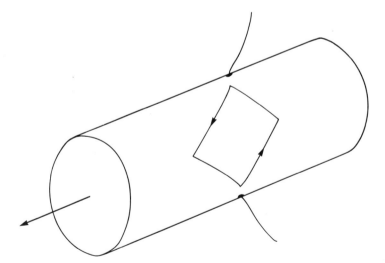

Figure 18. Approximate form of windings in Rummel and Ketelsen flowmeter.

carried out analytically, and resort must be had to numerical methods. For this reason the criterion used was

$$\epsilon = \left[\frac{1}{45} \sum_{i=1}^{45} (W_i - \overline{W})^2\right]^{1/2} \bigg/ \overline{W} \tag{12}$$

where $W_1, W_2, \ldots, W_{45}$ are values of W at 45 points nearly equally spaced in a quadrant of the flowmeter cross section. $\overline{W}$ is the mean value of W over a circle with radius 0.95 that of the flowmeter. Since it is generally the case that any change in the magnetic field designed to reduce the variation in weight function is accompanied by a need for greater power consumption, other things being equal, a constraint was placed on the flowmeter efficiency f and this in turn required consideration of a particular magnet design. This was taken to consist of copper strips laid on the inside surface of an iron tube concentric with the flow tube (Figure 19). The magnetic field was expressed in harmonics with coefficients a_{nm}. ϵ and f were expressed in terms of a_{nm}, and the values of a_{nm} for which ϵ was a minimum were then found while f was held constant. In this method, as in the two-dimensional optimization, the designer is free to choose a set of harmonics and thus to control the degree of complexity of the magnetic field and of the windings required to produce it. The weight function diagram for the field finally chosen is shown in Figure 20. It represents a substantial improvement over any other yet devised for the point-electrode flowmeter. The value of ϵ is 0.095. The axisymmetric weight function is shown in Figure 21 and this too is very good. In its present form the design has two disadvantages: it is 2.5 diameters long, and $f = 0.04$; that is, it requires 25 times as much power as a uniform-field flowmeter with the same sensitivity. The windings for producing the magnetic field are complex and have been prepared in the form of an

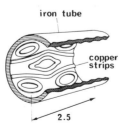

iron tube

copper strips

2.5

Figure 19. Form of magnet assumed by Hemp (Hemp, 1975) (reprinted by permission of Institute of Physics).

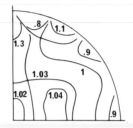

Figure 20. Weight function for Hemp's flowmeter (Hemp, 1975) (reprinted by permission of Institute of Physics).

etched copper sheet suitable for wrapping around the flowmeter tube, which is then placed in a suitable laminated iron tube. The artwork for the etching is shown in Figure 22. Note the regions of reversed magnetic field that appear either side of the electrodes. The main windings have a general shape similar to those in Rummel and Ketelsen's flowmeter. The component parts of a 2-cm-diameter flowmeter of this type are shown in Figure 23.

It is most convenient, both in medical and industrial applications, that a flowmeter be short in terms of its diameter. Although both the magnetic field and the virtual current then extend beyond the physical bounds of the flowmeter, these regions still contribute to the flowmeter signal. Designing the magnetic field is far more difficult, for the designer has the task of predicting the magnetic field beyond the physical bounds of the magnet. It is certain that those blood flowmeters that are most attractive to the surgeon and physiologist because of their very short length are also those that may give the most questionable results, both for velocity profile and other reasons (see below).

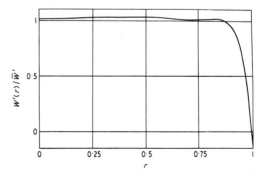

Figure 21. Axisymmetric weight function for Hemp's flowmeter (Hemp, 1975) (reprinted by permission of Institute of Physics).

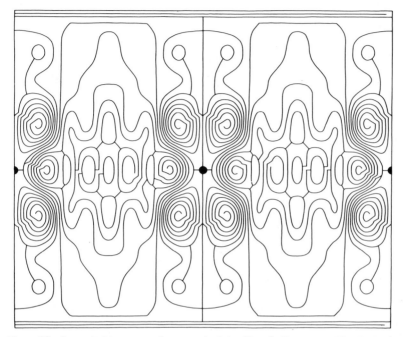

Figure 22. Artwork for current sheet required for Hemp's flowmeter. The electrode positions are shown as solid circles.

Effect of Blood Vessel, Hematocrit, and Surrounding Tissue

One of the main advantages of electromagnetic flowmeters in measuring blood flow is that the flowmeter can be constructed with a slot in its side, through which an intact artery or vein may be introduced (Kolin, 1960). In this situation (Figure 24) the voltage induced by the motion of the blood within the vessel is sensed by the electrodes through the conducting vessel wall, and one must inquire what effects are caused by the presence of the vessel that may change the sensitivity. These are of two kinds: the effect on velocity profile, and the effect of the electrical conductivity of the blood vessel wall. Consider first the effect on velocity profile. Figure 25 shows the weight function diagram of a two-dimensional point-electrode flowmeter employing a uniform magnetic field, superimposed on which is the inner boundary of the blood vessel wall. We suppose for the moment that the vessel has the same electrical conductivity as the blood. If the velocity profile of the flowing blood is axisymmetric, the blood vessel will

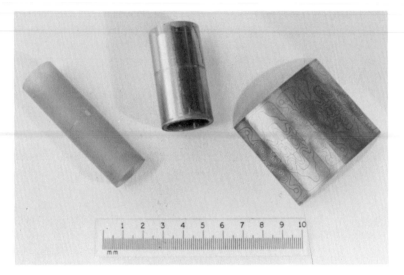

Figure 23. Component parts of Hemp's flowmeter: cannula, core, and field winding.

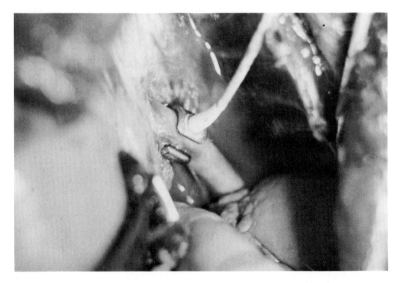

Figure 24. Toroid flowmeter on descending aorta of lamb.

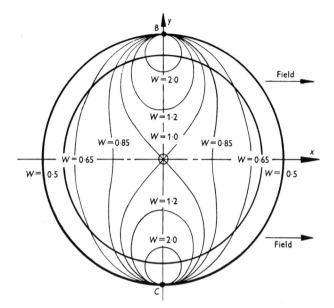

Figure 25. Weight function diagram of uniform field flowmeter with inner boundary of blood vessel superimposed.

not affect the sensitivity, since it can be regarded as a stationary annulus of blood and the axisymmetric condition is not violated. If, on the other hand, the velocity profile is asymmetric, the sensitivity will have been changed by introducing the vessel. In particular, we notice that the wall prevents the occurrence of flow in those peripheral regions where the weight function is most variable, and the flowmeter performance is therefore improved for asymmetric flows. The improvement is generally greater for arteries, because of their greater wall thickness, than it is for veins. Usually, the flowmeter does not have a uniform field; in this case the presence of a blood vessel changes the sensitivity, depending upon the wall thickness, even if the wall has the same conductivity as the blood and if the velocity profile is axisymmetric. As an example of this, Figure 26 shows the variation in response of a practical blood flowmeter (Clark and Wyatt, 1969) as the central region in which blood is assumed to flow with uniform velocity is changed in size. In practice, the introduction of a blood vessel would increase the sensitivity by up to 5%. This flowmeter is designed to have good uniformity of response for axisymmetric flow. The other curve is for another design (Bevir, 1971a) for which, although the

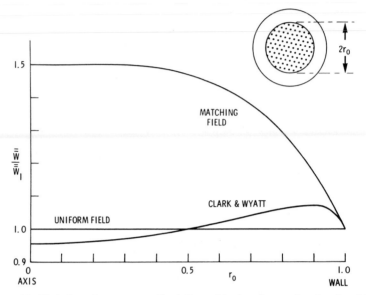

Figure 26. Variation of response to fixed flow with size of central region, in which the flow occurs with uniform velocity.

weight function is finite everywhere, the response to axisymmetric flows is very nonuniform. Here the introduction of a blood vessel could change the sensitivity by up to 25%. Even if some form of calibration were used with the vessel, in situ changes in it could cause significant error. Figure 27 shows a section of sheep carotid artery, with hematoma. The asymmetric flow would be expected to cause error of at least 10%. Figure 28 shows an axial section of the umbilical veins just inside the abdomen of the fetal lamb. A flowmeter around the common vein showed a change of 15% in response on rotating the flowmeter through 90°, a useful test for an asymmetric velocity profile.

We turn now to the effect of the electrical conductivity of the blood vessel. Figure 29 shows a cross section of the flowmeter tube, with electrodes at 0, 0' (Gessner, 1961; Wyatt, 1968a). The blood flows in the central region where the conductivity is σ_1 and we suppose the velocity profile is axisymmetric. Beyond the flowing blood is the vessel wall, which we suppose is uniform and isotropic, with conductivity σ_2; beyond that again is a thin layer of plasma of conductivity σ_3. We ignore the layer of

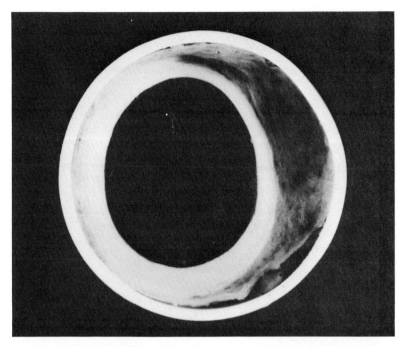

Figure 27. Carotid artery of sheep, with hematoma. Fixed at in vivo pressure in plastic tube simulating flowmeter.

plasma for the moment and consider only the effect of the vessel wall. Suppose now that $\sigma_2 = \sigma_1$ so the introduction of the vessel will not have disturbed the axisymmetric condition and the voltage between 0, 0' will be unchanged. Under this condition a certain potential difference will exist between the points i, i', determined by the flow and shunting effect of the vessel wall. Suppose now we reduce the conductivity of the wall: the shunting effect on i, i' will be reduced and the potential between these points rises. So too will the voltage between the electrodes at 0, 0', since this is determined solely by currents in the wall and the voltage at i, i'. Hence the introduction of a blood vessel with conductivity less than that of the blood will increase the flowmeter sensitivity (Figure 30). The best evidence is that σ_1/σ_2 is between two and four, and the graph shows that the effect of a blood vessel of thickness equal to 10% of the radius is to increase the sensitivity by about 8%. The situation is complicated by

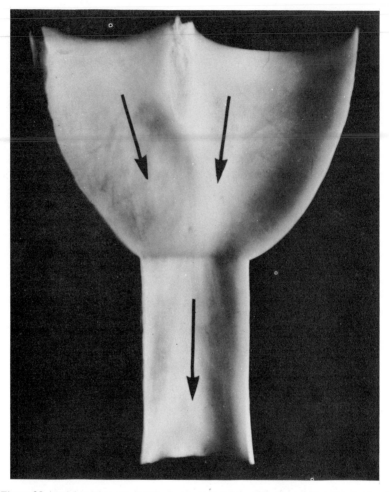

Figure 28. Axial section of umbilical vein just inside abdomen of foetal lamb, fixed at in vivo pressure with plastic tube around common vein.

the presence of the plasma layer around the blood vessel. Usually σ_3/σ_2 is between three and ten and a layer as thin as 0.001 in. can cause reduction of sensitivity in the order of % with small flowmeters.

Blood vessels are by no means uniform or isotropic, and further complication and error results from this. Edgerton (1968) and Bevir (1971b) have done analyses for anisotropic vessels. Edgerton gives experi-

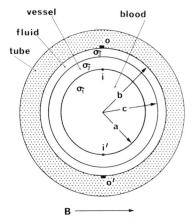

Figure 29. Cross section of transducer and contents (reprinted by permission of Institute of Physics). See text.

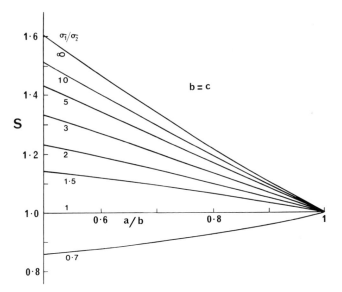

Figure 30. Variation of flowmeter sensitivity with wall thickness and conductivity ratio (reprinted by permission of Institute of Physics).

mental results obtained with a 2-mm flowmeter that show sensitivity differences as great as 50% with different blood vessels. Figure 31 shows results obtained with an undersized flowmeter used to measure flow in the abdominal aorta of a dog. Here simultaneous records of two flowmeters with equal sensitivities (without blood vessels) show a sensitivity ratio of 0.85, or 15% reduction caused by the blood vessel and fluid layer. Conductivity effects are less with veins, because of the smaller wall thickness.

Flowmeter response depends also upon hematocrit. Figure 32 shows the sensitivity variation observed when using a substantially uniform field flowmeter with laminar flow. The cause of the effect is uncertain. It has been ascribed to either nonuniform radial distribution of erythrocytes or to anisotropic conductivity of the blood due to orientation of the erythrocytes in laminar flow (Dennis and Wyatt, 1969; Bevir, 1971b). Hardly any change of sensitivity with hematocrit occurs when the flow is turbulent.

When a cuff flowmeter is immersed in an "ocean" of conducting material such as tissue or blood, its sensitivity changes because of partial short-circuiting of the electrodes. The effect is particularly noticeable in blood flowmeters of short geometric length where the magnetic field length approaches the geometric length. The error can amount to several percent. The Clark and Wyatt flowmeter was designed with the magnet length only one-half the geometric length, reducing the possible error to 3%. The effect was later analyzed by Bevir (1972), whose theoretical results are shown in Figure 33.

Calibration

The net effect on sensitivity of introducing a blood vessel into a flowmeter and implanting the flowmeter is due to

1. Effect of the vessel wall on velocity profile within the flowmeter;
2. Conductivity of vessel wall, and plasma layer, dependent on wall thickness and layer thickness;
3. Anisotropy of vessel wall;
4. Hematocrit, dependent on flow;
5. Conductivity of surrounding tissue.

The result is that the flowmeter sensitivity may increase, decrease, or even stay the same. It is not generally true that the introduction of a blood vessel into a flowmeter has a negligible effect on the sensitivity (Kolin, 1960). There is ample theoretic and experimental evidence to the contrary

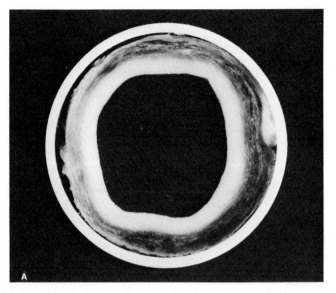

Figure 31. (a) Abdominal aorta of dog fixed at in vivo pressure in plastic tube simulating undersized flowmeter used to obtain the results in Figure 31(b), lower trace.

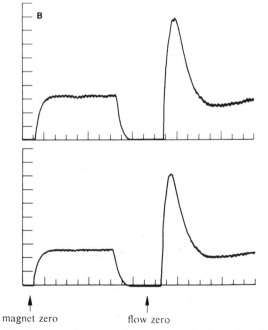

Figure 31. (b) Simultaneous flow records with cannular (*upper*) and perivascular (*lower*) flowmeter in vessel shown in Figure 31(a). Full vertical chart width represents 500 ml/min, neglecting vessel. 6 mm dia.

115

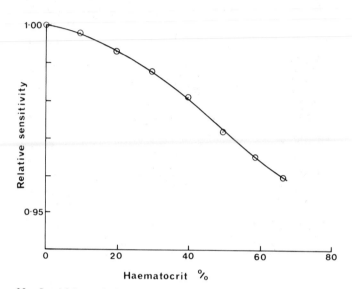

Figure 32. Sensitivity variation with hematocrit: 6-mm-diameter tube, laminar flow, 14.7 cm/sec mean, 37°C. (Reprinted by permission of the American Heart Association, Inc.)

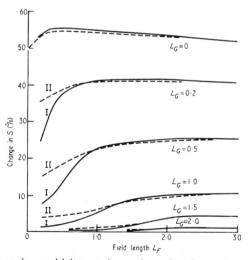

Figure 33. Change in sensitivity on immersion of a flowmeter in an ocean of conductivity equal to that of the flowmeter contents, assumed uniform. L_G, L_F are geometric and field lengths, respectively, in terms of flowmeter diameter (Bevir, 1972) (reprinted by permission of Institute of Physics).

(e.g., Figure 31 above; Dobson, Sellers, and McLeod, 1966; Ferguson and Landahl, 1966; Sellers and Dobson, 1967; Wyatt, 1968*a;* Edgerton, 1968; Bevir, 1971*b*). In addition to the above effects there is, of course, possible error from the velocity profile within the vessel, and this, if present, will depend upon flow. Now, provided all these effects are constant, it is in principle possible to calibrate the flowmeter in vivo. However (1), (2), and (3) above depend on blood pressure, vasoconstriction, vasodilatation, and chemical addition (Edgerton, 1968); (4) and the velocity profile depend on flow. In view of these variables it is not easy to recommend a calibration procedure, for there may be significant variations in sensitivity in the course of use, possibly in the order of tens of percent. This is particularly true of small arteries. If calibration is attempted, it can be useful only if done under in vivo conditions insofar as these can be defined.

Electromagnetic flowmeters, when used around large, stable, well-fitting blood vessels with flow that is axisymmetric or nearly so, can give accurate and consistent results. However, it is quite wrong generally to think of these devices, in their present form, as standard instruments. The reasons that have been given here for this view are fundamental to the flowmeter head. There are other sources of error, particularly in baseline, which are in part dependent on the electronic design and around which the main debate has formerly centered (see also Wyatt, 1968*b*).

DESIGN PROCEDURE

The process of designing a point-electrode flowmeter with reduced variation of sensitivity to velocity profile depends in part on the constraints placed on the velocity profile. Usually the profile is specified either as axisymmetric or rectilinear. The rectilinear weight function is

$$W(r,\theta) = \int_{-\infty}^{\infty} W_z \, dz \qquad (13)$$

and the axisymmetric weight function is

$$W'(r) = \frac{1}{2\pi} \int_0^{2\pi} W \, d\theta. \qquad (14)$$

Having obtained these, one can then assume some appropriate flow pattern of interest and calculate the signal that the flowmeter would give with this pattern; thus

$$U = \int_0^a \int_0^{2\pi} W(r,\theta)v(r,\theta)r \, dr \, d\theta \quad \text{(rectilinear flow)}, \tag{15}$$

where a is the tube radius, and

$$U = 2\pi \int_0^a W'(r)v(r)r \, dr \quad \text{(axisymmetric flow)}. \tag{16}$$

If the magnetic field and virtual current are known, it is possible to calculate W_z and thus W and W'. Bevir (1969) derived analytic functions for the virtual current and for the magnetic field produced by particular geometries of conductor within a cylindrical iron core. He produced tables from which it is possible to choose combinations of different rectangular coils to give a chosen small variation of axisymmetric weight function W'. Baker (1973) devised a numerical method for computing the rectilinear weight function of flowmeters employing a type of magnet similar to that assumed by Bevir, and thus for predicting the sensitivity to nonaxisymmetric as well as axisymmetric flows. Satisfactory designs for axisymmetric flow have also been achieved by direct flow testing of flowmeters employing both rectangular air-cored coils (Clark and Wyatt, 1968) and toroidal iron-cored magnets (Clark and Wyatt, 1969). The magnetic field of the toroidal magnets was modified near the electrodes by means of suitably shaped and positioned pieces of iron. The experimental and numerical methods are empirical since they give no indication of how to proceed to secure improvement. The optimization methods described in this paper, particularly the three-dimensional method developed by Hemp (1975), are not empirical. They automatically find the best field based on the criterion of mean-square deviation of weight function and they give results from which the sensitivity to any rectilinear flow can be calculated.

The analytic, numerical, and optimization procedures all have the disadvantage that a particular type of magnet has to be assumed at an early stage in the procedure. There are many "simple" magnets that are of interest but that are too complex either to analyze mathematically or to evaluate numerically. In such cases the magnet of interest is constructed and the normal component of magnetic field is measured at many points on the inside surface of the flowmeter. These values can be used to calculate the field anywhere within the flowmeter. Hence both W' and W can be found. This technique is useful not only as a semiempirical design procedure but also as a means of evaluating existing flowmeters. Figure 34 shows apparatus for recording the magnetic field by means of a small search coil (0.5 mm diameter) on the end of a vertical stem. It is fixed in

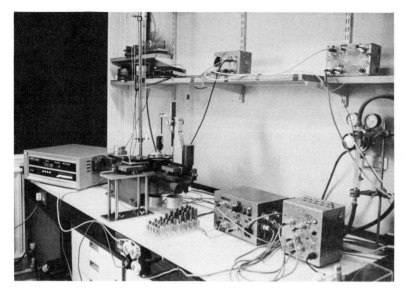

Figure 34. Apparatus for measuring magnetic field.

position while the magnet is automatically rotated about its own axis in steps of 6° or 3°. The readings are passed automatically to a computer. After each revolution the search coil is moved axially an appropriate amount and the magnet again rotated. 2,500 readings are taken, although it is planned to reduce this number substantially. At present the system can predict only axisymmetric weight functions (Bevir and Wyatt, unpublished), but work is in progress to enable asymmetric weight functions to be obtained (Satchell and Wyatt, unpublished).

Although it is very useful to know the rectilinear weight function distribution, it still leaves unanswered the question of how a given flowmeter responds to general, nonrectilinear flows. A method of determining this experimentally is under development by T. Cox, J. Hemp, and myself. It depends on the fact that if current is passed between the electrodes of a flowmeter that has its ends closed, resulting in current density $\underline{j}$ at some point within the flowmeter, then in general fluid motion will occur. The device is actually operating as a magnetic pump. However, it can be shown that no fluid motion will occur if curl $(\underline{B} \times \underline{j}) = 0$. Now this is just the condition that has to be satisfied for the device to be an ideal flowmeter. In fact, the flow produced in the pump role is that flow which would produce the worst error in the flowmeter role. It can be shown that if, shortly after the motion has been initiated, the pump role of the device is terminated and the flowmeter role instantly assumed, the voltage found between the electrodes is directly related to the mean-square deviation of the weight vector from the nearest curl-free vector field (Hemp, unpublished).

PRACTICAL ASPECTS OF HEAD DESIGN

In the early days of electromagnetic flowmeters the magnetic field was provided by a permanent magnet. The permanent magnet flowmeter has two advantages: it does not require a power source, and in practice it is about ten times more sensitive than a flowmeter of the same size using an A.C. magnetic field. However, these advantages are offset by two serious problems: first, nonpolarizable electrodes are required; second, a sensitive and stable low-noise D.C. amplifier is required. Therefore practically all subsequent development has proceeded using A.C. magnetic fields (see Wyatt, 1971). The signal from a flowmeter using a uniform magnetic field, with steady axisymmetric flow, is

$$U = \frac{0.0021 \, BQ}{d} + K\frac{\partial B}{\partial t} \ \mu V \tag{17}$$

where B is the field strength in gauss, Q the flow in milliliters per minute, and d the flowmeter diameter in millimeters. The term $K(\partial B/\partial t)$ is the so-called transformer e.m.f., or "quadrature voltage" in the case of sine-wave excitation. It is an artifact voltage, a consequence of using an alternating magnetic field. It produces an unwanted signal due both to flux linkage with the electrode connecting wires and to eddy currents produced in the blood, the blood vessel wall, and the surrounding tissues. It has to be separated from the flow-dependent signal. To give some indication of the relative magnitudes of the two parts of the signal, we can take the values of B and Q for a 10-mm-diameter cuff probe as 30 G and 2,000 ml/min, respectively, and obtain $U = 11 \ \mu V$ for the flow signal. Using a magnet frequency of 240 Hz we find experimentally that $K(\partial B/\partial t)$ does not exceed 50 μV. As is seen later, it is possible by electronic means to reduce the effect of $K(\partial B/\partial t)$ by a factor of 1,000, to the equivalent of 0.05 μV of "flow voltage." When sinewave excitation is used, the quadrature voltage is itself a sinewave but displaced in phase by 90° from the flow voltage.

The reduction of alternating flux from the circuit formed by the electrodes, the electrolyte, and the electrode connections is a geometric problem, and it is easy to reduce quadrature voltage from this cause to the order of microvolts. Fine electrode wires are used, located in grooves in the cannula. The plane containing these grooves is located in the magnetic field so that minimal flux crosses the plane. This requires a sufficiently symmetric magnetic field (Wyatt, 1961b, 1961c). Provided the effect of this quadrature can be further reduced electronically by a factor 1,000, it may be concluded that any error due to geometric misalignments in the head construction can be made quite negligible.

Suppose now that a blood vessel is in the flowmeter (Figure 35). An alternating electric field is caused in the fluid and blood vessel by the alternating magnetic flux and eddy currents flow as shown. As long as the system is electrically symmetric about the electrode axis, no quadrature voltage will appear between the electrodes. If a 10% asymmetry occurred caused, for example, by vessel movement or change of shape, a quadrature voltage of about 5 μV might appear between the electrodes. This in itself would not matter, but unfortunately tissue has a phase angle of ~0.01 rad and the result is that ~1% of the 5 μV, or 0.05 μV, is converted by the tissue into a signal indistinguishable from flow. It is one of many possible causes of baseline error (Wyatt, 1966a). It is easy to avoid the direct effects of quadrature voltage; it is the *indirect* effects due to small changes in phase of the quadrature voltage, caused by various mechanisms in the flowmeter head, which produce signals indistinguishable from flow and which can, if not avoided by proper design, cause serious baseline error.

One of the main sources of baseline error in an electromagnetic flowmeter is the electrodes. An interesting example of this is shown in Figure 36, where the response of two flowmeters in the same pipeline

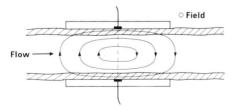

Figure 35. Eddy currents in flowmeter contents.

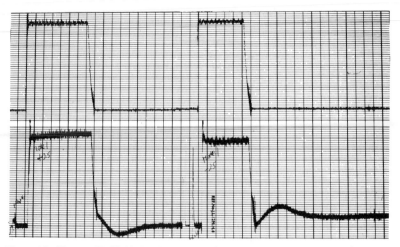

Figure 36. *Upper:* Nuffield Institute flowmeter. *Lower:* Biotronex Pulsed Logic flowmeter. Time scale, 7.5 sec per division.

is compared. The upper trace is taken with a Nuffield Institute flow-meter, the lower one with a commercial flowmeter. The flow was started and stopped abruptly. It was then again started in the reverse direction and stopped, the flowmeter output polarities having been changed, thus giving the same direction of deflection on the trace. The time scale is 7.5 sec per division. The slow periodic waves observed with the commercial flowmeter (Biotronex Pulsed Logic) were most probably caused by varying electrode impedance due to changing ionic concentrations at the electrodes after flow stopped, together with a very low amplifier input impedance of only 10,000 Ω (Roberts, 1969).

Electrodes in contact with an electrolyte behave electrically like a frequency-dependent combination of resistance and capacitance due to the charged Helmholtz layer at the interface (Wyatt, 1961*a, b*). The aim is to have low, uniform, and stable electrode impedance. Platinized electrodes are preferable to bright ones but have the disadvantage that the impedance rises about three-fold over a period of months of use, although bright electrodes can vary even more. A deposit of colloidal platinum produced by platinization can be removed by abrasion, although adherence can be improved by etching the electrode before platinization. We use electrodes of platinum on which finely divided platinum-iridium is deposited by a thermal process (Wyatt, 1971). Electrode surfaces are rarely uniform. As a result the functional electrode can change its position in the flowmeter if the electrode surface changes, thus altering the geometry of the electrode wiring loop and therefore the quadrature voltage induced in it. This is a minor matter. What is more troublesome is the interaction of the quadrature electric field in the flowmeter tube with the electrode. This causes current to flow through the electrode surface, producing at the electrode connection a potential the phase of which depends on the distribution of impedance over the surface of the electrode (Wyatt, 1964a, 1966a). The effect can be avoided by placing the electrode at the bottom of a recess, preferably equal in depth to the electrode diameter. This reduces the electric field at the electrode surface by a factor of 14. A small dimension of the electrode in the direction of the flowmeter axis also helps to reduce the effect. The electric field within the flowmeter that is responsible for this undesired electrode effect may be produced not only in the conducting blood and blood vessel between the magnet poles but also in the tissue surrounding the flowmeter if it is implanted. The magnitude of this additional field is dependent on the type of magnetic circuit used in the flowmeter (Wyatt, 1966a).

The ratio of the voltage across the magnet exciting coil to a typical voltage between the electrodes induced by flow is at least 10^7, and care must be taken to avoid coupling between the coil and the electrodes. If the electrode impedance is approximately 2 kΩ, it follows that the leakage impedance must be greater than 10^{10} Ω (Wyatt, 1961a). It is easy with epoxy resins and some other encapsulating materials to exceed 10^{10} Ω of resistance by several orders of magnitude, and there is no problem here. However, at 240 Hz, for example, an impedance of 10^{10} Ω is represented by only 0.05 pf capacitance. Adequate screening must be used in the flow head and in all plugs, sockets, and connecting leads to reduce its effect. Also it is preferable to make the exciting coil system balanced about ground. If the head is implanted, leakage can also take place from the coil through the outside of the transducer to the tissue and thence to the electrodes. Therefore it is necessary to screen the outside of the transducer or completely to screen the exciting coils.

The sensitivity (signal divided by flowrate) of an electromagnetic flowmeter of given size is determined by the desired signal-to-noise ratio and is therefore dependent on the bandwidth. Having determined the sensitivity, the designer then aims at small size and low power dissipation. A figure of merit that may be used for comparing the design efficiency of flowmeter heads of the same type and inside diameter is

$$K = \frac{S^2}{PV} \tag{18}$$

where S is the sensitivity, P is the power dissipation, and V is the volume. This illustrates how it is possible to trade power, volume, and sensitivity. The temperature rise of the flowmeter–tissue interface may be of greater interest than the power, as indicated by another figure of merit,

$$K' = \frac{S^2 A}{PV} \tag{19}$$

where A is the winding area from which heat is lost to the environment (Clark and Wyatt, 1969). Heat is lost by conduction to the tissues surrounding the flowmeter and by conduction and by forced and free convection to the flowing blood. We design our flowmeters so the temperature rise at the outer vessel wall does not exceed 2°C.

Flowmeters that are designed for use around a blood vessel require some means of access for the blood vessel. In practice, either a slot or some mechanical means of opening the flowmeter is necessary. This requirement may place quite a severe constraint on the magnet design and therefore on the extent to which error caused by asymmetric velocity profiles can be avoided. For this and other reasons it is possible that the best we can look forward to is a blood flowmeter with a nearly uniform weight function for rectilinear flow. Meanwhile, the least that manufacturers can do is to ensure that the flowmeter is sufficiently accurate with axisymmetric velocity profiles. Flowmeters are usually designed for convenience in use without any regard whatever for their sensitivity to velocity profile or other weaknesses.

Iron-cored flowmeters suffer power loss in the core due to eddy current and hysteresis loss. This causes a phase angle to exist between the exciting current and the magnetic field. It is important to keep this phase angle small so that variations in it due to heating or from head to head do not matter. Otherwise, quadrature voltage will be detected as a baseline variation. The phase angle, if sufficiently small and constant, can be allowed for in the electronic design.

The design features that have been described are illustrated in Figure 37. The field strength of this flowmeter is 136 G at the center of the flow

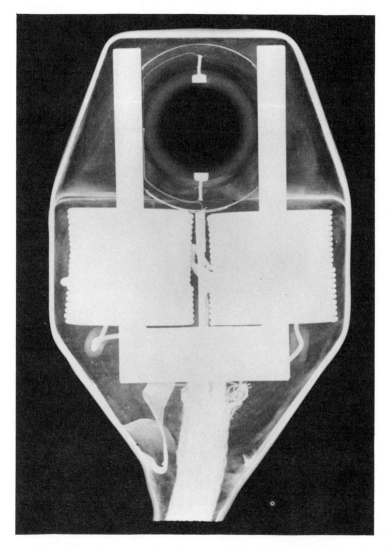

Figure 37. X-ray of 6-mm cannular flowmeter employing a nearly uniform magnetic field. (Reprinted by permission of the American Heart Association, Inc.)

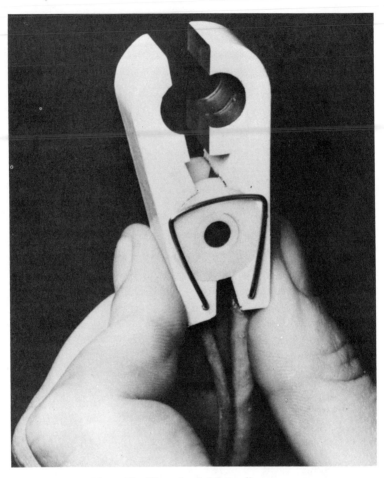

Figure 38. Clip-on head, 10 mm diameter.

tube and the sensitivity 46.4×10^{-3} μV/(ml)(min). The electrodes are recessed. The cannula is surrounded by a conducting screen to prevent coupling from the coils to the electrodes. The exterior is coated with silver paint, forming a grounded screen, to prevent coupling from the coils to any electrolyte around the flowmeter, or in the case of a cuff head of this type, to surrounding tissue when implanted. The quadrature voltage is not more than 10 μV, unless a very badly fitting blood vessel is present. The magnet is of laminated Permalloy to maintain a small phase angle (0.002 rad) and the pole pieces are high to provide good field uniformity. The

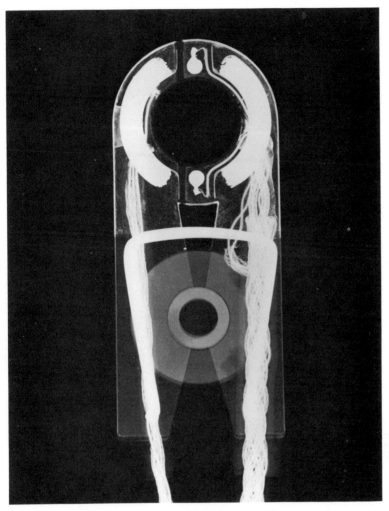

Figure 39. X-ray of clip-on head, 10 mm diameter.

change in sensitivity of this flowmeter due to change in axisymmetric velocity profile is 0.75% as the Reynolds number is changed from 1,000 to 8,000 using steady flow. This head dates from 1962 (Dennis and Wyatt, 1969).

Figure 38 shows an air-cored head of the clip-on type, 10 mm size. The central field strength is 27 G and the sensitivity 5.76×10^{-3} μV/(ml)(min).

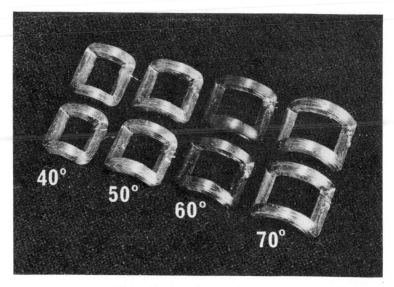

Figure 40. Curved rectangular coils.

In the x-ray (Figure 39) an end view of the curved rectangular exciting coils can be seen. The screening of the cannula and of the outside of the flowmeter is done with an extremely thin film of gold. The electrodes are recessed. The coils are interesting: they start as conical coils, which are calculated to distort in a mould under suitable pressure into almost perfect rectangular coils. The dependence of the sensitivity on axisymmetric velocity profile is due to the angle that the coil subtends at the center of the circle of which it forms an arc. Figure 40 shows four sets of coils the semiangles of which range from 40° to 70°. When each pair is mounted in turn on a suitable flow tube in a pipe line and the sensitivity recorded against Reynolds number (using salt water) the results shown in Figure 41 are obtained (Clark and Wyatt, 1968). Our clip-on flowmeters therefore use coils with a semiangle of 55° for which the response is practically independent of Reynolds number with steady axisymmetric flows. Our clip-on flowmeters date from 1965, and some years later Kanai confirmed theoretically the good profile characteristics of such coils (Kanai, 1969). The head phase angle is zero because it does not use iron.

A 10-mm-diameter toroid flowmeter (Clark and Wyatt, 1969) is shown in Figure 42. It has a central field strength of 27 G and a sensitivity of 5.76×10^{-3} $\mu V/(ml)(min)$. The electrodes, which cannot be seen in this picture, are recessed and also slot-like to increase the surface area and thus

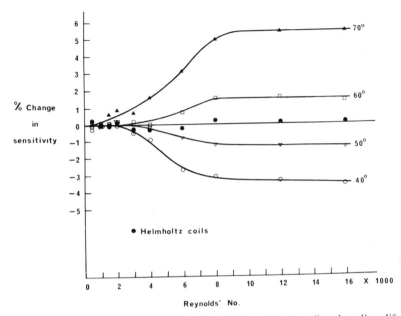

Figure 41. Sensitivity change versus Reynolds number using coils subtending different semiangles.

reduce the noise level. The magnet consists of a toroid wound on a laminated iron core and is completely encased in a screen of 0.0005 in. constantan foil. A suitably shaped piece of Permalloy is fixed between the magnet and each electrode (Figure 43). The function of these is to reduce the sensitivity to flow near the electrodes. The dependence of sensitivity on axisymmetric velocity profile is shown in Figure 44. The variation of sensitivity with Reynolds number (using salt water) is illustrated for different widths of the Permalloy strips over the electrodes. The flowmeter was 10 mm diameter and a 3.3-mm-wide Permalloy strip was chosen for this size. We have made many flowmeters of this type, ranging in size from 3 to 30 mm. The head phase angle is 0.006 rad.

All flowmeters made in this laboratory are encapsulated in epoxy resin at 80°C under vacuum (Wyatt, 1971).

ELECTRONIC DESIGN

The electronic requirements are as follows: to accept and amplify without distortion an alternating signal of the order of microvolts; to demodulate

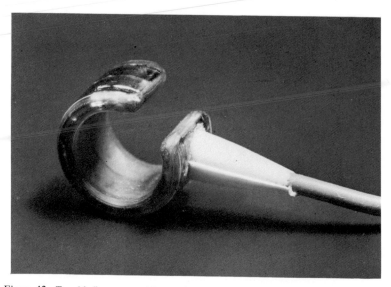

Figure 42. Toroid flowmeter, 10 mm diameter (reprinted by permission of *Medical and Biological Engineering*).

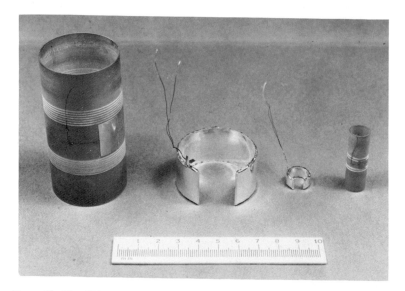

Figure 43. Toroid head: 40-mm and 10-mm cannulae and coils in early development. Note the Permalloy strips over the electrodes and the fully screened magnets.

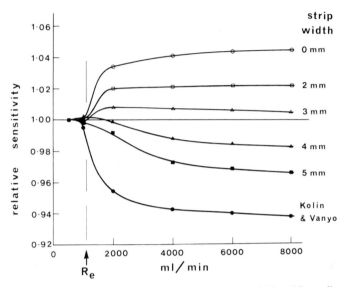

Figure 44. Sensitivity change versus flow using different widths of Permalloy strip over the electrodes. R_e indicates a Reynolds number of 2,000. The lowest curve refers to the head design of Kolin and Vanyo (1967) (reprinted by permission of *Medical and Biological Engineering*).

this so that a true facsimile of the signal envelope is obtained; to add as little amplifier noise as possible to the signal in transit; to eliminate the transformer e.m.f.; to be insensitive to electrode artifacts and interference; and to be insensitive to changes of electrode impedance. All this should be done without the need for instrumental adjustment to suit prevailing conditions. Expressed in its simplest form, the signal between the electrodes of a flowmeter of diameter d utilizing a magnetic field of peak value B_0 that varies sinusoidally with time is

$$U = \frac{B_0}{25\pi d} \left[Q_0 \sin \omega_c t + \frac{Q_m}{2} \left\{ \cos(\omega_c - \omega_m)t - \cos(\omega_c + \omega_m)t \right\} \right. \\ \left. + K \, B_0 \omega_c \cos \omega_c t \right] \mu V. \tag{20}$$

Q_0 is the mean flowrate, Q_m the phasic flow modulation amplitude, ω_c is $2\pi \times$ magnet frequency, ω_m is $2\pi \times$ modulation frequency. Notice the sidebands of frequencies $\omega_c - \omega_m$, $\omega_c + \omega_m$.

The preamplifier needs to be linear, low-noise, and with high input impedance. High input impedance renders the system less sensitive to common mode interference, whether this be at the magnet frequency or some other (Wyatt, 1961a, 1971). High input impedance is also necessary to prevent transformation of quadrature voltage into phase voltage, which is indistinguishable from that due to flow. Figure 45 shows how a phase voltage can be created across the amplifier input impedance RC by complex attenuation of the quadrature component in the signal U. The noise level at the amplifier output, referred to its input, is proportional to the factor $FR_s\Delta F_n$, where R_s is the equivalent noise resistance of the flowmeter, F the noise figure of the preamplifier, and ΔF_n the effective noise bandwidth of the system. ΔF_n depends not only upon the amplifier bandwidth and the bandwidth ΔF of the output filter, but also upon the type of demodulator used at the output of the amplifier. The reason is that noise that is contained in bands less than $2\Delta F$ wide around harmonics of the demodulator reference frequency (which is, of course, the magnet frequency) and that is passed by the amplifier, is converted to low-frequency noise by the demodulator (Wyatt, 1966b). A half-wave peak detector is most noisy, a full-wave average detector is least noisy (Figure 46). The factor $FR_s\Delta F_n$ has an enormous effect on flowmeter perfor-mance. With bad design it can be as high as $800\Delta F$; with good design it can be as low as $3\Delta F$. The ratio of these factors, 270, is the ratio of the powers that would have to be dissipated in the same transducers for a given signal-to-noise ratio. This is particularly important when complex wave excitation is used, e.g., square wave, when it is necessary to use an extended amplifier bandwidth with a limited demodulator detection period.

The preamplifier itself may have a low-noise FET or low-noise bipolar transistor as its input stage. Alternatively, a low-ratio, say 1:4, step-up transformer may be used. These have the disadvantages of size and cost, but they give excellent isolation for safety purposes, they increase design flexibility in the first stage, and they can be designed so the amplifier noise figure is lower than can be obtained any other way.

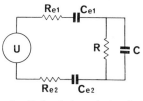

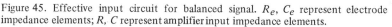

Figure 45. Effective input circuit for balanced signal. R_e, C_e represent electrode impedance elements; R, C represent amplifier input impedance elements.

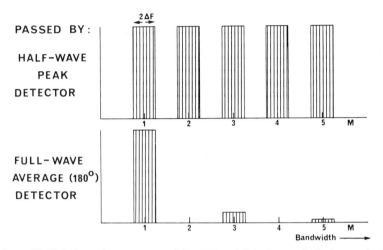

Figure 46. Relative noise power passed by different detectors. m is the harmonic of the magnet frequency.

A bandpass filter that passes the magnet frequency and appropriate sidebands reduces the noise level by a factor only $8/\pi^2$ and is not justifiable for this reason alone. However, amplifier swamping by electrode artifacts and line interference has to be guarded against, and a highpass filter early in the amplifier will do this. The alternative is to demodulate equally early, which has the disadvantage that a stable D.C. amplifier of fairly high gain is then needed. If a filter is used, it must have a linear phase-shift–frequency characteristic to avoid signal distortion, and this is most easily achieved by complementing the high-pass filter with a low-pass one. This has the additional advantage in that it reduces the possibility of amplifier swamping by high-frequency interference. The bandwidth must be able to accommodate the sidebands and the filter must have good transient response.

The detector is followed by a low-pass filter with variable switched bandwidth. It should have a linear phase-shift versus frequency characteristic to avoid distortion of a pulsatile flow wave. The filter bandwidth should be adjustable so that the information required can be obtained with as little noise as possible.

Because the flowmeter is to be used for measuring pulsatile flow, it must have a sufficiently large dynamic range. This should be at least 10 times the meter range.

Figure 47 illustrates the action of a full-wave phase-sensitive detector on phase and quadrature voltages when a small phasing error Δt is present. The error reduces the detected phase voltage by a negligible amount but may introduce significant error from the quadrature voltage if this is large enough. It is easy to maintain the phase stability of the amplifier and detector within $0.5°$, which would reduce the effect of quadrature by a factor 100. This factor is not large enough, but it is possible still further to reduce it.

Figure 48 shows how the direct and indirect effects of quadrature can be reduced. An input transformer is used and the center of the primary is fed with a quadrature voltage V_q' generated in proportion to the net quadrature voltage appearing at the amplifier output as determined by a quadrature-sensitive demodulator at the amplifier output. V_q' is connected so as to oppose the quadrature voltage V_q between the electrodes. In this way the net quadrature fed into the amplifier is reduced by a factor 50. Also, the transformer input impedance is raised for *quadrature* voltage by a factor 50, to about 50 MΩ. Thus the indirect effect of quadrature due to

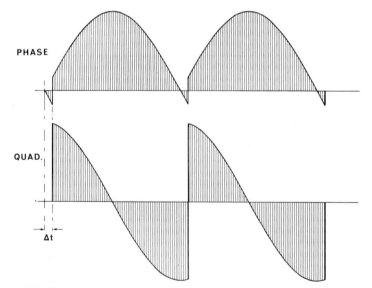

Figure 47. Phase and quadrature voltages at output of full-wave mean detector with phasing error Δt.

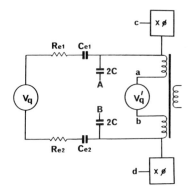

Figure 48. Quadrature suppression and neutralization of lead capacitance. R_e, C_e represent electrode impedance elements. *A, B* are connected to *c, d* rather than to ground. ϕ is nearly 1.

the potentiometer formed by the electrode impedances and the transformer input impedance is reduced by a factor 50. However, the connecting lead capacitances $2C$ could still cause error by similar potentiometering. This is avoided by using doubly screened leads and connecting the inner screens to the output of amplifiers with unity gain. This almost complete neutralization of the input lead capacitance operates for all signals, not just quadrature, and greatly improves rejection of common mode interference. Excellent stability is obtained so that after manufacture no phasing adjustments are necessary. Ten meters of connecting cable can be used between head and unit.

Figure 49 shows a block diagram of the Nuffield Institute unit that was designed in 1961. Three of these were built and are still in use. A feature is a GO/NOGO meter that records quadrature when the magnet is energized, and when the magnet is not energized records any interference that may be present. These units have no user-operated phasing controls and they go on working year after year without adjustments. It is very rare for the baseline error to exceed 0.2 μV referred to the input, even with high-sensitivity flowmeters employing high magnetic field strength (>100 G). A stable baseline is, of course, an essential property of a flowmeter. In general, the use of controls—such as a phasing control—to obtain a baseline corresponding to zero flow at the time of measurement is to be deprecated. It may be done only when it is known that the source of error affected by the control is stable and that other types of error are neg-

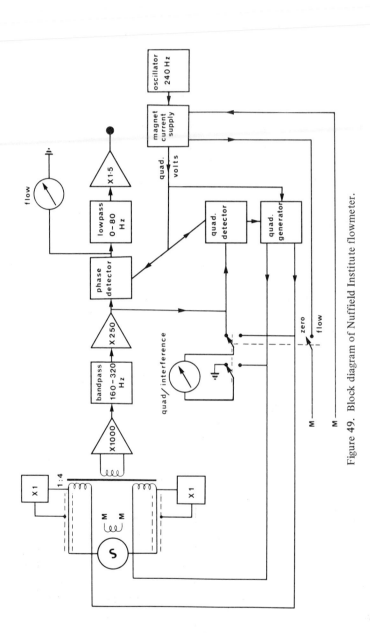

Figure 49. Block diagram of Nuffield Institute flowmeter.

ligible. Otherwise, there is a real danger of adjusting the control to compensate for other errors, thus making the instrument actually more sensitive to variations in the very error the control is intended to null.

Interference at a frequency equal to or at a harmonic of the magnet frequency will be partly transformed by the phase-sensitive detector to a change in level at the flowmeter output, corresponding to an alteration in baseline which, although an artifact, may go unrecognized as such. If the detector is a full-wave one, only odd harmonics of the magnet frequency will have this effect; if the detector is half-wave, both odd and even harmonics will cause error. Interference at a frequency less than the magnet frequency cannot cause baseline change. The most common source of interference in the magnet frequency range is the mains (line) voltage, both at its fundamental frequency and at harmonics thereof. Baseline error from this source can be altogether avoided by using a magnet frequency that is a few hertz removed from the nearest mains harmonic. If significant interference is present, it results in an easily recognizable difference frequency rather than a hidden baseline change. Harmonics are present in the mains voltage. They are generated also in other equipment, e.g., saturated reactor stabilizing transformers, which usually have high leakage fields that can couple electromagnetically with the flowmeter unit. Both odd and even harmonics of the mains frequency can be generated within the flowmeter amplifier itself if overloaded with interference at the mains frequency. It is advisable to use a magnet frequency high enough to permit a high-pass filter, with frequencies of high attenuation at both the mains and third harmonic frequencies, to be used at an early stage in the amplification system (Wyatt, 1966a, pp. 38, 41; 1968c, p. 59; 1971, p. 216). Too high a magnet frequency will cause excessive quadrature voltage and therefore baseline error from this cause. A good compromise would be 485 Hz.

Other Excitation Waveforms

Between 1955 and the present, a variety of magnet excitation waveforms have been used in addition to the sinewave: square wave, trapezoidal wave, triangular wave, and at least two forms of pulsed wave have all made their appearance (Figure 50). The reason for this proliferation of wave forms is that before 1959 (Kolin and Kado, 1959) neither Kolin nor those who tried to emulate him used phase-sensitive detection. Kolin had previously tried to *cancel* quadrature by introducing into the system a voltage manually adjustable in amplitude and phase. This was unsatisfactory for

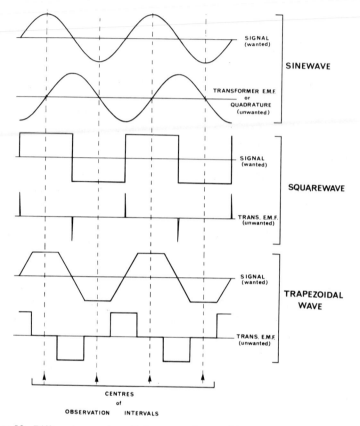

Figure 50. Different magnet excitation wave forms with the corresponding idealized transformer e.m.f.s.

use with intact arteries because the quadrature was too variable. Square-wave excitation was introduced in the mistaken belief that the trans-former e.m.f. was absent for 90% of the cycle (Denison, Spencer, and Green, 1955). However, it did lead to the introduction of phase-sensitive detection and an immediate substantial improvement in stability. Unfortunately, this was accomplished only by using a wide amplifier bandwidth and a very narrow detection pulse at the end of the transformer e.m.f. to record the flow voltage. This in turn was the cause of high noise level, and high magnetic field strengths were used to improve the S/N ratio. These involved large magnets with power dissipations exceeding 12 W and inductances so great that 100-W power supplies were used in the effort to pass a square current wave. The trapezoidal wave flowmeter was introduced (Yanof and Salz, 1961) because it appeared that it would have a region with a far smaller transformer e.m.f. than the square-wave type during which the flow induced voltage could be sampled. This is true, and it is a perfectly feasible flowmeter (Wyatt, 1971). However, it did not work satisfactorily as constructed by Yanof and Salz because the bandwidth of the input circuit was too narrow and the value of the wave shape was lost (Yanof, Salz, and Rosen, 1963). The pulsed flowmeter was introduced (Beck, Morris, and Assali, 1965) to overcome the power problems of the square-wave flowmeter. However, the noise level of this system is increased and the magnet power required for a given S/N ratio is unchanged. Kolin et al. (1974) have described an interrupted resonance system that is exceptionally well suited to the particular problems associated with the use of the catheter flowmeter in an external field. The system in effect gives a flat-topped current wave without the need for large power supply dissipation that would otherwise be called for by the large inductance of the external field coil. It is still necessary to detect over a brief period and the noise level is presumably high. However, this could be offset by using a larger magnetic field; the resultant increased magnet dissipation would be acceptable with an external coil.

There is an important distinction between the reduction of transformer e.m.f.s. by the use of complex waves and their reduction in the case of sinewave excitation by the use of phase discrimination with or without quadrature suppression, either manual (Kolin, 1953) or automatic (Hutcheon and Harrison, 1960; Wyatt, 1964b). The distinction is that with complex waves the transformer e.m.f. is reduced at the *source* whereas with sinewave excitation it is the *effect* of the transformer e.m.f. that is reduced. The importance of this distinction lies in the existence of the reactive impedance elements mentioned previously, both within and around the flowmeter, which convert a small but sometimes significant part of the transformer e.m.f. into a signal indistinguishable from that produced by flow. These complex impedances are in the blood vessel, the surrounding tissue, the electrode—electrolyte interface, and the combination of electrode resistance and lead capacitance (Wyatt 1966a, 1971). A reduction of transformer e.m.f. at the *source* might also be expected to reduce these indirect effects. However, this is not necessarily so, since the relaxation time of the complex impedances mentioned may be comparable to the cycle period of the magnetic field (e.g., Hognestad, 1968).

It has been shown (Wyatt, 1971) that the direct effect of transformer e.m.f. can best be reduced by using sinewave excitation with automatic quadrature suppression, because the signal-to-noise ratio is then higher, other things being equal. This conclusion has not been altered by the system used by Kolin et al. (1974). However, it may be possible to apply this system to perivascular flowmeters, using a far longer detection period than Kolin et al. have found necessary in their more demanding catheter flowmeter application, with a consequent reduction in noise level. Their system might then be preferable, although the need to tune individual probes might prove inconvenient.

Pulsed systems such as that devised by Westersten (e.g., Wyatt, 1971), in which opposing transformer e.m.f.s. of nearly equal amplitude are arranged to cancel, undoubtedly can be made to give a stable baseline although, like trapezoidal excitation, they yield a higher signal-to-noise ratio than sinewave excitation. The effectiveness of complex waves with iron-cored heads may be reduced through lack of linearity between the exciting current and the field, owing both to the shape of the $B-H$ curve and to iron losses. The use of ferrite as a core material may have some advantage here.

CATHETER VELOMETERS AND FLOWMETERS

The first catheter-tip velometer was described by Mills (1966) and similar devices have been described by Bond and Barefoot (1967) and others. They suffer from the disadvantage that they measure blood velocity only very near the exterior catheter wall over which the blood flows. In no practical sense do they have the property possessed by the perivascular flowmeter of integrating the velocity over the vessel cross section. They are capable only of measuring a highly localized velocity that is itself dependent on the boundary layer at the catheter wall and therefore on the Reynolds number (Bevir, 1971c). Their successful use in determining flow depends on knowing the relationship between flow and velocity at the point where the sensitive part of the velometer is positioned when an observation is made. In practice, this restricts the use of the instrument to those regions where the profile is flat or nearly so and where the anatomy permits positive location.

The first catheter-tip *flowmeter* was described by Kolin (1967) and Kolin, Archer, and Ross (1967). Its use is limited to the measurement of flow to specific branches of the aorta. A similar instrument has been described by Stein and Schuette (1969). These devices require great manipulative skill combined with radiography.

A far more promising approach to the problem of blood flow measurement using catheter devices is that of Kolin (1970*a*), who uses an external magnetic field. This not only permits the design of extremely small catheter instruments but also introduces a degree of flexibility in their application that is not possible with previous instruments (Kolin, 1970*b;* Kolin et al., 1970, 1971, 1974). However, there remain uncertainties connected with velocity profile and the shunting effects of surrounding tissue.

ULTRASONIC FLOWMETER VERSUS ELECTROMANETIC FLOWMETER

A contribution to the voltage between the electrodes of an electromagnetic flowmeter is produced at every point within the magnetic field where there is fluid movement and that is not too far from the electrodes. The total voltage between the electrodes is the sum of all these contributions. The electromagnetic flowmeter is inherently an integrating device and the art of electromagnetic flowmeter design consists in making the device integrate in the correct way.

The ultrasonic flowmeter does not inherently possess this property of integration and it is, strictly speaking, not a flowmeter but a velometer. As normally used (Hartley and Cole, 1974) it measures the blood velocity at a point in the blood vessel that has to be specified and in a direction that has to be specified. A measure of flow can be obtained only if the relationship between the measured velocity and the velocities parallel to the vessel axis at every other point in the same cross section of the vessel at the same instant is known. The simplest approach is to measure (by range gating the Doppler ultrasonic flowmeter) the maximum peak velocity in the vessel and then to assume some axisymmetric velocity profile, e.g., parabolic or flat. The internal diameter of the vessel is measured ultrasonically and a flow can then be calculated. However, the result is critically dependent on the assumptions as well as on the accuracy of the measurements, and everything can vary during the course of a pulse even when the velocity profile is axisymmetric. A change in axisymmetric profile from parabolic to flat could change the calculated instantaneous flow by 100%, whereas the corresponding error in even a poorly designed electromagnetic flowmeter would not exceed 10% and in a well-designed one about 2%. Uncertainty of the internal diameter of the vessel can cause error in the ultrasonic result amounting to 10% per 0.3 mm in a 6-mm-diameter vessel, with proportionately greater errors when using smaller vessels. The maximum corresponding error in the electromagnetic flowmeter would be 20%.

Calibration can be done in situ, but the ultrasonic flowmeter response depends not only on the state of the vessel wall (as the electromagnetic flowmeter does) but is also critically dependent on the velocity profile even when this is axisymmetric.

If the velocity profile is asymmetric, the error when using the ultrasonic flowmeter in the ways described above can be very large. In the hypothetical case of rectilinear flow constrained with uniform rectilinear velocity in a circular region of diameter equal to the vessel internal radius, with a vessel wall of thickness equal to 0.1 of the vessel external radius, the ultrasonic flowmeter would be in error by between 200 and 400%, depending upon the profile assumed, whereas the corresponding electromagnetic flowmeter error would be between −17% and +25%. The accuracy of the ultrasonic flowmeter can be greatly improved by scanning the velocity profile along a diameter at a given instant, thus obtaining the instantaneous velocity distribution. If this is symmetric and the velocity is axisymmetric, the flow can be calculated with an accuracy comparable to that of the electromagnetic flowmeter. However, it should be noted that a symmetric velocity distribution along a diameter does not necessarily mean that the velocity is axisymmetric. The ultrasonic equivalent of Hemp's flowmeter (assuming rectilinear flow) would measure the velocity at many points in the cross section at the same instant and carry out the necessary integration.

Ultrasonic flowmeters have the advantage that they operate in a less hostile environment than electromagnetic flowmeters both as regards electrical interference and electrical leakage. They also consume less power and are somewhat smaller and lighter in weight. However, their performance is not comparable and these factors would be much less favorable were it made so.

EVALUATING AN ELECTROMAGNETIC FLOWMETER

The important features to examine are presented in the following sections.

1 Baseline Stability

The buyer should request the value of the maximum baseline drift as a percentage of response on the most sensitive scale using specified probes (1) immersed in saline and (2) placed around an artery.

It should be possible to obtain a baseline of zero flow, within specified limits, by switching off the magnetic field.

Any user-operated control that is provided for the purpose either of altering the phase setting of the signal relative to the detector or of injecting a signal intended to offset any artifact produced in the head is to be condemned: it is a fruitless procedure, it is a confession of failure, and it unfairly places on the shoulders of the user the responsibility of (unnecessary) manipulation of the controls in the hope (often forlorn) of securing stable operation.

2 Noise

Noise could be requested as the r.m.s. noise voltage per $\sqrt{Hz}$ referred to the input at the magnet frequency (1) with the amplifier input shorted and (2) with specified probes connected and immersed in saline. The figures would allow the user to translate the noise into equivalent flow when the probe sensitivity was known.

Complex-wave flowmeters are inherently more noisy than sinewave flowmeters, but they can vary greatly in this respect. The effect of high noise can be offset by using probes that are larger or that attain a higher working temperature; alternatively, the bandwidth of the system can be restricted.

3   The Probe

Points to consider are bulk, shape, ease of application, and temperature rise at the outer wall of the blood vessel. In some situations (e.g., implantation in the fetus) the flowmeter lead will be stressed many thousands of times, so fatigue strength can be important. When implanted, the probe is immersed in salt water at 40°C, and it is imperative that the probes be constructed so as to avoid electrical leakage.

The probe sensitivity should be quoted in $\mu V/(ml)(min)$ and with no blood vessel present should be constant within ± 2% when using steady axisymmetric flows with velocity profiles ranging from parabolic to flat. This is a minimum requirement.

The ratio of geometric length to magnet length (L_G/L_F) should have a certain minimum value depending on the magnet length. The following table is a guide:

L_F diameters	L_G/L_F minimum
0.5	2
1	1.5
2	1

Note that L_F and L_G are expressed in terms of the flowmeter inside diameter.

4 Input Impedance

This should not be less than 100 kΩ and preferably in excess of 1 MΩ. The common mode impedance to ground should exceed 1,000 MΩ.

5 Frequency Response

The frequency response should be flat within ± 2% up to a stated frequency that should be selectable at convenient points in the range 0.1–80 Hz. The phase angle should be linear with frequency over the stated range.

6 Interference

The sensitivity to common mode interference with unbalanced source resistances at the amplifier input (say, no resistance in one lead, 2 kΩ in the other) should be requested over the frequency range 50 Hz to 10 kHz.

7 Magnet Frequency

This should not be less than about 480 Hz or greater than about 1 kHz. It should preferably not be locked to the mains frequency; such locking can cause baseline error. A frequency a few hertz removed from the nearest mains harmonic is suitable. It should be possible to couple together the magnet drives of similar units for the purpose of reducing interference between adjacent probes. (Note: error in sensitivity *may* then result, particularly with air-cored probes.)

8 Linearity

The system should be linear over a dynamic range at least 10 times the meter range.

9 Panel Controls

There should be as few as possible and they should be easy to use.
    The following controls are necessary and sufficient:

1. CAL/FLOW switch: changes amplifier input terminals from the probe to calibration signal generated from the magnet current.
2. CAL switch to alter calibration signal in 20% steps. Linked to RANGE to give output signal independent of RANGE.
3. RANGE switch.
4. ZERO/FLOW switch: turns magnet current on or off.
5. BANDWIDTH switch.
6. TEST push button to test the whole electronic system.

ACKNOWLEDGMENTS

I am grateful to Dr. J. Hemp and Mr. T. J. Cox for kindly reading the text and for their helpful criticisms. I am indebted to the British Heart Foundation for its support.

FIGURE CREDITS

I wish to acknowledge permission from the publishers to reproduce the following figures:

Figures 24, 27, 28, 31, 43, 45, 46, 47, and 49 taken from Wyatt, D. G., 1971. Electromagnetic blood-flow measurement. *In* B. W. Watson (ed.), IEE Medical Electronics Monograph I, pp. 181–243. Peter Peregrinus Ltd., London.

Figures 8, 13, and 26 taken from Wyatt, D. G., 1972. Velocity profile effects in electromagnetic flowmeters. *In* V. C. Roberts (ed.), Blood Flow Measurement, pp. 85–92. Sector Publishing Ltd., London.

Figures 38, 40, and 41 taken from Clark D. M. and D. G. Wyatt, 1968; also Wyatt, D. G. 1968. *In* C. Cappelen (ed.), New Findings in Blood Flowmetry, pp. 49–53 and 69–74. Universitetsforlaget, Oslo.

LITERATURE CITED

Arnold, J. S. 1951. An electromagnetic flowmeter for transient flow studies. Rev. Sci. Instrum. 22: 43–47.

Baker, R. C. 1973. Numerical analysis of the electromagnetic flowmeter. Proc. IEE 120: 1039–1043.

Beck, R., J. A. Morris, and N. S. Assali. 1965. Calibration characteristics of the pulsed-field electromagnetic flowmeter. Am. J. Med. Electronics. 4: 87–91.

Bevir, M. K. 1969. Induced voltage electromagnetic flowmeters. Ph.D. thesis, Warwick University, England.

Bevir, M. K. 1970. The theory of induced voltage electromagnetic flowmeters. J. Fluid Mech. 43: 577–590.

Bevir, M. K. 1971a. Long induced voltage electromagnetic flowmeters and the effect of velocity profile. Quart. J. Mech. Appl. Math. XXIV: 347–372.

Bevir, M. K. 1971b. The predicted effects of red blood cells on electromagnetic flowmeter sensitivity. J. Phys. D: Appl. Phys. 4: 387–399.

Bevir, M. K. 1971c. Sensitivity of electromagnetic velocity probes. Phys. Med. Biol. 16: 229–232.

Bevir, M. K. 1972. The effect of conducting pipe connections and surrounding liquid on the sensitivity of electromagnetic flowmeters. J. Phys. D: Appl. Phys. 5: 717–729.

Bond, R. F., and C. A. Barefoot. 1967. Evaluation of an electromagnetic catheter tip velocity-sensitive blood flow probe. J. Appl. Physiol. 23: 403–409.

Clark, D. M., and D. G. Wyatt. 1968. The effect of magnetic field inhomogeneity on flowmeter sensitivity. *In* C. Cappelen (ed.), New Findings in Blood Flowmetry, pp. 49–53. Unversitetsforlaget, Oslo.

Clark, D. M., and D. G. Wyatt. 1969. An improved perivascular electromagnetic flowmeter. Med. Biol. Eng. 7: 185–190.

Denison, A. B., M. P. Spencer, and H. D. Green. 1955. A square-wave electromagnetic flowmeter for application to intact blood vessels. Circ. Res. 3: 39–46.

Dennis, J., and D. G. Wyatt. 1969. The effect of haematocrit value upon electromagnetic flowmeter sensitivity. Circ. Res. 24: 875–885.

Dobson, A., A. F. Sellers, and F. D. McLeod. 1966. Performance of a cuff-type flowmeter in vivo. J. Appl. Physiol. 21: 1642–1648.

Edgerton, R. H. 1968. The effect of arterial wall thickness and conductivity on electromagnetic flowmeter readings. Med. Biol. Eng. 6: 627–636.

Ferguson, D. J., and M. D. Landahl. 1966. Magnetic meters: effects of electrical resistance in tissues on flow measurements, and an improved calibration for square-wave circuits. Circ. Res. 19: 917–929.

Gessner, U. 1961. Effects of the vessel wall on electromagnetic flow measurement. Biophys. J. 1: 627–637.

Goldman, S. C., N. B. Marple, and W. L. Scolnik. 1963. Effects of flow profile on electromagnetic flowmeter accuracy. J. Appl. Physiol. 18: 652–657.

Hartley, C. J., and J. S. Cole. 1974. An ultrasonic pulsed Doppler system for measuring blood flow in small vessels. J. Appl. Physiol. 37: 626–629.

Hemp, J. 1975. Improved magnetic field for an electromagnetic flowmeter with point electrodes. J. Phys. D: Appl. Phys. 8: 983–1002.

Hognestad, H. 1968. Some problems in square-wave electromagnetic flowmeter system design. *In* C. Cappelen (ed.), New Findings in Blood Flowmetry, pp. 55–59. Universitetsforlaget, Oslo.

Hutcheon, I. C., and D. N. Harrison. 1960. A transistor quadrature suppressor for a.c. servo systems. Proc. IEE 107B: 73–82.

Kanai, H. 1969. The effects upon electromagnetic flowmeter sensitivity of nonuniform fields and velocity profiles. Med. Biol. Eng. 7: 661–676.

Kolin, A. 1953. A method for adjustment of the zero setting of an electromagnetic flowmeter without interruption of flow. Rev. Sci. Instrum. 24: 178–179.

Kolin, A., and R. T. Kado. 1959. Miniaturization of the electromagnetic blood flow meter and its use for the recording of circulatory responses of conscious animals to sensory stimuli. Proc. Nat. Acad. Sci. U.S. 45: 1312–1321.

Kolin, A. 1960. Blood flow determination by electromagnetic method. *In* O. Glasser (Ed.), Medical Physics, Vol. 3, pp. 141–155. Year Book Publishers, Chicago.

Kolin, A., and J. Vanyo. 1967. New design of miniature electromagnetic blood flow transducers suitable for semi-automatic fabrication. Cardiovasc. Res. 1: 274–286.

Kolin, A. 1967. An electromagnetic intravascular blood-flow sensor. Proc. Nat. Acad. Sci. U.S. 57: 1331–1337.

Kolin, A., J. D. Archer, and G. Ross. 1967. An electromagnetic catheter flowmeter. Circ. Res. 21: 889–899.

Kolin, A. 1970a. A new approach to electromagnetic blood flow determination by means of a catheter in an external magnetic field. Proc. Nat. Acad. Sci. U.S. 65: 521–527.

Kolin, A. 1970b. An electromagnetic catheter blood flowmeter of minimum lateral dimensions. Proc. Nat. Acad. Sci. U.S. 66: 53–56.

Kolin, A., J. H. Grollmann, R. J. Steckel, and H. D. Snow. 1970. Determination of arterial blood flow by percutaneously introduced flow sensors in an external magnetic field. I. The Method. Proc. Nat. Acad. Sci. U.S. 67: 1769–1774.

Kolin, A., J. H. Grollmann, R. F. Steckel, and H. D. Snow. 1971. Determination of arterial blood flow by percutaneously introduced flow sensors in an external magnetic field. II. Implementation of the method in vivo. Proc. Nat. Acad. Sci. U.S. 68: 29–33.

Kolin, A., J. R. Steele, J. S. Imai, and R. N. Macalpin. 1974. A constant field interrupted resonance system for percutaneous electromagnetic measurement of blood flow. Proc. Nat. Acad. Sci. U.S. 71: 1294–1298.

Mills, C. J. 1966. A catheter tip electromagnetic velocity probe. Phys. Med. Biol. 11: 323–324.

Roberts, V. C. 1969. Haematocrit variations and electromagnetic flowmeter sensitivity. Bio-Med. Engn. 4: 408–412.

Rummel, T., and B. Ketelsen. 1966. Inhomogeneous magnetic field enables inductive flow measurement of all practical flow profiles. Regelungstechnik 6: 262–267.

Sellers, A. F., and A. Dobson. 1967. Some applications and limitations of electromagnetic blood flow measurements in chronic animal preparations. Gastroenterology 52: 374–378.

Shercliff, J. A. 1962. The Theory of Electromagnetic Flow Measurement. Cambridge University Press, Cambridge. 146 p.

Stein, P. D., and W. H. Schuette. 1969. New catheter-tip flowmeter with velocity flow and volume flow capabilities. J. Appl. Physiol. 26: 851–856.

Wyatt, D. G. 1961a. Problems in the measurement of blood flow by magnetic induction. Part I. Phys. Med. Biol. 5: 289–320.

Wyatt, D. G. 1961b. Problems in the measurement of blood flow by magnetic induction. Part II. Phys. Med. Biol. 5: 369–431.

Wyatt, D. G. 1961c. A 50 c/s cannulated electromagnetic flowmeter. Electron. Eng. 33: 650–655.

Wyatt, D. G. 1964a. Directional property of electrode surfaces. Nature 204: 1294–1295.

Wyatt, D. G. 1964*b*. Electromagnetic flowmeter for use with intact vessels. J. Physiol. 173: 8P.

Wyatt, D. G. 1966*a*. Baseline errors in cuff electromagnetic flowmeters. Med. Biol. Eng. 4: 17–45.

Wyatt, D. G. 1966*b*. Noise in electromagnetic flowmeters. Med. Biol. Eng. 4: 333–347.

Wyatt, D. G. 1968*a*. Dependence of electromagnetic flowmeter sensitivity upon encircled media. Phys. Med. Biol. 13: 529–534.

Wyatt, D. G. 1968*b*. The electromagnetic blood flowmeter. J. Sci. Instrum. 1: 1146–1152.

Wyatt, D. G. 1968*c*. Discussion. *In* C. Cappelen (ed.), New Findings in Blood Flowmetry, p. 59. Universitetsforlaget, Oslo.

Wyatt, D. G. 1971. Electromagnetic blood-flow measurements. *In* B. W. Watson (ed.), IEE Medical Electronics Monograph I, pp. 181–243. Peter Peregrinus, London.

Wyatt, D. G. 1972. Velocity profile effects in electromagnetic flowmeters. *In* V. C. Roberts (ed.), Blood Flow Measurement, pp. 85–92. Sector Publishing, London.

Yanof, H. M., and P. Salz. 1961. A trapezoidal-wave electromagnetic blood flowmeter. J. Appl. Physiol. 16: 566–570.

Yanof, H. M., P. Salz, and A. L. Rosen. 1963. Improvements in trapezoidal-wave electromagnetic flowmeter. J. Appl. Physiol. 18: 230–232.

ERRATA

The following are corrections to errors and omissions in earlier papers by the author.

Wyatt, D. G. 1964a. Nature 204: 1294–1295: The symbols ▲ and ■ in Fig. 2 should be interchanged.

Wyatt, D. G. 1966a. Med. Biol. Eng. 4: 17–45: (i) the symbols d, d' in Eqs. (2) should be interchanged; (ii) the next to the last figure in the last column of Table 2, referring to tissue phase angle, should read 0.15.

Wyatt, D. G. 1966b. Med. Biol. Eng. 4: 333–347:
p. 337:
  (i)   for detector input read amplifier input.
  (ii) for V_s read V_s^2.
  (iii) delete Kolin from Kolin, Spencer, and Denison (1959).
  (iv) for $(1 + 4)\phi$ read $(1 + 4\phi)$.
  (v)   insert A_1^2 after both Mean . . . Pulse formulae.
  (vi) for $(a/m)^2$ read $(a_m/m)^2$.
p. 340:
        for $2k^{1/2} BaA_1$ read $2k^{1/2} BaA_1/\epsilon$.
p. 344:
        for $A\mathrm{W}^2$ read $A_1{}^2\mathrm{W}$.

p. 345:

for $(\omega t+\phi)$ read $(m\omega t+\phi)$

Eq. (2): for $1/\omega T$ read $1/m\omega T$

for α_{pF}/α_F read α_{pF}

Dennis, J. and D. G. Wyatt. 1969. Circ. Res. 3: 39–46.

p. 877: Eq. (1):

for $(10-R_2)$ read $R_2(10-R_2)$.

p. 885:

(i)   delete T in equation for K.

(ii)   for $1.691 \cdot 10^{-3}$ read $3.382 \cdot 10^{-5}$.

Cardiovascular Flow Dynamics and Measurements
Edited by N. H. C. Hwang and N. A. Normann
Copyright 1977   University Park Press   Baltimore

chapter 3

NONINVASIVE ULTRASONIC FLOWMETRY

Donald W. Baker and Ronald E. Daigle

ABSTRACT

The development of quantitative techniques for the measurement of blood flow noninvasively is a difficult engineering, physiologic, and clinical problem. A rigorous approach requires the measurement of the primary variables of flow velocity, vessel area, and sound beam alignment in real time and in a practical manner applicable in a clinical situation. Flow disturbances analogous to turbulence, which may be produced by anatomic defects in the cardiovascular system, deserve special treatment. Instrument methods that are being developed to meet this need include pulse-echo real-time imaging and pulse Doppler flowmeters, all designed to work simultaneously in an integrated fashion to measure the primary variables. Computer-based systems will evolve to cope with the large amounts of data produced. Many engineering and medical considerations are involved in implementing these ideas into a clinically useful system. Opportunities and mechanisms for close collaboration between medicine and engineering must be established to develop these concepts.

INTRODUCTION

The physiologic variables that are used to characterize a particular disease state, and the diagnostic methods used to derive these variables, have generally been determined by the type of instrumentation that has been available to the clinician at the time. Much of the evaluation of the performance of the cardiovascular system has been based on data collected from x-ray techniques using contrast media injected into the blood, thus

Supported by NIH Grant HL-072 93.

obtaining images of blood vessels and of cardiac structures. Blood pressure can be recorded using indwelling catheters, and a limited type of blood pressure can be recorded using the Cuff and Kerotkoff sound technique. Certain cardiac variables can be evaluated using ultrasonic techniques, such as the motion patterns of the valves of the heart and the dimensions and motions of the ventricular chambers, as measured from selected acoustic windows. A more comprehensive and accurate characterization of the cardiovascular system, both in terms of its anatomy and in terms of the blood flow characteristics within it, awaits the development of more effective instrumentation techniques. The lack of such instrumentation has led to diagnostic techniques that rely on the use of *indirect* variables or variables that can be derived using invasive and potentially risky procedures.

A number of medical specialties are concerned with cardiovascular measurements: cardiology, cardiovascular surgery, neurology, obstetrics, and radiology. The two principal disease categories affecting the cardiovascular system are atherosclerosis and rheumatic heart disease, the latter affecting the performance of the heart valves. In only a few situations is the actual volume flow rate the most significant variable of interest. More often, the more significant variable of interest is the local anatomy of the blood vessel as it is altered by the formation of plaques or other lesions, causing impairment of blood flow. The performance of the heart as a pump may be impaired by altered characteristics of the valves, leading to stenosis (restricted opening of a valve), or to insufficiency (regurgitation through a leaky valve), or by septal defects that produce a shunting between the left and right heart. Alterations in the contraction patterns of the heart muscle due to impaired blood flow to the myocardial muscle is diagnostically important.

New instrumentation concepts for deriving new information or for measurement of important critical variables need to be developed in order to meet emerging, new, clinical criteria. These criteria relate as much to concept as to specific instrument characteristics. The ideal instrument is one that is able to selectively measure a particular physical variable among a combination of variables. Therefore, selectivity is an important characteristic. Reliability, i.e., reproducibility of a measurement, is also important. The required accuracy of measurements, whether it is 1, 5, or 20%, is usually very difficult to define because of the rather qualitative character of diagnostic medicine. Accuracy in the usual engineering sense, e.g. 1–5%, is frequently not a significant requirement even though most engineers strive for it.

The importance of a given measurement relates to the value of the particular variable in the overall diagnostic sequence. If the variable is crucial in a particular disease process, then changes in that variable will be directly related to changes in the disease process. The closer the measured changes can be related to these processes, the more significant the instrument concept will be. The cost-effectiveness of a measurement routine is very important in a health care delivery scheme. Ordinarily, a diagnostic instrument is most effective if the data can be acquired and reduced within an hour or less at a cost that is reasonable. The actual equipment cost needs to be included in the procedure costs and should, therefore, be realistic.

GENERAL CONSIDERATIONS

The ultimate goal of flowmeter developments should be the clinical application of these devices in quantitative measurements. Noninvasive flow measurements involve the detection of a set of primary variables. Any potential technique is required to accurately measure the instantaneous flow velocity and the cross-sectional area of the vessel at one particular site, and, for an ultrasonic Doppler flowmeter, the angle between the flow velocity vector and the sound beam axis must be known. It is also helpful to know the exact position of the flow measuring device with respect to the longitudinal axis of the flow channel. No single ultrasonic concept or method can make all of these measurements. As this chapter shows, each of these primary variables is a fundamental measurement requiring a specialized system optimized to produce those data. Once derived, the data can be combined in a variety of ways to produce a quantitative result. This sequence is required for measurements of flow acceleration, velocity, volume flow, and for investigations of turbulence. Other examples might include studies of the cross-sectional area of a vessel as a function of length, determination of the degree of stenosis or regurgitation through a valve, or the amount of blood flow through a septal defect. All of these can be defined in terms of these fundamental variables.

The characteristics of the biologic flow environment also place stringent requirements on instrument modalities. For example, the dimensional variability of the measurement site is a fundamental problem. The anatomy of every individual varies in subtle ways and sufficiently so that no general rules of thumb or "fudge factors" can be used. The exact and specific local anatomy must be evaluated in detail in order to arrive at the necessary numerical descriptions. Cardiovascular variables can be classified into three categories that relate to anatomic dimensions or structure as well as to dynamic flow properties. Category one deals with relatively static structures whose geometry or shape is relatively constant with time. The cross-sectional area of some peripheral arteries and veins falls into this class, where diameter variations may be less than 2%. The second category, which many peripheral vessels fall into, is a category defined as dynamic but nontranslating, meaning that the dimensions of the vessel may be functions of time. The flow velocity through the lumen is also a function of time. The blood vessel is usually tethered in tissues such that there is very little translational motion. The third category of measurement involves dynamic structures in which there is simultaneous translation. In these circumstances, vessel diameter, flow velocity, and location in three-dimensional space are all functions of time. These classes of variables include flow jets through septal defects and stenotic or regurgitant valves. The motion of the carotid artery might, for example, fall in this category.

The variations in blood flow patterns also specify or indicate various characteristics that must be incorporated into the instrumentation. Basically there are two categories of flow. The first, dealing with smooth or so-called well-behaved flow, involves relatively low Reynolds numbers. These usually occur where there are no anatomic defects such as altered valve characteristics or atherosclerotic plaques. The second category involves "disturbed" flows, of which there may be a whole range of values, from vortices, to eddies, to low levels of turbulence in the classic engineering sense. These flow patterns can result from jets produced in valvular stenosis, valvular regurgitation, or septal defects. They can also be produced as a result of calcification within the lumen of a vessel where there may be regions of narrowing or partial occlusion that produce Venturi-type jets, including vortices or eddies that can form downstream from the obstruction. These two classes of flow signals can and do produce distinctively different signal patterns when detected by Doppler flowmeters. These patterns are used diagnostically to evaluate altered anatomic situations.

TECHNIQUES AND TOOLS THAT HAVE POTENTIAL APPLICATION TO FLOW MEASUREMENT PROBLEMS

The measurement of volume or velocity flow rate involves an electronic system having several capabilities. The need to measure velocity, area, and angle has been discussed as a basic requirement to any type of quantitative flow measurement. Velocity can be measured using Doppler techniques (Baker and co-workers, 1968–1970). Vessel area can be determined using either Doppler techniques or pulse-echo techniques. To determine the angle between the Doppler beam and the flow velocity vector requires some combination of echo imaging and Doppler techniques.

Pulse Doppler

The operating principles of the pulse ultrasonic Doppler can be readily understood by referring to Figure 1. The pulse Doppler is a relative of the pulse-echo ultrasonic instrument. The signals that return from stationary and moving interfaces in a conventional echo device can be interpreted in two different ways. The most commonly used method involves detecting the envelope of the raw echo pattern to determine the location or position of particular acoustic interfaces. In Figure 1, the example shows a transducer aimed at a blood vessel in which there are raw echoes received from the near and far walls. The detection of the envelope of these echoes defines the location of the wall interfaces; the output then gives the position and diameter of the vessel. This is the basic signal detection technique used in all ultrasonic echo type machines. Returning to the original raw echo signal, we can process it in a different manner to separate off the Doppler-shifted components due to the moving blood in the lumen of the vessel. In the space between the two wall echoes in the figure, there are Doppler-shifted components in the return signal that may be 40–60 dB below the intensity of the nearby wall echo signals. These Doppler components have their frequencies shifted according to the velocity of the blood and the angle between the beam vector and the flow vector. If the frequency of the raw echoes is compared to a reference signal whose frequency is identical to the transmitted frequency, then it is possible to detect the Doppler frequency shift of these echoes as a function of depth along the beam axis. This is accomplished by comparing the raw echo with the reference frequency in a phase detector. The phase-detector output signal indicates the instantaneous phase difference between the echo and the reference signal as a function of depth. This function is called the range phase, $\Delta\phi$. If there is motion or velocity along the beam axis, the range phase, $\Delta\phi$, is modulated at that depth so that the variations in amplitude of the range phase correspond to the Doppler shift frequency. That is, if an interface is moving towards the transducer, the relative phase between the echo from that interface and the reference is advancing at a rate corresponding to the closing velocity. If the interface is moving away,

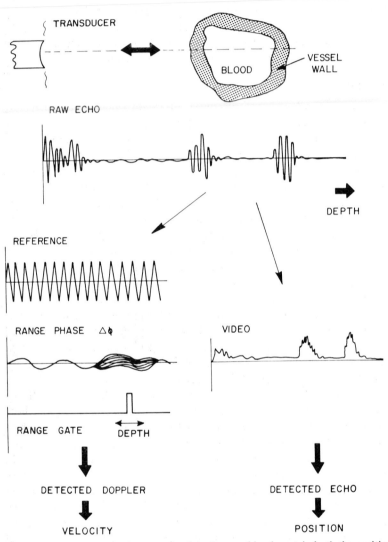

Figure 1. The raw echoes from moving interfaces or blood contain both the position and velocity information. Each can be derived simultaneously and independently using appropriate processing techniques.

the range phase is receding to produce a frequency difference corresponding to velocity away from the transducer. The Doppler modulation of the range phase is detected at the desired depth by a range gate. The output from this type of processing reveals the velocity component along the beam axis at that depth. Therefore, a pulse Doppler device can, within certain limits, function as both an echo device to indicate interface position and a velocity sensor, indicating the velocity of blood or an interface at a particular depth along the beam. Figure 2 shows a reasonably comprehensive block diagram of a pulse Doppler system.

The Doppler described here is a phase-coherent pulse Doppler. That means that each emitted burst is in phase with a master oscillator. This signal is generated by dividing the master oscillator frequency down to the pulse repetition frequency (PRF) via a PRF frequency divider. The output of this divider actuates a gated transmitter such that each transmitted burst is a short (1 μsec) replica of the master oscillator frequency. This signal is applied to the transmitting transducer element. Upon reception of the echoes from the tissue interfaces, these signals are then amplified some 30–60 dB depending upon the depth and the tissue interfaces. The receiving amplifier has its gain adjusted to increase the amplification for deeper interfaces to compensate for ultrasonic attenuation. The amplified raw echo is then compared to the master oscillator frequency in a pair of quadrature-phased detectors. The phase of the reference or master oscillator signal is shifted by $\pm45°$ to provide a reference for the amplified received signal. There are two outputs from the quadrature-phase detector. These signals both have similar frequency spectra but the phase of the components of each of these spectra is shifted $90°$ with respect to each other. When there is motion or velocity toward the transducer, the phase of one channel leads the phase of the other by $90°$. When there is motion away from the transducer, the phase relationship is reversed. The range phase signal from the quadrature-phase detectors is then sampled at a particular depth according to the location of the vessel of interest. At this point the Doppler difference frequency is in a form that must be filtered to remove the pulse repetition rate components and the low-frequency large-amplitude signals produced by the motion of interfaces such as vessel walls and myocardium. Once the signals are filtered, 100 Hz to 5 KHz typically, they are passed to a Doppler analyzer whose output may be the raw detected Doppler or an analog signal corresponding to the instantaneous mean frequency or mean velocity. A third output can be a real-time spectral analysis signal, which shows the instantaneous Doppler difference

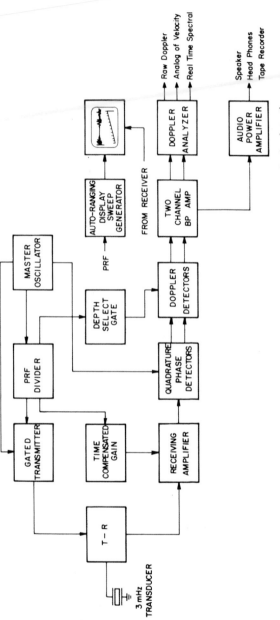

Figure 2. The functional block diagram of the pulsed Doppler shows the various steps in the detection process.

frequency as a function of time (Baker, Johnson, and Strandness, 1974). Other outputs are available and these are shown in Figure 3. Those outputs that can be derived simultaneously from the Doppler electronics include (1) the A-mode display, (2) the raw Doppler velocity spectra, (3) the time interval histogram or real-time spectral analysis, (4) the net analog velocity, (5) the analog velocity towards the transducer, and (6) the analog velocity away from the transducer (Nippa et al., 1975). It is also possible to have an M-mode type display from the Doppler that is used to indicate the position of the depth gate with respect to moving structures such as valves (Baker and Johnson, 1975).

Several characteristics of the pulse Doppler flowmeter need to be evaluated and described in order to outline its potential as a quantifiable device for flow measurement. The pulse Doppler is a type of sampled data system that must obey the sampling theorems. The basic equation defining

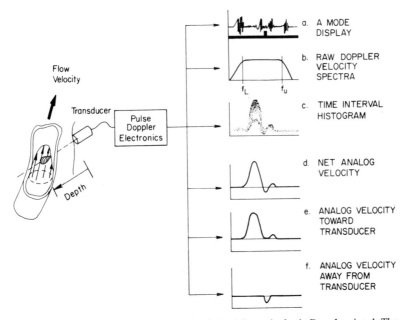

Figure 3. Several types of outputs can be derived from the basic Doppler signal. The A-mode display assists in aiming the transducer at the vessel of interest. The raw Doppler signal can be coupled to a speaker for oscillatory analysis. The remaining outputs are recorded for later analysis.

the measurement of Doppler shift for any Doppler, whether pulse or continuous wave, is given as

$$\Delta f = \frac{2 v f_0 \cos \theta}{c} \tag{1}$$

where

c = velocity of sound (cm/sec)
f_0 = center frequency (Hz)
θ = angle between velocity vector and beam vector
Δf = Doppler shift (Hz)
v = flow velocity (cm/sec)

Equation 2 states that the maximum Doppler shift that can be detected is equal to the pulse repetition rate divided by 2:

$$\Delta f_{max} = \frac{PRF}{2} \tag{2}$$

where

Δf_{max} = maximum Doppler shift (Hz)
PRF = pulse repetition frequency (Hz)

If one wishes to measure velocity and range unambiguously, then the maximum range that can be used is defined by Eq. 3:

$$R_{max} = \frac{1}{(1.3 \times 10^{-5}) \, PRF} \tag{3}$$

where R_{max} is the maximum range (cm). Here we see that for a given PRF, the maximum depth that the system can function over is the reciprocal of 13 times the PRF. The relationship between maximum Doppler shift and maximum range is given by Eq. 4:

$$\Delta f_{max} = \frac{1}{(2.6 \times 10^{-5}) \, R_{max}} \tag{4}$$

Equation 4 can be combined with Eq. 1 to give the maximum velocity that can be detected for a given range, center frequency, and angle:

$$v_{max} = \frac{c}{(5.2 \times 10^{-5}) R_{max} f_0 \cos \theta} \tag{5}$$

where v_{max} is the maximum detectable velocity at R_{max}.

These equations describe the basic limitations of a phase-coherent unambiguous pulse Doppler. In circumstances where the Doppler shift may exceed the pulse repetition rate limit, there is an aliasing or foldover of the detected Doppler spectrum. If one attempts to measure flows where the velocities exceed the sampling rate theorem, then one must resort to a pseudorandom code of noise-type Doppler that utilizes a type of auto-correlation detection. These devices are not hampered by the sampling rate theorem (Chethwa, 1975).

The spatial resolution of a pulse Doppler is determined by a number of factors illustrated in Figure 4. The typical resolution for a 5-MHz system, transmitting a 0.4-μsec-long burst with a transducer of a Q of 4 and a receiver band width on the order of 2 MHz, is on the order of 1.5–2.0 mm along the beam axis. The region of spatial sensitivity referred to as the sample volume is a teardrop shape as shown in Figure 5. The length of the teardrop, or sample volume, is determined by the applied burst duration and the transducer bandwidth. The sample volume width is determined by the beam width. The effect of this finite sample volume length is to skew the velocity profile in a direction away from the transducer. An example is shown in Figure 6 in which a parabolic profile is shown as a solid line and the measured profile is depicted by the curve through the circled points. The overrun, or skewing, of the measured profile to the right is due to the length of the sample volume; in this example it is 2 mm (Jorgensen, Campau, and Baker, 1973). It is possible to deconvolve the measures profile back to the true profile if the sample volume characteristics are known. This technique has been demonstrated by Jorgensen and Garbini (1974).

The detected output from a Doppler flowmeter may not be a single frequency even though there is a single velocity present in the sample volume region. There are a number of spectral broadening effects that can occur, causing the detected Doppler signal to have a spectral bandwidth that may not relate directly to the velocity of the fluid moving in the sample volume (Green, 1964). Basically there are four types of spectral broadening that can be readily identified. In Figure 7A is a type of spectral broadening due to the transit time effects of scatterers moving through a sample volume with a width corresponding to the beam width. A scatterer moving through this region at a velocity v produces an impulse function that may contain a single frequency but that has a duration T determined by the velocity and the beam width. The spectrum produced by this function has a width depending upon the duration of the transit time. A second type of spectral broadening, shown in Figure 7B, results from

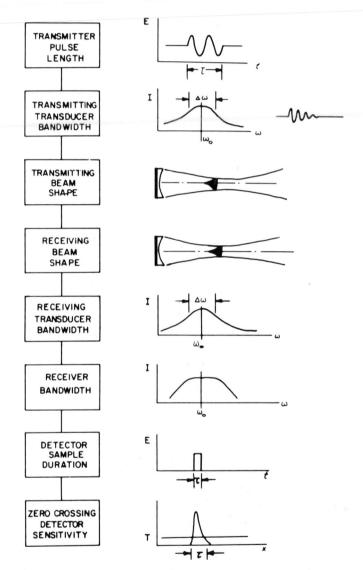

Figure 4. The resolution of a pulse Doppler depends on a sequence of constraints. The primary factors affecting this resolution are shown.

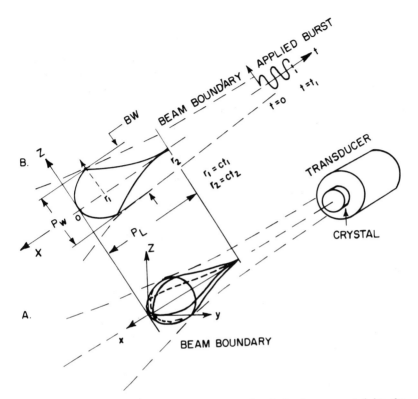

Figure 5. The sample volume of a pulse Doppler device is represented by the teardrop shape of the envelope of the transmitted burst.

velocity gradients within the sample volume. These occur when the sample volume is at the edge of a vessel in the flow shear area. Another type of broadening, shown in Figure 7C, results from the finite beam width of the transducer. In this example, scatterers moving through the beam subtend a slightly different angle as they go from one side of the beam to the other. Since the magnitude of the Doppler shift is dependent upon the angle, there is a band of Doppler frequency shifts generated as the particle passes through the beam width. The fourth identifiable type of spectral broadening, shown in Figure 7D, is due to disturbances, eddies, vortices, or turbulence in the flowing stream. This type of flow spectra often produces velocity components both toward the transducer and away from the transducer simultaneously within the sample volume. This causes the

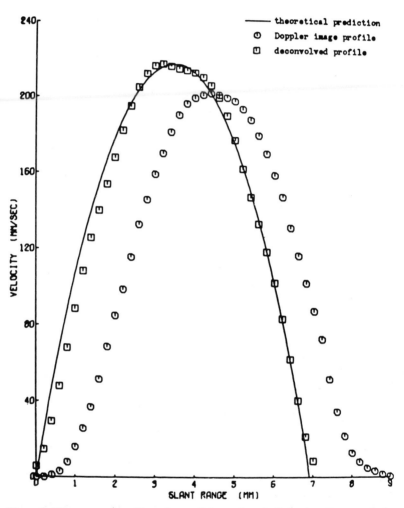

Figure 6. The measured profile under conditions of parabolic laminar flow reveals the skewing produced by the finite size of the sample volume. These errors can be corrected by deconvolution techniques.

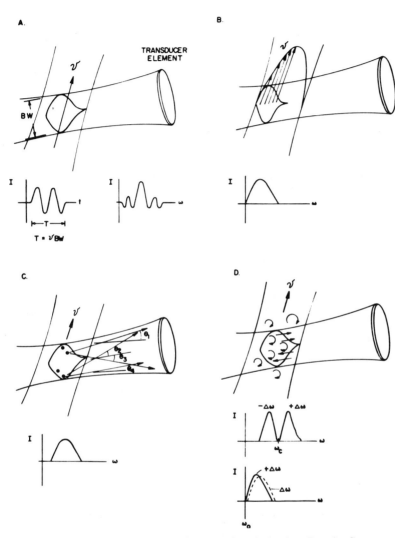

Figure 7. There are several sources of spectral broadening in a Doppler flowmeter. They include (a) transit time broadening as influenced by the velocity of the blood and the beam width; (b) velocity gradient broadening influenced by the size and location of the sample volume; (c) beam width broadening produced by the changing angle between scatterers and the transducer as they pass through the sample volume; (d) turbulence or disturbed flow produces many velocity components within the sample volume that lead to spectral broadening.

Doppler signal to be shifted simultaneously both above and below the carrier, ω_c. If a Doppler with a simple frequency detector is used, the lower sideband, $-\Delta\omega$, is folded over on top of the upper side band, $+\Delta\omega$. If a detection process is used that preserves the upper and lower sideband relationships, then the presence of disturbed or turbulent flow can be detected in the Doppler spectra. Tests have been made to show that a 4% turbulence causes the Doppler spectra to double its bandwidth; thus it is a relatively sensitive indicator of disturbed or turbulent flow (Forster, 1976).

Doppler Blood Flow Sensing

There have been no practical solutions, to date, to the problem of calibration of transcutaneous blood flow measurements. Because of the difficulty of this task, no method has come into routine use. Medicine has not made strong demands, until recently, for quantitative flow measurement techniques applicable to sites where this would be the easiest to accomplish. These "easy" sites include large vessels 3–5 mm in diameter and less than 5 cm in depth. There are, however, many demands for quantitation of cardiac blood flows, which is the most difficult measurement to accomplish. Progress in the development of quantitative methods for the deeper vessels has been very slow; instruments for this application have only recently been developed within one program. It is anticipated that even these new pulse Dopplers will require extensive redevelopment to meet fully the requirements for calibrated deep flow sensing.

Quantitation of blood flow, in the strictest sense, seems to involve only the measurement of a few variables defined by the basic Doppler equation. For the measurement of velocity one needs to rewrite the basic Doppler equation:

$$v = \frac{\Delta f c}{2 f_0 \cos \theta}. \tag{6}$$

For the measurement of volume flow Q, this output must be multiplied by the cross-sectional area A of the vessel:

$$Q = Av = \frac{A \Delta f c}{2 f_0 \cos \theta}. \tag{7}$$

The mean frequency shift (Δf) is the average over the total vessel lumen and θ is the average angle over the total lumen.

There are many hidden variables not appearing in the equations which nonetheless affect the measurement and determine whether calibration may even be feasible.

The flow chart in Figure 8 is the easiest way to depict the factors that can influence the final measurement. If a plan to quantitate blood flow noninvasively is ever to be carried out, it must consider the effects of all these inputs and devise a scheme to evaluate them or somehow include them in the measurement sequence.

Study of Figure 8 reveals that there are two pathways to volume blood flow. One approach is entirely dependent on the Doppler system for the measurement of velocity, angle, and cross-sectional area. The second approach mixes echo and Doppler together. Our experience suggests that the better resolution of the echo scanner system over Doppler imaging provides more accurate estimates of vessel area. No matter which path is followed, there are many potential pitfalls to evaluate and overcome.

Three different schemes for volume blood flow measurement have been evaluated by Daigle et al. (1974). A review of the error sources associated with each of these provides some additional insight into the quantitation problem. The various methods that have been pursued by investigators to develop a calibration scheme can be reduced to the following groups:

1. The uniform illumination method.
2. The diameter profile integration method.
3. The diameter gate average velocity method.

Uniform Illumination Method

This approach basically employs a continuous-wave Doppler that is capable of ensonifying (sonic illumination) the entire vessel lumen with a uniform field of acoustic energy. The Doppler shift is measured from the instantaneous back-scattered signal returning from the total lumen. This is different from a pulse Doppler, whose sample volume ordinarily is small compared to lumen dimensions. This approach suffers most from the inability to measure the angle θ and the diameter of the vessel for area determination.

The errors associated with this approach are outlined in Figures 9 and 10, and Table 1. Figure 9 shows the volume flow errors introduced for various velocity profiles by the zero-crossing meter output, with uniform ensonification of the vessel. These errors can be attributed to the fact that zero-crossing analyzers are not true first-moment processors. Their output

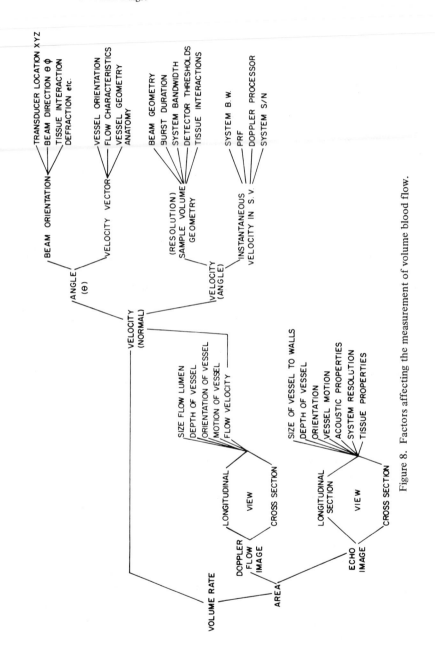

Figure 8. Factors affecting the measurement of volume blood flow.

VOLUME FLOW ERROR

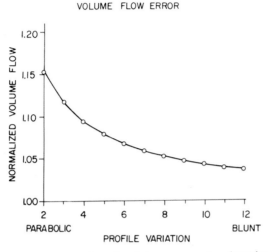

Figure 9. Volume flow error introduced by zero-crossing detection for uniform illumination method.

is not proportional to the instantaneous average Doppler shift but rather to the second moment, which skews the average higher than the true value. The solution to this problem lies in the development of a better first-moment processor, for example, the offset frequency readout being developed by Daigle et al. (1974).

A second source of error in this method stems from the necessity of an

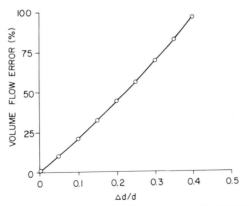

Figure 10. Percent error in volume flow due to error in diameter measurement.

Table 1. Principal volume flow errors associated with the uniform illumination method

Error source	Magnitude
Doppler angle errors	$\sim \dfrac{\cos\sigma}{\cos(\sigma+\Delta\sigma)} - 1$
Zero-crossing detection	see Figure 9
Noncylindrical vessel	$\sim$ distortion in diameter
Diameter measurement error	$\sim \dfrac{2\Delta d}{d} + (\dfrac{\Delta d}{d})^2$ (see Figure 10)

accurate measurement of the cross-sectional area of the vessel of interest. Figure 10 shows how the volume flow accuracy changes with small errors in the vessel diameter measurement. Continuous-wave Dopplers have no depth resolution, so they cannot be used to measure vessel diameter. Pulse Dopplers can measure vessel diameter, but resolution errors can affect the results. Real-time B-mode two-dimensional imaging appears to hold the best promise for determining vessel diameter and area.

There is no way to measure the angle between the sound beam axis and the flow vector with a continuous-wave Doppler. The best solution to this problem appears to be a combination of triangulation and "B-mode" imaging in order to view the vessel axis and the beam orientation in the same image.

Table 1 summarizes the errors associated with the uniform illumination method.

Diameter Profile Method

This approach requires the use of a pulse Doppler with a small sample volume to scan across the vessel and measure the velocity profile as a function of vessel diameter. This can be done by either a single or multigate instrument. A number of assumptions are necessary to complete the profile scan. The profile needs to be axial-symmetric, and the velocity vector needs to be parallel to the vessel wall at all times. If these conditions are met and the vessel does not move during the scan, it should be possible to integrate the velocity along the beam to arrive at an average value. This average is then extrapolated to the whole lumen.

Two categories of error can be readily identified: (1) experimental errors in applying the technique and (2) resolution errors in the measurement of local velocity and vessel diameter with the pulse Doppler.

The first group of errors involves the sound beam size and the accuracy of alignment with the vessel. There can be any number of reasons for misalignment errors. We would anticipate that real-time B-mode imaging should minimize these errors. Figure 11 shows this alignment problem and how it leads to a violation of the assumption of symmetry. Angle errors also fall in this category.

The second group of errors is dependent on the spatial resolution of the Doppler flowmeter. The sample volume or sample function has a finite length, which causes a broadening or skewing of the apparent profile. Examples of this skewing are shown in Figure 12. Deconvolution techniques have been developed for correcting these errors, but they have not been thoroughly evaluated. Figure 6 shows an example of the deconvolution-corrected profile.

Knowledge of the true vessel diameter is essential if the potential accuracy of the profile method is to be realized. Figure 13 shows the relative error range for computed volume flows when the exact diameter is known and when the diameter is estimated from the measured profile slopes.

The diameter profile method is more involved than the uniform

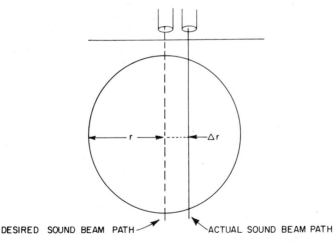

Figure 11. Transducer beam offset introduces error in velocity profile measurement and computed volume flow.

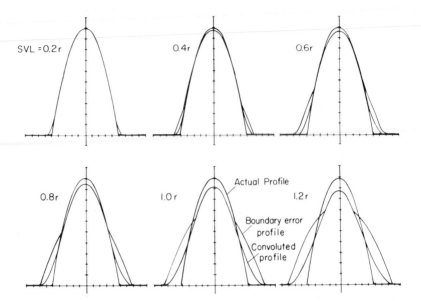

Figure 12. Convolution and boundary error for parabolic profiles. The sample volume length (SVL) increases for each successive set of profiles by 0.2r.

illumination method, but it potentially comes closer to making the volume flow measurement. Many factors have to be considered in order to minimize the errors that can come into the measurements and computations. These errors are summarized in Table 2. The primary limitations involve sound field alignment and Doppler resolution limitations. These difficulties could be overcome with real-time B-mode scanning and profile correction computations.

Diameter Gate Average

This approach is a combination of the uniform illumination and diameter profile integration method. A long-pulse Doppler gate is positioned to sample the flow velocity across the entire vessel lumen. This gate is adjusted to just fit inside the lumen of the vessel. If the flow characteristics are constant over the axial length of the vessel region under illumination, then the average velocity along this thin soundbeam represents the average velocity across the diameter of the vessel. If the gate is then narrowed and set to measure the peak velocity at the vessel centerline, the

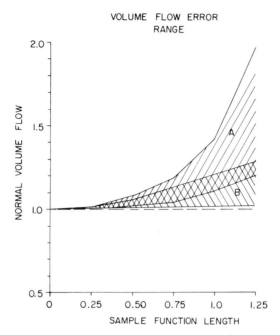

Figure 13. Error range for computed volume flow for a parabolic velocity profile. Error range B applies when the wall locations are known exactly; error range A applies if the wall locations are computed from the maximum and minimum profile slopes.

mean velocity for the whole vessel can be computed. A measurement of the diameter then allows calculation of total volume flow.

Experimental errors inherent in the diameter gate average velocity technique are much the same as those for the diameter profile integration method. The soundbeam must be oriented at a known Doppler angle and be located on the centerline of the vessel. The beam diameter must be smaller than 0.25 of the vessel radius or $\frac{1}{8}$ the diameter. The summary of the error contributions in this method is shown in Table 3.

The measurement of volume flow rate has been shown to be influenced by many factors in the measurement process. We have discussed the factors of angle and velocity as measured along the beam axis. We have not discussed ways to determine the angle between the velocity vector and the soundbeam axis, nor have we discussed methods for determining the cross-sectional area of the vessel of interest. There are two techniques

Table 2. Volume flow errors occurring in diameter profile integration method

Error source	Magnitude
Velocity profile not across true diameter	$\sim \cos$ (Doppler angle, σ)
Physiologic variation during scan	$\sim$ time required for scan
Noncylindrical vessel	$\sim$ distortion in diameter
Nonsymmetric velocity profile	$\sim$ degree of skewing
Blood velocity vector not parallel to vessel axis	$\sim$ function of off-axis angle, radius of vector, and duration of error during cardiac cycle
Beam diameter d too large for vessel radius r	function of d/r, small for d/r
Sound beam not aligned with vessel axis	$\sim (\frac{\Delta r}{r})^2$ for uniform velocity field
Doppler angle error	$\sim \dfrac{\cos\sigma}{\cos(\sigma+\Delta\sigma)} - 1$
Resolution errors	function of sample function length/radius and of wall location method

available for determining the area of a vessel: Doppler flow imaging and echo imaging.

Doppler Flow Imaging

Our ability to detect the velocity at a point in space using the pulse Doppler makes it possible to develop images of the vessel lumen by virtue of the location of the flow velocity. A scheme for doing this is shown in Figure 14 (Mozersky et al., 1971). The Doppler transducer is attached to an arm such that the transducer can be scanned in a fixed plane over the dimensions X and Y. The transducer can be rotated in the plane to line up with the vessel of interest. The principle involves mapping onto the face of a storage cathode ray tube the points in the scan plane where flow velocity is detected above a certain threshold value. To do this, the outputs from the sensors on the scan arm are fed to a cathode ray tube to position the trace on the oscilloscope screen. The depth of the sample volume is included in the display deflection signals so that those points along the beam where flow is detected are written on the face of the oscilloscope. When the transducer is scanned back and forth along the vessel in the

Table 3. Volume flow errors in the diameter gate average velocity method

Error source	Magnitude
Measured velocity not across true diameter	$\sim$ velocity variation along vessel
Noncylindrical vessel	$\sim$ distortion in diameter
Nonsymmetric velocity profile	$\sim$ degree of skewing
Blood velocity vector not parallel to vessel axis	$\sim$ function of off-axis angle, radius of vector and duration of error
Beam diameter d too large for vessel radius r	function of d/r; small for $d/r < 0.25$
Sound beam off vessel axis by Δr	$\sim (\frac{\Delta r}{r})^2$ for uniform velocity field
Doppler angle error	$\sim \dfrac{\cos\sigma}{\cos(\sigma+\Delta\sigma)} - 1$
Zero-crossing detection error	see Figure 9
Resolution error in diameter measurement	$\sim \dfrac{2\Delta d}{d} + (\dfrac{\Delta d}{d})^2$

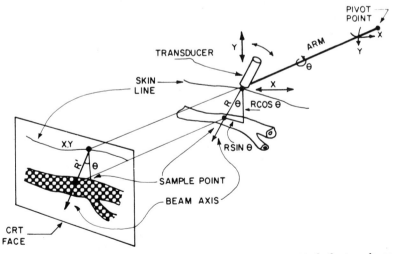

Figure 14. To produce Doppler flow images it is necessary to attach the transducer to an instrumented arm to develop the image on the face of a cathode ray tube.

plane, an image of the vessel is produced (Figure 15). The advantage of a vessel image produced by this technique, over echo imaging, is that the actual flow lumen is displayed. Frequently, the flow lumen may not coincide exactly with the vessel wall if there are plaques or other space-occupying lesions present in the vessel. The images produced by this technique can have various distortions or alterations in shape due to the resolution of the pulse Doppler system. Generally, the vessel images are slightly larger than the vessel by an amount equal to the length of the sample volume. In principle, these effects could be compensated for in the scale of the image. The possibility of imaging the jets that occur within the cardiovascular system, as a result of stenosis or partial occlusion, is quite feasible using this technique (Jorgensen, Senger, and Baker, 1975). An example of the potential is shown in Figure 16, in which a three-sided jet is imaged using the pulse Doppler technique. This example is similar to the type of jet one might expect in the stenotic aortic valve orifice. Longi-

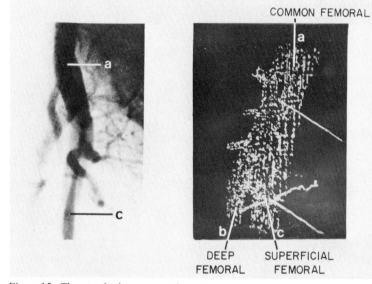

Figure 15. The standard x-ray arteriogram is shown on the *left*. A is the common femoral and C is the superficial femoral. The ultrasonic Doppler image is shown on the *right* in a plane normal to the plane of the picture on the left. The lines on the vectors on the flow image correspond to the position of the sound beam at particular instants in the scanning cycle.

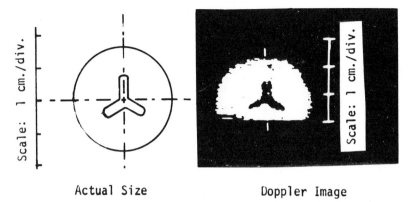

Actual Size   **Doppler Image**

Figure 16. Doppler imaging techniques can be used to show the cross sectional shape of irregular jets. This sample Doppler image of a "tri-legged" orifice simulates aortic stenosis.

tudinal and cross-sectional views of blood vessels can be made using this technique, and from these it is conceivable that the angle between the sound beam vector and the flow velocity vector might be estimated. This can be accomplished by superimposing on the longitudinal vessel image a line or vector corresponding to the beam direction.

Real-Time Two-Dimensional Imaging

In many cases it is more desirable to develop longitudinal and cross-sectional images of blood vessels using pulse *echo techniques*. The considerations or factors affecting echo image generation are shown in Figure 8. There are two different types of scanners used for developing real-time two-dimensional images. These include the mechanical scanners (Griffith and Henry, 1974) and the array-type electronic scanners (Thurstone and von Ramm, 1974). The array scanners involve no moving parts and can scan at very high rates. They are relatively complex in their construction and operation. This chapter limits its discussion to the mechanical scanners, which can be divided into two types. One is the oscillating sector scanner shown in Figure 17A, and the other is the rotating sector scanner, shown in Figure 17B.

Each of these scanner approaches has its own particular advantages and disadvantages. The oscillating sector scanner, placed directly on the skin, is most desirable when there is a small acoustic window providing access to the area of interest. This is particularly true when viewing the heart

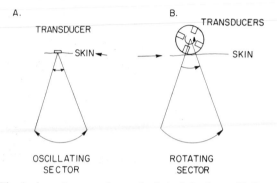

Figure 17. The basic sector scanning methods include the oscillating sector scan A with a single transducer and the rotating sector scan B in which a number of transducers mounted on a spinning disk sequentially scan over a region.

through one of the intercostal spaces. The rotating sector scanner could also be placed on the skin at this type of location; however, the origin of the sector is never directly on the skin because of the diameter of the rotor. Both the oscillating and rotating sector scanners can be mounted inside housings such that the transducer is back some distance from the skin line and the sound is transmitted through an acoustic window that is placed against the skin. This type of scanner is shown in Figure 18. The advantage of the type-B scanner is that it is possible to have a large or wide field of view at the skin surface. This is particularly advantageous in imaging peripheral vessels. It would have very little value in cardiac application

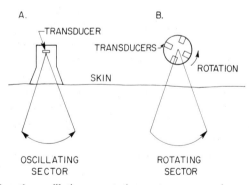

Figure 18. Either the oscillating or rotating sector scan can be positioned off the surface of the scan to produce a larger field of view at a skin surface.

because of the presence of ribs near the surface of the skin. Both types of sector scanners can produce images up to 50 frames per second or more; the frame rates are chosen according to the depth of penetration and the scan angle. In most cases it is not difficult to arrange the scanning rate to exceed the flicker fusion rate of the eye so as to produce stationary appearing images. The output from a rotating sector scanner is shown in Figure 19. The vessel shown is the bifurcation of the common carotid into internal-external carotid arteries. The resolution of this image is apparent when one considers that the vessel is no more than 5 mm in diameter.

Duplex Real-Time Imaging

Blood flow measurements, whether velocity or volume rates, can be made much more easily if the field of view or vessel of interest can be observed in real time and the flow measurement made simultaneously (Baker et al., 1974; Barber et al., 1974). A duplex concept has been developed whereby real-time two-dimensional images are produced in which there is super-imposed on the display a line corresponding to the location of the Doppler

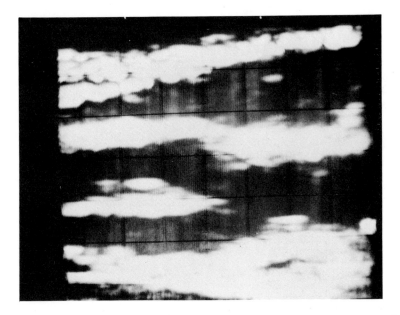

Figure 19. A rotating sector scanner can be used to produce longitudinal images of vessels such as the carotid artery shown here.

beam. The Doppler beam can be positioned in the field of view to intercept the vessel at the location of choice. This concept permits a real-time type of interactive operation for the measurement and quantitation of flow. Figure 20 shows a block diagram for a rotating sector type duplex system. The transducer is shown in the upper left corner of the diagram. It consists of a rotor having four transducers that are projecting the sound beam through an acoustic window corresponding to the type-B rotating sector scanner. As each echo transducer rotates into position, a small, magnetically actuated relay closes so that only one transducer at a time is energized to project through the acoustic window. The image plane in this example is approximately 4 cm by 5 cm deep. There are two Doppler transducers located on the housing, one aimed to image in the plane and the other aimed to intercept the image plane at an angle. The former position is used for flow detection in the longitudinal image and the latter is for flow detection in the cross-sectional image. The system consists of a complete pulse echo unit, a complete pulse Doppler unit, and associated timing and display circuitry. Figure 21 shows the duplex scanner transducer being used to image the carotid artery. One can observe

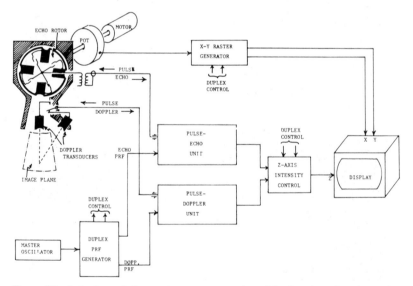

Figure 20. A duplex rotating sector scanner consists of both pulse echo electronics and pulse Doppler electronics for simultaneous, two-dimensional real-time imaging and flow detection.

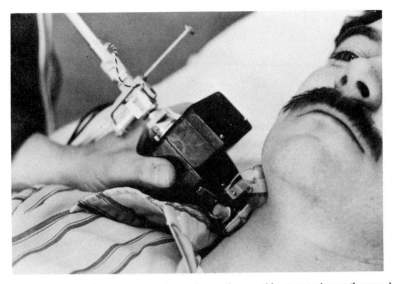

Figure 21. The duplex scanner can be used over the carotid artery to image the vessel and measure flow.

the Doppler transducers and the associated scan arm for detecting the position of the scanner.

Another type of duplex scanner is shown in Figure 22. This is an oscillating sector scanner designed for cardiac applications. A Doppler transducer is mounted adjacent to the echo transducer and is aimed by a steering rod to position the Doppler beam to intercept the sector scan plane. Figure 23 shows the scan format for the Cardiac Duplex Scanner. The oscillating sector scan covers an angle of approximately 30° and the adjacent Doppler transducer can be positioned anywhere in the field of view to intercept the sector scan plane. This type of scanner is particularly useful in cardiac examinations for detecting the specific location of stenotic or regurgitant flow jets produced by defective valves. Figure 24 is a simulation of the sector scan located at two sites of interest, with the Doppler beam brought in from the side to detect flow through valves or flows that might be produced by a septal defect. While it is possible to know the location of the Doppler beam with respect to the sector scan plane, it is important to be able to locate the scan plane as well as the Doppler beam with respect to some external reference so that measurements from one location to another can be related.

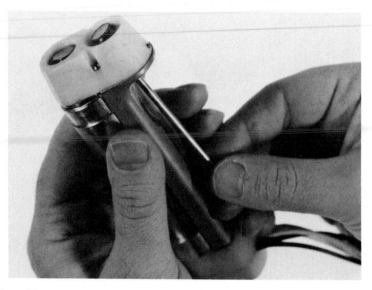

Figure 22. A cardiac version of the oscillating sector scanner has a separate Doppler transducer positioned by a short steering rod.

Three-Dimensional Transducer Position Sensors

The quantitation of blood flow frequently involves positioning the scan plane or Doppler transducer at a number of different angles or locations in order to complete a flow measurement. It is necessary to know the orientation of these locations with respect to each other in order to arrive at a measurement. The need to triangulate on a vessel to determine the flow velocity vector also indicates the need for a position-sensing system and a suitable coordinant reference base. There are basically two position-sensing methods available: the mechanical scan arms method and the noncontacting methods. Mechanical scan arms have frequently been used in ultrasound imaging for the purposes of sensing the transducer location. They are relatively simple and their cost is moderate. The disadvantages of the mechanical arms are (1) the arm is frequently in the way of the scanning routine, (2) the accuracy may be poor, and (3) they require a complicated mechanism that can easily come into misalignment. This is particularly true when the transducer is required to move with 5 or 6 degrees of freedom. An example of a mechanical scan arm is shown in Figure 25. This arm consists of a series of linkages and mechanical joints that are instrumented with potentiometers. Using a small analog processor

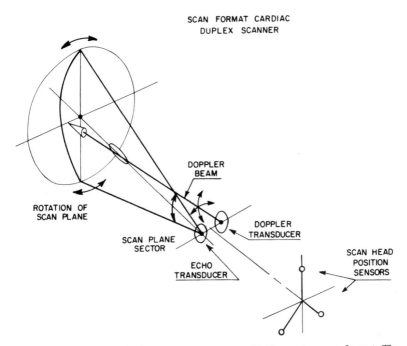

SCAN FORMAT CARDIAC
DUPLEX SCANNER

DOPPLER
BEAM

ROTATION OF
SCAN PLANE

SCAN PLANE
SECTOR

DOPPLER
TRANSDUCER

ECHO
TRANSDUCER

SCAN HEAD
POSITION
SENSORS

Figure 23. The cardiac duplex scanner uses an oscillating sector scan format. The adjacent pulse Doppler transducer can be steered to intercept this scan plane at any point in the field of view.

it is possible to determine the transducer axis and location at all times for connection into an oscilloscope display.

The noncontacting methods, involving either an acoustic system or optical tracking scheme, have a number of advantages over the mechanical arm (Moritz and Shreve, 1975). First, there is no connection or linkage between the transducer and the sensing apparatus; therefore, there is complete freedom of movement of the transducer head. The system developed by Moritz and Shreve, using a miniature acoustic spark-gap scheme, is shown schematically in Figure 26. In this device three spark-gaps are located on a disk attached to the transducer. These gaps are approximately 0.010 in. and each produces an acoustic shock wave that is propagated in all directions when excited with a high-voltage pulse. This shock wave is detected by an array of microphones located above the subject and the area of the procedure. By measuring the transit time from

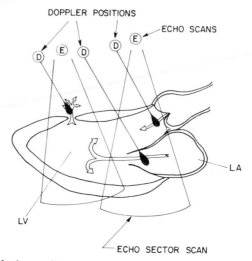

Figure 24. A duplex cardiac scanner permits the identification of important structures while being able to position the Doppler anywhere in the field of view.

each gap to the array of three microphones it is possible to compute the XYZ coordinants of each gap. Using the three gaps shown on the disk in the figure, it is possible to completely define the location and orientation of the scan plane. Since the location of the Doppler beam is known with respect to the scan plane, its location in space is also defined. This sensor apparatus is completely free to move about, and the accuracy is relatively high compared to the mechanical scan arm. For example, it is possible to locate a point approximately 15 cm from the transducer from a number of different angles with an accuracy of approximately 1 mm. This accuracy exceeds our knowledge of the diffraction effects in the tissue itself and is comparable to the resolution of the basic echo or Doppler systems. The noncontacting scheme described here is particularly reliable. There are no moving parts and the transducer is free to move in any of the 6 degrees of freedom. Several optical tracking techniques have been proposed, but these have not yet been developed to the point of producing a practical result for the medical flow measurement application.

Computer-Based Interactive Ultrasonic Systems

It is apparent that a great number of computations are necessary for the quantitation of flow velocity or volume flow rates derived transcutane-

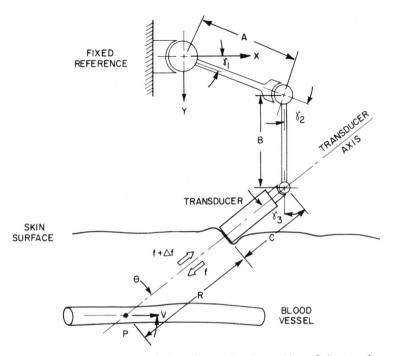

Figure 25. The conventional technique for sensing the position of the transducer with respect to a fixed reference involves the use of a mechanical arm with instrumented joints.

ously. It is relatively easy to visualize a computer-based ultrasound system consisting of the duplex scanner concept with interactive videographic displays. A schematic block diagram of such a system is shown in Figure 27. The system includes the three-dimensional acoustic position-sensing system, the echo and Doppler scanner, and the associated echo Doppler electronics, all centered around the central processor and timing control unit. In cases where the signal levels are very high and the system has high resolution, minimal computational support is probably necessary for optimization or smoothing of data. However, in cases of poor signal-to-noise ratio where resolution is traded for sensitivity, it is conceivable that computational support can compensate for system deficiencies. For example, in the pulse Doppler, in order to compensate for the lack of resolution due to the finite size of the sample volume, it may be necessary to deconvolute the velocity profile measurements with the actual sample

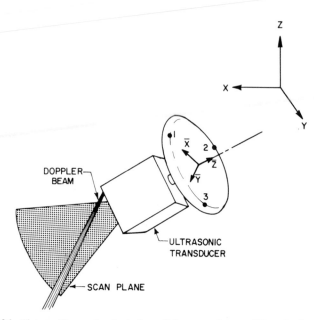

Figure 26. The position and orientation of the scan plane and Doppler beam can be more conveniently determined by sensing the transit time from a set of three spark-gaps, 1, 2, and 3 to an array of microphones positioned over the scanning area.

volume function for producing the real profile. The Doppler signals themselves can exhibit a poor signal-to-noise ratio and are not always able to produce a useful spectral plot. It may be possible to do a type of two-dimensional pattern averaging where the spectral pattern from each cardiac cycle is averaged with the next. The idea is based on the fact that the spectral pattern from a repeating coherent flow signal sums at a greater rate than the surrounding noise, which has a random nature. Also, one can expect to do more rigorous spectral analysis using Fast Fourier transform algorithms that require computational support. The calculation of the cross-sectional area of vessels or of flow jets requires the ability to identify these shapes on a suitable display and then to be able to use a light pen or other marker for outlining the shape of the area of interest. Once outlined, algorithms can be used to compute the area within the subscribed outlined shape. The computation required to determine the three-dimensional character of the flow vector involves triangulation and other calculations to produce a quantifiable result.

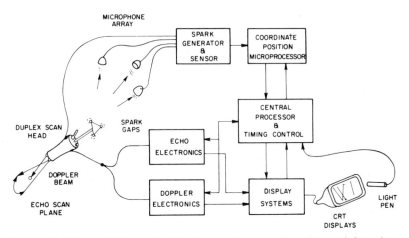

Figure 27. The acquisition and calibration of ultrasonic dimension and flow data require the development of a computer-based ultrasonic system. This system will consist of a duplex scan head and associated echo-Doppler electronics. Interactive graphic displays will be utilized to optimize the interaction between the user and the subject.

COLLABORATION REQUIRED FOR CONCEPT DEVELOPMENT

The measurement systems described in this paper cannot be realized by the engineering community without contact with the biological-medical problem area. The success of these devices requires a close liaison between the clinician, researcher, basic scientist, and instrumentation engineer. Model studies to evaluate and develop specifications for these systems have only been partially successful because the models seldom exhibit all of the acoustic properties and characteristics of the tissues encountered in the biologic situation. Interactive development with the medical problem is essential for achieving operational systems, and it is particularly crucial in the proper selection of variables for measurement.

LITERATURE CITED

Baker, D. W. 1970. Pulsed ultrasonic Doppler blood flow sensing. IEEE Proc. Sonics and Ultrasonics SU-17(3): 170–185.

Baker, D. W., and S. L. Johnson. 1975. Diagnosis of mitral valve disease using Doppler echocardiography. The Mitral Valve. Publishing Sciences Group, Paris, France.

Baker, D. W., S. L. Johnson, and D. E. Strandness. 1974. Prospects for quantitation of transcutaneous pulsed Doppler techniques in cardiology and peripheral vascular disease. *In* Robert S. Reneman (ed.), Cardiovascular Application of Ultrasound, pp. 108–124. North Holland, Amsterdam.

Baker, D. W., and D. W. Watkins. 1968. A phase coherent pulse Doppler system for cardiovascular measurement. Proceedings 20th Annual Conference on Engineering in Medicine and Biology 27: 2 (Abstract).

Barber, F. E., D. W. Baker, and A. W. Nation. 1974. Ultrasonic duplex echo Doppler scanner. IEEE Trans. Biomed. Eng. BME-21(2): 109–113.

Barber, F. E., D. W. Baker, D. E. Strandness, J. M. Ofstad, and G. O. Mahler. 1974. Duplex Scanner II: for simultaneous imaging of artery tissues and flow. Ultrasonics Symposium Proceedings, IEEE Cat. No. 74CHO 896-ISU: 774–748.

Chethwa, C. P. 1975. Blood flow measurement using ultrasonic pulsed random signal Doppler system. IEEE Trans. Sonics and Ultrasonics SU-22(1): 1–11.

Daigle, R. E., F. D. McLeod, D. W. Miller, M. B. Histand, and M. K. Wells. 1974. Transcutaneous measurement of volume blood flow. NASA Technical Report under Grant NS G-7009.

Forster, F. K. 1976. The applications and limitations of Doppler spectral broadening measurements for the detection of cardiovascular disorders. Proceeding. 1st. WFUMB, San Francisco.

Green, P. S. 1964. Spectral broadening of acoustic reverbation in Doppler shift fluid flowmeters. J. Acoust. Soc. Amer. 36(7): 1383–1390.

Griffith, J. M., and W. L. Henry. 1974. A sector scanner for real-time two-dimensional echocardiography. Circulation 49: 1147–1152.

Jorgensen, J. E., D. N. Campau, and D. W. Baker. 1973. Physical characteristics and mathematical modeling of the pulsed ultrasonic flowmeter. Med. Biol. Engineer. 404–421.

Jorgensen, J. E., and J. L. Garbini. 1974. Analytical calibration of the pulsed ultrasonic Doppler flowmeter. ASME Trans. J. Fluid Mech. 73-WA/B10-1: 158–167.

Jorgensen, J. E., R. D. Senger, and D. W. Baker. 1975. Assessment of accuracy in Doppler flow imaging.

McLeod, R. D., R. Daigle, and C. W. Miller. 1974. Doppler shift frequency to voltage conversion techniques. Proceedings of 19th Annual Conf. AIUM (Abstract).

Moritz, W. E., and P. L. Shreve. 1975. A microprocessor based spatial locating system for use with diagnostic ultrasound. IEEE Proc.

Mozersky, D. J., D. E. Hokanson, D. W. Baker, D. S. Sumner, and D. E. Strandness. 1971. Ultrasonic arteriography. Arch. Surg. 103: 663–667.

Nippa, J. H., D. E. Hokanson, D. R. Lee, D. S. Sumner, and D. E. Strandness. 1975. Phase rotation for separating forward and reverse blood velocity signals. IEEE Trans. Sonics and Ultrasonics SU-22(5): 340–346.

Thurstone, F. L., and O. T. Von Ramm. 1974. A new ultrasound imaging technique employing two-dimensional electronic beam steering. *In* P. Green (ed.), Acoustical Holography, Vol. 5., pp. 249–259. Plenum Press, New York.

Cardiovascular Flow Dynamics and Measurements
Edited by N. H. C. Hwang and N. A. Normann
Copyright 1977   University Park Press   Baltimore

chapter 4

HOT-FILM MEASUREMENTS OF ARTERIAL BLOOD FLOW AND OBSERVATIONS OF FLOW DISTURBANCES

Robert M. Nerem

ABSTRACT

Recent hot-film anemometer blood velocity measurements in the horse are used as the basis for a discussion of the flow characteristics in the major mammalian arteries. Anesthetized and conscious animal studies have been carried out using L-shape and catheter probes, respectively. These studies have included the following vessels: the ascending aorta and the aortic arch region, the abdominal aorta and some of the major branch vessels, and the coronary arteries. Based on these studies, the range of conditions to be encountered in the major arteries of the circulation system include peak Reynolds numbers from 100 to over 10,000 and values of the unsteadiness parameter from 2 to 30. The flow, although in many cases laminar and disturbance free, is

This research is supported by the National Science Foundation under Grant GK-31026 and the National Institutes of Health under Grant HL-16236.
Symbols used in this chapter are:

Re	Reynolds number, $\mathrm{Re} = VD/\nu$
α	Frequency or unsteadiness parameter, $\alpha = R(\omega/\nu)^{1/2}$
V	Mean velocity
R	Vessel radius
ω	Fundamental frequency of the flow pulsations
ν	Kinematic viscosity
$\hat{R}e$	Peak Reynolds number
$\hat{V}$	Peak systolic velocity
δ	Stokes layer thickness, $\delta = (2\nu/\omega)^{1/2}$

191

extremely varied in character. It may be asymmetric and certainly is not necessarily representative of fully developed Poiseuille flow. Furthermore, in the ascending aorta the flow may be highly disturbed and possibly even turbulent.

INTRODUCTION

The analysis of the flow of blood in major mammalian arteries presents a number of interesting and challenging problems. This is because the flow is pulsatile, commonly with a reversing phase, and passes through vessels that are both elastic and of complex geometry.

Unfortunately, until recently little information existed about the detailed nature of the viscous flow phenomena in the arterial system. This is at first sight surprising since the subject of viscous flow has been of continuing interest and importance in a wide range of engineering contexts. In general, however, engineering studies have examined both laminar and turbulent viscous flow primarily for steady-state conditions.

Furthermore, the problem in the arterial system has been uniquely difficult, partly because of the unsteady nature of the basic flow and partly because of limitations on instrumentation and access. Recently, however, point velocity and shear stress measurements within the arterial system have become possible with hot-film, constant-temperature anemometer systems (see Ling et al., 1968; Schultz et al., 1969; Seed and Wood, 1970a). These systems have been shown to have a frequency response adequate for turbulence measurements (Seed and Wood, 1970a; Nerem and Seed, 1972).

Initial in vivo studies using hot-film anemometer systems were carried out exclusively in animals smaller than humans, e.g., dogs and pigs. Limitations on the size of instrumentation precluded the resolving of certain important flow details in studies using these animals. Furthermore, in using these animals the observed values of the important flow similarity parameters, e.g., Reynolds number, Re = VD/ν, and the unsteadiness parameter, $\alpha = R(\omega/\nu)^{1/2}$ (V is mean velocity, D is vessel radius, ω is the fundamental frequency of the flow pulsations, and ν is the kinematic viscosity), differ from those associated with the human arterial system.

However, during the past several years and through the collaborative efforts of the Colleges of Engineering and Veterinary Medicine at Ohio State, hot-film anemometer velocity measurements of arterial flow have been carried out in horses. The use of this species has permitted the increased resolution of flow details and an extension of the range of in vivo animal studies to values of Reynolds number, Re, and the unsteadiness parameter, α, so as to encompass human arterial flow conditions.

Horses have aortic diameters of up to 5 cm, a brachiocephalic artery diameter on the order of 3 cm, intracostals 1 cm in diameter, iliac arteries with diameters up to 2 cm, and coronary arteries up to 1 cm in diameter. This size has offered the opportunity to obtain measurements in vessels and with a detail (in terms of instrumentation resolution versus vessel size) that was not previously afforded in animal studies.

It should be noted that the major motivation for this work lies in the fact that fluid mechanical factors have been identified in the literature as having an important influence on the location of sites showing preferential development of arterial disease (Bergel, Nerem, and Schwartz, 1976). For example, both Caro, Fitz-Gerald, and Schroter (1971) and Fry (1968) have identified arterial wall shearing stresses as a potentially important factor in the development of the atheroma. The results of Caro and Nerem (1973) using ^{14}C-cholesterol have shown that it is not an effect of wall shear on diffusion boundary-layer transport, but one considerably more subtle in terms of an effect of wall shear on the properties of the arterial wall. Similar steady-flow results have been obtained using ^{131}I-albumin, and data from experiments recently completed indicate that it is not only the mean component of arterial flow, but also the oscillatory components that have an important influence on the transport of albumin between blood and the arterial wall (Nerem, Mosberg, and Schwerin, 1975). Certainly the possible importance of such phenomena has provided a requirement for a more detailed knowledge of the properties of arterial blood flow.

HOT-FILM ANEMOMETER SYSTEM

The measurements to be used as the basis for the discussion here were carried out using a hot-film constant-temperature anemometer system with the film held at a temperature approximately 5°C higher than that of the blood. This system includes the Disa 55DO1 anemometer and the Disa 55D10 linearizer. The principle of operation of hot-film anemometer systems and some of the problems encountered in their use in blood velocity measurements have been discussed by Seed and Wood (1970b).

Both catheter probes and L-shape probes inserted by direct puncture through the vessel wall were used. These probes were manufactured in our own laboratory and are illustrated in Figure 1. The velocity probes were calibrated during each experiment using blood from the animal. At the start of each experiment, a 200-ml sample of blood was taken, anticoagulated with heparin, and placed in the calibration turntable channel (Seed and Wood, 1969). Here it was maintained at a temperature of 38°C with a thermostatically controlled water heater—circulator. The probe was immersed in the blood, and by controlling the speed of the turntable channel, the probe was calibrated at various known constant velocities. Output signals were passed through the linearizer, which was adjusted to provide a linear output voltage—velocity relationship.

Although only a steady-state flow calibration was performed, there

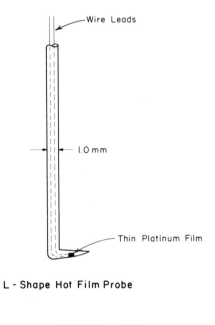

L - Shape Hot Film Probe

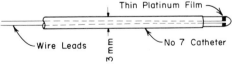

Catheter Hot Film Probe

Figure 1. Hot-film velocity probes used in investigations at Ohio State University.

have been previous evaluations of the performance of hot-film anemometer systems under unsteady flow conditions. Certainly, the demonstration of flow disturbances and turbulent velocity fluctuations, which may extend up to several hundred hertz in frequency, imposes more stringent demands on the frequency response of the measurement system than normal phasic recording of blood flow. The response of the hot-film system, tested electrically (Seed and Wood, 1970*a*), has been shown to be sensibly flat to over 400 Hz. This test does not entirely define the behavior of the system, however, since heat transfer from the film is ultimately dictated by the form of the boundary layer over the probe surface, and small-amplitude, high-frequency fluctuations in the stream velocity may not be reflected instantaneously within the boundary layer. This topic was examined in detail by Seed and Wood (1970*b*); their results suggest that at a stream velocity of 100 cm/sec small fluctuations are recorded faithfully up to a frequency of about 70 Hz but show some amplification beyond this.

The ability of such a system to respond to turbulent velocity fluctuations has been checked by mounting a calibrated probe in a pipe rig and exposing it to a water flow that was accelerated to a supercritical Reynolds number velocity and then decelerated and stopped (Nerem and Seed, 1972). The probe signal is displayed in Figure 2 and illustrates that

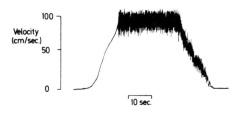

Figure 2. Signal from hot-film needle probe in pipe flow. The flow was increased until turbulence occurred, and then stopped. Peak Reynolds number 9,500.

turbulence, once established, may persist in a decelerating flow to quite low velocities.

The L-shape probes manufactured in our laboratory are physically quite similar to those used by Seed and Wood (1970*a, b*) and by Nerem and Seed (1972), and thus would be expected to have the same frequency response characteristics. This is also supported by the more recent experiments by Clark (1974) and the theoretical analysis of Pedley (1972). For the catheter probes, similar performance characteristics exist for forward flow, i.e., flow coming in over the tip of the catheter; however, for reverse flow the catheter probes are rather unresponsive. None of the probes used in the present series of experiments had a direction capability.

EXPERIMENTAL PROCEDURE

The measurements of local velocity waveforms discussed here were carried out in horses that varied in weight between 136 and 410 kg. The animals were preanesthetized with Acepromazine maleate (0.05 mg/kg body weight) given intravenously, approximately 30 min before anesthesia. Anesthesia was induced with a single bolus of pentobarbital sodium, approximately 15 mg/kg body weight. The animals received a continuous drip of glycerol gyacolate at the rate of approximately 50–200 mg/min depending on the assessed conditions of the preparation. Additional pentobarbital sodium was administered as required. Ventilation was maintained with a Mark 9 servorespirator (Bird Corporation, Palm Springs, California) driven with 100% oxygen through an endotracheal tube. After the thoracotomy was performed, the respirator output was adjusted to provide adequate distension of both lungs.

For thoracic measurements, the thorax was opened via a left or right thoracotomy with resection of 4–6 ribs depending upon the exposure required. Abdominal measurements were made via a laporatomy incision from the paralumbar fossa ventral to the midline and cranial to the xiphoid cartilage. The left carotid artery was exposed and a number 8 French catheter was passed into the aorta and attached to a Statham P23Aa pressure transducer. This system was used to monitor aortic pressure. An axial lead, ECG, demonstrating a marked R wave, was attached and the ECG recorded for timing synchronization of velocity and pressure recordings.

In the coronary artery studies, the left common coronary artery and the area of the bifurcation into the left circumflex and anterior descending

coronary arteries were dissected. A superficial branch of the left circumflex coronary artery was dissected free and an eighteen gauge telgon
catheter approximately 15 cm long was placed in this superficial branch
and advanced into the left circumflex artery. The catheter was then
attached to a Statham P23Aa pressure transducer to measure pressure
within the coronary artery.

L-shape probe measurements were carried out with the probe inserted
by direct vessel puncture. After insertion, the probe was aligned as nearly
as possible on a diameter normal to the vessel wall. A micrometer device,
which was attached to the probe after puncture of the vessel wall, allowed
for graduated changes in probe position. The internal diameter of the
vessel at each site was measured by traversing the probe from the near wall
to the far wall and adding this distance to the probe width. The probe was
then traversed across the vessel in approximately 1-mm steps. Local
velocity waveforms were thus recorded at a series of positions across the
vessel. By keying on the ECG, the instantaneous velocity profile could
then be reconstructed. It should be noted that velocity waveforms were
measured repeatedly at the centerline station to check changes in flow
conditions as well as for probe fouling due to fibrin deposition. If a drift in
probe output was noted, the film was wiped gently against the vessel wall
to remove any deposition on the sensor surface. In addition, the film cold
resistance was repeatedly checked in order to ensure the repeatability of
the velocity probe measurements.

In the coronary flow studies a rubber positioning device, which also
helped seal the imposed wound, was attached to the probe prior to
puncture of the vessel wall. This device consisted of a rubber disk, 15 mm
in diameter and 5 mm thick, with a hole in its center through which the
probe shaft snugly fit. The probe was inserted into the lumen of a vessel to
a depth such that this rubber disk rested against the top of the artery wall.
By changing the position of the disk along the length of the probe,
graduated changes in probe position could be obtained. Because of the
light weight of the probe and the attached rubber positioning device, the
probe was free to move with the heart as it beat, although the position of
the probe within the vessel lumen remained fixed relative to the outer
wall.

Catheter measurements of aortic flows in conscious horses were also
conducted. The horses were tranquilized with Acepromazine maleate (0.05
mg/kg of body weight). The area of the jugular furrow was then instilled
with lidocaine HCl 2% and the jugular vein and carotid artery were

dissected. The hot-film catheter was taped to a Pieper pressure transducer (Pieper, 1967), and the tip of the hot-film catheter always extended at least 1–2 cm beyond the pressure catheter. The two catheters were then passed down the carotid artery, through the ascending aorta and aortic valve into the left ventricle. The various positions were verified by typical pressure waveforms. The catheter was then withdrawn and at selected positions velocity waveforms were recorded. In all catheter measurements, recordings at various positions were repeated in order to guard against any probe fouling going undetected.

RESULTS AND DISCUSSION

Velocity Distribution

In this section the results obtained by Nerem et al. (1974, 1975), using the procedures and instrumentation previously described, are used to discuss the nature of the flow in the aorta and its major branch vessels. The primary similarity parameters of interest will be (1) the peak Reynolds number, $\hat{R}e = \hat{V}D/\nu$ ($\hat{V}$ is the peak systolic velocity, D the vessel diameter, and ν the kinematic viscosity, which equals approximately 0.035 cm^2/sec for blood with a normal hematocrit), (2) the unsteadiness or frequency parameter, α, and (3) the ratio of the peak centerline velocity to the mean velocity. Particular attention is paid to entrance effects, asymmetries in the velocity profile that may be ascribed to vessel curvature or branching, and whether or not any flow disturbances are present. A discussion of the possible existence of blood flow turbulence is left to the next section. It should be emphasized that hot-film anemometer measurements have been carried out in nearly 40 horses and that the few figures included here have been selected as being representative.

   The Ascending Aorta and the Aortic Arch   Hot-film anemometer measurements have been carried out in the ascending aorta and the aortic arch region in both anesthetized and conscious horses.

   Peak centerline flow velocities of nearly 100 cm/sec were obtained and the corresponding peak Reynolds number, $\hat{R}e$, was on the order of 10,000. The range of values of the unsteadiness parameter, α, was 10–30, and the estimated ratio of peak velocity to mean velocity at the centerline ranged from 3.5 to 7.

   Disturbed flows were frequently encountered in the conscious animals. This is illustrated in Figure 3 where a series of measured velocity wave-

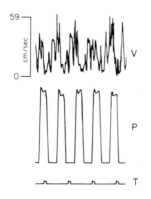

Catheter within Ventricle

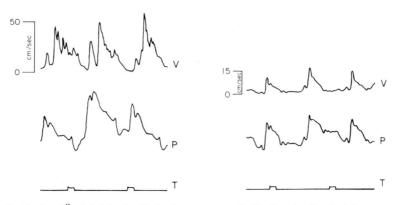

Catheter 1" Distal to Aortic Valve   Catheter in Carotid Artery

Figure 3. Hot-film catheter velocity probe recordings in conscious horse (no. 10) as catheter is withdrawn from left ventricle and out into the carotid artery; *P,* pressure waveform; *V*, velocity waveform; *T*, time marks.

forms are presented for three positions: the left ventricle, just distal to the aortic valve, and the carotid artery. Also shown are the measured pressure waveforms. It should be emphasized that these pressure measurements were uncalibrated and the crude waveform obtained was only used to determine the catheter location. However, the mean arterial pressure was estimated to be between 85–105 torr. It should also be noted that the tip of the hot-film catheter was located approximately 5 cm proximal to the tip of the pressure transducer.

It is obvious from Figure 3 that the flow in the left ventricle has a reasonably high velocity and considerable high-frequency content. Unfortunately, the orientation of the catheter probe and the flow within the ventricle is not known in these conscious animal measurements. Thus, because differences in probe orientation may cause as much as a factor of 2 change in calibration characteristics, the peak velocities measured may range from a low of 30 cm/sec to the indicated value in Figure 3 of approximately 60 cm/sec.

The high-frequency content is of interest because these disturbances are undoubtedly convected into the aorta itself and are thus important if one is to understand the nature of and conditions necessary for the presence of highly disturbed aortic flows. This is considered in detail in the next section.

In addition to this possible presence of high-frequency disturbances, the most striking feature of the flow in the ascending aorta and the aortic arch is the flatness of the profile in the center region of the vessel. In what must be characterized as an entrance region, the flow here is composed of an inviscid core and a thin wall boundary-layer region within which viscous effects are generally confined. Based on steady-state pipe-flow data and for the Reynolds numbers characterizing the mean aortic flow (Goldstein, 1938), the entrance length, i.e., the distance required for a fully developed viscous flow to be attained, would be approximately 30–40 tube diameters. The aortic arch measurements performed as part of this study were obtained within 15 cm of the aortic valve (3–5 vessel diameters) and thus the presence of an inviscid core and a thin wall boundary layer was not surprising. The nature of the boundary layer, of course, must be a combination of the properties due to a steady-state mean flow and the unsteady, pulsatile flow. In terms of unsteady effects, for pulsatile flow in an infinite cylindrical tube the viscous effects in the limit of α becoming large are confined to a thin wall boundary layer (Nerem, 1969). Thus this also would suggest that the velocity profile should appear flat, as observed.

The measurements obtained in these studies were not performed in the plane of aortic arch curvature, because of limitations on access. Thus no skewing due to a curvature effect was anticipated. However, even in the plane of curvature any such effect may have been small because of the gradual curvature of the horse's aortic arch. However, in dogs and humans there is a rather sharp curvature to the aortic arch, and Seed and Wood (1971) in their canine studies found a noticeable skewing of the velocity profile with, on the average, the lower velocity being at the outer, anterior wall of the aorta and the higher velocity at the inner, posterior wall. This is as would be expected for inviscid flow in a curved pipe. Seed and Wood (1971) also observed skewing of the velocity profile due to outflow from the aorta into branch vessels. The extent of any such outflow varied with time through the cardiac cycle and it would appear that any such effect in the aortic arch region should be considered as superimposed on top of the skewing associated with the curvature of the aorta itself.

The Abdominal Aorta and its Major Branch Vessels Hot-film velocity waveform measurements have also been obtained in the abdominal aorta, both proximal to the mesenteric artery, between the mesenteric and renal arteries, and distal to the position where the renal artery branches off. In addition, profiles have been measured in the terminal aorta and the internal and external iliac arteries. In the horses used, the distal aorta usually gave off paired external iliac arteries and within 1–3 cm bifurcated into the internal iliac arteries. Limited velocity waveform measurements also were obtained in the mesenteric and renal arteries. In these measurements the peak Reynolds number, $\hat{R}e$, ranged from just under 100 to over 2,500 (the smaller values correspond to branch vessels and the terminal aorta); the unsteadiness parameter, α, varied from 2 to 16, and the ratio of peak centerline velocity to mean velocity 1.5 to 7.

Velocity profiles measured in the abdominal aorta and selected branch vessels are presented in Figures 4, 6, and 7; Figure 5 shows centerline waveforms for the aorta and for two selected branch vessels. Included in Figures 4, 6, and 7 is a centerline velocity waveform, and indicated on each waveform is the time corresponding to the associated velocity profiles. It is obvious that these profiles are in many cases complex and not necessarily indicative of a fully developed Poiseuille flow. Only the profiles presented in Figure 4, corresponding to a position proximal to where the mesenteric artery branches off of the abdominal aorta, show anything like a relatively flat, slug type of flow character.

Before discussing these velocity profiles further, the development of the velocity wave along the aorta should be commented on. In general, slightly higher velocities (on the order of 125 cm/sec) are observed in the abdominal aorta, proximal to the mesenteric artery branch point, as compared to the ascending aorta and aortic arch region. However, the mesenteric and renal arteries branch almost immediately adjacent to one another, and the large diversion of blood into these branches results in low velocities at distal points in the abdominal aorta and in the iliac arteries. Although the velocity profile in the mesenteric artery could not be

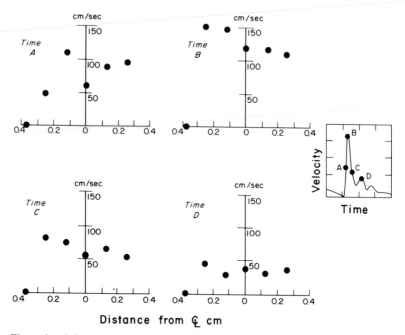

Figure 4. Abdominal aorta velocity profile in anesthetized horse (no. 25) at various times during cardiac cycle as indicated; measurements performed proximal to branching of mesenteric artery in plane orthogonal to plane of branching.

resolved because of the small vessel size, an approximate midstream velocity waveform was recorded; this is compared in Figure 5 with center-line waveforms for the aorta, both proximal to the mesenteric artery and distal to the renal artery, and for the external iliac artery. As is evident, the higher velocities are observed proximal to where the mesenteric artery branches and in the mesenteric artery itself.

Returning to a discussion of the velocity profiles, of interest is the fact that the profiles distal to the renal artery are no longer necessarily flat, but demonstrate a more fully developed viscous flow character. In addition, there is a skewing of the profile that is illustrated in Figure 6 and is believed to be associated with the effects of the branching of the mesenteric and renal arteries. The profile shown in Figure 6 was obtained in a plane such that the near wall was closer to the side where the renal artery branches than the far wall side, and the skewing is believed to be associated with the development of a new boundary layer distal to the renal

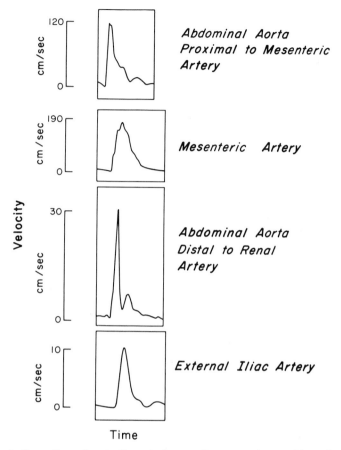

Figure 5. Recordings of centerline velocity waveforms at various positions along the abdominal aorta and in branching vessels for anesthetized horse (no. 25).

artery branch point. Thus, although the velocities are relatively low in this region, there seem to be marked profile characteristics associated with branching effects.

Within 10–20 cm distal to the renal artery (depending upon the size of the horse) the abdominal aorta branches into the iliac arteries. The profiles in the terminal aorta and in the external iliac artery, just before branching into the internal iliac arteries, are characterized by the same low velocities as in the abdominal aorta just proximal and by profiles, though dissimilar,

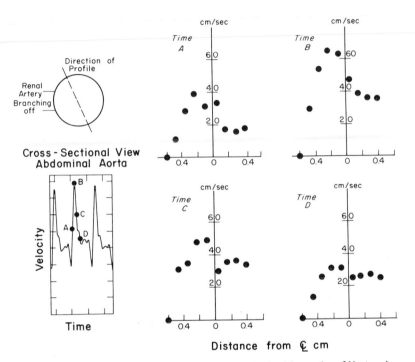

Figure 6. Abdominal aorta velocity profile in anesthetized horse (no. 21) at various times during cardiac cycle as indicated; measurements performed distal to branching of renal artery, proximal to iliac bifurcation in plane indicated.

indicative of a somewhat fully developed viscous flow. The terminal aorta profile is of particular interest because of the much lower velocity on the centerline than in the region further out near either wall. This is illustrated in Figure 7 for an animal where, because of the high heart rate, the velocities and thus Reynolds numbers were reduced. Based on measurements in a limited number of animals, there is an indication of a centerline dip in the profile, the magnitude of which decreases with increasing Reynolds number. The general shape of these profiles is in agreement with previously reported measurements in branching air flows (Schroter and Sudlow, 1969).

It should be noted that high-frequency disturbances have not been observed in the abdominal aorta and its branch vessels. However, no conscious animal measurements have been performed in these vessels, and thus no definite conclusions can be stated. Low-frequency disturbances on

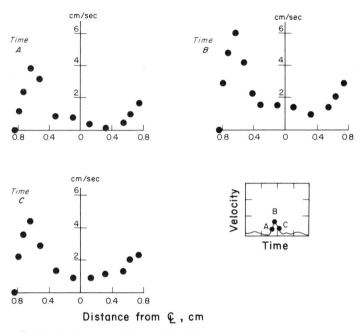

Figure 7. Terminal aorta velocity profile in anesthetized horse (no. 23) at various times during cardiac cycle as indicated; measurements performed in plane orthogonal to plane of branching.

the order of 5–10 Hz have been observed in certain animals in the abdominal aorta distal to the renal artery branch point. This appears to be a laminar flow, but with a low-frequency oscillation that may be the result of complexities associated with the bifurcation at the renal artery branch point.

The Coronary Arteries Hot-film velocity measurements have also been carried out in the left common, the left anterior descending (LAD), and the left circumflex coronary arteries of the horse. Here the peak centerline velocities have been observed to range from 10 to 80 cm/sec. The corresponding range of peak Reynolds number, $\hat{Re}$, is 200–1,500 although generally less than 1,000. The value of the unsteadiness parameter, α, was between 3 and 8 and the estimated ratio of peak centerline velocity to mean velocity ranged from slightly in excess of unity to almost 7.

Based on these conditions and the velocity profiles measured, the flow appears to rapidly become fully viscous, i.e., viscous effects will make themselves manifest across the entire lumen of the vessel, and the entrance length is thus extremely short. This is true both in terms of the pulsatile component of the flow as well as for the mean flow conditions. With regard to the latter, in the left common coronary artery the mean center-line Reynolds number is on the order of 100; this means that any entrance effects associated with the mean flow are limited to within a distance of approximately 3 diameters from the entrance at the coronary ostium. This is in general less than the distance to the LAD-left circumflex bifurcation point.

The fully viscous behavior of the flow is also borne out by the skewing of the velocity profile in the left common coronary artery as is illustrated in Figure 8. This skewing was in general observed to be toward the near wall, i.e., the wall opposite the myocardium, through which the probe was inserted. This is the outer wall as this vessel curves over the base of the heart, and for a fully viscous flow, the skewing should be toward the outer wall because of the secondary flow effects introduced by the vessel curvature.

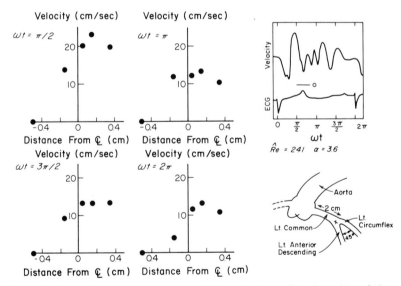

Figure 8. Centerline velocity waveform, ECG, velocity profiles for indicated time, and the location of measurement in the left common coronary artery of an anesthetized horse (no. 43). Measurements were performed in the plane of curvature of the artery.

In the left anterior descending and left circumflex coronary arteries the skewing appears to be also influenced by secondary flow effects. Some measurements were carried out just distal to the LAD-circumflex bifurcation. Normally, one might expect that downstream of a bifurcation the flow will be skewed toward the flow divider side. However, the opposite has, as often as not, been observed here, and this is illustrated in Figure 9. This suggests a strong secondary flow effect that may tend to warp the profile, and it well may be that the effects associated with the vessel curving around the base of the heart dominate any effects due to branching. Further downstream of the bifurcation, there appears to be a more fully developed flow character with little profile skewing being evident.

Taken as a whole, there is an indication from these studies that the pattern of coronary flow is strongly dependent on local geometric details. Furthermore, there appears to be a large systolic flow component, particu-

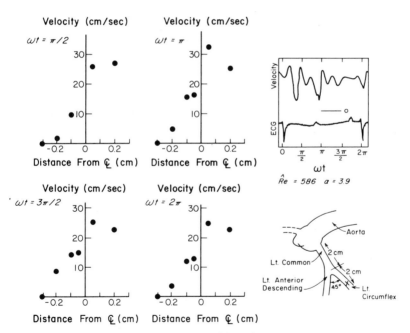

Figure 9. Centerline velocity waveforms, ECG, and velocity profiles for indicated time and the location of measurement in the left circumflex coronary artery of an anesthetized horse (no. 47). Measurements were performed perpendicular to the plane of the bifurcation.

larly in the left common coronary artery. This in a sense is not too surprising since the vessels being discussed here lie on the surface of the myocardium and are presumably filled to capacity during systole. The role of systole in this filling process may be all-important to the health of the heart.

It should be noted that from such velocity profile measurements as these an estimate of the level of arterial wall shear stress can be made. Such an estimation is only very approximate because of inaccuracies in determining the profile shape near the wall. However, using the measured profiles, the wall shear rate appears to be on the order of 500 sec^{-1} and the wall shear stress approximately 20 dynes/cm^2.

Finally, all observed velocity waveforms have appeared to be laminar and free of the high-frequency disturbances that in many cases typify the flow in the aorta. However, there often appeared relatively large-amplitude, low-frequency flow pulsations, as may be seen in Figures 8 and 9. These were primarily present during systole but often maintained themselves throughout the cardiac cycle. The frequency of these pulsations was on the order of 5–10 Hz, which is not unlike the natural vibration frequency of the heart.

This seems to be a result of a surging of the flow as a whole and not a result of vortex shedding or any flow instability that would demonstrate a radial dependence. This is because points at various positions across the lumen of the vessel appear to move in phase. Thus it is possible that these low-frequency oscillations manifest themselves through a coupling with some solid mechanical event associated with the heart and are not purely fluid mechanical in origin.

This phenomenon is not believed to be an artifact of the measurement technique since Wells et al. (1974) have recently observed similar oscillations using a pulsed Doppler velocity meter. Such oscillations have also been observed in our coronary pressure waveforms and in preliminary electromagnetic flow meter measurements. Although such oscillations have not in general been observed in smaller animals, it may well be that they are also present in the human coronary system.

Blood Flow Turbulence?

The possible existence of turbulence in arterial flows has long been of interest; however, until recently, any consideration of the conditions necessary for its occurrence has been largely speculative. The first systematic attempt to examine the conditions necessary for the appearance of turbulence, i.e., random high-frequency flow disturbances, in the aorta was that of Nerem and Seed (1972). In their study the in vivo flow conditions in anesthetized dogs were altered through the use of drugs and vagal stimulation with the purpose of covering a range of cardiac outputs and heart rates so as to include normal conscious animal flow conditions. These studies recently have been extended by both Seed and Nerem working independently. Seed and Thomas (1972) have reported studies in conscious human patients, both normal and with cardiac abnormalities, while Nerem et al. (1974) have carried out additional animal studies using both dogs and horses, both anesthetized and conscious.

Although from the viewpoint of flow disturbances a wide variety of flow conditions have been reported in the previously cited references on hot-film measurements, in general, measured velocity waveforms can be characterized as one of three types: undisturbed, disturbed, and highly disturbed. In this characterization the undisturbed velocity waveform is one that exhibits negligible high-frequency content and is representative of laminar flow; the disturbed velocity waveform is one that has high-frequency components only at peak systole and is thought to be representative of a transitional flow condition; and the highly disturbed velocity waveform is one with high-frequency disturbances persisting all the way through the deceleration phase of systole. It is thought to be representative of at least the initiation of turbulence in blood flow. All three of these general types of flow characterizations were observed by Nerem and Seed (1972) and also have been observed in the more recent studies.

The most striking feature of the measurements reported by Nerem and Seed (1972) is the fact that within a given animal both undisturbed and disturbed flow conditions could be observed by simply changing the animal's heart rate and cardiac output (the peak systolic velocity, $\hat{V}$, and not the cardiac output was actually measured). This indicates that Reynolds number is not the sole criterion for flow instability and the possible transition to turbulence in such a highly pulsatile flow (the peak-to-mean velocity ratio may vary from 3 to 8). In fact, the data of Nerem and Seed (1972) were found to best correlate, in terms of a criterion for the onset of disturbances, using two parameters: the peak Reynolds number, $\hat{Re}$, and the unsteadiness or frequency parameter, α. For the dog ascending thoracic aorta, it was found that the equation:

$$\hat{Re}_{cr} \cong 150 \qquad (1)$$

served as a reasonable dividing line between those conditions corresponding to observations of disturbed and highly disturbed flow and those conditions corresponding to undisturbed flow. This is termed a critical

Reynolds number criterion since it corresponds to the onset of (observable) disturbances and not necessarily to transition itself. Obviously, as $\alpha \to 0$, the steady-flow Reynolds number criterion must be approached asymptotically. However, when α is large, the unsteady nature of the boundary layer must dominate any stability considerations.

The results of the conscious horse studies previously discussed suggest that the appearance of disturbed and highly disturbed ascending aortic flows are the rule and not the exception. Because of the basic unsteady nature of such flows, it is both appropriate and convenient, in comparing these results with those of Nerem and Seed (1972), to present the data in the form of a peak Reynolds number based on the Stokes layer thickness, $\hat{R}e_\delta$, where:

$$\delta = (2\nu/\omega)^{1/2} . \tag{2}$$

ω is taken as the heart rate or the fundamental frequency, and although there are major harmonics that contribute to the velocity waveform, these are here ignored.

In Figure 10 the conscious horse measurements of Nerem et al. (1974) and the dog data of Nerem and Seed (1972) are presented in this form. Here it may be seen that for the ascending aorta a single critical Reynolds number, $\hat{R}e_{\delta \ cr} = 100$, can be defined which, at least within the limits of

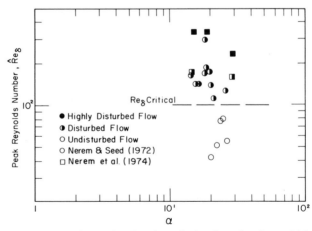

Figure 10. Peak Reynolds number based on Stokes boundary-layer thickness and frequency parameter for dog and horse ascending aorta data indicating character of flow disturbances.

the data scatter, has little dependence on the parameter α. For $\hat{Re}_\delta < \hat{Re}_{\delta\ cr}$, no observations of disturbed waveforms have been noted. It was noted earlier that Seed and Thomas (1972) have observed highly disturbed flow conditions in the ascending aorta of a conscious human who was judged by conventional cardiology tests to be normal. Calculating a value of $\hat{Re}_\delta$ from this experimental condition results in a value of 550. This is obviously well above the critical value indicated in Figure 10. In fact, flow conditions in conscious man normally correspond to a value of $\hat{Re}_\delta > 100$, and thus the occurrence of highly disturbed or even turbulent aortic flows should not be unexpected.

In a similar way the dog descending aorta data of Nerem and Seed (1972) can be represented, and these data indicate a value of $\hat{Re}_{\delta\ cr} = 150$, again with little apparent dependence on the unsteadiness or frequency parameter. This difference between the values of $\hat{Re}_{\delta\ cr}$ for the ascending and descending aorta is more than likely due to the effect of disturbances emanating from the heart on the stability of the ascending aorta flow. These finite-amplitude flow disturbances in the left ventricle (see Figure 3), although convected into the ascending aorta, should damp out during diastole (this has not been conclusively demonstrated to date) and thus would not reappear in the second beat flow in the descending aorta.

von Kerczek and Davis (1974) have summarized the results of existing experimental studies on the stability of oscillatory flows, and the values of the $\hat{Re}_{\delta\ cr}$ determined here for the ascending and descending aorta may be compared with the results of these experiments and theoretical stability calculations. The Stokes layer, both on an oscillating flat plate and on the wall of a circular pipe with a pulsating flow (where α is large), has an experimentally determined value for $\hat{Re}_{\delta\ cr}$ of approximately 500. This is somewhat larger than that deduced here from in vivo aortic flow measurements. On the other hand, the modified Stokes layer on the bottom of a water channel over which small surface waves travel has been found experimentally to be in the range of 110–160. The discrepancy between the values of $\hat{Re}_{\delta\ cr}$ for these different experiments could be due to experimental difficulties, due to the effects of finite amplitude disturbances, or due to the fact that in the free surface wave experiments the boundary layer is modified from that associated with a pure Stokes layer. In the aorta the wall boundary layer is also certainly modified, because of both the influence of the higher harmonics of the basic waveform and the mean flow; this may be the reason that the in vivo measurements suggest values in better agreement with the free surface wave experiments.

Calculations of the stability of Stokes layers have included the use of both the energy theory for finite amplitude disturbances (von Kerczek and Davis, 1972) and linear theory for small disturbances (von Kerczek and Davis, 1974). The former provides $\hat{Re}_{\delta cr}$ values of 19 for three-dimensional disturbances and 38.9 for two-dimensional disturbances, both of which are well below those deduced from experiment. The linear theory has only been carried out for the finite Stokes layer where a second parallel but stationary plate is placed at a distance h from the first one. For $\beta = h/\delta = 8$ where δ is the Stokes layer thickness, $Re_{\delta cr}$ was calculated to be 800. However, the trend is that as β increases, $Re_{\delta cr}$ also increases. This suggests that for the pure Stokes layer ($\beta = \infty$), $\hat{Re}_{\delta cr}$ may be quite large or even infinite.

Available experimental results, including those obtained for in vivo aortic flows, are thus bounded by the predictions of the energy and linear theories. The fact that the values deduced in vivo for $\hat{Re}_{\delta cr}$ are so bracketed and are also in general agreement with results from other related experiments suggests that a Stokes layer type instability is a plausible explanation for the occurrence of high-frequency disturbances in aortic flows.

Returning to the analysis of in vivo velocity waveforms, the characterization of observed velocity waveforms as undisturbed, disturbed, or highly disturbed on a visual basis is admittedly somewhat crude. However, Nerem and Seed (1972) frequency-analyzed their recorded velocity waveforms, and from this analysis of the data, it appears that the onset of disturbances occurs just after peak systole and that the disturbances are then damped out during diastole. The former is consistent with the deceleration phase providing the greatest instability. A crude calculation of amplification rates suggests that only after deceleration with the accompanying velocity profile inflection will the amplification rate be great enough that appreciable disturbance content could be generated in a time on the order of the duration of systole and for typical aortic flow conditions. This is also borne out by the more detailed stability considerations of Nerem, Seed, and Wood (1972). In this sense the dependence of an experimentally measured critical Reynolds number, $\hat{Re} = \hat{V}D/\nu$, on the frequency parameter, α, or the use of the Reynolds number based on Stokes layer thickness, $\hat{Re}_{\delta}$, can be explained from the viewpoint that as the heart rate increases, there is a decrease in the duration of systole, and thus a decrease in the time available for disturbance amplification. Only with a larger

Reynolds number, $\hat{R}e$, will the flow then be sufficiently unstable to result in the appearance of observable disturbances within the duration of systole.

Once the velocity waveform is broken down into frequency components, an energy spectrum can be computed. This was done by Nerem and Seed (1972) for that part of the cycle corresponding to the region of peak systole, and the increase in high-frequency content from the undisturbed to the highly disturbed flow was found to be approximately one to two orders of magnitude at the higher frequencies. It also should be noted that Nerem and Seed (1972) reported that for highly disturbed flow conditions a loud, low-pitched systolic murmur was audible.

Finally, in this discussion I have tried to be somewhat careful to talk about the degree of disturbance and not turbulence and transition to turbulence. This is because measurement limitations preclude one from saying what the exact properties of a highly disturbed aortic flow are. If not turbulent, the flow would appear to certainly be highly transitional. If turbulent, it is not a fully developed turbulence that persists through both systole and diastole but one that is generated anew with each beat, during systole, and then damps out, only to be regenerated on the next beat.

CONCLUSIONS

As is apparent from the results discussed here, the flow conditions in the major arteries cover a wide range. Considering just two basic fluid mechanical parameters, the range of conditions encountered includes peak Reynolds numbers ranging from 100 to 10,000 and unsteadiness parameter values from 2 to 30. Associated with these widely different conditions are markedly different velocity waveforms, velocity profiles, and flow disturbance characteristics. Although much of what has been said here has been based on in vivo studies in the horse, the flow in man and animals of comparable size would not be expected to be significantly different from a qualitative viewpoint. It is thus obvious from these results that the flow in the arterial system, although in many cases laminar and disturbance free, is extremely complex in character. Furthermore, in the ascending aorta the flow is certainly highly disturbed and may even be turbulent.

Further studies will provide additional insight into the details of these fluid mechanical characteristics, and it appears that the horse, because of the size of its vessels, offers itself as an excellent experimental animal for such studies. Although certain phenomena observed may possibly be species dependent, equine studies certainly are complementary to studies in dogs such as reported previously in the literature and serve to help bracket the range of flow conditions that would be expected in man.

LITERATURE CITED

Bergel, D. H., R. M. Nerem, and C. J. Schwartz. 1976. Fluid dynamic aspects of arterial disease. Atherosclerosis 23: 253–261.

Caro, C. G., J. M. Fitz-Gerald, and R. C. Schroter. 1971. Atheroma and arterial wall shear: observation, correlation and proposal of a shear dependent mass transfer mechanism for atherogenesis. Proc. Roy. Soc. (London B) 117: 109–159.

Caro, C. G., and R. M. Nerem. 1973. Transport of ^{14}C-4-cholesterol between serum and wall in the perfused dog common carotid artery. Circulation Res. 32: 187–205.

Clark, C. 1974. Thin film gauges for fluctuating velocity measurements in blood. J. Phys. E: Sci. Instr. 7: 548–556.

Fry, D. L. 1968. Acute vascular endothelial changes associated with increased blood velocity gradients. Circulation Res. 22: 165–197.

Goldstein, S. 1938. Modern Developments in Fluid Dynamics, Vol. 1. Clarendon, Oxford, p. 301.

Ling, S. C., H. B. Atabek, D. L. Fry, D. J. Patel, and J. S. Janicki. 1968. Application of heated film velocity and shear probes to hemodynamic studies. Circ. Res. 23: 789–801.

Nerem, R. M. 1969. Fluid mechanical aspects of blood flow. In Proceedings of the 8th International Symposium on Space Technology and Science, Tokyo, Japan, pp. 1201–1216.

Nerem, R. M., and W. A. Seed. 1972. An in vivo study of the nature of aortic flow disturbances. Cardiovasc. Res. 6: 1–14.

Nerem, R. M., W. A. Seed, and N. B. Wood, 1972. An experimental study of the velocity distribution and transition to turbulence in the aorta. J. Fluid Mech. 52: 137–160.

Nerem, R. M., J. A. Rumberger, Jr., D. R. Gross, R. L. Hamlin, and G. L. Geiger. 1974. Hot-film anemometer velocity measurements of arterial blood flow in horses. Circ. Res 4: 193–203.

Nerem, R. M., A. T. Mosberg, and W. E. Schwerin. 1975. Transendothelial transport of ^{131}I-albumin. Biorheology 12: 81–87.

Nerem, R. M., J. A. Rumberger, Jr., D. R. Gross, and G. L. Geiger. 1975. Hot-film coronary artery velocity measurements in horses (in preparation).

Pedley, T. J. 1972. On the forced heat transfer from a hot-film embedded in the wall in two-dimensional unsteady flow. J. Fluid Mech. 55: 329–357.

Pieper, H. 1967. Catheter-tip manometer for measuring blood pressure during G-changes. J. Appl. Physiol. 22: 352–353.

Schroter, R. C., and M. F. Sudlow. 1969. Flow patterns in models of the human bronchial airways. Resp. Physiol. 7: 341—355.

Schultz, D. L., D. S. Tunstall-Pedoe, G. de J. Lee, A. J. Gunning, and B. J. Bellhouse. 1969. Velocity distribution and transition in the arterial system. *In* G. E. W. Wolstenholme and J. Knight (eds.), Circulatory and Respiratory Mass Transport. A CIBA Foundation Symposium, pp. 172—199. Churchill, London.

Seed, W. A., and N. B. Wood. 1969. An apparatus for calibrating velocity probes in liquids. J. Sci. Instr. 2: 896—898.

Seed, W. A., and N. B. Wood. 1970a. Development and evaluation of a hot-film velocity probe for cardiovascular studies. Cardiovasc. Res 4: 253—263.

Seed, W. A., and N. B. Wood. 1970b. Use of a hot-film probe for cardiovascular studies. J. Phys. E: Sci. Instr. Series 2, 3: 377—384.

Seed, W. A., and N. B. Wood. 1971. Velocity patterns in the aorta. Cardiovasc. Res 5: 319—330.

Seed, W. A., and I. R. Thomas. 1972. The application of hot-film anemometry to the measurement of blood flow velocity in man. *In* Proceedings of DISA Conference on the Industrial and Medical Environments, pp. 298—304. Leicester University Press, England.

von Kerczek, C., and S. H. Davis. 1972. The stability of oscillatory Stokes layers. Stud. Appl. Math. 51:239—252.

von Kerczek, C., and S. H. Davis. 1974. Linear stability theory of oscillatory Stokes layers. J. Fluid Mech. 62: 753—773.

Wells, M. K., D. C. Winter, A. W. Nelson, and T. C. McCarthy. 1974. Hemodynamic patterns in coronary arteries. *In* R. M. Nerem (ed.), Fluid Dynamic Aspects of Arterial Disease, pp. 36—38. Ohio State University, Columbus, Ohio.

Cardiovascular Flow Dynamics and Measurements
Edited by N. H. C. Hwang and N. A. Normann
Copyright 1977   University Park Press   Baltimore

chapter 5

METHODS FOR MEASUREMENT OF CEREBRAL BLOOD FLOW IN MAN

Niels A. Lassen

ABSTRACT

A survey of currently available methods for measurement of cerebral blood flow in man is given. Many of the clinically important brain diseases such as tumors, stroke, brain trauma, or epilepsy entail focal or regional flow alterations. Therefore special emphasis is laid on methods allowing measurements of regional cerebral flow, rCBF. The intra-arterial ^{133}Xe injection is now widely used as standard method for rCBF measurement. It affords a good two-dimensional resolution when using a suitable dynamic gamma camera that allows a high counting rate to be recorded. But, because of superposition of tissues, the three-dimensional resolution is limited. This, in particular, means that smaller areas of ischemia (low flow) tend to be overlooked whereas local hyperemia is readily discerned. The ^{133}Xe inhalation method is less accurate, contaminated by extracerebral uptake, and insensitive both for detecting regional ischemia and regional hyperemia. Spatial resolution is also much more limited. For these reasons great caution must be exercised in interpreting the results.

Methods yielding three-dimensional rCBF data are needed in order to gain more precise information on spatial localization, especially ischemic areas. The most promising is computer-assisted axial tomography with freely diffusible radioactive isotopes or with x-rays using intra-arterial contrast injection. But the available techniques are still too slow: in order to measure blood flow, one "exposure" must be taken over 2–5 seconds.

INTRODUCTION

Only a few methods give quantitative information about blood flow in the human brain. This is mainly due to the inaccessibility of the brain within the skull and to the complexity of the cerebral arterial and venous systems.

Before reviewing the various methods used in man, it should be mentioned that much of the fundamental knowledge has been gained by methods only applicable to animals. Measurements of the diameter of the small arteries on the surface of the brain antedate even the classical studies of Roy and Sherrington (1890). This technique continues to be useful. Modern technical improvements involve the use of micropipettes and stereo microscope in combination with an image splitter and a TV camera that allows us to accurately assess diameter variations of a few percent (Kuschinsky et al., 1972). Autoradiography of brain slices using diffusible indicators is the best quantitative method for measuring local blood flow in a great many parts of the brain (Reivich et al., 1969; Eklöf et al., 1974). Microspheres are also being used, but it is still not quite clear if this technique gives reliable quantitative data in small tissue masses (Pannier and Leusen, 1973; Shulman, Furman, and Rosende, 1975; Meyer and Klassen, 1975).

FLOW MEASUREMENTS AT LEVEL
OF LARGE ARTERIES OR VEINS

Electromagnetic flowmeters applied to the surgically exposed great vessels on the neck have been widely used to record flow before and after reconstructive vascular surgery. A direct flow measurement on a single cerebral artery does not, however, permit conclusions about brain tissue blood flow (Boysen et al., 1970) because the four large arteries anastomose in the circle of Willis at the base of the brain and in the arterial network on the brain surface. In fact, in special disease states one may find that all four arteries are occluded, and yet the cerebral blood flow remains at its normal level because it is kept up by collateral arterial supply.

On the venous side, cerebral blood flow measurements in man have been carried out from thermovelocity probes inserted in one of the two large cerebral veins, the internal jugular veins (Meyer and Gotoh, 1964). However, the drainage pattern of these veins is not constant. Indeed, one may readily obliterate one or even both by manual compression without compromising the cerebral blood flow. Only a moderate rise in pressure of intracerebral veins and intracranial pressure results with venous blood draining only via other exits through the cranium and along the spinal channel.

Currently a variety of noninvasive methods, mainly based on ultrasound principles, are being applied to the study of the neck vessels. Such methods may well yield some information as to the patency of these vessels, but cannot be used for measuring cerebral blood flow.

IMPEDANCE PLETHYSMOGRAPHY

Some years ago considerable effort was devoted to the study of the electrical impedance of the cranial tissues to a high-frequency alternating current, applied with scalp electrodes. This so-called rheoencephalographic technique records pulse synchronous impedance changes that are due mainly to blood volume variations. Quantitative data on blood flow are not obtainable, and the information is influenced by blood volume variations in the extracranial tissues. The method is noninvasive and can readily be combined with routine electroencephalography (Jenkner, 1962). However, the information gained is of little scientific or clinical value (cf. Meyer and Perez-Borja, 1964; Geddes et al., 1964), and now the method has practically been abandoned.

INDICATOR METHODS

Indicator methods constitute the only useful group of methods. In principle, the indicator is supplied to the brain tissue and then removed by the blood stream. The blood flow is measured by recording the rate of indicator clearance, or by its dilution, either directly in the tissue, or by sampling arterial and venous blood. There are two groups of indicator methods; they differ in a most important respect, namely, whether the indicator substance is (1) nondiffusible, remaining within the cerebral vascular bed because it cannot cross the brain capillary wall, the so-called blood-brain barrier, or (2) freely diffusible across this barrier.

Nondiffusible Indicators

Cerebral angiography is the classic method based on nondiffusible indicators. It affords excellent anatomic detail, vessels down to an inner diameter of about 0.1 mm being visible. Using several projections, three-dimensional information becomes available. The transit time of the bolus from the arteries to local veins yields a rough measure of local blood flow. Attempts to use quantitative densitometric recording of the bolus passage have also been made (Hilal, Resch, and Amplatz, 1966). With computerized axial tomography it might be possible to measure the mean transit time passage of the bolus in a much more precise way (height-over-area approach; see below), using the steady-state "equilibrium" value as a measure of the local plasma pool. This demands, however, that the scanning of a slice of brain tissue be made every second as opposed to the 10-sec exposure now necessary with the fastest instruments.

The passage of a nondiffusible radioactive indicator through the head can conveniently be followed by the use of external detectors. The method has been taken up and given up again a number of times. Currently, the intravenous injection of 10–15 mCi of ^{99m}Te pertechnetate, combined with rapid exposures on a single-crystal Anger-type gamma camera, is enjoying popularity in some centers as an adjunct to the subsequent static brain imaging. The resulting crude isotope angiogram hardly justifies the effort in routine cases; it yields only a qualitative measure of cerebral blood flow affording only gross localization. Its most precise clinical usage is perhaps as a substitute for four-vessel angiography in cases of so-called brain death, where objective documentation is wanted (e.g., if the kidneys are to be used for transplantation) (Braunstein et al., 1973). In this situation ^{133m}In seems to offer some advantage (Hoop et al., 1973).

Nondiffusible indicators can also be used for cerebral blood flow measurements in accordance with the Stewart-Hamilton principle: injecting a known quantity of indicator in the internal carotid artery of one side, total cerebral blood flow can be calculated from the area under the two venous dilution curves (Nylin et al., 1960). This is indeed a cumbersome and invasive method demanding in principle sequential injection of both internal carotids.

Freely Diffusible Indicators

Heat Clearance In this context, heat may be considered an inert, freely diffusible indicator that can be applied locally to the cerebral tissue and then cleared by the blood stream. This approach, involving heated thermistors implanted in brain tissue, is used widely in studies in experimental animals and has also been used in humans (Seylaz, 1973). The invasive nature of the method limits its applicability.

Hydrogen Clearance By polarography, a continuous record of tissue H_2 concentration is obtained using a platinum electrode inserted in the tissue. The indicator gas is best supplied by inhalation. This method is as traumatic as heat clearance, but has the advantage that quantitative cerebral blood flow (CBF) data can readily be obtained from the half-time, $t_{1/2}$, of the washout curve (Pasztor et al., 1973):

$$CBF = 100 \times 0.693/t_{1/2} \text{ ml}/100 \text{ g/min} \tag{1}$$

Kety–Schmidt Nitrous Oxide Method This classic method, published in 1945, was the first method allowing quantitative measurement of cerebral blood flow in man (Kety and Schmidt, 1945, 1948). It is based on estimating the rate at which the brain saturates (or desaturates) with an inert gas inhaled at constant concentration. The input to the brain is the inert gas concentration in arterial blood, sampled at the femoral or brachial artery. The output from the brain is followed by sampling cerebral venous blood in the internal jugular vein at the level of the superior bulb at the base of the skull.

In the terminology of the frequency function of transit times, $h(t)$, it follows that if the arterial curve is a perfect step function (i.e., if it reached a constant level of concentration 1.0 at the moment the inhalation starts) then the venous curve is the cumulative distribution function $H(t) = \int_0^t h(\tau) \, d\tau$. Thus the *area* between the constant level and the venous curve is $\int_0^\infty (1 - H(t)) \, dt$, and this equals the mean transit time for the tracer used, $\bar{t} = \int_0^\infty t \cdot h(t) dt$. This result is readily obtained by partial integration. Thus, because we have to normalize the curves to unit height by dividing with the equilibrium concentration, i.e., the *height* at equilibrium, we obtain

$$\text{mean transit time } \bar{t} = \frac{\text{area}}{\text{height}} \text{ min} \tag{2}$$

The area is not altered if the arterial curve deviates from a perfect step function, provided the arterial curve reaches a constant level (the height). This is seen by applying the elementary convolution theorems. The above derivation of the basic information, obtainable by the arteriovenous difference method of Kety and Schmidt, is presented to emphasize its relation to the intra-arterial injection method discussed in the next section; in fact, the two methods are basically the same, viz., they measure the mean transit time, $\bar{t}$.

The mean transit time is, as first shown by Meier and Zierler (1954), the volume/flow ratio of the system. Expressed per gram of brain tissue, the Meier–Zierler theorem becomes:

$$\bar{t} = \frac{\lambda}{f} \text{ min} \qquad (3)$$

λ is the volume of distribution per gram of brain, i.e., it is the equilibrium ratio of the amount of indicator in 1 g of brain and the amount in 1 ml of blood. Thus, λ is the partition coefficient of Kety. f is the blood flow per gram of tissue.

The conventional unit of tissue mass for cerebral blood flow (CBF) measurement is 100 g: i.e., CBF = 100 × f. Inserting this into Eqs. 2 and 3 and solving for CBF we get:

$$CBF = 100 \times \lambda \times \frac{\text{height}}{\text{area}} \text{ ml/100 g/min} \qquad (4)$$

This is the fundamental height-over-area equation first derived by Kety by applying the Fick principle. Kety's derivation is more simple to follow, but it illustrates less well the essence of the experimental observation, viz., that the measured parameter is the mean transit time $\bar{t}$.

The partition coefficient λ is, as stated, defined as the equilibrium concentration ratio $c_{\text{tissue}}/c_{\text{blood}}$. When using inert gases as tracers, this ratio equals the ratio of the solubility coefficients, using 1 g and 1 ml as the unit of mass for tissue and blood, respectively. The solubility for many inert gases in brain tissue is somewhat less in gray matter (cortex) than in white matter. But within either of these two tissues no great variability of solubility can be expected, because this would entail gross alteration in water percentage or percentage of neutral triglyceride fat (which does not exist in the brain at all). More variation must be expected with respect to the inert gas solubility in blood because the volume of red cells (hematocrit) influences this factor. This effect is, however, easy to measure and to correct for.

Two further comments regarding λ should be made. First, it is precisely the relative constancy of λ for inert gases that constitutes the essence of the Kety–Schmidt method. When using nondiffusible indicators that remain inside the brain vessels, all the same equations hold, but in this case λ is the fractional plasma volume in brain tissue divided by that in the blood (plasmatocrit = 1 – hematocrit). In addition, the local plasma volume in brain tissue cannot, with any certainty, be assumed a priori to remain practically constant. Second, because we only know λ, the volume of distribution of the inert gas per gram of tissue, and not V, the volume of distribution in the whole brain, we can only measure blood flow per gram of tissue, not total cerebral blood flow. One does not, to be quite explicit, first measure total flow and then divide by the weight of the tissue: flow is directly obtained per unit weight.

Kety and Schmidt used nitrous oxide. Currently, radioactive inert gases or argon are often used in order to facilitate the analysis of blood samples. Usually, the duration of the procedure is 10 min; Kety demonstrated that in normal brains, for practical purposes, this length of time is sufficient for saturation of brain tissue. This changes Eq. 4 to:

$$\text{CBF} = 10 \times \lambda \times \frac{\text{venous curve height at 10 min}}{\text{area to 10 min}} \text{ ml/100 g/min} \qquad (5)$$

A slight overestimation of CBF results from this procedure, but it has the considerable advantage that extrapolation is avoided. In very accurate studies bilateral sampling of internal jugular blood is recommended (Munck and Lassen, 1957), and desaturation may be advantageous (McHenry, 1964).

The arteriovenous sampling method retains its position as reference method for studies in man. A major advantage is that the cerebral metabolism can readily be assessed by multiplying the flow with the corresponding arteriovenous differences of O_2, CO_2, glucose, lactate, etc.

The Intra-Arterial ^{133} *Xe Method*   This method is based on principles developed by Lassen and Ingvar (1961) (Lassen et al., 1963; Høedt-Rasmussen, Sveinsdottir, and Lassen, 1966). The isotope is supplied directly to the brain and its passage through various brain regions is followed by external gamma detection. The method is currently the standard method for obtaining quantitative data on regional cerebral blood flow (rCBF) in man and in animals. Hence a somewhat detailed description is given in order properly to expose its advantages and disadvantages.

The Isotope   Any freely diffusible gamma-emitting radioisotope may in principle be used. The inert gases have the advantage that their rapid elimination through the lung reduces recirculation to the brain and also reduces the radiation exposure. For this reason one would prefer to avoid the use of nongaseous tracers like radioiodine-labeled iodoantipyrine or radioactive water (labeled with ^{15}O-oxygen).

Of the many radioactive inert gases, only ^{133}Xe is used to any extent. It has a 5.5 day half-life and emits an 81-keV primary gamma ray as well as a 31-keV x-ray. It is commercially available dissolved in saline at a suitable strength of 5–10 mCi/ml. We, however, make this solution ourselves from gaseous ^{133}Xe in order to reduce the costs.

Compton scatter constitutes a serious problem when using ^{133}Xe. Soft electromagnetic radiation, as that of ^{133}Xe, is deflected ("scattered") with only a slight decrease in its energy. Hence one cannot effectively eliminate Compton scatter from ^{133}Xe. In order to do so, one would have to cut away sharply (using a lower-level discriminator) all energies below approximately 78–80 keV. This would in turn mean not only a severe reduction in counting rate, but it would also introduce unavoidable fluctuations in the sensitivity of the photomultipliers and would thus critically influence the equivalent discriminator level.

A higher-energy gamma-emitting xenon isotope is the 250-keV ^{135}Xe. Its 9-hr half-life renders its use quite cumbersome and expensive. While in theory it should be advantageous to use ^{135}Xe because Compton scatter could be reduced, we have, in a limited number of studies comparing ^{135}Xe to ^{133}Xe, found almost the same absolute values of rCBF as well as almost the same resolution. The 36-day half-life ^{127}Xe with gamma energy of 203 keV may soon become commercially available and would presumably be the indicator of choice. (With higher energies, as with position-emitting, freely diffusible emitting indicators, the necessity of heavy shielding and thick crystals reduces the spatial resolution.)

Discriminator Setting of the Counting System   It follows from the above discussion that with ^{133}Xe one cannot, for practical reasons, use a narrow discrimination. We follow Potchen's recommendation of including all energies from below 31 keV to above 81 keV (Potchen et al., 1969). A high counting rate is thereby obtained, and the stability of the system is much better than with a narrow window.

Collimation and Spatial Resolution   We use cylindrical lead tubes with a length of 40 mm, with an inner diameter of 7–12 mm, and with a wall thickness of 2 mm, as collimators for ^{133}Xe. The excitation radiation of lead has almost the same energy as the primary radiation of ^{133}Xe. However, this source of spurious counts is negligible since its incidence is very low. Hence the use of another material (e.g., brass) would not offer any advantages.

Since the aim is to record regional clearance curves of a tracer, one might consider the use of a focusing collimator design. However, since the brain constitutes an extensive three-dimensional source of radiation, a focusing device is not very effective. The situation is not the same as when one scans for a brain tumor. In that case, a hot point source is to be detected in a tissue with a low counting rate, and here focusing does have some depth-resolving power. In rCBF studies, on the other hand, a large part of the brain (usually one hemisphere) is relatively evenly labeled and focusing only renders the tissue area counted from less well defined since, as seen through the collimator, it includes the tissues both in front of and behind the focal plane.

In practice, therefore, only a two-dimensional resolution is obtained by the parallel or 20-cm-in-radius converging collimators used (the latter yielding a considerable magnifying effect).

Concerning the possibilities for three-dimensional resolution, the reader is referred to the discussion on radiation detection systems.

The superposition of radiation from the different tissue layers defies any hope of a truly localized measurement. Using ^{133}Xe, the softness of the radiation means that photons from deeper brain tissue layers are absorbed to a greater extent than those from more superficial layers. The half-thickness of tissue absorption is approximately 4 cm; i.e., when counting from the side of the head, the convexity of the brain is recorded more than twice as efficiently as the midline structures. This means that a gross depth resolution exists.

With cylindrical collimation, the brain tissue mass counted from has the form of a truncated cone. Thus, if layers of equal thickness are considered at different distances from the crystal, then a larger tissue mass of the more distant layers is seen by the crystal. Since the mass seen is directly proportional to the square of the distance, and since the counting efficiency is inversely proportional thereto, then it follows that

1. The counting rate is relatively insensitive to variations of the distance from the crystal to the head.
2. The inverse-square law of decreasing counting efficiency does not operate to render superficial structures better recorded; one simply sees so much more of the deeper tissues that this compensates for the greater distance.

We have discussed above the rather poor depth resolution of the rCBF methods in some detail since it is essential, and since it applies also to other types of recording systems in use, e.g., gamma camera systems. With regard to resolution in the other two dimensions, i.e., the resolution in the plane of the detector head, we have to confine the comments to the ^{133}Xe systems we currently use, consisting of 254 individual scintillation crystals, each with its own photomultiplier. Using the Dynamic Gamma Camera (Medimatic, Inc., Dk-2000 Copenhagen F, Denmark) and the high-resolution converging collimator, the resolution at a plane 4 cm from the surface of the converging collimator (corresponding roughly to the plane of the cortex of the convexity of the hemisphere) is 2 cm. This corresponds to half-maximum—full-width for a point source.

Radiation Detection Systems In order to obtain adequate temporal resolution, a maximum counting rate of 500—1000 cps is necessary for each surface element studied. This means that for most commercial gamma cameras the number of regions one can study is actually quite limited. The multiple-crystal scintillation camera can accommodate a higher counting rate, and thus each of the 294 crystals can apparently yield an adequate curve (Cannon et al., 1974). We use the computer-based 254-detector Dynamic Gamma Camera (Sveinsdottir and Lassen, 1975), Figure 1. It allows strictly parallel processing and admits more than 4,000 cps per detector without significant coincidence loss ($<1\%$).

The use of the section scanning technique devised by Kuhl et al. (1973) seems to offer the only realistic means of three-dimensional flow studies. Perhaps advantage can be taken of positron annihilation coincidence counting (Ter-Pogossian et al., 1975). The technique consists of computer-assessed axial tomography, but it is still too slow to yield the one-exposure-per-second temporal resolution required for quantitative rCBF studies. A quantitative "map" using ^{13}N-labeled ammonium is the best so far achieved (Ter-Pogossian et al., 1975). The importance of the three-dimensional approach is not only that it is the only realistic way of detecting smaller areas of low blood flow (ischemia), but, in addition, it is the most promising way of improving the rCBF technique based on inhalation or intravenous injection of radioactive tracers; it should allow the exclusion of extracerebral contamination.

Calculation of Regional Cerebral Blood Flow, rCBF A typical ^{133}Xe clearance curve as obtained by external counting is shown in Figure 2, which also outlines the basic principles of calculation of rCBF. The clearance curve recorded over the head $C(t)$ is the residue curve: the entire bolus is initially deposited in the region and it is then washed out by nonlabeled arterial blood; thus, at any time, what is recorded is what remains (the residue) of the bolus. This residue is therefore equal to the

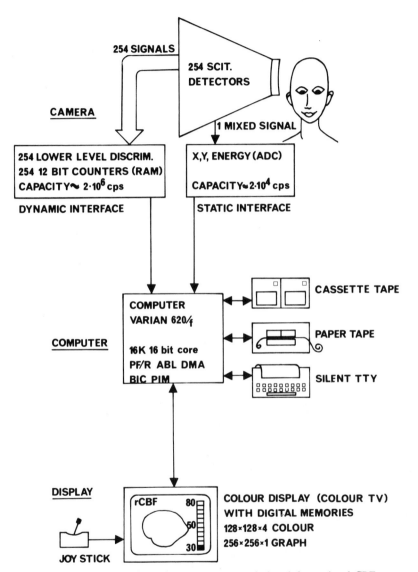

Figure 1. A 254-detector dynamic gamma camera designed for regional CBF measurement and for conventional static isotope scintigrams (Medimatic Inc., Copenhagen).

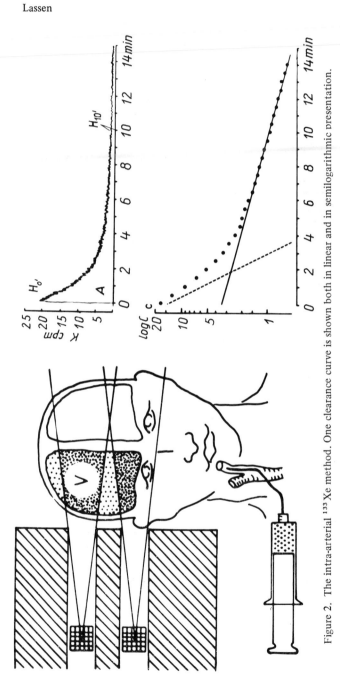

Figure 2. The intra-arterial ^{133}Xe method. One clearance curve is shown both in linear and in semilogarithmic presentation.

bolus minus the cumulative loss. In the terminology of frequency function of transit times, $h(t)$, it follows that, for a unit of radioactivity,

$$\text{Residue for one}$$
$$\text{unit of activity} = 1 - \int_0^t h(\tau)\, d\tau$$
$$= 1 - H(t) \qquad (6)$$

As was commented on in the previous section, the mean transit time, $\bar{t}$, is $\int_0^\infty (1 - H(t)\, dt)$. Thus $\bar{t}$ is the total area under the residue curve normalized for unit height. Assuming that the maximum counting rate (the height of the curve) is a measure of the entire bolus and integrating on both sides of Eq. 6 yields, as first shown by Zierler (1965),

$$\bar{t} = \frac{\text{area}}{\text{height}} \text{ min} \qquad (7)$$

This is precisely the same equation as Eq. 2, but it should be recalled that in Eq. 2 we are concerned with a saturation experiment recording from inlet (artery) and outlet (vein); in Eq. 7 we are concerned with a bolus experiment with recording over the tissue—the difference between cumulative inflow and cumulative outflow.

As previously shown, since $\bar{t} = \lambda/f$ and CBF = $100 \times f$, Eq. 7 gives:

$$rCBF = 100 \times \lambda \times \frac{\text{height}}{\text{area}} \text{ ml}/100 \text{ g/min} \qquad (8)$$

This is the same as Eq. 4, thus reemphasizing the method for obtaining the data from the experimental curves (see also Lassen and Ingvar, 1972).

λ is found in a table based on the measured hemoglobin concentration and taking the value corresponding to the whole brain. "Height" corresponds to the initial height of the curve, i.e., its maximal counting rate in cpm, minus the background counting rate. "Area" is the total number of impulses recorded during 15 min (minus the background) and extrapolated to infinity. This extrapolation is performed by plotting the curve on semilogarithmic paper and estimating the $t_{1/2}$ of the tail part of the curve. The extrapolated area from 15 min to infinity is then given by (height at 15 min) $\times t_{1/2 \text{ tail}}/0.693$. Because of the extrapolation one may use the term $rCBF_{\text{infinity}}$ to designate the flow value obtained by Eq. 8.

The derivation of the basic equation, viz., $\bar{t}$ = area/height, used for obtaining Eq. 8 is related to the approach to certain statistic (stochastic) considerations of probabilities, viz., the use of frequency distribution and of cumulative distribution of transit times, [$h(t)$ and $H(t)$, respectively, in Zierler's terminology (Meier and Zierler, 1954)]. For this reason the $rCBF_{infinity}$ is also called the $rCBF_{stochastic}$. The term stochastic is, however, not clear. Its meaning is not obvious to those unfamiliar with statistics and its application is imprecise because it conveys an erroneous concept of randomness; in theory, $\bar{t}$ is derived for infinitely many tracer molecules and $C(t)$ is therefore, in principle, "deterministic" (precisely defined) and not "stochastic" (subject to some degree of random statistical fluctuations).

An approximate value of rCBF (a slight overestimation; see Lassen and Klee, 1965) may be obtained after 10 min of clearance using, as Kety did, the height/area ratio until the tenth minute:

$$rCBF_{10} = 100 \times \lambda \times \frac{\Delta \text{ height}}{\Delta \text{ area}} \text{ml}/100 \text{ g/min} \qquad (9)$$

where λ has the same value as indicated above, Δ height is the difference between the counting rates in cpm at zero time and at 10 min, and Δ area is the total number of impulses recorded over the region in the 10 min (minus the background).

Another approximation of the rCBF may be obtained (Olesen, Paulson, and Lassen, 1971) by taking the $t_{1/2}$ of the initial almost monoexponentially decreasing curve segment. We usually employ the curve segment from 15 to 75 sec for calculating the $t_{1/2}$ of the initial slope (Figure 3):

$$rCBF_{init} = 100 \times \lambda_g \times \frac{0.693}{t_{1/2}} \text{ml}/100 \text{ g/min} \qquad (10)$$

where λ_g is the tissue:blood partition coefficient of the gray matter of the brain (this coefficient is used since the rapidly perfused gray matter dominates the initial part of the clearance curve). One may conveniently use a fixed value of λ_g of 0.87, since the initial slope on the logarithmically recorded curve (D_o) is related to $0.693/t_{1/2}$ as follows: $0.693/t_{1/2} = \ln (10) \times D_o \simeq 2.30 \times D_o$ and consequently,

$$rCBF_{init} = 200 \times D_o \text{ ml}/100 \text{ g/min} \qquad (11)$$

The initial slope calculation represents an estimation of the blood flow in the gray matter of the region studied. Because of the effect of the white matter, $rCBF_{init}$ underestimates $rCBF_{gray}$ matter to such an extent that values approaching $rCBF_{10}$ are obtained.

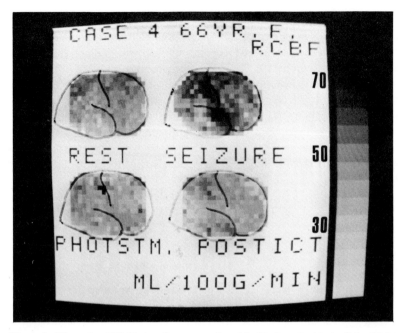

Figure 3. The color TV display (here reproduced in black and white) of the Multidetector Scintillation Camera. The code gives the rCBF in ml/100 g/min as calculated from the initial slope of each of the 254 ^{133}Xe wash-out curves.

The patient was a 66-yr-old woman with motor epilepsy of the left hand and some hallucinations. During photostimulation the epileptic focus is seen. During a spontaneous seizure the same area—and much more widespread areas as well—become activated. The electroencephalogram could not localize the focus.

The importance of the initial slope value resides in the fact that the duration of the steady-state condition of cerebral blood flow is correspondingly short. The most important abnormalities of the ^{133}Xe clearance curves are seen in the early curve segment (Palvölgyi, 1969; Paulson, Lassen and Skinhøj, 1970); these are abnormalities that may well tend to be obscured by the averaging inherent in evaluating the entire curve to infinity. Direct inspection of the early (2 min or so) part of all clearance curves is for this reason an absolute necessity; one cannot just use calculated numbers.

Biexponential resolution of ^{133}Xe clearance curve yields estimates of the $rCBF_{(white\ matter)}$, the $rCBF_{(gray\ matter)}$, and of the percentage of grey matter of the region (Høedt-Rasmussen, Sveinsdottir, and Lassen,

1966). This analysis is based on a simple model in which the two compartments are coupled in parallel. It also assumes diffusion equilibrium for ^{133}Xe between each tissue and its corresponding venous blood throughout the wash-out. Computer programs for this form of curve resolution are available. Recently, we have described a fast algorithm based on finding the four unknowns from the initial *S*lope, the maximal *H*eight, the *A*rea, and the first time *M*oment, the SHAM method (Caprani, Sveinsdottir, and Lassen, 1975). It is, however, also quite easy to perform the curve resolution manually.

Since $\bar{t}$ of a monoexponential curve equals $t_{1/2}/\ln(2) \simeq t_{1/2}/0.693$, it follows that:

$$\text{rCBF}_{\text{gray}} = 100 \, \lambda_{\text{gray}} \times \frac{0.693}{t_{1/2} \text{ fast component}} \quad \text{ml/100 g/min} \qquad (12)$$

$$\text{rCBF}_{\text{white}} = 100 \, \lambda_{\text{white}} \times \frac{0.693}{t_{1/2} \text{ slow component}} \quad \text{ml/100 g/min} \qquad (13)$$

whereas the relative weight of the cortex and the white matter is given by

$$w_{\text{cortex}} = 100 \, \frac{I_{\text{cortex}}/\text{rCBF}_{\text{cortex}}}{I_{\text{cortex}}/\text{rCBF}_{\text{cortex}} + I_{\text{white}}/\text{rCBF}_{\text{white}}} \quad \text{percent} \qquad (14)$$

$$w_{\text{white}} = 100 \, (1 - w_{\text{cortex}}) \, \text{percent} \qquad (15)$$

where I_{cortex} and I_{white} are, respectively, the zero time intercept of the fast and the slow components of the biexponential resolution. The theory and the limitations of the biexponential approach have been discussed in detail elsewhere (Høedt-Rasmussen et al., 1966). It suffices here to state that it appears to be valid in normal man as well as in most chronic diffuse brain disorders.

Comments It must be emphasized that the ideal study cannot be made, i.e., one cannot follow the clearance curve until the entire bolus has traversed the region under steady-state conditions. In practice, one makes use of the observation that after about 7–9 min of ^{133}Xe wash-out, usually only one major, fairly homogeneous, tissue component (the white matter of the region) still contains radioactivity, and that this radioactivity is washed out monoexponentially until the cessation of the recording at 15 min. It cannot be doubted, however, that in pathologic states there may be tissue elements with still lower flow rates than the white matter. The ^{133}Xe clearance from such tissues can only dominate the curve at a much later time than 5–9 min (and it will then tend to be obscured by the small amount of recirculating tracer). With this in mind, one may state that contributions from very slowly clearing brain tissues tend to be inadequately taken into account. The extreme case of low flow is that of a brain infarct with no circulation. Because there is no arterial inflow, ^{133}Xe does not enter such an area. Hence such an infarct is completely overlooked. Fast flow components corresponding to hyperemic tissues are, on the other hand, readily recognized in the early part of the curve.

As a final comment, the close relation between the arteriovenous and the intra-arterial methods may again be stressed. Both measure the mean transit time $\bar{t}$ of inert gas molecules traversing the brain. For both methods the measurement is essentially free from extracerebral contamination. Using the $\bar{t}$ analysis, the same height-over-area equation is derived for the average flow. The two methods also give the same values for CBF in normal man (Table 1).

The [133]Xe Inhalation Method (Figure 4) This method was first outlined by Conn (1955) and subsequently further developed by Mallett and Veall (1965). The method is atraumatic, and the inhalation of rather high doses of ^{133}Xe results in only a small radiation exposure (Lassen, 1965).

The method is based on an inhalation period of 1–5 min (or an IV

Table 1. Cerebral blood flow in normal man

	Method		
Parameter	Kety and Schmidt[a] N$_2$O inhalation a-v sampling 1948 (n=14)	Lassen et al.[b] [85]Kr inhalation a-v sampling 1960 (n=11)	Ingvar et al.[c] [133]Xe injection external recording. 1965 (n=7)
CBF calculated to 10 min of saturation or desaturation	53.8 ± 12.0 (ml/100 g/min)	50.4 ± 4.9 (ml/100 g/min)	49.8± 4.1 (ml/100 g/min)
CBF calculated by extrapolating to infinity	—	43.0 ± 3.7 (ml/100 g/min)	44.7 ± 4.5 (ml/100 g/min)

[a]Kety, S. S. and C. F. Schmidt, J. Clin. Invest. 27: 476 (1948).
[b]Lassen, N. A., I. Feinberg, and M. H. Lane, J. Clin. Invest. 39: 491 (1960).
[c]Ingvar, D. H., S. Cronqvist, R. Ekberg, J. Risberg, and K. Høedt-Rasmussen, Acta Neurol. Scand., Suppl. 14: 72 (1965).

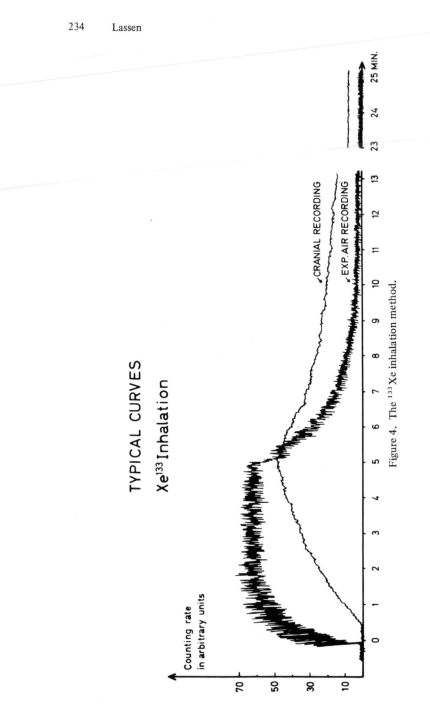

Figure 4. The ^{133} Xe inhalation method.

injection of ^{133}Xe dissolved in saline) followed by a clearance wash-out period of up to 40 min. The uptake and subsequent clearance are followed by externally placed scintillation detectors; up to seven are now being used on either side of the head.

The input curve to the brain is the ^{133}Xe curve in the arterial blood. A good estimate of its shape is obtained by sampling alveolar air, using end-expiratory air samples. Only in patients with severe lung disease is this relationship invalid.

We can consider the ^{133}Xe inhalation as a series of intra-arterial injections, each subsequent injection being of different size depending on the height of the end-expiratory air curve at that time. In mathematical terms this means that as measured by the external detectors, the inhalation curve is the convolution of the bolus response and the end-expiratory curve. Cerebral blood flow is calculated by a deconvolution procedure, viz., one attempts to estimate the bolus response that one would have seen had an intra-arterial injection been made. The deconvolution procedure represents, so to speak, a division of the air curve into the head curve. For this reason it is clear that in order to get a reliable result, both curves must be recorded with high accuracy (Figure 4). It is recommended that the maximal counting rate should be in the order of 1,000 cps.

The duration of the inhalation is in most studies 2 min. With shorter duration the influence of ^{133}Xe in the airways becomes more important. Owing to Compton scatter, the radioactivity in these regions unavoidably influences the head curves. For the same reason the intravenous injection approach can hardly be recommended: it represents a very brief inhalation.

The discriminator setting is actually best made to include both the 31- and the 81-keV radiation; this gives a good counting rate. Mallett and Veall (1965) have proposed to use the 31-keV (which mainly stems from the extracerebral tissues) to correct the 81-keV signal, resulting in a "pure" brain curve. This ingenious proposal, however, markedly reduces the statistical accuracy of the head curve. In addition, the approach cannot be expected to afford a perfect correction because some 31-keV radiation originating from the brain does, nevertheless, penetrate the skull.

The detector system must comprise a head detector and an end-expiratory air detector. Because the counting rate is lower than with the intra-arterial ^{133}Xe injection method, it is possible to use a conventional single-crystal camera as head detector. The fairly low maximal counting rate over the head means that the section scanning technique for three-dimensional pick-up (see the previous section) cannot be used. One would probably have to go to an isotope with higher energy, such as ^{127}Xe, and then use a much higher dose.

The extracerebral contamination constitutes the largest source of error. It can be estimated that only about 50% of the counts recorded stem from the brain (Oldendorf, 1969). Soft tissues outside the skull, airways, and scattered radiation from more distant sources all contribute to this contamination. When comparing the curves from the two sides of the head it must be remembered that counts originating in one hemisphere cross the central line; despite the absorption of the radiation in the tissue, a considerable "cross talk" does exist that reduces side-to-side differences by a factor of about four (Risberg et al., 1975).

The calculation of the cerebral blood flow has been made in a number of different ways, all of which are based on a distinct model of the system. (By contrast, the height-over-area equations used in the arteriovenous and intra-arterial injection methods are not based on a model.)

Originally a three-compartment model was employed, yielding a three-exponential $h(t)$ curve (Mallett and Veall, 1965) on clearance curves recorded for 40 min. Then it was suggested to lump together the two slowest compartments and only record the clearance curves for 12 min (Obrist et al., 1971). This approach gives results that compare quite well with those of the intra-arterial ^{133}Xe method (Reivich et al., 1975). Recently a mono-compartment model assuming an initial monoexponential clearance has been applied to the first few minutes of the clearance curve (Risberg et al., 1975; Wyper, Lennox, and Rowan, 1975). Although the development tends to emphasize the fastest components (cerebral cortex) and to reduce the influence of extracerebral influences, the basic limitations of the method are not circumvented. In particular, the use of the model precludes the recording of smaller fast blood flow components, as often seen in trauma or tumor cases. The method is also insensitive to detection of tissue ischemia, because low flow areas are poorly represented—as previously discussed in relation to the intra-arterial ^{133}Xe method.

In summary, the two methods (intra-arterial and inhalation) give about the same overall CBF values over a wide flow range (Reivich et al., 1975), but the resolution of the inhalation method is so poor that it is best to regard the values as averages for large parts of the hemispheres (almost as with the Kety-Schmidt method). Particular caution must be exercised with the inhalation method under conditions when alterations of blood flow in extracerebral tissues may occur.

The problem of the clinical use of the ^{133}Xe inhalation procedure is almost, one might say, a philosophic one: Why not use it since it does no harm? The fact is, however, that the data are difficult to make use of in terms of rCBF. Often one hears the thought expressed that the inhalation method (or the method based on the intravenous injection of ^{133}Xe) might be used as an atraumatic, semiquantitative screening procedure. This presupposes that one might be able to differentiate fairly sharply between various brain diseases—preferably even in their preclinical stage—by such techniques. There is no evidence available to support this contention.

CONCLUDING REMARKS

To discuss methods without mentioning results or commenting on the serious diseases where cerebral blood flow is abnormal is misleading. It suggests a "l'art pour l'art" attitude of studying an object simply because it is there. In order to put the present topic in its proper perspective, these topics must briefly be commented upon.

In man, the normal blood flow of the brain is about 50 ml/100 g/min. Calculated for the whole 1,400 g of brain tissue, the flow is 700 ml/min; i.e., about 15% of the cardiac output of resting man goes to the brain, which is only 2% of total body weight. This is indicative of the high metabolic rate of the brain tissues. rCBF measurements by intra-arterial ^{133}Xe injection have revealed regional differences in flow within the brain, probably reflecting differences in functional and metabolic activity. Of special interest is the finding that rCBF changes locally in a meaningful manner with functional changes in the region recorded from. An outstanding example of local rCBF changes elicited by functional activation is afforded by the focal flow increase recorded over the appropriate brain cortex areas during hand movements, mouth movements, and foot movements, respectively. More complex patterns of rCBF increase have been found to accompany other types of brain work such as visual perception, verbal perception, perception of music, or memorization of numbers (Brain Work, 1975). Studies of this type performed in normal man and in patients with brain tissue lesions of known localization may contribute to the elucidation of the classic problem of where in the brain various functions are localized.

In elderly patients with senile brain dysfunction characterized by intellectual impairment, so-called dementia of old age, the cerebral blood flow is reduced in parallel with the reduced metabolic rate of the brain.

The best correlation is seen in left-sided CBF decreases. This may be considered "meaningful" because the left side of the brain (the left hemisphere) is the localization of speech and of speech-related intellectual functions in most subjects. In addition, Ingvar et al. found more discrete focal rCBF alteration within the hemispheres, alterations that correlated with the clinical manifestations (Ingvar and Gustafson, 1970; Ingvar, 1975). In most cases these observations cannot be used for diagnostic purposes. An exception is perhaps the peculiar chronic brain syndrome called Korsakoff's psychosis, which can arise in patients with chronic alcoholism. The syndrome is characterized by marked forgetfulness for recent events and by confabulations "designed" to fill the memory gaps. Here the CBF is normal, in consonance with the selective memory impairment that leaves the intellectual functions intact (Simard et al., 1971).

Apoplexy (stroke) is an acute disease of the central nervous system caused by occlusion or rupture of a brain artery. In many cases, particularly in milder ones, the brain arteries appear quite normal when studied by conventional x-ray techniques a few days after the onset of symptoms. But with the rCBF method using ^{133}Xe, abnormal tissue perfusion is usually demonstrable; such abnormalities in animal studies are typically seen *after* a temporary brain artery obstruction has been disobliterated.

Brain tumors characteristically cause alterations of cerebral blood flow both locally, around the tumor, and globally, and in remote regions as well.

rCBF studies by ^{133}Xe injection may be of clinical value in diagnosing brain tumors. In our experience, cerebral tumors alter brain blood flow even at a very early stage. In several of our cases involving small tumors, the whole battery of conventional diagnostic tools had all failed.

In most patients with epileptic seizures, the attack starts in deep brain structures and spreads symmetrically to the superficial part of the brain, the brain cortex. But seizures can also start in a focus localized within the cortex. In many such cases rCBF can identify the focus by revealing local hyperemia (sometimes during a provocation test). The impression gained so far is that the focus is better localized in this manner than by electroencephalography (Hougaard and Oikawa, 1975).

The above examples do not by far exhaust the number of medical problems of relevance. Of practical importance have been the contributions made regarding neuroanesthesia in regard to critical cases of severely brain injured patients in general. In such patients the risk of vasodilator drugs acting upon the brain vessels, and thereby increasing intracranial pressure, is now generally acknowledged.

So, in ending, let it be stated that, while previously inaccessible, cerebral blood flow is today known in more detail than flow in other body organs. This is because of the development of appropriate methods. Much effort is directed toward making new variations of existing methods; these efforts often would serve a better purpose by simply extending the employment of existing methods. The major limitation of the existing methods lies in the difficulty in accurately recording low cerebral blood flow (ischemia). That is unfortunate because it is often precisely what one wants to know: Is rCBF adequate, i.e., above the ischemia threshold?

For this purpose, three-dimensional rCBF methods are necessary; otherwise, superposition of high and low flow areas tends to obscure the ischemia. The most promising techniques are those that are based on the computer-assisted axial tomography principle, either using x-rays from an external source or gamma rays from radioisotopes. As has been pointed out previously, currently available techniques are, unfortunately, too slow.

LITERATURE CITED

Boysen, G., H. J. Ladegaard-Pedersen, N. Valentin, and H. C. Engell. 1970. Cerebral blood flow and internal carotid artery flow during carotid surgery. Stroke 1: 253–261.

Brain Work. 1974. Proceedings of VIII. Alfred Benzon Symposium, Copenhagen 1974. D. H. Ingvar and N. A. Lassen (eds.). Munksgaard, Copenhagen.

Braunstein, P., I. Kricheff, J. Korein, and K. Corey. 1973. Cerebral death: a rapid and reliable diagnostic adjunct using radioisotopes. J. Nucl. Med. 14: 122–124.

Cannon, J. J., R. R. Sciacca, J. C. M. Brust, P. M. Johnson, and S. K. Hilal. 1974. Measurement of regional cerebral blood flow with [133] Xenon and a multiple-crystal scintillation camera. Stroke 5: 371–383.

Caprani, O., E. Sveinsdottir, and N. A. Lassen. 1975. SHAM, a method for biexponential curve resolution using initial slope, height, area, and moment of the experimental decay type curve. J. Theor. Biol. 52: 299–315.

Conn, H. L., Jr. 1955. Measurement of organ blood flow without blood sampling. J. Clin. Invest. 34: 916–917.

Eklöf, B., N. A. Lassen, L. Nilsson, K. Norberg, B. K. Siesjö, and P. Torlöf. 1974. Regional cerebral blood flow in the rat measured by the tissue sampling technique; a critical evaluation using four indicators

240   Lassen

C^{14}-Antipyrine, C^{14}-Ethanol, H^3-water and Xenon[133]. Acta Physiol. Scand. 91: 1–10.

Geddes, L. A., H. E. Hoff, C. W. Hall, and H. D. Millar. 1964. Rheoencephalography. Cardiovasc. Res. Bull. 2: 112.

Hilal, S. K., J. A. Resch, and K. Amplatz. 1966. Determination of the carotid and regional cerebral blood flow by a radiographic technique. VII. Symp. Neurorad., New York, 1964. Acta Radiol. 5, part I: 232.

Hoop, B., Jr., A. Amer III., R. G. Ojemann, W. H. Sweet, and R. H. Ackerman. 1973. A technique for the assessment of cerebral circulation. In Cerebral Death, Symposium Abstracts, Stroke 4: 344.

Hougaard, K., T. Oikawa, E. Sveinsdottir, E. Skinhøj, D. H. Ingvar, and N. A. Lassen. 1976. Regional cerebral blood flow in focal cortical epilepsy. Arch. Neurol. 33: 527–535.

Høedt-Rasmussen, K., E. Sveinsdottir, and N. A. Lassen. 1966. Regional cerebral blood flow in man determined by intra-arterial injection of radioactive inert gas. Circulat. Res. 18: 237–247.

Ingvar, D. H. 1975. Brain work in presenile dementia and in chronic schizophrenia. *In* Brain Work. Alfred Benzon Symposium VIII. 1974. Munksgaard, Copenhagen, pp. 482–496.

Ingvar, D. H., and L. A. Gustafson. 1970. Regional cerebral blood flow in organic dementia with early onset. Acta Neurol. Scand. 46, suppl. 43: 42–73.

Ingvar, D. H., and N. A. Lassen. 1961. Quantitative determination of regional cerebral blood flow in man. A preliminary communication. Lancet ii: 806–807.

Jenkner, F. L. 1962. Rheoencephalography. Charles C Thomas, Springfield, Ill., p. 73.

Kety, S. S., and C. F. Schmidt. 1945. The determination of cerebral blood flow in man by the use of nitrous oxide in low concentration. Amer. J. Physiol. 143: 53–66.

Kety, S. S., and C. F. Schmidt. 1948. The nitrous oxide method for the quantitative determination of cerebral blood flow and cerebral oxygen consumption of normal young men. J. Clin. Invest. 27: 484–492.

Kuhl, D. E., R. Q. Edwards, A. R. Ricci, and M. Reivich. 1973. Quantitative section scanning using orthogonal tangent correction. J. Nucl. Med. 14: 196–200.

Kuschinsky, W., M. Wahl, O. Bosse, and K. Thurau. 1972. Perivascular potassium and pH as determinants of local pial arterial diameter in cats. Circulat. Res. 31: 240–251.

Lassen, N. A. 1965. Assessment of tissue radiation dose in clinical use of radioactive inert gases, with examples of absorbed doses from $H_2{}^3$, Kr^{85} and Xe^{133}. V International Symposium, Bad Gastein 1964. Urban & Schwarzenberg, München and Berlin, pp. 37–47.

Lassen, N. A., K. Høedt-Rasmussen, S. C. Sørensen, E. Skinhøj, S. Cronqvist, B. Bodforss, and D. H. Ingvar. 1963. Regional cerebral blood flow in man determined by Krypton-85. Neurology 13: 719–727.

Lassen, N. A., and D. H. Ingvar. 1961. The blood flow of the cerebral cortex determined by radioactive Krypton-85. Experientia 17: 42–45.

Lassen, N. A., and D. H. Ingvar. 1972. Radioisotopic assessment of regional cerebral blood flow. Progr. Nucl. Med. 1: 376–409.

Lassen, N. A., and A. Klee. 1965. Cerebral blood flow determined by saturation and desaturation with Kr^{85} : An evaluation of the validity of the inert gas method of Kety and Schmidt. Circulat. Res. 16: 26–32.

Mallett, B. L., and N. Veall. 1965. The measurement of regional cerebral clearance rates in man using xenon-133 inhalation and extracranial recording. Clin. Sci. 29: 179–191.

McHenry, L. C., Jr. 1964. Quantitative cerebral blood flow determination. Application of a Krypton-85 desaturation technique in man. Neurology (Minnesota) 14: 785–793.

Meier, P., and K. L. Zierler. 1954. On the theory of the indicator dilution method for measurement of blood flow and volume. J. Appl. Physiol. 6: 731–743.

Meyer, J. S., and F. Gotoh. 1964. Continuous recording of cerebral metabolism, internal jugular flow and EEG in man. Trans. Amer. Neurol. Assn. 89: 151–163.

Meyer, J. S., and C. Perez-Borja. 1964. Critical evaluation of rheoencephalography in control subjects and proven cases of cerebrovascular disease. J. Neurol. Neurosurg. Psychiat. 27: 66–78.

Meyer, M. W., and A. C. Klassen. 1975. Regional brain blood flow during sympathetic stimulation. In Cerebral Circulation and Metabolism. Proc. VI. Internal Symposium on Cerebral Blood Flow, Philadelphia 1973. Springer Verlag, New York, pp. 459–461.

Munck, O., and N. A. Lassen. 1957. Bilateral cerebral blood flow and oxygen consumption in man by use of [85] Krypton. Circulat. Res. 5: 163–168.

Nylin, G., B. P. Silfverskiöld, S. Löfstedt, O. Regenström, and S. Hedlund. 1960. Studies on cerebral blood flow in man using radioactive-labelled erythrocytes. Brain 83: 293–298.

Obrist, W. D., H. K. Thompson, H. S. Wang, and S. Cronqvist. 1971. A simplified procedure for determining fast compartment rCBF's by [133] Xenon inhalation. In Brain and Blood Flow. Proc. of IV. International Symposium on the Regulation of Cerebral Blood Flow, London 1970. Pitman Medical and Scientific, London, pp. 11–15.

Oldendorf, W. H. 1969. Absolute measurement of brain blood flow using non-duffusible isotopes. In Cerebral Blood Flow. Clinical and Experimental Results. Proc. of III. International Symposium on Cerebral Blood Flow, Mainz 1969. Springer Verlag, New York, pp. 53–55.

Olesen, J., O. B. Paulson, and N. A. Lassen. 1971. Regional cerebral blood flow in man determined by the initial slope of the clearance of intraarterially injected [133] Xe. Stroke 2: 519–540.

Palvölgyi, R. 1969. Regional cerebral blood flow in patients with intracranial tumors. J. Neurosurg. 31: 149–163.

Pannier, J. L., and I. Leusen. 1973. Circulation to the brain of the rat during acute and prolonged respiratory changes in the acid base balance. Pflügers Arch. 338: 347–359.

Pasztor, E., L. Symon, N. W. C. Dorsch, and N. M. Branston. 1973. The hydrogen clearance method in assessment of blood flow in cortex, white matter and deep nuclei of baboons. Stroke 4: 556–564.

Paulson, O. B., N. A. Lassen, and E. Skinhøj. 1970. Regional cerebral blood flow in apoplexy without arterial occlusion. Neurology (Minneap.) 20: 125–138.

Potchen, E. J., D. O. Davis, R. Wharton, R. Hill, and M. Taveras. 1969. Regional cerebral blood flow in man. Arch. Neurol. Chicago 20: 378–383.

Reivich, M., J. Jehle, L. Sokoloff, and S. S. Kety. 1969. Measurement of regional cerebral blood flow with antipyrine-14C in awake cats. J. Appl. Physiol. 27: 296–300.

Reivich, M., W. Obrist, R. Slater, and H. Goldberg. 1975. A comparison of the Xe^{133} intracarotid injection and inhalation techniques for measuring regional cerebral blood flow. Presented at the VII. International Symposium on Cerebral Blood Flow and Metabolism, Aviemore, Scotland, 1975.

Risberg, J., J. H. Halsey, E. L. Wills, and E. M. Wilson. 1975. Hemispheric specialization in normal man studied by bilateral measurements of the regional cerebral blood flow. A study with the 113-Xe inhalation technique. Brain (in press).

Roy, C. S., and C. S. Sherrington. 1890. The regulation of the blood supply of the brain. J. Physiol. (London) 11: 85.

Seylaz, J. 1973. Techniques for continuous measurement of local cerebral blood flow, Pa_{O_2}, Pa_{CO_2} and blood pressure in the non-anesthetized animal. Pflügers Arch. 340: 175–180.

Shulman, K., M. Furman, and R. Rosende. 1975. Regional cerebral blood flow. Evaluation of the microsphere technique. In: Cerebral Circulation and Metabolis. Proc. VI. International Symposium on Cerebral Blood Flow, Philadelphia 1973. Springer Verlag, New York, pp. 148–151.

Simard, D., J. Olesen, O. B. Paulson, N. A. Lassen, and E. Skinhøj. 1971. Regional cerebral blood flow and its regulation in dementia. Brain 94: 273–288.

Sveinsdottir, E., and N. A. Lassen. 1975. A 254-detector system for measuring regional cerebral blood flow. In Cerebral Circulation and Metabolism. Proc. of VI. International Symposium on Cerebral Blood Flow, Philadelphia 1973. Springer Verlag, New York, pp. 415–417.

Ter-Pogossian, M. M., M. E. Phelps, E. J. Hoffman, and M. E. Raichle. 1975. A positron emission transverse tomograph (Pett) for the three dimensional and non-invasive measure of cerebral hemodynamics and metabolism. Presented at the VII International Symposium on Cerebral Blood Flow and Metabolism, Aviemore, Scotland, 1975.

Wyper, D. J., G. A. Lennox, and J. O. Rowan. 1975. A ^{133}Xe inhalation technique for rCBF measurement: Theory and normal responses. Presented at the VII International Symposium on Cerebral Blood Flow and Metabolism, Aviemore, Scotland, 1975.

Zierler, K. L. 1965. Equations for measuring blood flow by external monitoring of radioisotopes. Circulat. Res. 16: 309–321.

Cardiovascular Flow Dynamics and Measurements
Edited by N. H. C. Hwang and N. A. Normann
Copyright 1977   University Park Press   Baltimore

chapter 6

FLOW-RELATED PROBLEMS IN CARDIOVASCULAR SURGERY

George P. Noon

ABSTRACT

Many congenital and acquired cardiovascular problems that require surgical palliation or correction are accompanied by or result from abnormal blood flows. The qualitative and quantitative definition of these flows are important for adequate clinical evaluations; they should provide: (1) precise data to help formulate a decision on the best mode of therapy, (2) a base line for evaluating immediate and long-term therapeutic results, and (3) a comparison of the therapeutic results and the natural history of the disease.

Flow patterns are of primary concern in the development and employment of cardiovascular prosthetic devices, materials, and support systems. It is mandatory that stringent standards be established. Despite exacting engineering design, devices may fail because biologic alterations detrimental to organ functions and/or to the total organism may occur following short- or long-term usage. These biologic interactions compound the problems we face.

Biomedical engineering, combined with the efforts of medical clinicians and basic science researchers, have made possible the rapid and profound evolution within cardiovascular surgery. Only through their continued collaborative work will we be able to solve the many remaining problems.

INTRODUCTION

Many congenital and acquired vascular disorders that require surgical palliation or correction are accompanied by or result in abnormal flows. An estimation of the physiologic effects upon the organism is important.

Appropriate measurements provide information necessary for making a decision regarding the best mode of therapy and also give a baseline for comparison of immediate and long-term results of treatment and the natural history of the disease. Flow patterns are of primary concern in the development of cardiovascular prosthetic devices, materials, and support systems. Biologic alterations detrimental to the organism and/or device function may occur following short- or long-term usage. The limits of acceptable ranges must be studied and established for successful application. Biomedical engineering combined with efforts of medical clinicians and basic science researchers is providing us with more and more of this vital information.

This chapter presents a series of illustrations to demonstrate some of the flow-related problems encountered in surgery. The schematic diagram of the arterial tree in Figure 1 shows common sites of occlusive disease and aneurysm resulting most commonly from atherosclerosis, although there are other acquired and congenital disorders that can produce similar abnormalities. The patient's symptoms from occlusive disease depend upon the site where the process occurs and its severity: the coronary arteries produce angina pectoris and myocardial infarction, the arteries supplying the brain can produce transient neurologic disorders and stroke, and arteries to the intestine can produce intestinal malfunction and infarction or death of the intestine. Hypertension may result from narrowing of the renal arteries. Stenosis in the abdominal aorta, iliac, femoral, or distal arteries in the extremities produces difficulty with walking, rest pain, or gangrene of the extremities.

There are a variety of techniques used in the reconstruction of diseased or injured arteries. Primary repair is used in localized injuries. An aneurysm or ballooning out of the artery is treated with resection and replacement with a graft. Segmental areas of narrowing can be removed by an endarterectomy, and closure with a patch graft or primary suture, depending upon the size and location of the artery. Bypass grafts provide distal flow to an occlusive segment without removing and replacing the diseased artery. In patients with arterial occlusion from an embolus or thrombus, balloon catheters are used to remove the occluding material (Figure 2). Flow studies have influenced the development of techniques of vascular anastomosis that minimize the possibility of stenosis at the suture line. In large vessels such as the aorta, end-to-end anastomosis may be used without significant change in the arterial circumference or flow pattern. In smaller arteries, however, stenosis may occur at the anastomosis when

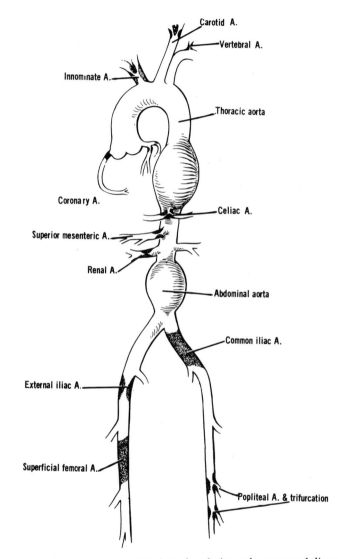

Figure 1. Arterial tree and common sites of occlusive and aneurysmal disease from the atherosclerosis.

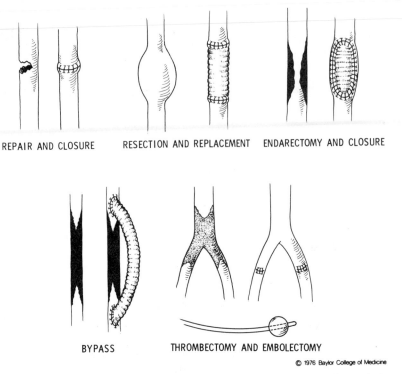

REPAIR AND CLOSURE   RESECTION AND REPLACEMENT   ENDARECTOMY AND CLOSURE

BYPASS   THROMBECTOMY AND EMBOLECTOMY

© 1976 Baylor College of Medicine

Figure 2. Reconstructive techniques used in surgical treatment of lesions of the arteries.

vessels are sutured end-to-end without beveling the cut end, the vessels, and/or graft (Gibson, 1910, 1911–1912; Phelan and Herrick, 1958).

Dacron grafts are the most commonly used prostheses in vascular surgery (Figure 3); however, the use of Dacron is limited to larger arteries with high flows. When smaller arteries such as coronary, upper extremity, or the peripheral vessels in the leg below the knee are involved, the saphenous vein is the graft of choice. Bovine heterografts are also used in the peripheral vessels.

When occlusive disease involves the coronary arteries, the primary technique used to improve the flow to the distal vessels is saphenous vein grafts from the ascending aorta to the artery distal to the occlusion. In Figure 4A arteriograms demonstrate the extent of the disease preoperatively, and in Figure 4B, bypass grafts are shown functioning several years after surgery. In follow-up studies, it has been found that blood flow of 40

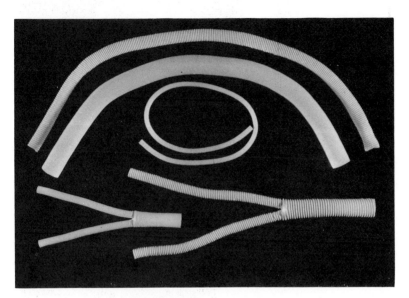

Figure 3. Photograph of several types of Dacron grafts.

ml/min or greater results in the highest patency. The internal mammary artery anastomosed to the left anterior descending (Figure 5) or other coronary arteries has a patency somewhat higher than the venous bypass; however, blood flow is less. A small percentage of veins develop areas of occlusion or narrowing from subintimal fibroplasia, which is rarely seen in the internal mammary artery. This most likely results in the difference in patency.

In cerebral circulation, the most common site of occlusive disease is the carotid artery. The vertebral and proximal aortic arch vessels are less frequently involved. The symptoms with which the patient presents vary from frank stroke to transient neurologic deficits, or nonlocalizing symptoms such as lightheadedness, dizziness, loss of memory, and confusion. These vessels each supply specific areas of the brain, but, as shown in Figure 6, through collateral channels they also provide blood flow to other regions of the brain. Stenosis of the extracranial internal carotid artery is treated by endarterectomy and closure usually with a patch. This removes the stenotic plaque and establishes normal blood flow. Operative pressure studies in patients with atheromatous lesions of the carotid artery demonstrate gradients when a stenosis of 50% or greater is present. Operative correction of stenotic lesions invariably results in a proportionate increase

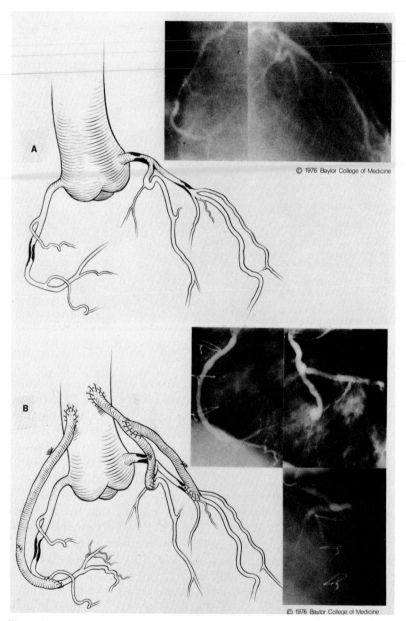

© 1976 Baylor College of Medicine

© 1976 Baylor College of Medicine

Figure 4. *A*, Drawing and preoperative arteriogram illustrating several stenotic lesions of the coronary arteries. *B*, Drawing and postoperative arteriogram showing vein bypass grafts to the coronary arteries, functioning satisfactorily (same patient). Reprinted by permission of Baylor College of Medicine.

250

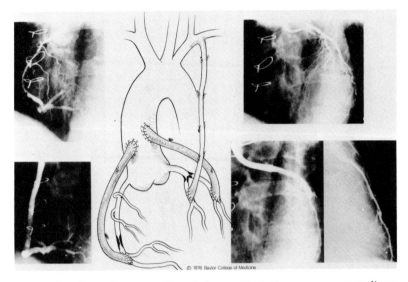

© 1976 Baylor College of Medicine

Figure 5. Drawing and postoperative arteriogram illustrating coronary artery disease treated successfully with combination of vein bypass grafts from ascending aorta to right and circumflex coronary arteries and internal mammary artery bypass to left anterior descending coronary artery. Reprinted by permission of Baylor College of Medicine.

in blood flow from 50–450% of the preoperative level (Crawford et al., 1960; Crawford, Wukash, and DeBakey, 1962). All patients who have symptoms of cerebrovascular insufficiency do not necessarily have an occlusive lesion. Atherosclerosis also causes ulceration of the carotid artery from which debris may break away and embolize to the brain. In this instance, measurement of flows or pressure gradients would not help in determining the cause of symptoms because they would not be altered. The arteriogram in Figure 7 demonstrates a patient having symptoms of cerebrovascular insufficiency from ulceration and emboli but with normal blood flows. An embolus in the retinal artery of this patient is seen in Figure 8.

Nature accommodates for occlusions in arteries by development of collateral circulation and also by a "steal." Figure 9 illustrates an occlusion of the right subclavian artery in which blood flows from the left vertebral to basilar artery and then retrograde through the right vertebral artery, filling the right subclavian artery. This produces a "steal" of blood from the brain, giving rise to symptoms of intermittent cerebral ischemia. To

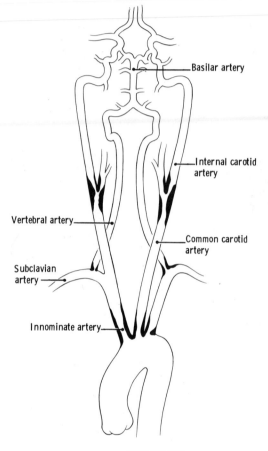

© 1976 Baylor College of Medicine

Figure 6. Sites of occlusive disease in the extracranial arteries and the collateral circulation in the brain.

correct this, a right carotid subclavian bypass is performed and blood then flows in the normal direction.

A patient with occlusive disease of all the main vessels to the brain is demonstrated in Figure 10. This is corrected with bypass grafts from the ascending aorta to the right carotid and left carotid arteries and both subclavian arteries. All these grafts are shown functioning well 2 years after operation. A segmental occlusion of the brachial artery is illustrated

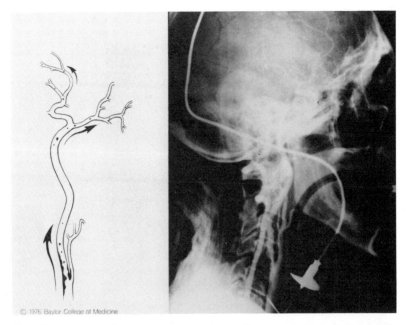

Figure 7. Drawing and preoperative arteriogram illustrate ulcerative lesion of the internal carotid artery and the pathway of embolization to the brain. Reprinted by permission of Baylor College of Medicine.

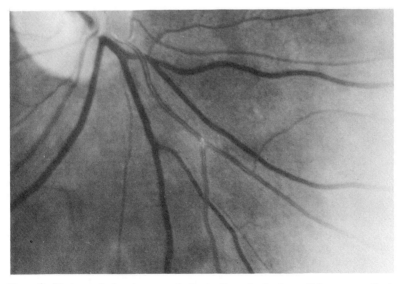

Figure 8. Photograph showing an embolus in the retinal artery of the same patient.

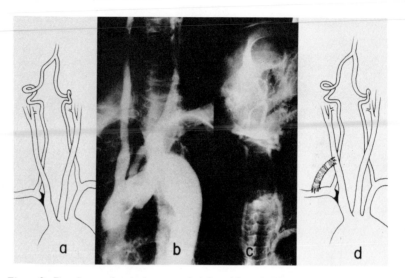

Figure 9. Drawing and arteriograms showing (*a*) and (*b*) occlusion of the right subclavian artery and (*c*) resultant subclavian "steal" syndrome with blood flow to the right subclavian artery by retrograde flow in the right vertebral and (*d*) operative correction with carotid subclavian bypass.

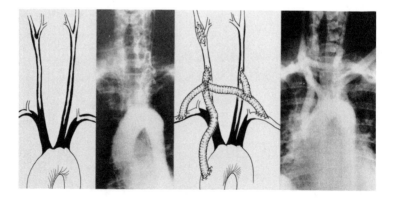

Figure 10. Diagram and preoperative arteriogram illustrating occlusions of the innominate artery, left carotid, and left subclavian arteries. Drawing and postoperative arteriograms demonstrating satisfactory functioning bypass grafts to the right carotid, left carotid, and both subclavian arteries. Reprinted by permission of Baylor College of Medicine.

in Figure 11. This was treated with an autogenous vein bypass graft instead of Dacron, which would not function as well in this position.

Occlusive disease of the renal artery can result in hypertension. This is illustrated in a case of bilateral fibromuscular disease of the renal arteries (Figure 12). This was treated with bypass grafts from the abdominal aorta to both renal arteries. Arterial pressure measurements demonstrated a preoperative pressure gradient; following operation this was relieved. Patients with aneurysms of the main renal artery or its branches may have no stenosis, but still develop hypertension from an altered flow pattern. With correction of the aneurysm these patients become normotensive.

Narrowing of the abdominal aorta decreases the circulation to the lower extremities. These patients develop pain in the legs and buttocks with walking, which is relieved with rest. Dacron grafts can be used to bypass the occlusive lesions with good long-term results.

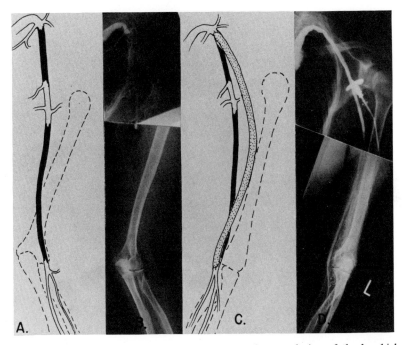

Figure 11. Drawing and preoperative arteriogram of an occlusion of the brachial artery. Drawing and postoperative arteriogram of satisfactory functioning vein bypass graft to brachial artery.

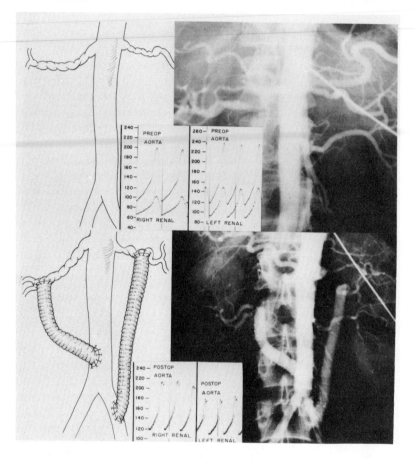

Figure 12. Drawing, preoperative arteriogram, and arterial pressure graph illustrating stenosis of the renal arteries due to fibromuscular disease. Drawing and postoperative arteriogram illustrate successful bypass graphs from aorta to both renal arteries. Graph shows arterial and aortic pressure now superimposed. Reprinted by permission of Baylor College of Medicine.

A patient with a localized occlusion of the right iliac artery is illustrated in Figure 13. Circulation was reestablished with a bypass graft from the opposite femoral artery. It was thought that this operation might produce a "steal" in the noninvolved extremity, but experience has shown that a "steal" does not occur.

Occasionally, bypass grafts become infected and have to be removed. Alternative routes of blood flow must be constructed to maintain per-

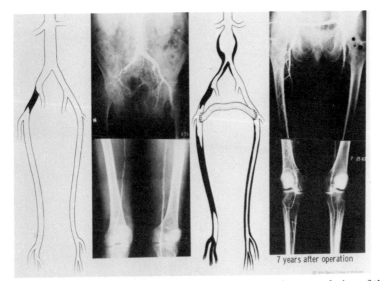

7 years after operation

Figure 13. Drawing and preoperative arteriogram demonstrating an occlusion of the right iliac artery. Drawing and postoperative arteriogram demonstrating satisfactory appearance of right femoral to left femoral bypass graph. Progressive atherosclerotic changes are noted 7 yr later in follow-up study with development of an aneurysm of the abdominal aorta and bilateral femoral and popliteal arteries. Reprinted by permission of Baylor College of Medicine.

fusion. This is demonstrated in Figure 14, which illustrates a patient who had an abdominal aorta and iliac graft replacement removed because of infection. Distal circulation was maintained with bypass graft from the right axillary artery to both common femoral arteries. In this situation, it is the usual practice to insert the new bypass graft before removing the old infected graft. Flow competition occurs if there is normal blood flow through the old graft. Unless this flow is diminished, the new graft quickly occludes. The blood flow is reduced by partial or complete ligation of the old graft or host artery.

The arterial system of the lower extremity is illustrated in Figure 15. The profunda femoris artery has many branches that can form collateral circulation in the extremity. In patients with occlusions of the superficial femoral, the popliteal, or tibial vessels, it is often possible to maintain a viable extremity by preserving flow through the profunda artery because of the rich collateral it can provide. When it is necessary to perform a bypass graft from common femoral to popliteal artery for superficial

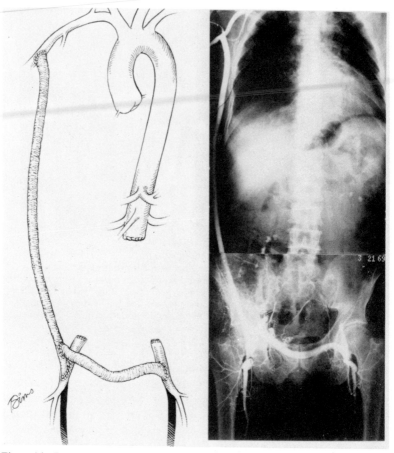

Figure 14. Drawing and postoperative arteriogram illustrating satisfactorily functioning axillary femoral bypass graft and femerofemoral bypass graft. Previous aorto bilateral iliac graft is removed.

femoral artery occlusion, Dacron and venous grafts work equally well if the distal anastomosis is above the knee. However, when the graft is extended across the knee joint, the Dacron graft is less effective because the blood flow is less than above the knee and the flexion of the knee may kink the graft. As in other small arteries where there is low flow, the venous graft must be used in replacement and bypass surgery. A bypass

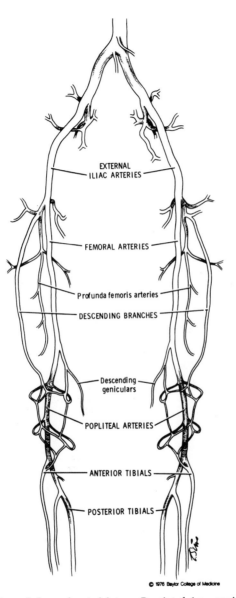

EXTERNAL
ILIAC ARTERIES

FEMORAL ARTERIES

Profunda femoris arteries

DESCENDING BRANCHES

Descending
geniculars

POPLITEAL ARTERIES

ANTERIOR TIBIALS

POSTERIOR TIBIALS

© 1976 Baylor College of Medicine

Figure 15. Drawing of femoral arterial tree. Reprinted by permission of Baylor College of Medicine.

from the common femoral artery to the distal anterior tibial artery at the
level of the ankle is shown in Figure 16. A bypass graft from the aorta to
femoral arteries has a 5-yr patency of approximately 90%. Bypasses to the
popliteal artery above the knee have a 5-yr patency close to 70%; bypass
to the tibial arteries have a 5-yr patency of about 50%. This illustrates that
the patency of bypass grafts is progressively worse as one extends them to
more distal and smaller vessels.

Another common vascular disease is aneurysms, which are a dilatation
and ballooning out of the arterial wall. The main problem with aneurysms,
especially in the abdominal and thoracic cavities, is rupture and death.
Aneurysms in the extremities often thrombose or have pieces break off
and embolize, producing distal ischemia, while rupture and death are rare.

There are several types of aneurysm, the most common etiology being

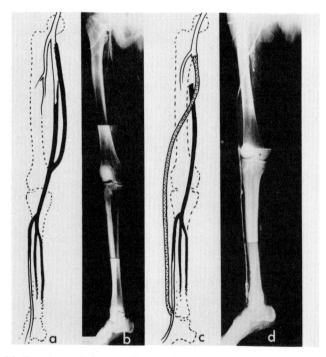

Figure 16. Drawing and preoperative arteriogram showing occlusion of femoral,
popliteal, and posterior tibial arteries. Drawing and postoperative arteriogram demonstrating satisfactory vein bypass graft from femoral artery to anterior tibial artery at
the ankle.

atherosclerosis. Atherosclerotic aneurysms are generally fusiform in shape. Syphilitic aneurysms may be fusiform or saccular. When an artery is ruptured by injury, the surrounding tissues may contain the hemorrhage and form a traumatic aneurysm. Before the development of artificial arteries, homografts were used to replace diseased vessels. A small percentage of these homografts developed aneurysms. False aneurysms may occur at the suture line between a graft and host artery primarily because of deterioration of the suture. Another type of aneurysm is the dissecting

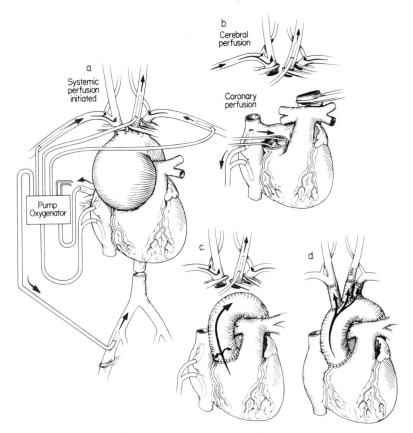

Figurre 17. Drawing of an aneurysm of the ascending aorta and aortic arch with scheme of cardiopulmonary bypass with arterial cannulation of both axillary, left common carotid, femoral, and both coronary arteries are demonstrated. (a) The aneurysm is resected and replaced, following which cardiopulmonary bypass is discontinued (b–d).

262   Noon

aneurysm. It develops when a tear in the inner lining of the artery occurs and blood dissects through the layers of the arterial wall. They are classified according to their location and the distance they extend in the arterial tree. Dissecting aneurysms can shear off major branches from the aorta, resulting in impaired or absent blood flow to vital structures. Blood

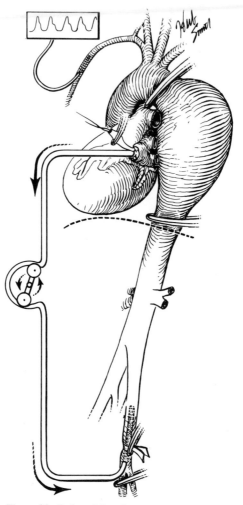

Figure 18. Left atrial to femoral artery bypass.

flow through aneurysmal vessels is often slow because of eddies formed proximal to the aneurysmal dilatation (Holman, 1954).

The location of aneurysms can present special flow problems during operation. In order to resect an aneurysm of the ascending aorta and replace it with graft, total cardiopulmonary bypass must be used to maintain total body perfusion and oxygenation during the operation. When the aneurysm involves the aortic arch, additional arterial return

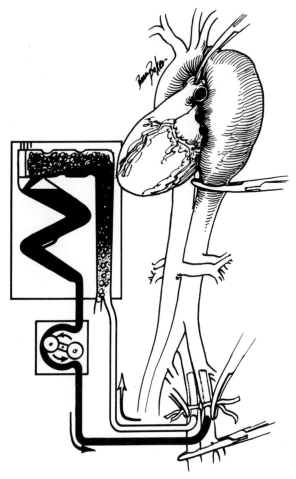

Figure 19. Femoral vein femoral artery partial cardiopulmonary bypass.

cannulas are necessary to provide cerebral circulation because these vessels must be clamped temporarily. This is illustrated in Figure 17.

Aneurysms of the descending thoracic aorta utilize different methods of extracorporeal bypass. One method is from the left atrium to the common femoral artery. It provides (1) distal perfusion during clamping

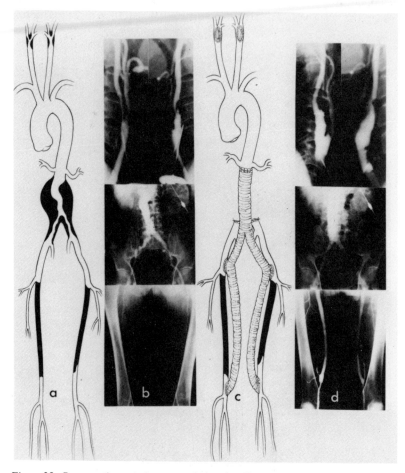

Figure 20. Preoperative arteriogram and drawing illustrate stenosis of both carotid arteries, aneurysm of the abdominal aorta, and occlusions of both femoral arteries. Drawing and postoperative arteriograms show patch grafts to both carotid arteries, resection, and Dacron graft replacement of aneurysm of abdominal aorta and bilateral femoral bypass grafts, all functioning well.

and (2) control of blood pressure proximal to the clamp by removing the blood from the left atrium to reduce the amount of blood pumped by the heart. Thus the extracorporeal bypass minute volume is carefully controlled to maintain optimum distal flow and proximal pressure control (Figure 18). An alternative method used with similar effects is to remove venous blood from the vena cava before it reaches the heart, oxygenate, and return it via the femoral artery (Figure 19).

A patient with atherosclerosis may have several concomitant blood flow problems because of the segmental nature of the disease. A patient with occlusive disease of the carotid arteries, an aneurysm of the abdominal aorta, and occlusive disease of the lower extremities is illustrated in Figure 20. These conditions are treated in the order of their importance: if there is rupture, or impending rupture of the aneurysm, it is treated first; otherwise, the carotid artery circulation is restored first to avoid the possibility of a stroke. Bypass grafts in the lower extremities are a first priority only if there are severe ischemia and impending gangrene. An aneurysm of the abdominal aorta and narrowing of both renal arteries in Figure 21 are treated with resection and Dacron graft replacement of the aneurysm and bypasses to both renal arteries. In renal artery surgery a vein graft is used if the bypass is beyond the bifurcation.

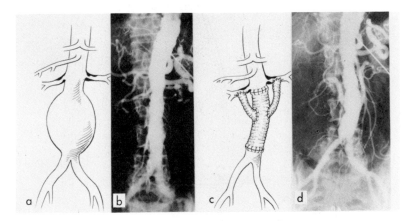

Figure 21. Drawing and preoperative arteriogram illustrate aneurysm of the abdominal aorta and stenosis of both renal arteries. Drawing and postoperative arteriogram illustrate Dacron graft replacement of the aneurysm of the abdominal aorta and functioning bypass grafts to both renal arteries. Reprinted by permission of Baylor College of Medicine.

Even though operations like this can be performed and normal flows established, atherosclerosis is a progressive disease and may result in future problems. Disease may develop causing aneurysm or occlusion proximal or distal to the grafts. Thus, in operating on these patients, consideration must be given to both the current situation and what may be anticipated in future years.

An arteriovenous fistula is an abnormal communication between the arterial and venous systems. The hemodynamic consequences depend on the size of the fistula and the vessels involved. In small or peripheral vessels, arteriovenous fistulas are usually of no hemodynamic consequence. In some patients with chronic renal failure we take advantage of this fact and create an arteriovenous fistula to enlarge the veins and increase their blood flow to form an easy access for hemodialysis. When larger vessels are

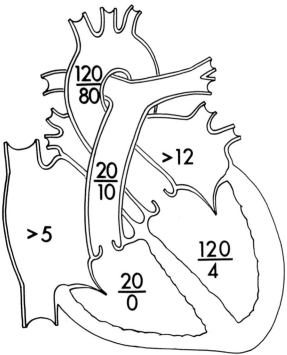

© 1976 Baylor College of Medicine

Figure 22. Chambers of the heart and the great vessels, with normal pressures noted. Reprinted by permission of Baylor College of Medicine.

involved, high output cardiac failure may develop from the high flow through the fistula. The surgical treatment of an arteriovenous fistula is closure.

Congenital abnormalities of the heart produce changes in flow dynamics by abnormal communications between the chambers of the heart and/or systemic and pulmonary circulations; there may also be stenotic lesions of the valves and great vessels. Some of the common congenital cardiovascular malformations are atrial septal defect, ventricular septal defect, tetralogy of Fallot, patent ductus arteriosus, aortic valvular stenosis, pulmonary valvular stenosis, and coarctation of the thoracic aorta. A schematic diagram of the heart and great vessels with normal pressures is shown in Figure 22.

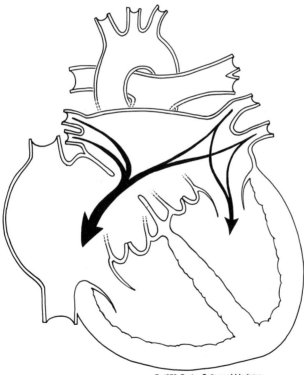

© 1976 Baylor College of Medicine

Figure 23. Atrial septal defect demonstrating abnormal blood flow pattern. Reprinted by permission of Baylor College of Medicine.

An atrial septal defect is an opening in the septum that separates the right and left atria (Figure 23). The size of the defect may vary from a minute hole to total absence of the septum. Normally, the left atrial pressure is higher than the right; therefore, a left to right shunt of blood usually develops. This increases the total volume of blood pumped by the right atrium and ventricle and results in an overload of the pulmonary circulation and eventually pulmonary hypertension and increased pulmonary resistance. These patients may exhibit exercise intolerance, frequent respiratory tract infections, and congestive heart failure. A small defect is nearly always well tolerated. Larger defects produce complications. Treatment is surgical closure of the defect either by primary suture or patch graft utilizing total cardiopulmonary bypass.

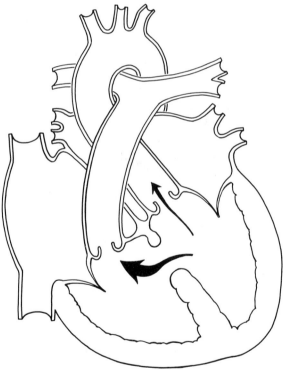

© 1976 Baylor College of Medicine

Figure 24. Drawing illustrates ventricular septal defect and consequent abnormal blood flow pattern. Reprinted by permission of Baylor College of Medicine.

A ventricular septal defect also usually results in a left to right shunt of blood because the left ventricular pressure is usually higher than the right. Blood flow is increased in the pulmonary circulation and left heart (Figure 24). The patient's symptoms depend upon the size of the defect and the magnitude of the shunt. Fatigue, dyspnea, respiratory tract infections, and congestive heart failure may all occur. Banding of the pulmonary artery with a constricting tape is performed in infancy as a palliative procedure if there is congestive heart failure; it decreases the shunting and pulmonary blood flow. Total correction by surgical closure of the defect is performed usually at 4–5 yr of age. If pulmonary banding has been previously performed it is repaired at this time of complete correction.

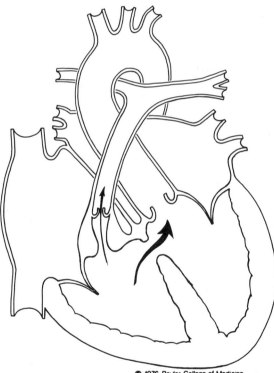

© 1976 Baylor College of Medicine

Figure 25. Tetralogy of Fallot with ventricular septal defect, infundibular stenosis and overriding of the aorta. Abnormal blood flow pattern is demonstrated. Reprinted by permission of Baylor College of Medicine.

Tetralogy of Fallot is defined as a ventricular septal defect combined with infundibular pulmonic stenosis, hypertrophy of the right ventricle, and overriding of the aorta (Figure 25). The infundibular and pulmonary valve stenosis results in increased right ventricular pressure and a right to left shunt through the ventricular septal defect. Systemic oxygenation is poor as a result of the decreased pulmonary flow. Signs and symptoms are usually cyanosis, syncopal attacks, and exercise intolerance. A character-istic feature of this disease is squatting, which helps the child obtain relief of symptoms. It is thought that squatting decreases the arterial blood flow to the legs and thereby increases systemic resistance. The increased left ventricular pressure tends to equalize the right to left shunt and allows better flow to the lungs and increased oxygenation of the blood.

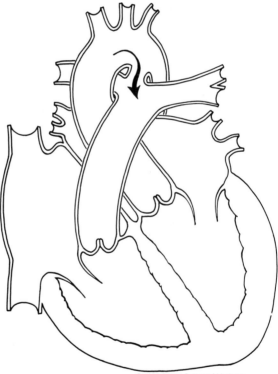

© 1976 Baylor College of Medicine

Figure 26. Drawing illustrates patent ductus arteriosus and flow pattern. Reprinted by permission of Baylor College of Medicine.

Ideal surgical treatment is complete repair of the defect; however, palliative procedures may be performed in small infants to temporize until their condition and size improve enough to tolerate a complete repair. The aim of these procedures is to increase the pulmonary circulation and oxygenation by creating a systemic to pulmonary artery shunt. The most common sites used for these shunts are a side-to-side anastomosis of the

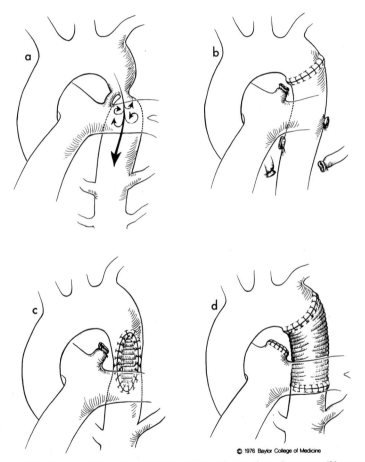

© 1976 Baylor College of Medicine

Figure 27. Drawing illustrating (a) coarctation of the thoracic aorta, (b) resection and end to end anastomosis of the aorta, (c) incision and patch graft angioplasty of the coarctation, and (d) resection and Dacron graft replacement of the coarctation. Reprinted by permission of Baylor College of Medicine.

ascending aorta to right pulmonary artery, and end-to-side subclavian artery to pulmonary artery. The ascending aorta to pulmonary artery shunt is not without potential flow problems; precise measurement of the anastomosis is imperative. If the anastomosis is too large, blood flow through it will be excessive and cardiac failure will follow. The shunts are closed when complete correction of the tetralogy is performed. Complete correction consists of closing the ventricular septal defect and relieving the right ventricular outflow obstruction.

The ductus arteriosus connects the pulmonary artery with the aortic isthmus. Its function in the fetus is to carry blood from the pulmonary artery to the aorta, thus bypassing the lungs, which are not used for oxygenation until after birth. The ductus normally closes at birth or shortly after. When the ductus remains patent after birth, a left to right shunt develops (Figure 26) because of the higher pressure in the aorta. Symptoms vary with the size of the shunt. Surgical treatment is to ligate the ductus.

Congenital stenosis of the pulmonary valve impedes the flow of blood from the right ventricle to the pulmonary artery. There is a subsequent

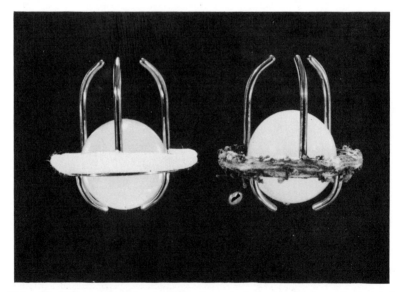

Figure 28. Photograph of a normal ball valve and a ball valve that has undergone ball variance resulting in improper seating.

increase in right ventricular pressure and hypertrophy of the right ventricular wall. In these patients the severity of the symptoms may vary greatly from fatigue and dyspnea to right heart failure. Definitive treatment is relief of the stenosis by incising the valve.

Aortic valvular stenosis increases the work load of the left ventricle as it strives to provide adequate systemic pressure and flow. The ventricle hypertrophies as a result of this extra work. The blood supply to the ventricle itself may be compromised as the ventricular muscle thickens or if systemic pressure is decreased. These children are relatively symptom free. Dyspnea, fatigue, and occasional syncopal attacks may occur. Surgical correction of the stenosis is by valvulotomy or valve replacement.

Coarctation of the thoracic aorta is a localized congenital narrowing of the aorta usually immediately distal to the left subclavian artery near the level of the insertion of the ductus arteriosus. This stenosis causes proximal hypertension. To improve distal circulation, collateral circulation through the intercostal arteries develops. The child with coarctation may be asymptomatic but eventually develops complications from the hypertension. Common methods of repair of the coarctation are illustrated in Figure 27.

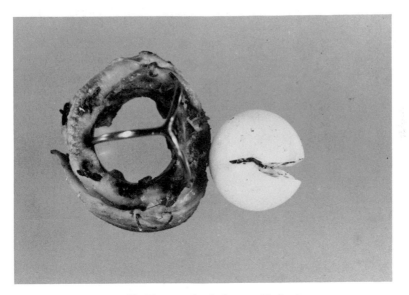

Figure 29. Photograph of a fractured ball valve.

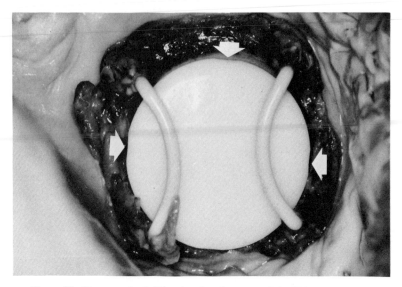

Figure 30. Photograph of disk valve showing wear of the disk at the edges.

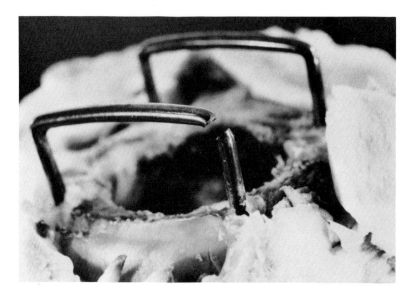

Figure 31. Photograph of disk valve with broken strut.

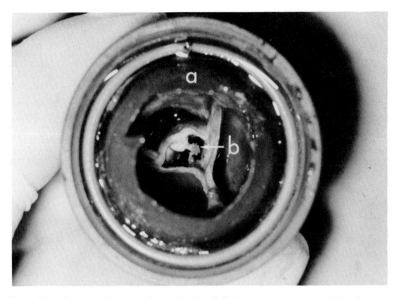

Figure 32. Photograph of porcine valve in a left heart bypass pump with (*a*) thrombus and (*b*) stenosis.

Prosthetic cardiac valves are studied and stress tested in the flow dynamics laboratory before they are made available for patient use. We are still, despite this testing, unable to predict some of the problems that occur after implantation. Significant alterations may develop, such as ball variance from absorbed lipid materials causing serious flow problems from abnormal movement or seating of the ball (Figure 28). Ball fracture has occurred (Figure 29). A disk valve tested in a pulse duplicator for periods equivalent to 60–90 yr had no evidence of wear; however, after 5 yr in a patient, the disk had become deformed by wear (Figure 30). Strut breakage has also occurred (Figure 31). These complications arise despite extensive laboratory testing. Alterations that are not anticipated may occur months to years after biologic implantation; therefore it takes many years to develop, test, and evaluate prosthetic valves. Another problem associated with prosthetic valves is thromboembolism. From the valves used 10 to 15 yr ago thromboembolism occurred in approximately 75% of the patients; presently it is seen in less than 5%.

Biologic valves are excellent hemodynamically and are virtually free of thromboembolism; however, in implantation a significant percentage become deformed in time by scar or degeneration resulting in malfunction. A porcine valve that works perfectly well as a heart valve replacement developed clot formation and stenosis in an artificial heart pump (Figure 32). Presumably, the difference in flow patterns in the heart and the pump resulted in the malfunction of the valve.

The illustrations presented here represent a few of the flow-related problems that face the surgeon and those related disciplines that provide the basic understanding of flow-related diseases and problems and the research and development of devices and methods of diagnosis and treatment.

LITERATURE CITED

Crawford, E. S., M. E. DeBakey, F. W. Blaisdell, G. C. Morris, and W. S. Fields. 1960. Hemodynamic alteration in patients with cerebral arterial insufficiency, before and after operation. Surgery 18: 1–76.

Crawford, E. S., D. Wukash, and M. E. DeBakey. 1962. Hemodynamic changes associated with carotid artery occlusion: an experimental and clinical study. Cardiol. Res. Bull. 1: 1–3.

Gibson, A. H. 1910. On the flow of water through pipes and passages having converging or diverging boundaries. Proc. Roy. Soc. London 83A: 366.

Gibson, A. H. 1911–1912. On resistance of flow of water through pipes and passages having diverging boundaries. Trans. Roy. Soc. Edinburgh 48: 97.

Holman, E. 1954. The obscure physiology of post stenotic dilation: its relationship to the development of aneurysms. J. Thor. Surg. 28: 2–109.

Phelan, J. T., and J. F. Herrick. 1958. Some applied rheological principles as to vascular surgery. Mayo Clin. Proc. 33: 5–108.

Cardiovascular Flow Dynamics and Measurements
Edited by N. H. C. Hwang and N. A. Normann
Copyright 1977   University Park Press   Baltimore

chapter 7

BLOOD FLOW STUDIES
IN VASCULAR SURGERY

Ruben Cronestrand

ABSTRACT

The aim of vascular surgery is the normalization of blood flow. The best way to determine whether blood flow is adequate is to measure it, which requires a knowledge of the normal flow. Blood flow at operation is influenced by many factors. The pelvic and lower limb blood flow is very dependent on the loading of the vascular system. Blood loss is most often underestimated, resulting in a hypovolemic patient with an increased sympathetic tone in the limb arteries. Blood flow studies in that situation give low basal flow values and do not reflect the capacity of the vessel to conduct blood. A more appropriate study is to test the maximal flow by releasing the sympathetic tone. The basal and maximal flows together give better information about the capacity of the vessel and also about the volemic state. Adequate blood flow values in the lower limb arteries and blood flow changes in the early postoperative hours and days are given. The flow-increasing effects of different exercises are reported. Also, postural changes at rest and during exercise, some rheologic changes in the vascular bed of the leg during exercise, as well as the collateral function after vascular reconstruction at rest and during exercise are discussed.

PREOPERATIVE BLOOD FLOW
STUDIES IN PELVIC AND LOWER LIMB ARTERIES

Introduction

The aim of vascular surgery in patients with occlusive disease is to restore an adequate blood flow through the reconstructed vessel. The surgeon should be obliged to prove that an adequate blood flow exists after ending the reconstructive procedure. Various methods have been used for that purpose, for example, pulse palpation in the operative region, studies of distal pulses, intra-arterial measurements of pressure differences, preoperative arteriography, toe oscillometry, and blood flow measurements. Only blood flow measurements give information about the blood volume that is flowing through the reconstructed vessel. Of the methods for measuring blood flow, the electromagnetic flowmeter is most suitable for measurements during surgery when the vessel in question is dissected free.

The electromagnetic flowmeter, based on Faraday's law of electromagnetic induction, was developed independently by Kolin (1936) and Wetterer (1937). For almost two decades it was used in animal experiments; Spencer et al. (1955) seem to have been the first investigators to use the electromagnetic flowmeter in man to check results after vascular surgery. Since then a great number of publications have shown the value of the method. Many vascular surgeons have reported cases with small flow rates through the reconstructed vessel, in which extension of the operation or correction of technical faults has resulted in success of the operation. These efforts should be made at the initial operation when they are most easily performed and when the chance for success is best. Blood flow at operation is influenced by many factors such as anesthesia which, in itself, can decrease cardiac output (CO) up to 50%. The various anesthetic agents have very different effects upon CO and regional blood flow. Other factors regulating the flow are arteriosclerotic changes in the vessels, variations in blood pressure, variations in $PaCO_2$, and general or local hypothermia. Last but not least, the blood flow (basal flow) in the extremities is very dependent on the loading of the vascular system.

Femoro-popliteal Vein Bypass Flow

Flow values after reconstruction reported from different centers vary considerably, as do the values within the same material, as shown in Table 1 and Figure 2, below. Thus Mannick and Jackson (1966) reported blood flow in 14 femoro-popliteal vein bypasses ranging from 15 to 90 ml/min with a mean of 50 ml/min, while Cronestrand and Ekeström (1970a) in 16 bypasses reported flows ranging from 105 to 505 ml/min with a mean of 215 ml/min. The latter value is more than 4 times higher than that of Mannick and Jackson. The other data are grouped between those two extremes. From this great variation arises one question: "What is a 'normal' basal flow in a femoro-popliteal vein bypass and in the pelvic and lower limb arteries?"

Aksnes, Cappelen, and Hall (1966) left an electromagnetic flow probe on the common femoral artery after open heart surgery and studied the blood flow as well as CO in the early postoperative period. They found that blood flow in the femoral artery ceased at low values for CO. They stressed the necessity of transfusions far exceeding the volume calculated from the blood loss, in order to maintain an adequate circulating blood volume. Cronestrand and Ekeström (1970a) found an unsatisfactory perioperative blood flow in seven femoro-popliteal vein bypasses, which increased an average of 90–215 ml/min after further blood transfusions. Evidently, the lower limb blood flow is very dependent on the loading of the vascular system. In a hypovolemic state the circulation is hypokinetic with a low CO. In order to maintain an adequate central circulation, the flow in the periphery (in the arms and the legs) is decreased by an increased sympathetic tone. Studies of the peripheral blood flow in that situation result in low flow values corresponding to the grade of hypovolemia.

It is very difficult to measure the blood loss during an operation. The routine method is to calculate the blood loss; this calculation is usually too low, resulting in a hypovolemic patient with strangled circulation in the pelvic and lower limb arteries. Thus the great variation in reported blood flow values is explained. Ekeström and the present author have always tried to obtain hypervolemia in these patients by transfusing at least one bottle more than indicated from the calculated blood loss. That explains our high blood flow values.

Studies of the basal blood flow after vascular reconstruction in the pelvic and lower limb arteries give appropriate information only if the patients are normovolemic. A low flow value could give evidence of bad surgery, but also of hypovolemia in the patient. In that situation a study of the maximal flow capacity could give more information, which could be achieved by pharmacologic vasodilatation. A vasodilator is given intra-arterially in the vessel concerned, thus decreasing the effects of sympathetic tone. Such a pharmacologic test of the peripheral resistance was introduced by Cappelen and Hall (1964), who used 40 mg of papaverine. Many vascular surgeons perform that test and use papaverine in doses of 5–40 mg. Papaverine is a potent vasodilator that acts on all smooth muscles and thus opens the physiologic arteriovenous shunts also. It seems logical to use a β-stimulator that opens the precapillary sphincters and mimics exercise. That is why we used 1 ml of Vasculat, which has been shown by Mellander (1966) to be a β-stimulator. The dilatation is rapid and reaches its maximum after about 30 sec; it then levels off during the following 3–5 min. The combined values of the basal and the maximal flows give an appropriate estimate of the result of surgery as well as of the vascular and volemic state of the patient. In seven patients with reconstructed pelvic and lower limb arteries, the basal and maximal flows were measured before and after transfusion of 500 ml of blood. In the first situation the relative flow increase was 170%, and in the latter only 70% (Figure 1). The relative flow increase decreased with increasing volemia. A low basal flow and large flow increase during vasodilatation indicate hypovolemia, and the patient has to be transfused (Cronestrand and Ekeström 1970a).

A low basal flow and a small increase during vasodilatation can be associated with bad surgery if the calf arteries have been classified as good on the preoperative angiogram. If they have been classified as bad, it is more likely to be associated with a bad prognosis (Cronestrand, Ekeström, and Hambraeus, 1968a). It must be noted, however, that preoperative estimation of the calf arteries is sometimes hazardous, particularly in those

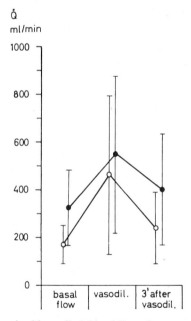

Figure 1. Basal and maximal lower limb blood flow after reconstruction (after 50 mg of Vasculat) and following declination before (○) and after (●) transfusion of 500 ml of blood (mean of seven patients). Mean ± SD.

patients with bad collaterals. The angiography could be more reliable if a vasodilator were given 30 sec before the contrast.

Many authors have tried to predict the prognosis regarding graft patency from preoperative blood flow studies. Cappelen and Hall (1964) reported a 50% incidence of thrombosis during the first postoperative month in eight patients with basal vein bypass flows below 100 ml/min, but only 10% in bypasses with flows exceeding 100 ml/min. Later, Hall (1969) reported three cases of early thrombosis in a series of 11 cases with preoperative basal flow below 100 ml/min. Little et al. (1968) found an 80% failure rate when flows were less than 60 ml/min, while the flow in those remaining patent beyond 3 mo was 100 ml/min or more. Terry, Allan, and Taylor (1972) found in 80 limb cases that the incidence of failure within 3 mo was 32% if the flow was less than 100 ml/min and only 6% if the flow exceeded 100 ml/min. In 90 limb cases, Dedichen (1973) obtained similar basal flow figures. He also reported 36% primary failures after maximal blood flows less than 250 ml/min; the failure rate fell to 3.8% after maximal flow rates of 250 ml/min or more. Primary failures were not seen in vessels with basal and maximal flow rates of 150 and 400 ml/min or above. Pagé et al. (1973) had two cases of early thrombosis in 20 femoro-popliteal vein bypasses with high flows. One had a basal flow of 140 ml/min and maximal of 225 ml/min, and the other one had basal flows of 80 and 160 ml/min, respectively; this implies 50 and 100% increase, respectively, during vasodilatation. In four bypasses with flows less than 60 ml/min they had graft patency after 10 mo. Those four cases, however, had maximal flows that were 4 times the basal flows. Accordingly, the patients were hypovolemic, and that is the reason for the lack of correlation between the basal flow and patency rate. Mannick and Jackson (1966), Barner et al. (1968), and Mundth et al. (1969) reported femoro-popliteal bypass flows ranging from 15 to 90, 17 to 130, and 13 to 190 ml/min, respectively; these values compare well with each other but are less than those reported by others. They were unable to find a positive correlation between graft patency and preoperative blood flow values. The patient with the lowest flow in Barner's material increased from 17 to 325 ml/min during vasodilatation, which means an increase of 1,800%, and most of the patients increased several hundred percent. These values indicate hypovolemia in the patients and thus do not reflect the normal (normovolemic) situation, and that is the reason for the lack of correlation. Mannick and Jackson, and Mundth et al. did not study the maximal flow, but because of the good correlation between the basal flows in those three materials it appears very likely that their patients were hypovolemic as well, and that hypovolemia was the reason for the lack of correlation between preoperative flow rates and graft patency.

Vein Bypass Flow at Various Loadings of the Circulatory System

In order to further elucidate the importance of the loading of the vascular system for pelvic and lower limb blood flows, we (Cronestrand et al., unpublished data) have studied a group of claudication patients, operated on with femoro-popliteal vein bypass during various loadings of the circulatory system. Central hemodynamics were studied during the whole procedure, and the vein bypass flow as well as the common femoral artery blood flow were measured at various loadings of the circulatory system. During reconstruction the patients lost blood, but they were not transfused in order to produce hypovolemia. The blood loss ranged from 500 to 1,300 ml/min with a mean of 900 ml/min. When the reconstruction was completed, the basal mean blood flow in the vein bypass was on the average 53 ml/min (range 25–90), and augmented to 145 ml/min on the average during acute vasodilatation (range 70–270) according to Figure 2. After transfusion with 450 ml of blood, the bypass flow increased significantly to an average basal flow of 92 ml/min (range 60–175), and the maximal flow increased to 185 ml/min (range 110–300). After transfusion with 900 ml of blood (total) there was a further significant increase of the basal flow to 150 ml/min (range 70–250) and of the maximal flow to 230 ml/min (range 110–350). After transfusion with 1,350 ml, there was still a significant increase of the basal flow to 200 ml/min (range 80–350), and of the maximal flow to 260 ml/min (range 110–400). The basal flow values after reconstruction, in the most hypovolemic state, ranging from 15 to 90 ml/min, are comparable with those of Mannick and Jackson (1966) (15–90 ml/min), Barner et al. (1968) (17–130 ml/min), and Mundth et al. (1969) (13–190 ml/min). The values after the first transfusion, 92 ml/min (range 70–175 ml/min), are comparable to those of Golding and Cannon (1966), Little et al. (1968), Hall (1969), Pagé et al. (1973), and Dedichen (1973).

After transfusion with 900 ml of blood the patients were normovolemic according to blood loss estimations, and in that situation the blood flow values are comparable to those of Sako, Woyda, and Ferguson (1960), Cappelen and Hall (1964), Cronestrand (1971), Terry et al. (1972), and Bliss (1973). After the third transfusion the patients were

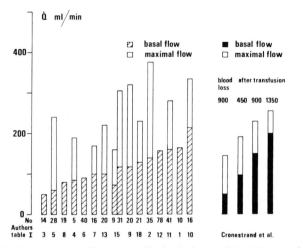

Figure 2. Basal preoperative femoro-popliteal vein bypass blood flow (ml/min) and maximal after different doses of papaverine according to different authors. To the right basal femoro-popliteal vein bypass blood flow and maximal after 100 mg of Vasculat at various loadings of the circulatory system, mean of nine patients. Cronestrand et al. (unpublished data).

hypervolemic according to blood loss estimations; in that situation the basal flow of 200 ml/min (range 80–350) is only comparable with our own data (1970a) presented in Figure 2.

It is obvious from Figure 2 that many patients leave the operating room in a hypovolemic state and that hypovolemia is the reason for the lack of correlation between basal flow levels and graft patency. The maximal flow is a better measure for prediction of graft patency, as shown by us, Cronestrand et al. (1968a), Hall and Fjeld (1973), and Dedichen (1973). In a series of 31 patients we had a good correlation between the maximal preoperative flow and the clinical result.

Hall and Fjeld (1973) had 100% graft patency after 2 yr in patients with maximal flow, after papaverine, of more than 300 ml/min, and Dedichen (1973) had only 3.8% primary failures after maximal blood flow of 250 ml/min or more.

Superficial Femoral Artery Flow

Many authors have reported superficial femoral artery (sup fem art) flow together with the femoro-popliteal bypass flow and popliteal flow so there are only a few reports dealing separately with that flow. The difference in flow between the proximal portion of the sup fem art and the proximal portion of the popliteal artery is small because only a few small branches leave between those two points. In 41 femoro-popliteal vein bypasses the average basal flow was 160 ml/min and the maximal flow was 280 ml/min (Table 1 and Figure 3), and in 59 sup fem art the average basal flow was 170 ml/min after reconstruction and the maximal flow was 310 ml/min (Table 2; Cronestrand, 1971; Figure 4). Dedichen (1973) studied the sup fem art flow in 30 patients subjected to operation and varicose veins. The mean basal flow in the upper portion of this artery was 140 ml/min and the maximal flow averaged 650 ml/min. Cronestrand et al. and Brismar et al. (unpublished data) studied the sup fem art flow in a group of nine elderly and nine young people in connection with operation for varicose veins. The patients were under neuroleptic anesthesia. The blood flow measurements were done before the veins were extirpated. In the elderly group, similar to the group of patients operated on for arteriosclerotic changes in the limbs, the average flow was 158 ml/min (range 90–375) and in the young group the average flow was 190 ml/min (125–325) and increased to 310 ml/min (225–400) after 100 mg of Vasculat. The difference between the elderly and the young group was statistically without significance.

Common Femoral Artery Flow

Cronestrand and Ekeström (1970c) reported common femoral artery (com fem art; see Table 3) blood flow of 390 ml/min, an average in eight patients after reconstruction for occlusive disease in the femoro-popliteal region. During vasodilatation with 50 mg of Vasculat, the average maximal

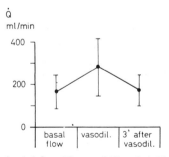

Figure 3. Basal and maximal (after 50 mg of Vasculat) blood flow (ml/min) in 41 femoro-popliteal vein bypasses and following declining. Mean ± SD.

Table 1. Preoperative vein bypass blood flow (ml/min) according to different authors

		No. of cases	Basal Mean	Basal Range	Maximal Mean	Maximal Range	Vasodilator
(1) Sako et al.	1960	10	165	60–266			40 mg papav. mainly
(2) Cappelen and Hall	1964	35	140	50–300	375	200–600	
(3) Mannick and Jackson	1966	14	50	15– 90			
(4) Golding and Cannon	1966	5	85		190		30 mg papav.
(5) Barner et al.	1968	28	60	17–130	240	60–450	15 mg papav.
(6) Little et al.	1968	40	90	20–180			
(7) Bernhard et al.	1968	16	100	15–185	170	23–315	5 mg papav.
(8) Mundth et al.	1969	19	80	13–190			
(9) Hall	1969	20	118	30–480	320	120–700	40 mg papav.
(10) Cronestrand and Ekeström	1970a	16	215	105–505	335	150–670	50 mg Vasculat
(11) Cronestrand	1971	41	160	± SD 80	280	± SD 135	50 mg Vasculat
(12) Terry et al.	1972	78	157	20–445			
(13) Pagé et al.	1973	20	101	35–240	220	110–400	15 mg papav.
(14) Bliss	1973	21	128		230		40 mg papav.
(15) Dedichen	1973	31	118	± SD 45	305	± SD 31	40 mg papav.
		9	72	± SD 23	160	± SD 98	40 mg papav.

285

Table 2. Preoperative sup fem art blood flow (ml/min) according to different authors

| | | No. of cases | Preoperative blood flow (ml/min) | | | | Vasodilator |
| | | | Basal | | Maximal | | |
			Mean	Range	Mean	Range	
Thurau	1963	3	120				
Delin and Ekeström	1965	3	180	100–300			
Golding and Cannon	1966	3	100		235		30 mg papav.
Cronestrand and Ekeström	1970a	5	210	100–295	340	215–420	50 mg Vasculat
Cronestrand and Ekeström	1970b	13	175	85–410	285	140–535	50 mg Vasculat
Cronestrand	1971	59	170	± SD 95	310	± SD 130	50 mg Vasculat
Controls							
Schenk et al.	1960	2	156	144–168	450		50 mg priscolone
Dedichen and Kordt	1974	50	140	± SD 50	625	± SD 190	40 mg papav.
Cronestrand et al.	(unpubl. data)	9 (old)	158	90–375			
Brismar et al.	(unpubl. data)	9 (young)	190	125–325	310	225–400	100 mg Vasculat

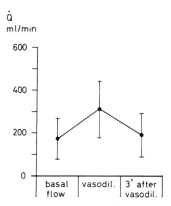

Figure 4. Basal and maximal (after 50 mg of Vasculat) blood flow (ml/min) and following declining after reconstruction in 59 superficial femoral arteries. Mean ± SD.

flow was 720 ml/min. Similar flow values were reported by Cronestrand (1971); in 33 patients, after reconstruction in the iliac-femoro-popliteal region, basal flow was 340 ml/min and maximal flow was 600 ml/min (Figure 5). Those flow values are much higher than those reported by Barner et al. (1968) (basal 116 ml/min and maximal 313 ml/min after 15 mg of papaverine) and by Austen et al. (1964), who measured the com fem art flow in 19 adults suffering from different types of heart disease and reported an average basal flow of 170 ml/min. Patients with heart disease are frequently hypokinetic, and that might explain the low values. As I suggested regarding the vein bypass flow, Barner's patients were most likely hypovolemic, and, similarly, that might be the reason also for the low flow values in the com fem art in his material. Dedichen and Kordt (1974) measured the com fem art blood flow in 50 patients undergoing operation for varicose veins and hernias. Thirty were operated under local anesthesia and 20 under general anesthesia. There was no difference between the two groups, and the average basal flow was 250 ml/min and the maximal flow 1,000 ml/min after 40 mg of papaverine. Cronestrand et al. and Brismar et al. (unpublished data) measured com fem art blood flow in nine elderly and nine young patients in connection with operation for varicose veins. The blood flow measurements were performed before the veins were extirpated, and the dissection of the artery concerned was done without any blood loss at all, so the patients were normovolemic. The patients were under neuroleptic anesthesia. The average basal flow in the elderly group was 280 ml/min and in the young group 455 ml/min,

Table 3. Preoperative com fem art blood flow (ml/min) according to different authors

		No. of cases	Preoperative blood flow (ml/min)				Vasodilator
			Basal		Maximal		
			Mean	Range	Mean	Range	
Barner et al.	1968	20	116	22–230	313	120–700	15 mg papav.
Cronestrand and Ekeström	1970c	8	390	240–650	720	345–1440	50 mg Vasculat
Cronestrand	1971	33	340	± SD 190	600	± SD 330	50 mg Vasculat
Controls							
Austen et al.[a]	1964	19	170	100–360	1013	± SD 265	40 mg papav.
Dedichen and Kordt[b]	1974	30	253	± SD 82	975	± SD 300	40 mg papav.
Dedichen and Kordt[c]	1974	20	240	± SD 70	745	475–1230	100 mg Vasculat
Cronestrand et al.[c]	(unpubl. data)	9 (old)	280	150–450			100 mg Vasculat
Brismar et al.[c]	(unpubl. data)	9 (young)	453	250–950	730	400–1400	100 mg Vasculat

[a]Patient with heart disease.
[b]Local anesthesia.
[c]General anesthesia.

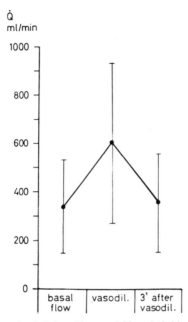

Figure 5. Basal and maximal (after 50 mg of Vasculat) blood flow (ml/min) and following declining in 33 common femoral arteries after reconstruction. Mean ± SD.

which was statistically insignificant, and the average maximum flows were 745 and 730 ml/min, respectively. These control values by Dedichen and Kordt (1974) and Cronestrand et al. (unpublished data) are somewhat lower than those reported by Cronestrand and Ekeström (1970c) and Cronestrand (1971). The control values by Brismar et al. (unpublished data) are somewhat higher. The young group is hyperkinetic compared to the elderly group (Table 3). The higher flow values in our patients from 1970 and 1971 are probably explained by hypervolemia, which we strived to attain by some overtransfusion in order to increase pelvic and lower limb blood flow and avoid early thrombosis.

Dedichen and Kordt (1974) found the same blood flow value in the group operated under local anesthesia as in the group under general anesthesia and had a slight increase in pelvic and lower limb artery blood flow by induction of anesthesia. Most anesthetic drugs decrease CO significantly. In a recent study (Cronestrand et al. and Brismar et al., unpublished data), we found that neuroleptic anesthesia decreased CO from 6.7 to 4.9

liters/min in young healthy controls, and from 5.1 to 3.2 liters/min in elderly, arteriosclerotic patients ($p < 0.001$). We did not study pelvic and lower limb blood flow before induction of anesthesia, so we do not know how it changed. It seems logical, however, to assume that leg blood flow decreased also. However, the anesthetic drugs act in different ways. In the work of Dedichen and Kordt (1974) the type of anesthesia is not reported. If Halothane was used, it might explain the slight increase in pelvic and lower limb blood flow after induction of anesthesia. Halothane is known to be a sympaticolytic drug (Black and McArdle, 1962); thus it decreases the sympathetic tone also in the leg vessels. Despite a decreased blood pressure, the pelvic and lower limb blood flow might increase under Halothane anesthesia. Halothane anesthesia was used in the patients reported by Cronestrand and Ekeström (1970a–c) and by Cronestrand (1970a–c, 1971), and the anesthesia might be another reason for the high flow values, as well as the overtransfusion.

Iliac Artery Flow

Golding and Cannon (1966) reported an average basal blood flow of 710 ml/min in common iliac arteries (com iliac art; Table 4) and 510 ml/min in the external iliac (ext iliac art) in 21 aorto-iliac reconstructions, with an average increase of 75% after 30 mg of papaverine. These values are higher than those in my reports (Cronestrand, 1970a, 1971): average basal flows of 490 and 450 ml/min in the com iliac art after reconstruction and maximum flow of about 900 ml/min; basal flow of 340 and maximum flow of 640 ml/min in the ext iliac art (Figures 6 and 7). Dedichen and Kordt (1974) measured the common iliac flow in 20 controls and reported a basal flow of 390 ml/min and a maximal flow of 1,300 ml/min. Our somewhat higher basal flow values might again be explained by hypervolemia in our overtransfused patients.

"Normal" Basal Flow Values in Pelvic and Lower Limb Arteries

The question posed earlier, namely, what is a "normal" basal flow in a femoral-popliteal vein bypass and in the pelvic and lower limb arteries, can now be answered. The basal flows in a normovolemic state have to be, in milliliters per minute,

Vein bypass	100–150
Sup fem art	150–200
Com fem art	200–300
Ext iliac art	250–350
Com iliac art	300–500

Table 4. Preoperative com iliac art and ext iliac art blood flow (ml/min) according to different authors

	No. of cases	Preoperative blood flow (ml/min)				Vasodilator
		Basal		Maximal		
		Mean	Range	Mean	Range	
Com iliac art						
Golding and Cannon 1966	21	710		1.240		30 mg papav.
Cronestrand 1970[a]	23	490	260–1.300	925	400–1.800	50 mg Vasculat
Cronestrand 1971	42	450	± SD 260	870	± SD 450	50 mg Vasculat
Controls						
Dedichen and Kordt 1974	20	390	± SD 80	1.300	± SD 220	40 mg papav.
Ext iliac art						
Golding et al. 1966	21	510		1.200		30 mg papav.
Cronestrand 1971	19	340	± SD 240	640	± SD 330	50 mg Vasculat

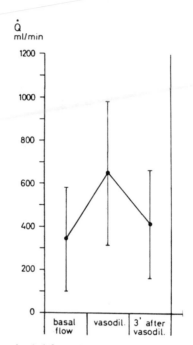

Figure 6. Basal and maximal (after 50 mg of Vasculat) blood flow (ml/min) and following declining in 19 external iliac arteries after reconstruction. Mean ± SD.

POSTOPERATIVE BLOOD FLOW
STUDIES IN PELVIC AND LOWER LIMB ARTERIES

Introduction

"There is a hope that in the future it may be possible to implant probes or some type of probe device which can be removed without difficulty so that flow measurements may be made not only in unanesthetized patients, but even in patients exercising on a tread mill. This is looking into the future" (Schenk et al., 1960).

Blood flow values measured preoperatively are influenced by many factors, as mentioned above. Postoperative studies have been desired for a long time, and implantation of flow probes has been proposed. Twenty years ago, when the electromagnetic flowmeter began to be used in man, the flow probes were too big for implantation. Small probes suitable for implantation were developed 10 yr later by Cappelen and Hall (1964) in Norway and by Denison, Spencer, and Green in the United States. Aksnes,

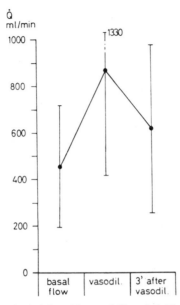

Figure 7. Basal and maximal (after 50 mg of Vasculat) blood flow (ml/min) and following declining in 42 common iliac arteries after reconstruction. Mean ± SD.

Cappelen, and Hall (1966) were the first to report on blood flow studies by implanted flow probes in man. Aksnes et al. left probes on the com fem art, after open heart surgery, for the purpose of determining the correlation between CO and femoral artery blood flow. They found, however, that at low cardiac outputs, the femoral blood flow was close to zero. They also found that in order to maintain an adequate CO it was necessary to transfuse well above the calculated blood loss.

Reifel, Tytus, and Spencer (1966) reported implantation of flow probes on the carotid artery; the probes were left in situ for 10 days. For the same reason Nornes (1963) left probes on the carotid artery for up to 3 wk.

Changes in Basal Flow in the First
Postoperative Days (Postoperative Hypervolemia)

Electromagnetic blood flow studies during the first postoperative days after vascular reconstruction in lower limb arteries were reported by Renwick et al. (1968), Cronestrand et al. (1968b, 1970a–c), Cronestrand (1971), and Hall (1969).

Renwick et al. and Hall reported that with this method they were able to detect vessel occlusions caused by thrombosis, resulting in immediate reoperation and restoration of blood flow. Renwick et al. reported one patient with clinical signs of hypovolemia; a very low flow in the vein graft increased after rapid transfusion of blood and fluid. They also reported a steady rise of flow in the early postoperative hours. In two cases with profunda femoris reconstruction, the maximum flow was reached during the first 2–8 hr. In the femoro-popliteal vein bypasses, the average basal flow was 55 ml/min (range 25–75) in nine cases, and maximal basal flow occurred at the tenth hour, averaging 260 ml/min (range 100–250); it declined to 195 ml/min at 20 hr after the operation. Hall (1969) implanted flow probes on 20 femoro-popliteal vein bypasses and made flow studies up to 4 days after the operation. Hall found a general reduction of the peripheral resistance, calculated as pressure divided by flow, during the first hours after the operation. The average postreconstructive basal flow was 120 ml/min (range 30–480) and the maximum flow after 40 mg of papaverine was 320 ml/min (range 120–700). The last measurement was 210 ml/min (range 90–540), i.e., almost a doubling of the initial postreconstructive flow. Cronestrand et al. reported an initial average postreconstructive flow of 215 ml/min in 16 vein bypasses. During vasodilatation the maximum flow was 335 ml/min. In the afternoon of the day of operation, the average flow was 220 ml/min and rose to 320 ml/min at noon on the first postoperative day. Hall does not report on the maximal postoperative basal flow. Only the figures of Renwick et al. and the present author can be compared in that respect. The maximal postoperative basal flows of 260 and 320 ml/min, respectively, compare well. In Renwick et al., patients increased their flows almost 500%, from 55 to 260 ml/min, and my patients about 50% from 215 to 320 ml/min. In Renwick et al., patients were very hypovolemic, according to the above discussion, and that is the reason for the very marked increase during the early postoperative hours (Table 5).

Hall studied the effect of foot exercise on flow. He found a positive correlation between the maximum flow during the operation, induced by papaverine, and the postoperative maximal flow caused by foot exercise. Cronestrand, Ekeström, and Hambraeus (1968b), Cronestrand and Ekeström (1970a–c), Cronestrand (1970a–c) as well as Cronestrand, Ekeström, and Holmgren (1971) and Cronestrand, Juhlin-Dannfeldt, and Wahren (1973) made more extensive studies of the blood flow in different lower limb arteries during the early postoperative days, under different

Table 5. Blood flow in femoro-popliteal vein bypass at operation and in the early postoperative course according to different authors

		Postreconstructive flow (ml/min)	Maximal flow during vasodilatation	Maximal postoperative flow (ml/min) at rest
Renwick et al.	1968	55		260
Hall	1969	120	320	(210)
Cronestrand and Ekeström	1970[a]	215	335	320

circumstances. Flow probes were implanted on the femoro-popliteal vein bypass, sup fem art, com fem art, ext iliac art and com iliac art (Figure 8). The probes were left in situ up to 6 days postoperatively; in most patients they were left for 3–4 days. Readings were made from occlusion zero performed with an occlusion string. Probes produced by Nycotron (Drammen, Norway) were used. The probes were spool shaped with the slot rather wide and placed diametrically to the cable so that it was possible to remove the probe by gentle traction. In some patients the probe was

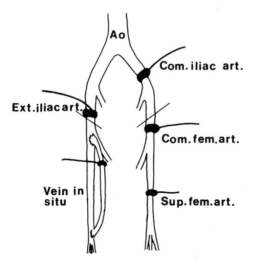

Figure 8. Flow probes placed on common iliac artery, external iliac artery, common femoral artery, superficial femoral artery, and femoro-popliteal vein bypass.

dislodged, and, in fact, the problem was to avoid dislocation and not to remove the probe. The resting blood flow was studied in supine and upright position. In all four groups (Figure 9) there was an increase of blood flow during emergence from anesthesia in the final phase of the operation. Three to four hours later the resting blood flow had decreased about 25%. It then rose 50% in the bypass group and in the sup fem art, which was significant; the maximum of the postoperative hyperemia was on the first postoperative day. It persisted in the bypass group and declined in the sup fem art group. In the com fem art and com iliac art there was an increase of the resting blood flow, too, but that increase was without significance (Figure 9).

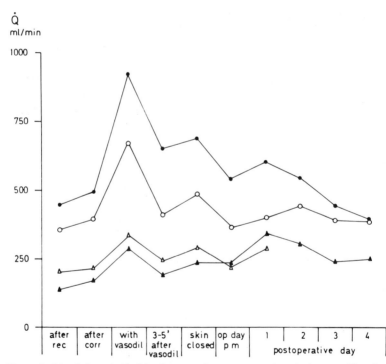

Figure 9. Blood flow (ml/min) after vascular reconstruction, during vasodilatation, and following declination during operation, at the end of operation, and at rest during the first 1–4 postoperative days; mean values of 13 bypasses (△), 13 superficial femoral arteries (▲), 7 common femoral arteries (○), and 18 common iliac arteries (●). Reproduced with permission from Scand. J. Thorac. Cardiovasc. Surg. (Suppl. 4) (1970).

Blood Flow Increase in Pelvic and
Lower Limb Arteries by Different Exercises

Effect of Passive Exercise   Passive exercise did not increase blood flow.

Effect of Active Exercise   The blood flow was almost doubled in all vessels by active unloaded movements of the feet. The foot exercises were easily performed even on the day of operation and required only minor effort by the patient. Another efficient, flow-increasing exercise was heel raising, which was used from the first postoperative day. This exercise increased the sup fem art flow to the same degree as fast walking, almost 400%, and the iliac art flow was trebled. Heel raising engages mainly muscles below the knee and is thus a very suitable exercise for those patients with distal occlusions not amenable to surgery.

The major flow-increasing muscular exercise studied was fast walking, which was used from the second postoperative day. This exercise was more efficient in increasing flow in all vessels studied than cycling with a load of 300 kpm/min. It was also more easily performed and better tolerated than cycling (Figure 10).

Cycling was cumbersome for those patients with incisions in the groin or close to the knee. It was efficient in increasing blood flow in the proximal vessels, but the superficial and popliteal flows were only doubled. Obviously, the calf muscles do not contribute much to the work performed on the bicycle. Heel-raising and walking are much more discriminating than the exercise on a cycling ergometer for preoperative testing of patients with intermittent claudication.

Blood flow increased markedly at the onset of exercise and then gradually for 1 min; it reached a fairly steady level during the second minute. Figure 11 shows a recording of com iliac art blood flow in a patient on the fourth postoperative day while walking on a treadmill at 100 steps/min. After 1 min of exercise the flow was 3,200 ml/min, which represented 90% of the maximum flow obtained during that exercise period of 3 min.

Postural Blood Flow Changes

Hall (1969) studied the effect of postural changes with the patient lying in the horizontal supine position. When the table was tilted 15° with the head down and later with the feet down, there were only small changes in pelvic and lower limb blood flow, and they were soon brought back to

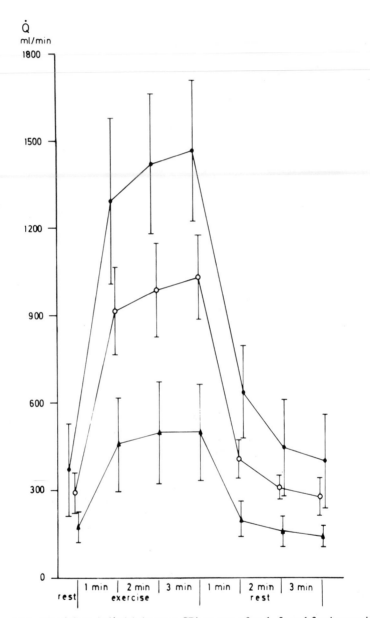

Figure 10. Blood flow (ml/min) (mean ± SD) at rest, after 1, 2, and 3 min exercise (treadmill walking 72 steps/min) and 1, 2, and 3 min after exercise in superficial femoral artery (▲) (7 patients, 16 exercise periods), common femoral artery (○) (4 patients, 12 exercise periods) and common iliac artery (●) (5 patients, 16 exercise periods).

298

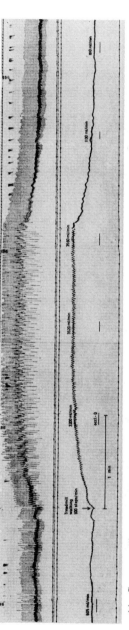

Figure 11. Common iliac artery blood flow (ml/min) at rest, during 3-min exercise period (walking on a treadmill 100 steps/min) and 2 min after exercise (patient no. 63). Reproduced with permission from Scand. J. Thorac. Cardiovasc. Surg. 4 (1970).

control values. When the operated limb alone was elevated 30°, the bypass flow decreased markedly, and this state lasted as long as the leg was elevated. Hall also showed that the maximum systolic flow was the same throughout, but the diastolic flow was reduced during the elevation of the limb.

Com iliac art blood flow (Cronestrand, 1970*b*) was significantly lower (23%) in the sitting position than in the supine position, both at rest and during exercise (Figure 9). Heart rate, blood pressure, and oxygen uptake were somewhat higher in the sitting than in the supine position at rest. Oxygen uptake and heart rate during exercise did not differ significantly between the two postures (Figure 12).

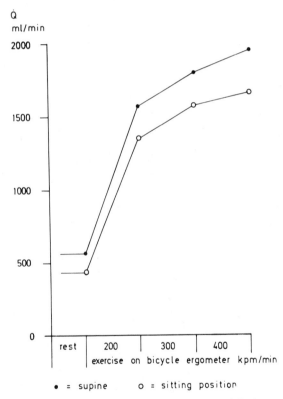

Figure 12. Leg blood flow in common iliac artery at rest and during exercise on a cycling ergometer in supine and sitting position. Mean values of eight legs. Reproduced with permission from Scand. J. Thorac. Cardiovasc. Surg. (Suppl. 4) 1970.

Rheologic and Metabolic Studies

Seven patients (Cronestrand et al., 1971) with flow probes left in situ on the com iliac art were catheterized via a cubital vein and a brachial artery, and the catheter tips were positioned just proximal to the flow probe (Figure 13). The patients were examined in the supine position at rest and during two-legged exercise on a cycling ergometer on the fourth day after operation. Blood was sampled for determination of gas tension, pH, oxygen saturation, and lactate. Oxygen uptake, blood pressure, and blood flow were measured.

The total mechanical efficiency was 23%. Com iliac art blood flow at rest averaged 320 ml/min and was linearly related to total oxygen uptake. Pressure difference over the vascular bed averaged 92 mm Hg at rest and was unchanged during exercise because of a slight parallel increase in iliac

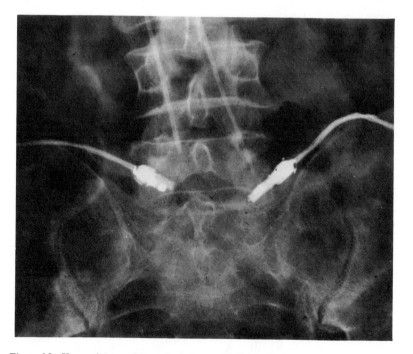

Figure 13. X-ray picture of two electromagnetic flow probes placed on the common iliac arteries and the position of the venous and arterial catheters. Reproduced with permission from Scand. J. Thorac. Cardiovasc. Surg. 5:52 (1971).

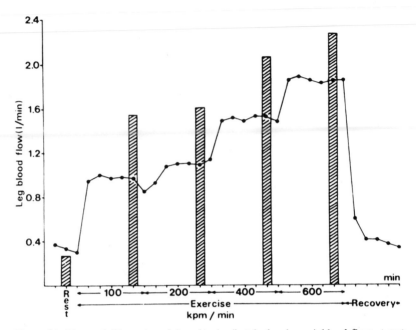

Figure 14. External iliac artery (●) and vein (hatched columns) blood flow at rest and during exercise of stepwise increased workloads in patient M. L. Reproduced with permission from Scand. J. Clin. Lab. Invest. (Suppl. 128) 31:170.

arterial and iliac venous pressure. The vascular resistance of the leg decreased hyperbolically with increasing leg oxygen uptake and blood flow. That marked decrease took place before the blood flow had increased to 1 liter/min. The venous oxygen saturation decreased from 63% to 22%. The arteriovenous oxygen difference across the leg increased from 65 to 140 ml/liter. The leg oxygen uptake increased linearly with total oxygen uptake.

Leg blood flow increased linearly with leg oxygen uptake and the arteriovenous difference over the leg varied as a hyperbola with an asymptote at a value of 160 ml/liter.

Leg blood flow calculated from the increase in oxygen uptake during exercise and the iliac arteriovenous oxygen difference, using the equation suggested by Donald et al. (1957) was, on an average, 300 ml higher than that obtained with the electromagnetic flowmeter.

The mechanical efficiency of the leg averaged 43% for all loads

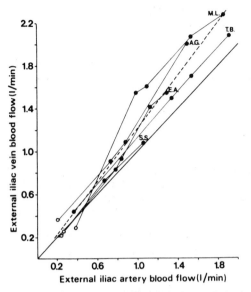

Figure 15. Relationship between external iliac artery blood flow measured with electromagnetic flowmeter and external iliac vein blood flow determined using an indicator dilution procedure at rest (○) and during cycling exercise (●). The regression (y = 1.36, x − 0.11, r = 0.98, p < 0.001) deviates significantly from the line of identity (p < 0.02). Reproduced with permission from Scand. J. Clin. Lab. Invest. (Suppl. 128) 31:171.

studied. This value for mechanical efficiency seems too high, indicating an underestimation of blood flow or the existence of a significant collateral circulation.

Studies of Persistent Collateral Flow after Reconstruction

In order to study the possible existence of a collateral flow after pelvic and lower limb artery reconstruction (Cronestrand, Juhlin-Dannfeldt, and Wahren, 1973), five patients with complete occlusions of the iliac artery were studied 4–6 days after desobliteration. An electromagnetic flow probe was left on the ext iliac art, and the external iliac vein blood flow was determined by indicator dilution technique. Simultaneous measurements gave similar values in the resting state, but a significantly larger venous flow during exercise, suggesting postoperative persistence of collateral circulation to the leg (Figure 14). During exercise of increased intensity there was a progressive rise in the absolute difference between the two flow measurements. The regression of venous flow versus arterial suggests that a fixed fraction of about 35% of leg blood flow during exercise was supplied via collateral arterial pathways (Figure 15). Leg mechanical efficiency was 28–30% calculated from the venous flow, which is a more reliable value, indicating a significant collateral flow even after reconstruction of total occlusions in the pelvic and lower limb arteries.

LITERATURE CITED

Aksnes, E. G., Ch. Cappelen Jr., and K. V. Hall. 1966. Cardiac output and regional (femoral) blood flow in the early postoperative period after heart surgery. Acta Chir. Scand. (Suppl. 357): 299–305.

Austen, W. G., A. G. Morrow, D. J. Patel, and H. W. Bender. 1964. The direct measurement of femoral blood flow in man. J. Thorac. Cardiovasc. Surg. 47: 230–237.

Barner, H. B., D. R. Judd, G. C. Kaiser, V. L. Willman, and C. R. Hanlon. 1968. Blood flow in femoropopliteal bypass vein grafts. Arch. Surg. 96: 619–627.

Black, G. W., and L. McArdle. 1962. The effects of halothane on the peripheral circulation in man. Brit. J. Anaesth. 34: 2.

Bliss, B. P. 1973. Pressure, flow and peripheral resistance measurements during surgery for femoro-popliteal occlusion (preliminary observations on 21 limbs). Scand. J. Clin. Lab. Invest. 31 (Suppl. 128): 179–183.

Cappelen, Chr., Jr., and K. V. Hall. 1964. The great saphenous vein used in situ as an arterial shunt after vein valve extirpation. Acta Chir. Scand. 128: 517–525.

Cronestrand, R. 1970a. Measurements on the common iliac artery. Scand. J. Thorac. Cardiovasc. Surg. (Suppl. 3): 17–27.

Cronestrand, R. 1970b. Effect of body position on leg blood flow at rest and during exercise. Scand. J. Thorac. Cardiovasc. Surg. 4: 173–177.

Cronestrand, R. 1970c. Leg blood flow at rest and during exercise after reconstruction for occlusive disease. Scand. J. Thorac. Cardiovasc. Surg. (Suppl. 4): 1–24.

Cronestrand, R. 1971. Blood flow after carotid, subclavian, renal, and leg artery reconstruction. In V. C. Roberts (ed.), Blood Flow Measurement, pp. 111–114. Sector Publishing Ltd., London.

Cronestrand, R., and S. Ekeström. 1970a. Blood flow after peripheral arterial reconstruction. Scand. J. Thorac. Cardiovasc. Surg. 4: 159–171.

Cronestrand, R., and S. Ekeström. 1970b. Measurements on the superficial femoral artery. Scand. J. Thorac. Cardiovasc. Surg. (Suppl. 3): 1–8.

Cronestrand, R., and S. Ekeström. 1970c. Measurements on the common femoral artery. Scand. J. Thorac. Cardiovasc. Surg. (Suppl. 3): 9–16.

Cronestrand, R., S. Ekeström, and G. Hambraeus. 1968a. The value of blood flow measurements in acute arterial surgery. Scand. J. Thorac. Cardiovasc. Surg. 3: 48–51.

Cronestrand, R., S. Ekeström, and G. Hambraeus. 1968b. Pre- and postoperative flow measurements after femoral-popliteal arterial reconstructions. Scand. J. Thorac. Cardiovasc. Surg. 2: 128–132.

Cronestrand, R., S. Ekeström, and A. Holmgren. 1971. Rheologic and metabolic studies in the vascular bed of the leg after arterial reconstruction, at rest and during exercise. Scand. J. Thorac. Cardiovasc. Surg. 5: 51–60.

Cronestrand, R., A. Juhlin-Dannfeldt, and J. Wahren. 1973. Simultaneous measurements of external iliac artery and vein blood flow after reconstructive vascular surgery: Evidence of increased collateral circulation during exercise. Scand. J. Clin. Lab. Invest. (Suppl. 128) 31: 167–172.

Dedichen, H. 1973. Prognostic significance of intraoperative flow and pressure measurements in reconstructive vascular surgery. Scand. J. Clin. Lab. Invest. 31 (Suppl. 128): 189–192.

Dedichen, H., and K. F. Kordt. 1974. Blood flow in normal human ileo-femoral arteries studied with electromagnetic techniques. Acta Chir. Scand. 140: 371–376.

Donald, K. W., P. N. Wormald, S. H. Taylor, and J. M. Bishop. 1957. Changes in the oxygen content of femoral venous blood and leg blood flow during leg exercise in relation to cardiac output responses. Clin. Sci. 16: 567–591.

Golding, A. L., and J. A. Cannon. 1966. Application of electromagnetic blood flowmeter during arterial reconstruction. Results in conjunction with papaverine in 47 cases. Ann. Surg. 164: 662–677.

Hall, K. V. 1969. Postoperative blood flow measurements in man by the use of implanted electromagnetic probes. Scand. J. Thorac. Cardiovasc. Surg. 3: 135–144.

Hall, K. V., and N. B. Fjeld. 1973. Preoperative assessment of run-off by electromagnetic flowmetry. Scand. J. Clin. Lab. Invest. 31 (Suppl. 128): 185–188.

Kolin, A. 1936. An electromagnetic flowmeter. Principle of the method and its application to blood flow measurements. Proc. Soc. Exp. Biol. Med. 35: 53.

Little, J. M., A. G. R. Sheil, J. Loewenthal, and A. H. Goodman. 1968. Prognostic value of intraoperative blood-flow measurements in femoropopliteal bypass vein-grafts. Lancet 2: 648–651.

Mannick, J. A., and B. T. Jackson. 1966. Hemodynamics of arterial surgery in atherosclerotic limbs. I. Direct measurement of blood flow before and after vein grafts. Surgery 59: 713–720.

Mellander, S. 1966. Comparative effects of acetylcholine, butyl-nor-synephrine (Vasculat), noradrenaline, and ethyl-adrianol (Effontil) on resistance, capacitance, and precapillary sphincter vessels and capillary filtration in cat skeletal muscle. Angiologica 3: 77–99.

Mundth, E. D., R. C. Darling, J. M. Moran, M. J. Buckley, R. R. Linton, and W. G. Austen. 1969. Quantitative correlation of distal arterial outflow and patency of femoropopliteal reversed saphenous vein grafts with intraoperative flow and pressure measurements. Surgery 65: 197–206.

Nornes, H. 1963. Long-term implanted electromagnetic probes in man. Observations during graded occlusion for internal carotid artery aneurysms. *In* New Findings in Blood Flowmetry, p. 215. Universitetsforlaget, Norge.

Pagé, A., M. Brais, R. Cossette, L. Dontigny, R. Lévy, Cl. Mercier, and L. C. Pelletier. 1973. Mesure du débit sanguin dans les pontages fémoropoplités. Union Med. Can. 102: 1277–1281.

Reifel, E., J. S. Tytus, and M. P. Spencer. 1966. Monitoring internal carotid blood flow during graded occlusion for aneurysm. Bull. Mason Clin. 20: 29–36.

Renwick, S., I. T. Gabe, J. P. Shillingford, and P. Martin. 1968. Blood flow after reconstructive arterial surgery measured by implanted electromagnetic flow probes. Surgery 64: 544–553.

Sako, Y., W. C. Woyda, and D. J. Ferguson. 1960. Direct flow measurements in evaluation of surgery for arteriosclerosis. Surg. Forum XI: 479–484.

Schenk, Jr., W. G., A. D. Menno, M. Anderson, and Th. Drapanas. 1960. Application of the electromagnetic flowmeter to vascular studies in human patients. Surgery (St. Louis) 48: 211–218.

Spencer, M. P., A. B. Denison Jr., W. F. McGuire, and R. I. Myers. 1955. Electromagnetic measurement of blood flow through intact human arteries. Am. J. Med. 19: 153.

Terry, H. J., J. S. Allan, and G. W. Taylor. 1972. The relationship between blood flow and failure of femoropopliteal reconstructive arterial surgery. Brit. J. Surg. 59: 549–551.

Wetterer, E. 1937. Eine neue Methode zur Registrierung der Blutströmungsgeschwindigkeit am uneröffneten Gefäss. Z. Biol. 98: 26–36.

Cardiovascular Flow Dynamics and Measurements
Edited by N. H. C. Hwang and N. A. Normann
Copyright 1977   University Park Press   Baltimore

chapter 8

FLOW DYNAMICS IN CIRCULATORY PATHOPHYSIOLOGY

D. Eugene Strandness, Jr.

ABSTRACT

Atherosclerosis results in progressive arterial narrowing, which leads to problems when the demands for flow either at rest or during exercise cannot be met. At low flow rates, the arterial cross section must be reduced by 80–90% before there is a fall in flow and a decrease in systolic and mean pressure distal to the stenosis. Resting flow levels are usually maintained within a normal range even with complete arterial occlusion by a compensatory reduction in peripheral resistance.

With complete arterial occlusion, blood is forced to follow the alternate pathways, the collaterals, which are high-resistance vessels, particularly in their midzone, leading to the loss of potential energy. The collateral arteries can usually accommodate the flows required for the nutritive needs of the tissue at rest, but functionally they cannot accommodate the flow requirements of the exercising limb. The hemodynamic changes that become apparent with the higher flow rates observed with exercise are (1) a further increase in the pressure drop across the collaterals, (2) a reduction in the peak flows normally required to meet the metabolic requirements of the muscle, (3) a prolongation in the period of postexercise hyperemia, and (4) changes in the arterial velocity pattern proximal and distal to the site of involvement. Based on these physiologic changes, it is possible to quantitatively assess the magnitude of the functional abnormalities produced by atherosclerosis.

INTRODUCTION

Diseases involving the arterial system commonly produce problems when the pathologic process either acutely or chronically occludes the involved vessel, thus interfering with the delivery of blood to the part. Survival of the tissue depends entirely upon the rate at which the occlusion occurs, the immediately available collateral circulation, and the metabolic requirements of the ischemic tissue. While there are many disease entities that can result in arterial obstruction, atherosclerosis is by far the most common and important disease of the Western World. Furthermore, because of its importance, the pathophysiology of the circulatory changes that accompany the disease has been studied extensively.

At the outset, it must be recognized that most studies dealing with the pressure and flow changes occurring secondary to atherosclerosis have largely described the changes at a far-advanced stage of the disease. The physiologic changes that follow acute and chronic arterial occlusions, particularly involving the extremities, are well known. However, very little information is available concerning the very early changes that may occur with pressure and flow as the intimal surface becomes roughened, but the artery is not yet narrowed. As will be mentioned, intensive efforts under way to study the effects of preclinical disease on flow dynamics will hopefully lead to earlier recognition of the disease before irreversible changes have taken place.

The arterial system, with a pulsatile pump at its inlet, with a series of branching tubes of differing wall properties, and carrying a complex fluid medium, poses great analytic problems for even the most sophisticated fluid dynamicist. When the effects of atherosclerosis on the artery are added, the problem becomes even more complex. Irregularities of the intima—blood interface, narrowing of the lumen, changes in vessel wall properties, the development of collateral circulation, and changes in flow velocity in response to stress—all greatly add to the complexity of the problems. In addition, the arterioles that are not involved by atherosclerosis serve as a point of variable resistance to flow and are therefore extremely important in maintaining tissue perfusion at a level necessary for viability of the part.

PRESSURE—FLOW RELATIONSHIPS ACROSS ARTERIAL STENOSES

It is well known that at some point in the development of an arterial plaque, the degree of narrowing becomes sufficient to interfere with blood flow. Viscous energy losses are increased because of the narrowed segment and are manifested by a decrease in pressure and/or flow. The body attempts to keep blood flow at a constant level by dilatation of the peripheral arterioles to compensate for the increased resistance of the stenotic segment. Only when the arterioles have reached a state of maximal vasodilatation does a further reduction in the cross-sectional area result in an impairment of blood flow.

The observation that not all stenoses in the arterial system are hemodynamically significant, has led to the concept of the so-called critical arterial stenosis. This is usually defined as the percentage by which the cross-sectional area of the vessel must be reduced to produce a decrease in blood flow. Before considering the case of the arterial stenosis, it is necessary briefly to review those factors responsible for energy losses in a steady-flow system.

Although the application of Poiseuille's law to the arterial system is a gross oversimplification, it does serve to remind us of the major factors that contribute to the pressure drops which occur, at least in a laminar flow system.

$$\Delta P = Q \cdot \frac{8L\eta}{r_i^4} \tag{1}$$

$$\Delta P = \bar{V} \cdot \frac{8L\eta}{r_i^2} \tag{2}$$

where

ΔP = mean pressure gradient between two points A and B
L = length of the segment
Q = flow per unit time
$\bar{V}$ = mean velocity of fluid
r_i = inside radius
η = fluid viscosity.

The effect of inside radius on the pressure drop is self-evident. This is graphically shown in Figure 1, which shows that when the tube radius gets below 0.2 cm, flows in the range of 300 cm^3/min (normal limb blood flow) result in a very large mean pressure drop of about 35 mm Hg over a 10-cm segment. Also, the effect of increasing the mean velocity $\bar{V}$ is apparent from Eq. 2. The inside radius of the artery and the flow velocity become of great importance in understanding the pressure–flow changes that occur with arterial narrowing.

May et al. (1963a and b) studied, experimentally, the effects of a short (1 cm), fixed stenosis on flow through the iliac arteries of dogs.

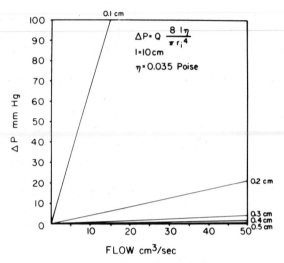

Figure 1. The relationship between blood flow and the mean pressure drop across tubes varying in diameter from 0.1 to 0.5 cm. Tube length is 10 cm. From D. E. Strandness, Jr., and D. S. Sumner, Hemodynamics for Surgeons. Grune and Stratton, Inc., New York, New York, 1975. Reprinted with permission.

These authors found no reduction in pressure and flow until the cross-sectional area of the artery was reduced by 80%; likewise, the mean pressure drop was less than 10% of the value in the prestenotic segment until this level of lumen reduction was achieved (Figure 2). To express some of these important relationships, the authors arrived at the following formulation:

$$\Delta P = \frac{8\eta L}{r_1^2}\, V_1\left(\frac{A_1}{A_2}\right)^2 + \frac{4.8\eta}{r_1}\, V_1\left(\frac{A_1}{A_2}\right)^{3/2} + pV_1^2\left(\frac{A_1}{A_2}\right)^2 \qquad (3)$$

where

A_1 and r_1 represent the cross-sectional area and radius of the pre- and poststenotic arterial segments.

A_2 is the area of the stenotic segment.

L is the length of the stenotic segment.

From Eq. 3 it is possible to calculate the relationship between the radius of the stenotic segment and velocity in the prestenotic segment on the measured mean pressure drop. It must be stressed that the pressure drops must always exceed those predicted by Poiseuille's law, which is based only on the viscous losses. Some variables that are known to affect

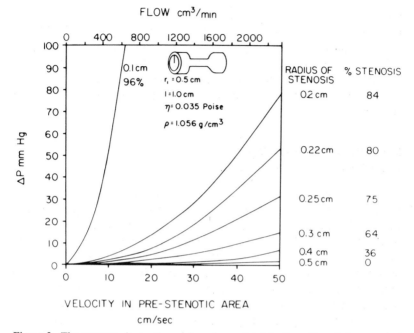

Figure 2. The pressure drop across a stenosis as related to the radius of the narrowed segment. Curves based upon Eq. 3. From D. E. Strandness, Jr., and D. S. Sumner, Hemodynamics for Surgeons. Grune and Stratton, Inc., New York, New York, 1975. Reprinted with permission.

both pressure and flow include arterial geometry, entrance and exit effects, roughness elements, flow profile, and pulsatile nature of the input to the system (Berguer and Hwang, 1974; Byar et al., 1965; Roos, 1962; Young and Tsai, 1973).

The formulation proposed by May et al. (1963a and b) has been justifiably criticized by Berguer and Hwang (1974). They properly indicated that Poiseuille's law cannot be applied to pulsatile flow through a stenotic segment and, second, that the portion of the equation dealing with the pressure loss due to expansion,

$$\Delta P_E = p V_1^2 \left(\frac{A_1}{A_2}\right)^2,$$

cannot be derived from the classical equations. Although these criticisms are well taken, Eq. 3 can be used effectively to illustrate some important points concerning critical stenoses. For example, in the idealized stenosis in Figure 3, at low flow rates equivalent to volume flows of 200–300 cm^3/min (mean velocity approximately 5 cm/sec), a greater than 95% reduction in cross-sectional area would be required for a 10 mm Hg pressure drop. With a flow rate approximately eight times that, with a velocity of 50 cm/sec, the same pressure drop would occur with a 60% stenosis.

PRESSURE-FLOW CHANGES
WITH COMPLETE ARTERIAL OCCLUSION

As the arterial plaque gradually enlarges to the point of completely obstructing the vessel, a new set of considerations is brought into play. First, without some set of alternate pathways around the obstruction, the ischemic part would die. Second, the extent of the problems produced by the occlusion is dependent on the resistance of the alternate pathways, the collaterals, and that offered by the arterioles. Third, it is not adequate to discuss the function of the collaterals in terms of resting flow rates alone, because these channels do vary in their ability to respond to the needs of increasing flow requirements. Also, there is now good evidence that collateral artery function can improve with time and under the influence of such programs as exercise.

It is important briefly to consider, in general terms, the anatomy of the collateral arteries (Longland, 1953). These arteries are preexisting channels and are not formed de novo in response to ischemia. The vessels themselves can be described in terms of their location referable to the site of occlusion as shown in Figure 4. The stem and reentry channels are the largest and least critical in terms of resistance to flow. Those vessels that constitute the midzone are the smallest and are the channels that undergo the greatest transformation when called on to assume the major transport role for blood bypassing the area of occlusion. Experimental studies in the dog have shown that with acute occlusion, the midzone collaterals may not be visible initially on angiographic studies. However, with the passage of time, they increase in size as they carry more blood to the ischemic areas.

Hemodynamically, the problem with collateral channels generally is their small size and therefore increased resistance to flow. The extent to which they can vary in size and add to the resistance to flow is extremely variable, as illustrated in Figure 5. Each of these patients had chronic arterial occlusion with differing degrees of disability.

% STENOSIS A_2/A_1 x 100

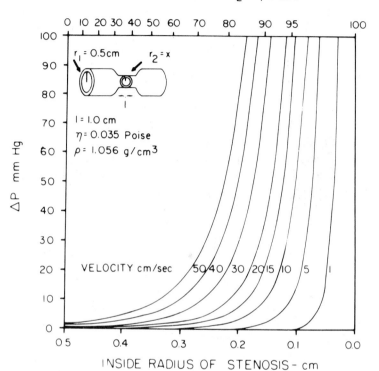

Figure 3. The effect of increasing flow velocity through stenoses of varying diameter on the mean pressure drop. From D. E. Strandness, Jr., and D. S. Sumner, Hemodynamics for Surgeons. Grune and Stratton, Inc., New York, New York, 1975. Reprinted with permission.

Figure 6 schematically illustrates the relationship between pressures and resistances with one single stenosis and one collateral bed. Using this type of electrical analog, it is possible to express its effect on total limb blood flow by the following relationship:

$$Q_T = \frac{P_A - P_B}{R_{CS} + R_D} \tag{4}$$

where

Q_T = total limb flow

P_A = mean pressure proximal to disease

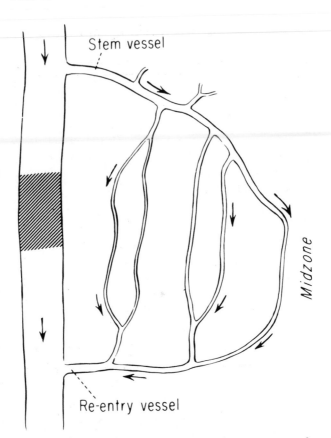

Figure 4. Schematic diagram indicating the three major components of a collateral bed.

P_B =   mean pressure distal to disease

R_{CS} =   the combined resistance to flow of the stenosis and the collateral channels

R_D =   resistance of all vessels distal to the diseased area.

Since R_{CS} is usually abnormally high, total limb blood flow, Q_T, can remain constant only if R_D decreases. The resistances summed in the R_D term constitute the medium-sized small arteries and the arterioles. It is presumed, and probably true, that the greatest decrease in resistance

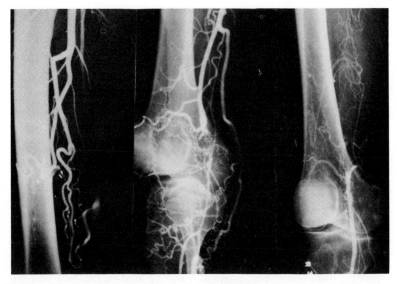

Figure 5. Three examples of the marked variation that can occur in the extent of the collateral artery development about an area of occlusion involving the same arterial segment. The patients in the left and middle panel were essentially asymptomatic with no measurable pressure drop across the involved area. The patient illustrated in the right panel had intermittent claudication with a large pressure gradient even at rest.

occurs at the level of the arterioles that is essential in maintaining resting flow at a normal level. As is pointed out later, resting blood flow, even with multiple levels of occlusion, i.e., multiple collateral channels in series, is usually within the normal range.

For the most part, the inefficiency of the collateral channels becomes obvious when there is a marked demand for flow that occurs during periods of stress, such as exercise or reactive hyperemia. Because exercise increases the metabolic requirements of muscle, there is a further decrease in R_D as the intramuscular arteries become widely dilated in an attempt to increase flow to meet the needs of the tissue. This initiates a whole series of complex events that affect the hemodynamic performance of the diseased arterial system. These can be summarized as follows:

1. Cardiac output increases to an extent determined by the workload.
2. The resistance to flow offered by R_{CS} probably remains fixed although there is some indirect evidence that it may acutely decrease slightly.

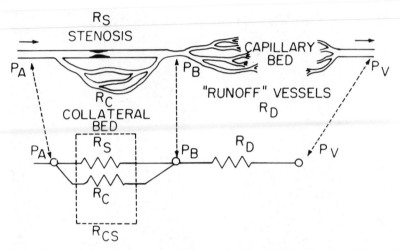

Figure 6. Electrical analog of an arterial stenosis, the parallel collateral arteries and the arteries distal to the site of disease. See text. From D. E. Strandness, Jr., and D. S. Summer, Hemodynamics for Surgeons. Grune and Stratton, Inc., New York, New York, 1975. Reprinted with permission.

3. R_D falls to very low levels, increasing the flow and flow velocity through the very small collateral arteries in the midzone.

4. As flow increases across the midzone collaterals, the pressure drop, P_A-P_B, increases even further.

5. The pressure P_B is countered by the pressure generated by the contracting muscle, further reducing the perfusion of the ischemic muscle.

The problem that occurs is related to the relatively fixed collateral resistance R_{CS}. This bypassing network is simply unable to accommodate the large flows required to prevent muscular ischemia and leads to many of the hemodynamic changes that are so well documented. Another factor of great importance is that multiple levels of occlusion bring into play additional collateral beds that add to the total resistance to flow. In fact, the resistances in series are indeed additive, thus further compounding the ischemic problem of the most distal part of the limb (Sumner and Strandness, 1969). This fact is of great importance in understanding the pressure–flow changes that occur with advancing disease, particularly when limb viability is in question; it is well known that removal of or bypassing the most proximal level of collaterals can greatly improve pressure and flow through more distant collateral circuits (Strandness, 1969).

REVIEW OF HEMODYNAMIC
CHANGES ASSOCIATED WITH ATHEROSCLEROSIS

The human arterial system is unique, as it relates to the effects of atherosclerosis, since there is no animal model, at least not yet studied, that accurately mimics the disease seen in man. Although it is possible to use invasive methods in an animal model to quantitate the fluid dynamics associated with arterial occlusion, it is very difficult to continue these studies longitudinally over a period of months to years. This is of great practical importance because it is now known that atherosclerosis progresses at variable rates, making it dangerous to draw meaningful conclusions from either acute or short-term experiments.

Although it is not within the scope of this chapter to review the methods available for studies in humans, it is necessary at least to consider the type of information that can be obtained. Ideally, it would be necessary directly to measure volume flow, flow velocity, vascular dimensions, wall properties, and pressure changes in order to describe the hemodynamic events more completely. This would require, at least at the present time, anesthesia, exposure of vessels proximal and distal to the vascular bed of interest, and the employment of a variety of measuring devices to obtain the necessary data. This is obviously impossible in the human and for this reason most studies tend to examine those variables that can be estimated by using noninvasive devices, such as plethysmographs (Dahn, 1965; Hillestad, 1963a and b), Doppler flowmeters (Strandness and Sumner, 1975; Yao, 1970), pulse volume recorders (Darling et al., 1972; Strandness and Bell, 1965), and some systems that permit an estimation of at least systolic blood pressure (Strandness and Bell, 1965; Strandness and Sumner, 1975). Although the data are not at all inclusive of all the desired hemodynamic information, a great deal has been accomplished in understanding the pressure and flow changes which take place.

Normal Pressure—Flow Changes at Rest

The normal lower extremity has a resting blood flow somewhere in the range of 300–600 cc/min, which is accommodated with a drop of only a few mm Hg in mean arterial pressure. In terms of the pulsatile pressure and flow, there is a gradual amplification of the systolic pressure so that at the level of the distal limb, it exceeds that recorded from the central aorta (McDonald, 1960). Also, the shape of the pressure pulse waveform is gradually transformed from one that is roughly triangular shaped in the central aorta to a wave with prominent dicrotic wave on the downslope (Figure 7). Although there is gradual amplification in the systolic blood pressure, there are also changes in both flow velocity and direction that are important to recognize since they are altered by atherosclerosis. These pressure and flow changes are a consequence of the nonuniform characteristics of the normal arterial system and are not considered further in this chapter. For technical reasons, most measurements of pressure and flow in the human have been limited to estimation of systolic pressure and regional blood flow. With regard to pressure, a variety of sensors can be used to measure the systolic pressure at any level of the limb and compare it to that recorded from the arm (Strandness and Bell, 1965; Strandness and Sumner, 1975). Normally, the ankle systolic pressure should be equal to, or exceed that, recorded from the arm (Carter, 1969). This fact is of great importance in recognizing hemodynamically significant arterial lesions proximal to the ankle.

Blood flow in the limbs can be measured regionally (finger, foot, calf)

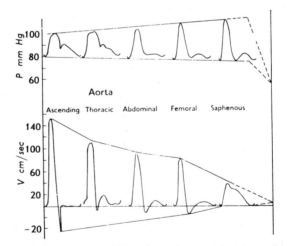

Figure 7. Changes in pressure and flow from the central aorta to the level of the saphenous artery in the dog. Redrawn, with permission, from D. A. McDonald, Blood Flow in Arteries. Baltimore, Williams and Wilkins, 1960.

or in specific tissues, such as muscle, fat, and skin. The regional blood flows are usually measured by plethysmographic techniques, which, of course, do not permit a separation of flows in the various tissues or compartments of the limb. Flows to specific tissues can be accomplished by the use of isotope clearance techniques where the tag is deposited in the tissue of interest.

The level of blood flow to the calf under resting conditions is usually in the range of 1.5—6.5 ml/100 ml/min depending upon such factors as the ambient temperature (Elsner and Carlson, 1962; Livingstone, 1961; Ludbrook, 1966; Snell, Eastcott, and Hamilton, 1960). The magnitude of the blood flow to the foot or toes is considerably less on a volume basis than it is to the hand and the fingers (Allwood and Burry, 1954; Conrad, 1968). Flow, particularly to the digits, can vary over a wide range depending upon the environmental conditions and emotional state of the patient. For example, fingertip flow, which is primarily skin, may vary from 1.0 ml/100 ml/min to as much as 300 ml/100 ml/min (Mead and Schoenfeld, 1950). As is pointed out below, the level of resting blood flow determined either for a region or a specific tissue is rarely altered significantly even with rather extensive arterial disease. This is because the resistance R_D, shown in Figure 6, may be reduced sufficiently to maintain flow at normal resting levels.

Normal Pressure—Flow Changes With Stress

The pathophysiology of arterial narrowing and occlusion is most completely described by noting the response when large increases in flow are required by either exercise or reactive hyperemia. For this reason, it is important briefly to review some of the normal responses. While there are some differences between the changes that occur with reactive hyperemia and exercise, the latter best serves as an example for discussion.

Total limb blood flow increases dramatically with exercise, the final level depending upon the severity of the stress (Figure 8). A fivefold increase with moderate exercise is not at all unusual (Pentecost, 1964). Flow measured by ^{133}Xe in the gastrocnemius muscle has shown that flow rises to 10—20 times its resting level when normal subjects walk 160 meters at 4.8 km/hr (Lassen and Kampp, 1965). The flow generally remains at a constant level during the exercise period. The normal response after cessation of exercise is for flow to very rapidly return to the preexercise level, often within the first minute.

The changes in systolic blood pressure of the lower limbs have also

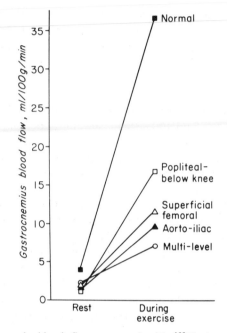

Figure 8. Calf muscle blood flow measured with ¹³³Xe in normal subjects and patients with arterial disease at different levels.

been studied extensively. If the ankle systolic pressure is expressed as a ratio to the arm systolic pressure, it provides an ankle/arm index which is normally greater than or equal to 1. When a normal subject is stressed maximally by graded exercise, the ankle pressure falls immediately post exercise to a variable degree but within 1–2 min it returns to near its preexercise level (Stahler and Strandness, 1967). However, at the lower work loads that are commonly used to evaluate the pressure–flow changes in patients, the ankle systolic pressure either remains unchanged or increases slightly (Figure 9).

Pressure–Flow Changes at Rest in Patients With Atherosclerosis

Systolic Pressure–Calf Blood Flow   It has been well established that the amount of blood flow delivered to skin and muscle under resting conditions is usually within normal levels even in the presence of multiple levels of occlusion (Sumner and Strandness, 1969). This is, of course, possible only by a reduction in peripheral resistance below that normally

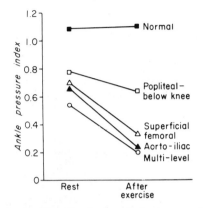

Figure 9. Ankle pressure index for the same patient groups shown in Figure 8.

present. However, even with tissue blood flow at normal levels, there is a reduction in the systolic pressure distal to the disease resulting from energy losses as the blood traverses the high-resistance collateral bed. The extent of the decrease in systolic pressure at the ankle accurately reflects the extent of the added resistance by either single or multiple collateral beds in series. As shown in Figure 9, there is a progressive fall in ankle pressure with more severe disease. In general, if the ankle systolic pressure is greater than 50% of arm systolic pressure, there is only one level of occlusion.

A point of considerable importance is that there are patients with arterial stenoses who have essentially normal ankle systolic pressures at rest. For example, in the study by Carter (1972) (see Figure 10), there were some patients with mild stenoses discovered on angiographic studies who had essentially normal ankle systolic pressures. An example of such a case is shown in Figure 11. As is pointed out later, the presence of disease in this group of patients can often be brought out by increasing the flow across the stenosis, accentuating the energy losses, thus "unmasking" the arterial narrowing (Carter, 1972; Brener et al., 1974).

One of the more difficult problems in assessing the hemodynamic effects of arterial disease is the great variation from patient to patient, even with complete arterial occlusion. In Figure 5, collateral pathways that developed in response to complete occlusions involving the superficial femoral-popliteal area in three patients are shown. The collaterals that are apparent in the left and middle panels were of sufficient size to keep the

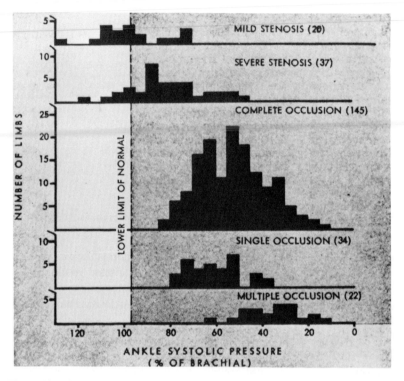

Figure 10. The relationship between the ankle systolic pressure (expressed as percent of brachial) in 202 patients with peripheral arteriosclerosis. All patients had arteriography for verification and classification of the extent of disease. From S. A. Carter, Clinical measurement of systolic pressures in limbs with arterial occlusion. JAMA 207:1869, 1969. Reprinted with permission.

patient essentially normal, hemodynamically, with daily activity. However, the patient shown on the right panel had a significant reduction in systolic pressure at rest and was disabled with intermittent claudication. For this reason, it is important to understand that each patient has his or her own hemodynamic response to atherosclerosis that is dependent upon many factors such as location and extent of the disease, functional characteristics of the collateral circulation, cardiac function, level of sympathetic activity, and coexisting diseases such as diabetes mellitus.

Limb Volume Pulse—Arterial Flow Velocity

The manner in which the limb, foot, or digit volume changes with each cardiac cycle does provide some useful information with regard to the

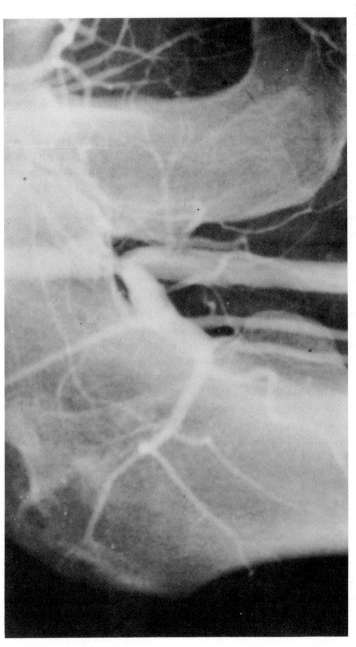

Figure 11. The stenosis in the common femoral artery was not hemodynamically significant at rest. However, with exercise, a fall in pressure distal to this lesion did occur.

presence of arterial disease. These can be recorded with a mercury strain gauge (Strandness and Bell, 1965), segmental pulse volume recorder (Darling et al., 1972), or impedance plethysmograph (Van De Water and Mount, 1973). The observed changes that occur with atherosclerosis include a delay in the rise time of the pulse and a loss of the dicrotic wave on the downslope. The pulse is highly damped because some of the higher harmonics are lost, owing to the arterial disease.

With the development of the ultrasonic velocity detector, it has become possible noninvasively to investigate in a qualitative fashion the effect of arterial disease on the velocity pattern. Depending on the artery being examined, most peripheral arteries have a relatively constant velocity pattern of the type shown in Figure 12. The normal velocity pattern has essentially three separate phases that characterize the waveform (Strandness and Sumner, 1975; Yao, 1970). First, there is the most prominent, high-velocity component associated with systole. Second, during early diastole as flow deceleration occurs, there is often a very brief period when flow entirely reverses. This is a normal finding in the femoral artery and brachial artery and can be observed as far peripherally as the tibial arteries. Third, just before systole, there is a small but definite late forward flow component. When this type of velocity pattern is observed, there is no significant arterial disease proximal to the recording site.

With the development of arterial narrowing and occlusion, several changes take place. If the recording is made downstream from the stenosis, there is a reduction in the peak velocity, the rise time (foot to peak) of the velocity is prolonged, flow reversal disappears, flow does not return to zero, and the late forward flow pattern is also not seen (Figure 12).

Gosling and King (1974) have placed two Doppler probes successively and simultaneously at specific points in the lower extremity to evaluate transit time and a term, which they refer to as the pulsatility index. The pulsatility index is defined as shown in Figure 13. The index (PI) is independent of the ordinate scale factor, and therefore vessel-probe geometry, and may be used to compare waveforms between different sites of the same subject or between patients.

Pressure–Flow Changes With Exercise in Patients With Atherosclerosis

As previously mentioned, the arterial system, even when involved with extensive disease, is able to compensate and satisfy the resting requirements for blood flow in most cases. A more complete description of the pathophysiology is possible when the response to stress is examined. The

Brachial artery flow

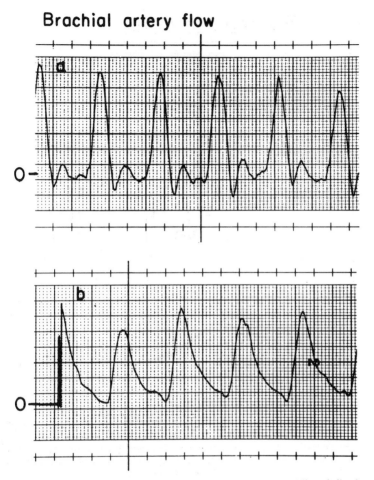

Figure 12. The velocity tracings from a normal brachial artery (A) and distal to a subclavian artery occlusion (B). See text for explanation.

diseased arterial system, particularly with stenoses and occlusions, cannot accommodate the large flow demands of the exercising muscle.

Before considering in some detail the hemodynamic changes, a few general points should be made. First, profound changes in pressure and flow occur at very low work loads which produce only a minimal response in the normal subject (Strandness and Bell, 1964). Second, the primary abnormality that is responsible for the pressure–flow changes is the abnor-

$$PI = \frac{Peak\ to\ Peak}{mean}$$

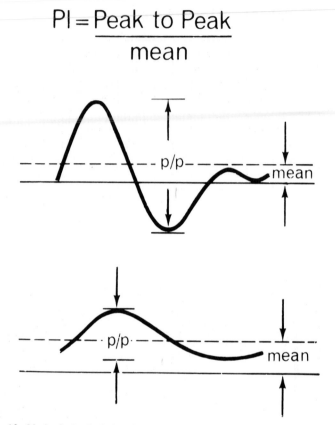

Figure 13. Method of calculating the pulsatility index from a velocity waveform. The examples indicate how this is accomplished with varying waveform shape. From R. G. Gosling and D. H. King, Ultrasonic Angiology in Arteries and Veins. Edinburgh, Churchill Livingstone, 1974. Reprinted with permission.

mally high resistance offered by the collateral channels. Third, since many of the patients with atherosclerosis involving the peripheral arteries also have coexisting coronary artery disease, changes in myocardial performance may affect the peripheral vascular response.

Most of the studies done of the peripheral vascular response have been carried out immediately before and after exercise. The flow response has usually been measured at the calf level by using a plethysmograph or the measurement of isotope clearance with the injectate deposited in skeletal muscle. Limb blood pressures (systolic) are made at the ankle level. Patients with chronic atherosclerosis have as their most common complaint muscle pain brought on by exercise and promptly relieved by rest—so-called intermittent claudication.

The work loads employed to characterize the pressure—flow response are minimal. In our laboratory, a treadmill set at 2 mph and a 12% grade has been the standard exercise procedure. This is a comfortable walking speed that produces no problems even with elderly patients.

As exercise proceeds, flow to muscle occurs during two phases: muscle contraction and muscle relaxation. During contraction, the muscle generates a pressure that tends to counter the transmural pressure in those arteries supplying the exercising unit (Lassen and Kampp, 1965; Walder, 1958). This counter pressure is, of course, absent during relaxation so that the greatest flow increment occurs during this time. Muscular ischemia may rapidly develop because of a combination of the following: (1) the perfusion pressure distal to the disease and that available for the muscle are already reduced even at rest; (2) as exercise proceeds with a marked fall in intramuscular resistance due to the ischemia, the perfusion pressure tends to fall even further; (3) the collateral network, because of its high resistance and the small size of the midzone arteries, cannot accommodate the increased flow; (4) because flow, and therefore flow velocity, increase through the midzone arteries, energy losses are increased, thus adding to the problem of the pressure fall that is so important for perfusing the intramuscular arteries; and (5) a vicious cycle is initiated by exercise that can be reversed only by stopping walking.

The flow delivered to the limb with arterial disease varies in two major ways: (1) the peak flows achieved immediately after exercise are often lower than normal; and (2) the time required for the flow to return to baseline is prolonged (Sumner and Strandness, 1969; Snell et al., 1960). This time period is commonly referred to as the period of postexercise hyperemia. Although it is true that in some patients with minimal disability the peak postexercise flows achieved with limited exercise may fall in the normal range, the period of postexercise hyperemia is delayed. Hillestad (1963a) showed that with 1 min of supine exercise, 73% of the total postexercise flow occurred within the first minute after exercise, as compared to only 33% in patients with intermittent claudication.

When the entire spectrum of postexercise flow patterns is examined, it is possible to characterize in general terms essentially three types of responses (Figure 14) (Sumner and Strandness, 1969). With the type-I

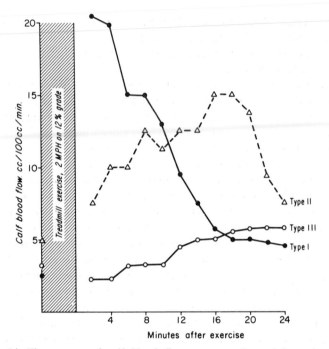

Figure 14. Three types of calf blood flow patterns observed in patients with atherosclerosis and intermittent claudication. See text for explanation.

response, peak calf blood flows are reached within the first 2 min but there is pronounced delay in recovery. This type of flow pattern is most often observed with disease confined to a single level and an excellent collateral network. In the type-II response, the peak calf blood flow may be markedly delayed even though the initial postexercise values exceed the resting level. This pattern is most often observed with disease at two levels, such as aortoiliac and femoropopliteal. The most abnormal pattern is the type-III response, where the postexercise levels are below even the resting level. This pattern is seen only in patients with the most far-advanced disease whose perfusion even at rest is inadequate to meet the nutritional needs of the feet and toes. A more complete description of the hemodynamic changes can be made if the measurement of calf blood flow can be combined with determination of ankle systolic pressure. The pattern observed in a patient with iliac artery occlusion is shown in Figure 15. As noted, there is an inverse relationship between pressure and flow. When

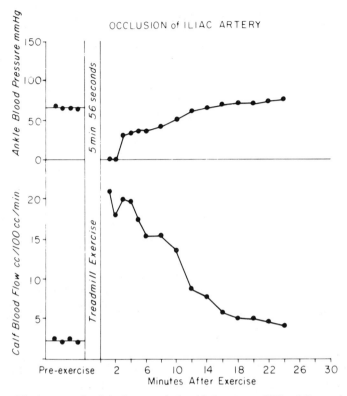

Figure 15. An example of the inverse relationship between calf blood flow and ankle systolic pressure after walking to the point of claudication.

the calf blood flows and ankle pressures are compared, as related to the level and extent of occlusion, there is an excellent correlation (Figure 16). Although this should not be surprising, this observation has important clinical implications. Because there is such a good correlation, it is possible using the ankle blood pressure response alone to predict the pattern of the calf blood flow response and thus, indirectly at least, to assess the severity of the disease.

Another factor of great importance that has emerged from studies of this type is that any changes in collateral artery resistance can be objectively assessed by examining both the resting ankle systolic pressure and, most importantly, its response to exercise. This has great practical importance in evaluating the results of both operative and nonoperative therapy

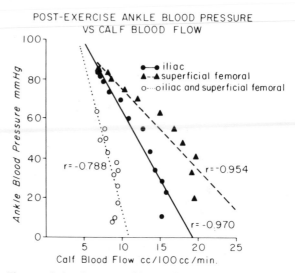

POST-EXERCISE ANKLE BLOOD PRESSURE
VS CALF BLOOD FLOW

Figure 16. The correlation between ankle systolic pressure and calf blood flow when the patients are subdivided according to the level of the arterial occlusion. From D. S. Sumner and D. E. Strandness, Jr., The relationship between calf blood flow and ankle blood pressure in patients with intermittent claudication. Surgery 65:763, 1969. Reprinted with permission.

(Skinner and Strandness, 1967; Strandness, 1970). If an occluded artery has been successfully replaced or bypassed, the ankle systolic pressure and exercise response should be restored to normal. Furthermore, if new disease develops or the arterial reconstruction fails, the newly added resistance is reflected in a return of the pressure–flow changes to a more abnormal state.

It is also becoming apparent that collateral artery resistance may not be static and may change because of factors not yet understood. While physicians have long been aware that, particularly following an acute arterial occlusion, collateral artery resistance can and does decrease, allowing better perfusion of the limb, it is not generally appreciated that with time (months, years), these changes can continue. An example of this is shown in Figure 17. The ankle pressure, when expressed as the arm/ankle ratio, is normal if it is 1.0 or less. This patient received no treatment; nevertheless, between 6 mo after an occlusion and 2 yr, the ratio decreased from over two to slightly above one.

There is also good evidence that exercise training, if regularly and

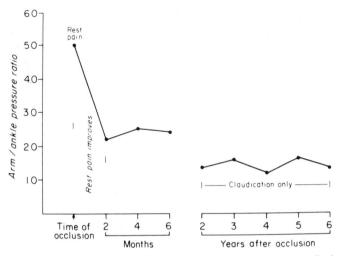

Figure 17. The changes in the arm/ankle pressure ratio ($\leqslant 1$ is normal) that can occur following acute arterial occlusion.

rigorously pursued, can result in an increase in ankle systolic pressure without a concomitant change in central pressure, an increase in walking time and, most importantly, an improvement in the postexercise pressure–flow changes (Skinner and Strandness, 1967). The mechanisms responsible for these apparent changes in collateral artery resistance remain unexplained.

WHAT OF THE FUTURE?

It is clear that many of the pressure and flow changes that occur secondarily to atherosclerosis are well understood. However, it must be emphasized that these changes, with few exceptions, are the results of a disease that has already reached an advanced stage. The question that remains to be answered is whether it is feasible to detect changes, particularly in such variables as the velocity profile, at a stage when disease is certainly at the preclinical level and is hopefully reversible if and when the appropriate treatment is found.

The measurement of instantaneous flow changes throughout the pulse cycle and across the arterial cross section is a formidable undertaking; it requires the sophistication of pulsed ultrasonic techniques that can then be applied transcutaneously at selected sites to actually measure the velocity profile. Initial progress has already been demonstrated, but the only results in humans so far reported are by Brunner et al. (1974). These authors, using a pulsed Doppler with 14 gates, have been able to map the velocity distribution in 11 normal subjects and 13 patients with peripheral atherosclerosis. In the normal common femoral artery, the velocity profile is symmetric except for the brief phase of late systolic flow deceleration. It is of interest that there was a steep rise near the vessel wall, but a flat distribution across the remainder of the diameter. However, in patients with atherosclerosis, the early reversal of flow disappeared and the profiles were asymmetric when there was definite intimal disease in the region of the velocity measurement. The extent to which studies of this type may be useful in identifying the earlier changes brought about by atherosclerosis remains to be demonstrated.

LITERATURE CITED

Allwood, M. J., and H. S. Burry. 1954. The effect of local temperature on blood flow in the human foot. J. Physiol. (Lond) 124: 345.

Berguer, R., and N. H. C. Hwang. 1974. Critical arterial stenosis. A theoretical and experimental solution. Ann. Surg. 180: 39.

Brener, B. J., J. K. Raines, R. C. Darling, and W. G. Austen. 1974. Measurement of systolic femoral arterial pressure during reactive hyperemia. An estimate of aortoiliac disease. Circulation Suppl. II: II-259.

Brunner, H. H., A. Bollinger, M. Anliker, H. J. Zweifel, and W. Rutishauser. 1974. Bestimmung instanter strömungsgeschwindigkeits profile in der A. femoralis communis mit gepulstem Doppler-ultraschall bei stenosen und verschlüssen der beckenarterien. Deutsch. Med. Wschr. 99: 3.

Byar, D., R. V. Fiddian, M. Quereau, J. T. Hobbs, and E. A. Edwards. 1965. The fallacy of applying Poiseuille equation to segmental arterial stenosis. Am. Heart. J. 70: 216.

Carter, S. A. 1969. Clinical measurements of systolic pressures in limbs with arterial occlusive disease. JAMA 207: 1869.

Carter, S. A. 1972. Response to ankle systolic pressure to leg exercise in mild or questionable arterial disease. N. Engl. J. Med. 287: 578.

Conrad, M. C. 1968. Abnormalities of the digit vasculature as related to ulceration and gangrene. Circulation 38: 568.

Dahn, I. 1965. On clinical use of venous occlusion plethysmography of calf. II. Results in patients with arterial disease. Acta Chir. Scand. 130: 61.

Darling, R. C., J. K. Raines, B. J. Brener, and W. G. Austen. 1972.

Quantitative segmental pulse volume recorder. A clinical tool. Surgery 72: 873.

Elsner, R. W., and L. D. Carlson. 1962. Post-exercise hyperemia in trained and untrained subjects. J. Appl. Physiol. 17: 436.

Gosling, R. G., and D. H. King. 1974. Ultrasonic Angiology in Arteries and Veins. Churchill Livingstone, Edinburgh.

Hillestad, L. K. 1963a. The peripheral blood flow in intermittent claudication. V. Plethysmographic studies. The significance of calf blood flow at rest and in response to timed arrest of the circulation. Acta Med. Scand. 174: 23.

Hillestad, L. K. 1963b. The peripheral blood flow in intermittent claudication. VI. Plethysmographic studies. The blood flow response to exercise with arrested and free circulation. Acta Med. Scand. 174: 23.

Lassen, N. A., and M. Kampp. 1965. Calf muscle blood flow during walking studied by the Xe^{133} method in normals and in patients with intermittent claudication. Scand. J. Clin. Lab. Invest. 17: 447.

Livingstone, R. A. 1961. Blood flow in the calf of the leg after running. Am. Heart J. 61: 219.

Longland, C. J. 1953. The collateral circulation of the limb. Ann. Roy. Coll. Surg. Eng. 13: 161.

Ludbrook, J. 1966. Collateral artery resistance in the human lower limb. J. Surg. Res. 6: 423.

May, A. G., J. A. DeWeese, and C. G. Rob. 1963a. Hemodynamic effects of arterial stenosis. Surgery 53: 513.

May, A. G., L. Van de Berg, J. A. DeWeese, and C. G. Rob. 1963b. Critical arterial stenosis. Surgery 54: 250.

McDonald, D. A. 1960. Blood Flow in Arteries. Williams and Wilkins, Baltimore, p. 328.

Mead, J., and R. C. Schoenfeld. 1950. Character of blood flow in the vasodilated fingers. J. Appl. Physiol. 2: 680.

Pentecost, B. L. 1964. The effect of exercise on the external iliac vein blood flow and local oxygen consumption in normal subjects and in those with occlusive vascular disease. Clin. Sci. 27: 437.

Roos, A. 1962. Poiseuille's law and its limitation in vascular systems. Med. Thorac. 19: 224.

Skinner, J. S., and D. E. Strandness, Jr. 1967. Exercise and intermittent claudication. II. Effect of physical training. Circulation 36: 23.

Snell, E. S., H. H. G. Eastcott, and M. Hamilton. 1960. Circulation in the lower limb before and after reconstruction of obstructed main artery. Lancet 1: 242.

Stahler, C., and D. E. Strandness, Jr. 1967. Ankle blood pressure response to graded treadmill exercise. Angiology 18: 237.

Strandness, D. E., Jr. 1969. Peripheral Arterial Disease: A Physiologic Approach. Little, Brown, Boston, Chapter 9.

Strandness, D. E., Jr. 1970. Exercise testing in the evaluation of patients undergoing direct arterial surgery. J. Cardiovasc. Surg. 11: 192.

Strandness, D. E., Jr., and J. W. Bell. 1964. An evaluation of the hemo-
dynamic response of the claudicating extremity to exercise. Surg.
Gynecol. Obstet. 119: 1237.
Strandness, D. E., Jr., and J. W. Bell. 1965. Peripheral vascular disease:
Diagnosis and objective evaluation using a mercury strain gauge. Ann.
Surg. 161 (Suppl).
Strandness, D. E., Jr., and D. S. Sumner. 1975. Ultrasonic Techniques in
Angiology. Hans Huber, Berne, p. 146.
Sumner, D. S., and D. E. Strandness, Jr. 1969. The relationship between
calf blood flow and ankle blood pressure in patients with intermittent
claudication. Surgery 65: 763.
Van De Water, J. M., and B. E. Mount. 1973. Impedance plethysmography
in the lower extremity. J. Surg. Res. 15: 22.
Walder, D. N. 1958. A technique for investigating the blood supply of
muscle during exercise. Brit. Med. J. 1: 255.
Yao, S. T. 1970. Experience with the Doppler ultrasound flow velocity
meter in peripheral vascular disease. In J. A. Gillespie (ed.), Modern
Trends in Vascular Surgery, Chap. 15. Butterworths, London.
Young, D. F., and F. W. Tsai. 1973. Flow characteristics in models of
arterial stenoses. II. Unsteady flow. J. Biomech. 6: 547.

Cardiovascular Flow Dynamics and Measurements
Edited by N. H. C. Hwang and N. A. Normann
Copyright 1977   University Park Press   Baltimore

chapter 9

CARDIOVASCULAR STUDIES OF U.S. SPACE CREWS:
An Overview and Perspective

G. Wyckliffe Hoffler

ABSTRACT

Early concerns for adverse effects upon man from exposure to the weightlessness of space have proved to be largely unfounded. Nevertheless, significant symptomatology and physiologic alterations do occur, apparently as adaptive phenomena, both upon entry into orbit and upon return to earth gravity. The cardiovascular system figures prominently in much of the observed changes, which include weight loss, decrements in leg mass, cephalad shift of body fluids, decreased blood volume and heart size, and variations in orthostatic tolerance and exercise capacity.

Accumulation of sufficient data, from which a composite picture can be pieced and by which reasonable hypotheses could be formulated, has required multiple investigative teams working with crews of many and varied space missions. Development of special and unusual procedures and techniques has become necessary. Parallel ground-based studies designed to reproduce as nearly as possible inflight findings have greatly aided integration and understanding of the space data. Challenges continue, however, and await more sophisticated, or perhaps orthodox, investigations which the Space Shuttle era promises.

INTRODUCTION AND BACKGROUND

Well before orbital space flight became a reality, much conjecture and hypothesizing had dealt with possible and probable effects of weightlessness upon man's cardiovascular system (Berry, 1973). This concern was in large part due to, and perhaps justified by, the very mobile character of the contents of the vascular tree. Accompanying early experience with manned flights, significant consequences of exposure to the space environment were seen in clinical symptomatology and in physiologic test observations, generally demonstrating a reduced postflight orthostatic tolerance (Catterson et al., 1963; Berry and Catterson, 1967). Orthostatic tolerance may be defined as the ability of primates to stand and function in the upright position by means of developed and adapted anatomic structures and physiologic mechanisms of the cardiovascular system for countering hydrostatic forces imposed by gravity.

Since man functions usually in the erect stance with the long axis of his body oriented parallel to the gravitational force vector at the surface of the earth, this position may be considered his normal state. The price, however, is a continuous contest against fluid drift or pooling into the dependent end of the body, the ultimate consequences of which produce syncope. Routine and habitual departures from erect posture, such as horizontal sleep, induce significant cyclical internal alterations, and a diurnal pattern has been determined for human orthostatic tolerance (Aschoff and Aschoff, 1969).

Because the cardiovascular system conforms to many aspects of a closed hydraulic design, redistribution of hydrostatic pressures accompanies changes in body posture. A teleological objective of the primate circulatory system is to maintain adequate cerebral blood pressure, circulation, and perfusion, which normally operate at the low-pressure, or cephalad, end of the long axis of the body.

For a rigid system, internal hydrostatic pressures would be a function of the angle this long axis makes with the horizontal and the distance from a pivotal or zero reference point. This latter hydrostatic indifference point has been measured to be slightly below the diaphragm in erect human beings (Gauer and Thron, 1965). Since human beings, and certainly their vascular systems, are not rigid, this transitional zone shifts headward with head-down tilt or headward acceleration stress. It may be presumed to shift, at least qualitatively, in like fashion in space where no acceleration forces impinge on the total organism. In any case, all mechanisms and functions normally combatting the inexorable force of gravity on earth suddenly become unopposed upon entry into the weightlessness of orbital flight. The net result is the symptomatology and postflight consequences noted above, apparently sequelae of whatever adaptive processes take place during this non-natural state (Gauer and Henry, 1963; Klein et al., 1969).

So simple and certain a finding as reduced postflight orthostatic tolerance has not proved as easily explained. A plausible etiology for reduced orthostatic tolerance has been sought in diminished circulating blood volume, plasma, and/or red cell mass; in increased peripheral venous compliance, altered central pump dynamics; disturbed neurologic control of the cardiovascular system; and in renal-hormonal changes induced by varying gravity vector and pressure forces. In actuality, the truth probably encompasses a little of them all, and relates directly and/or indirectly to the peculiar hypodynamia attendant exposure to weightlessness (Berry, 1973).

This overview examines currently relevant data and their permissible interpretations as of the present moment, viz., after Skylab and the Apollo–Soyuz Test Project (ASTP) missions. Much effort has been expended by many medical, physiology, and engineering teams in attaining this current level of accomplishment. The amassed data are literally astronomic and only the more obvious and pertinent determinations have received open publication. No distinctive integrative work has yet taken place. This paper is an attempt to put into perspective from available information one major physiologic area. Documented, factual returns are accorded priority. Consideration then turns to selected extrapolations that may be reasonably surmised. Finally, questions that may become grounds for important early Shuttle investigations are entertained. This summation must necessarily fall short of adequate comprehension and represents only the present step, based on incomplete knowledge, toward fully understanding physiologic functions in this newly experienced space environment.

FACTUAL DATA

Weight Loss

One of the most consistent determinations following space flight has been weight loss. Because this entity bears importantly on much of the succeeding development for cardiovascular findings, the following details are to be emphasized. The astronaut pilot lost nearly 8 lb (3.5 kg, 5.3%) during the 34-hr Mercury 9 flight in 1963 (Catterson et al., 1963). Of 18 Gemini crewmen on flights from 5 to 331 hr duration, only one returned without weight loss and the group mean loss was 5.6 lb (2.5 kg) or 3.4% of preflight weight (unpublished data, Johnson Space Center, Houston, Texas). A virtual duplication of this picture was seen in 33 Apollo crewmen flying missions from 6 to 12.6 days duration. Based on launch day weights, only two showed no decrement in weight postflight, with the group mean loss being 6.2 lb (2.8 kg) or 3.7%. Using preflight mean weights from several measurements as early as 30 days before launch, all lost weight and the mean decrement was even larger (7.8 lb, 3.5 kg, or 4.5%) (Hoffler, Wolthuis, and Johnson, 1974).

Data from the Skylab missions appear to offer further corroboration with a mean weight loss for the nine crewmen of 3.5 kg (4.9%) (unpublished data, Johnson Space Center, Houston, Texas). However, for these missions, widely varying in durations (28, 59, and 84 days), another interpretation may be legitimate, namely, an inverse relationship between weight loss and mission duration. The three Skylab crewmen of each mission averaged 5.7, 3.8, and 1.1 kg weight loss, respectively. The three ASTP crewmen in a 9-day mission averaged 2.0 kg (2.5%) weight loss (unpublished data, Johnson Space Center, Houston, Texas).

Figure 1 presents graphically the percentage weight loss versus mission duration for all U.S. space fliers. The average overall weight loss has been 2.8 kg or 3.8%. This plot allows several significant statements. Whatever may be the etiology of weight loss in the space environment, the disturb-

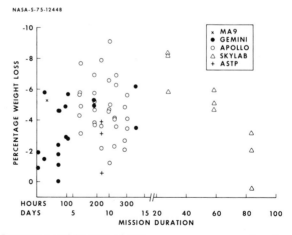

Figure 1. Percentage weight loss of U.S. space crewmen as a function of mission duration, based on preflight (usually the mean of multiple values) and immediate postflight weights.

ing stressors are at work very early after launch and they persist for several weeks. It is not possible to determine if this weight loss is wholly a function of deficit intake. However, it does appear that a stabilizing effect, or perhaps even reversing trend, has begun in the longer duration missions.

Leg Volume Decrements; Headward Mass Shift

Nearly as well documented as weight loss is the fact of a headward migration of body mass while in weightlessness. Early hypotheses of centripetal displacement of blood to the thoracic region led to predictions that a relative blood volume excess would be appreciated by volume receptors or indirectly by baroreceptors (Gauer and Henry, 1963). This in turn would evoke circulatory, hormonal, and renal responses in order to reequilibrate intravascular volume. Participation by other body fluid compartments in these adjustments to the absence of gravity has apparently received little consideration.

Measurements of maximal calf girth during early Apollo missions revealed invariably large decrements postflight. This finding was firmly quantitated throughout the Apollo program with an average calf girth decrease for 24 crewmembers of almost 3%. At that time it was reasoned that this loss represented, at least in part, atrophy of a muscle group prominently employed for human movement in 1 g, but relatively little used in weightlessness (Hoffler et al., 1974).

This type of measurement was amplified on crewmen of the last two Apollo missions in order to approximate true volume determinations. On the supine crewmen multiple circumferences were taken pre- and postflight from above the malleoli to as high on the thigh as practicable, using bony landmarks for repetitive accuracy (Figure 2). Accuracy of the method is about 1%. Calculated lower limb volumes based on assumed circular geometry showed an average loss per crewman of nearly a liter for the combined volume of both legs, or 5%; the largest loss of these six crewmen was 10%. This is more than the total preflight leg blood volume; it is, therefore, clearly obvious that the leg volume deficit must be accounted for by other than vascular contents.

Skylab provided not only confirmation of this change in leg size with even greater postflight size deficits, but also a time course of the alteration inflight. Maximal calf girths measured preceding every orthostatic tolerance test (Lower Body Negative Pressure, *v.i.*) revealed rapid, early (by fourth day) inflight decrements with very gradual flattening of the regression curve. Even in the 84-day flight, it is not fully clear that maximal calf

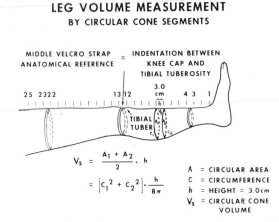

NASA S 74 3274

LEG VOLUME MEASUREMENT
BY CIRCULAR CONE SEGMENTS

Figure 2. The method of leg volume measurement by obtaining multiple circumferences. Calculation is based on assumed circular geometry and summation of multiple, trucated, conical volumes.

girth has reached a stable plateau (Figure 3). Inflight loss in calf girth averaged well over 7%. This approximates a 3.5% volume decrement for that immediate anatomic region.

Actual limb volume determinations by the previously described method, employing multiple circumferences, yielded postflight combined losses averaging for all nine Skylab crewmen 1.5 liters (9.1%); the largest loss was 2.3 liters (13.2%) on the SL2 pilot. Inflight left leg volumes obtained only on the three Skylab 4 crewmen were considerably lower than those obtained shortly after recovery. These three averaged for the left leg alone 1.1 liters (14.6%) deficit inflight, but only 0.7 liter (9.4%) immediately after recovery. Approximately 80% of the net inflight decrement occurred by the third or fifth day in orbit when their first leg volume measurements were obtained (Figure 4).

Further information on this rather significant migration of body mass cephalad was acquired by the Apollo–Soyuz (ASTP) crewmen. The left leg of the Command Module Pilot showed a half liter (6%) decrease in volume by 6 hours in orbit. All three averaged 0.7 liter deficit (8.3%) by 32 hr; the last inflight volumes obtained at 205 hr averaged 0.9 liter (11.3%) below preflight mean values. Earliest recovery values yielded a mean deficit of only 0.5 liter (5.9%) (Figure 5).

In conjunction with almost universal inflight symptoms of head full-

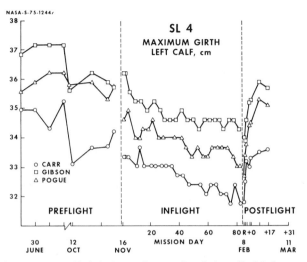

Figure 3. Maximal left calf girths in centimeters for all three Skylab 4 crewmen. Pre-, in-, and postflight mission phases are indicated. Variation in individual measurements does not obscure the exponential decrease in calf size during the flight, nor the rapid restitution of size after return to earth gravity. Time course and magnitude of this measurement are important in assessing fluid shifts headward.

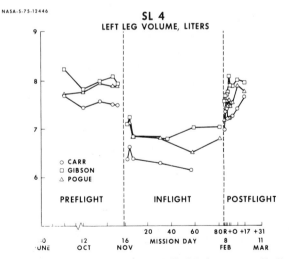

Figure 4. Left leg volume in liters for all three Skylab 4 crewmen. Earliest inflight values for two crewmen are on Mission Day 3. Volume decrement seems more abrupt and of greater magnitude than the single maximal calf measurement in Figure 3.

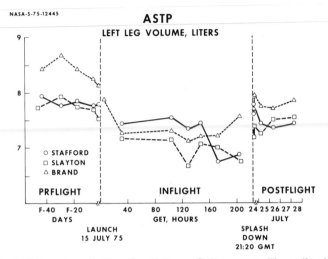

Figure 5. Left leg volume in liters for all three ASTP crewmen. The earliest inflight value for one crewman is at 6 hr mission elapsed time and 32 hr for all three. In this, as in Figure 4, immediate postflight leg volumes are considerably greater than the corresponding last inflight value.

ness and nasal stuffiness, crew observations and photographs of facial plethora and distended neck and scalp veins, the foregoing data on leg mass changes confirm rather voluminous fluid shifts headward. This no doubt involves interstitial and lymphatic as well as vascular compartments. Perhaps even intracellular fluids might undergo a redistribution in weightlessness, but there is little factual support as yet.

Blood Volume Decrements

Special hematologic data obtained on the three longer Gemini missions (4, 8, and 14 days duration) initially presaged a hemolytic process (Fischer, Johnson, and Berry, 1967). Red cell mass deficits up to 20% measured by radioisotope dilution were observed postflight. This has subsequently been attributed to the pure oxygen atmosphere of the Gemini vehicle. Somewhat smaller decreases in plasma volume were seen in four of the six crewmen evaluated by the isotope technique. The 14-day mission yielded converse results in plasma volume, i.e., increased postflight plasma volume.

More extensive blood studies were conducted on 21 Apollo crewmen of seven missions (Johnson, 1975). Again, postflight blood volume changes varied widely. Red cell mass changes ranged from +2.3% to −17.0% of preflight values, but the 21-crewman average of −7.5% is a highly significant decrement ($p < 0.001$). Curiously, a statistically significant difference between the average change for the six crewmen of Apollo 7 and 8 (mean, −2.2%) and the 15 other crewmen (mean, −9.5%) can be shown. This has been attributed to the fact that atmosphere in the 7 and 8 Apollo vehicles never was purged to pure oxygen content, which was the case on all the other Apollo missions, and, of course, was the launch status of Gemini vehicles.

Plasma volume measured on 18 Apollo crewmen was likewise significantly decreased by an average of 6%. No difference between the crewmen exposed to the two types of cabin atmospheres could be demonstrated, however. Likewise, total blood volume significantly decreased by 6.3% and no difference for atmosphere effect occurred (Johnson, 1975).

For the much longer Skylab missions, nine crewmen averaged postflight 11.1% loss in red cell mass and 10.8% loss in plasma volume, both highly significant decrements. In these missions a two-gas atmosphere prevailed most of each mission but periodic exposures to 100% oxygen occurred. An unexpected finding was obtained, however, in that the mean difference in red cell mass loss between the three crewmen of the 28-day mission and the three of the 84-day mission was significantly less for the longer mission, while their losses in plasma volume showed a reverse effect. Three astronauts in the 56-day Skylab Medical Experiments Altitude Test (SMEAT, a ground-based chamber test designed to simulate many aspects, including atmospheric, of the Skylab) showed a mean plasma volume change of +1.6% and mean red cell mass change of −2.7%, in no way comparable to changes of either Skylab crew (Johnson, 1975).

The etiology and complexity of intravascular volume losses are poorly understood, but it must be clear that intravascular volume decrements are an integral element accompanying space flight.

Decreased Orthostatic Tolerance

Since decreased blood volume would be expected to lower orthostatic tolerance, the former alteration has been considered a paramount factor in lessened orthostatic tolerance observed almost universally after space flight. A tendency toward spontaneous syncope has, in fact, occurred in several crewmen immediately after their recovery. In virtually all cases where specific orthostatic stress testing was employed, decreased tolerance has become evident (Shvasty, 1972).

During Gemini missions tilt table testing from a supine control position to 70° head-up tilt utilized heart rate, blood pressure, and change in leg volume as evaluation criteria (Figure 6). Comparison of pre- and postflight results yielded a simple but meaningful and quantitative assessment of orthostatic tolerance from cardiovascular responses to this form of controlled orthostatic stress. For the 18 Gemini crewmen with available pre- and postflight data, supine resting heart rates increased an average of 29% and tilt-stressed heart rates 51% after flight (unpublished data, Johnson Space Center, Houston, Texas).

By means of a special apparatus enclosing the lower half of the body and with an adequate waist seal, reduced atmospheric pressure can be applied to this isolated region. The effect of the differential pressure is to displace blood and other body fluids footward with much the same cardiovascular effects as erect posture in earth gravity. The level of lower body negative pressure (LBNP) may be varied; the LBNP protocol shown

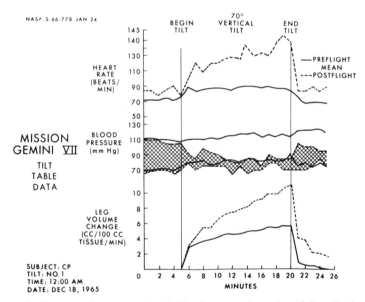

Figure 6. Heart rate (beats per minute), blood pressure (systolic and diastolic, in mm Hg), and change in leg volume (in percentage) during a 25-min, 70° tilt test protocol, the first and last 5 min being in the horizontal, supine position. Preflight mean curves are solid lines and the first postflight test values are dashed (or hatched). The crewman was Command Pilot of the 14-day Gemini 7 flight. (After Berry and Catterson, 1967.)

in Figure 7 has been determined to produce orthostatic stress comparable to that of one gravity. Eighteen Apollo crewmen underwent this slightly unorthodox orthostatic test; six other Apollo crewmen were tested by simple passive standing. A typical LBNP response is depicted in Figure 8, and a direct comparison of heart rate response to LBNP and tilt table orthostatic stresses in the same crewman is graphically demonstrated by Figure 9. Overall Apollo results yielded average immediate postflight elevations of 11% ($p < 0.02$) in supine resting heart rate and 42% ($p < 0.001$) during orthostatically stressed heart rate. Postflight pulse pressure was reduced in the supine resting state by 8% (N.S.) and by 25% ($p < 0.02$) during orthostatic stress, with at least seven crewmen experiencing presyncopal symptoms during their immediate postflight test.

Apollo plethysmographic measurements of the change in calf size as a function of fluid shifts into the legs during LBNP stress have provided additional physiologic information. Maximal change in calf size during postflight LBNP was surprisingly 12% (N.S.) less than preflight values. This has been a troublesome determination, for similar measurements during Gemini tilt tests had indicated a larger leg volume expansion postflight. Skylab revealed an amplifying detail. LBNP stress inflight produced an

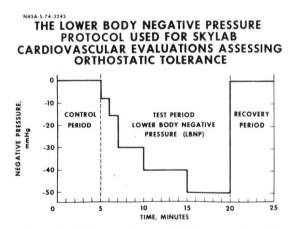

Figure 7. The Lower Body Negative Pressure (LBNP) protocol used for Apollo and Skylab assessments of orthostatic tolerance. Like the tilt test used for Gemini crew evaluations, this is 25 min in duration with the first and last 5 min being at supine rest, ambient pressure conditions. Stepwise decreases in the lower body stressing pressure provide multiple levels of orthostatic stress.

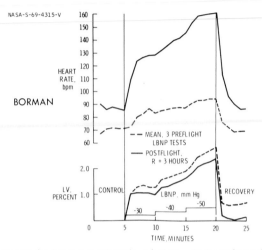

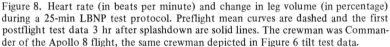

Figure 8. Heart rate (in beats per minute) and change in leg volume (in percentage) during a 25-min LBNP test protocol. Preflight mean curves are dashed and the first postflight test data 3 hr after splashdown are solid lines. The crewman was Commander of the Apollo 8 flight, the same crewman depicted in Figure 6 tilt test data.

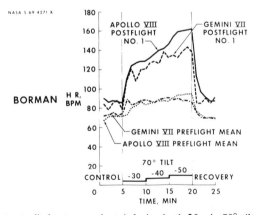

Figure 9. Heart rate (in beats per minute) during both 25-min 70° tilt and LBNP test protocols. Preflight mean curves and immediate postflight curves are differentiated and labeled accordingly. The same crewman flew both named space missions. See Figures 6 and 8.

average 83% greater calf volume increment than the same stress preflight. Immediately after flight this measurement was only 10% greater than preflight, not too unlike the postflight Apollo average.

Moreover, during Skylab missions, LBNP was employed inflight as well as postflight for assessing orthostatic tolerance (Figure 10). Inflight tolerance decreased quite comparably to that seen immediately postflight as determined by heart rate elevations (Figure 11); postflight findings were again like data on Apollo crews. Compared to preflight reference responses, Skylab heart rates further increased during inflight LBNP tests an average of 30% ($p < 0.01$) and 33% ($p < 0.005$) immediately on recovery. Resting heart rate elevations in both phases of the missions averaged only 10% and 3%, respectively, and were not statistically different from

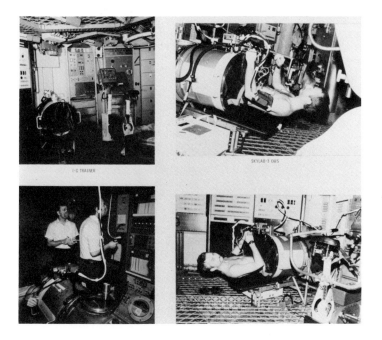

Figure 10. Operational set-up for performing the Skylab LBNP test protocol in the 1 g trainer where most preflight tests occurred, in the Cardiovascular Mobile Laboratory where most postflight tests were performed, and in the orbiting Skylab itself where the crew conducted all such tests.

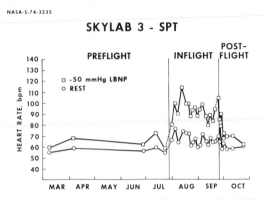

Figure 11. Composite plot of supine resting and −50 mm Hg LBNP stressed (the maximal level) heart rates (in beats per minute) for the Skylab 3 Science Pilot for every LBNP test over all three mission phases. Vertical lines delineate launch and recovery dates. Elevations in both resting and orthostatically stressed heart rates during the flight and in the immediate postflight period are clearly apparent.

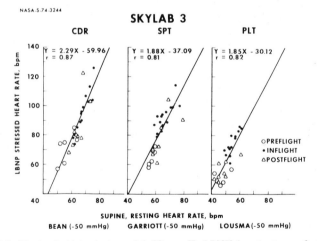

Figure 12. Maximal attained stressed (−50 mm Hg LBNP) heart rate as a function of the corresponding and immediately preceding supine, resting heart rate (both in beats per minute) for all three crewmen of the Skylab 3 mission. Regression equations obtained from multiple tests during all three mission phases have significant r values.

preflight values. An apparent exception, however, was that resting heart rate actually decreased inflight for the three Skylab 2 crewmen. An interesting and significant positive correlation has been shown to exist between LBNP stressed heart rate and the preceding supine resting heart rate (Figure 12). Average pulse pressure, however, although encompassing great individual variability, was not significantly reduced. Even so, there were 15 inflight episodes of presyncope occurring among six of the nine crewmen and their total 139 inflight LBNP assays; one episode occurred on recovery day (Johnson et al., 1974).

Decreased Heart Size
The only other discrete data available from which regional body or organ volumes may be derived are chest x-rays and echocardiographs. Standard

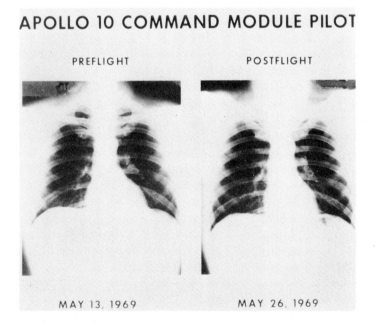

Figure 13. Standard 6-ft posterior–anterior chest roentgenograms of the Apollo 10 Command Module Pilot taken 5 days before launch and on recovery day. The change in heart size is visually apparent. Both films were randomly exposed with respect to the cardiac cycle.

posterior-anterior chest x-rays have been taken as a clinical routine before and after each U.S. space flight on every crewman. A review of these films provides a large base for assessing heart size in this planar projection (Figures 13 and 14). The simplest determination, with some experiential sanction is perhaps the cardiothoracic (C/T) ratio. Figure 15 tabulates C/T ratio measurements on the basis of diametral and areal dimensions for eight Skylab crewmen. Summing data from four Mercury crewmen making orbital flights, 18 Gemini, 30 Apollo, and 9 Skylab crewmen, a postflight decrement in the C/T ratio of −0.018 is shown to be statistically significant at $p < 0.001$ (unpublished data, JSC, Hoffler et al., 1974 and Nicogossian et al., 1974).

Pre- and postflight echocardiograms were obtained only on Skylab 4 and ASTP crews, but postflight data on the latter were compromised by the noxious gas episode. Two of the three Skylab crewmen showed modest postflight decrements in resting left ventricular end-diastolic volume and

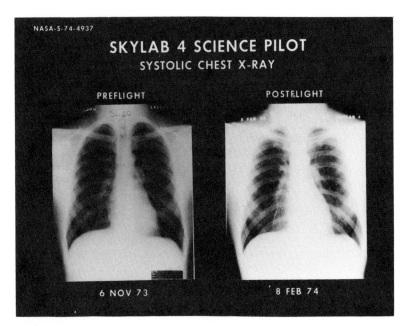

Figure 14. Standard 6-ft posterior–anterior chest roentgenograms of the Skylab 4 Science Pilot taken 10 days before launch and on recovery day. Both films were exposed by electrocardiographic signal triggering to correspond in time to peak systole.

NASA-S-74-4549

DETERMINANTS OF CARDIAC SIZE
FROM ROENTGENOGRAMS

CARDIAC PHASE	MEASUREMENT	PREFLIGHT		POST FLIGHT (R+0)		STATISTICAL SIGNIFICANCE
		MEAN	STANDARD DEVIATION	MEAN	STANDARD DEVIATION	
SYSTOLE	C/T_D [A]	0.416	0.029	0.390	0.018	$p^E < 0.05$
	C/T_A [B]	0.180	0.019	0.166	0.018	$p < 0.01$
	$D_1 \times D_2$ [C]	238.87(cm^2)	38.13(cm^2)	221.90(cm^2)	40.82(cm^2)	N.S. [F]
	PLAN. [D]	123.81(cm^2)	13.31(cm^2)	114.22(cm^2)	12.74(cm^2)	$p < 0.05$
DIASTOLE	C/T_D	0.403	0.018	0.399	0.021	N.S.
	C/T_A	0.177	0.015	0.164	0.020	$p < 0.01$
	$D_1 \times D_2$	248.41(cm^2)	28.28(cm^2)	212.27(cm^2)	34.09(cm^2)	$p < 0.05$
	PLAN.	121.71(cm^2)	7.74(cm^2)	111.67(cm^2)	12.20(cm^2)	$p < 0.01$

N = 8 (R+0 FILM UNSATISFACTORY ON SL-3 PILOT)
[A] CARDIOTHORACIC RATIO BASED ON THE RESPECTIVE DIAMETERS
[B] CARDIOTHORACIC RATIO BASED ON THE RESPECTIVE AREAS
[C] CARDIAC AREA DETERMINED FROM THE PRODUCT OF THE MINOR AND MAJOR DIAMETERS
[D] CARDIAC AREA DETERMINED BY PLANIMETRY
[E] PROBABILITY
[F] N.S. = NOT SIGNIFICANT

Figure 15. Determinants of cardiac size by diametral and areal cardio-thoracic ratios averaged from eight Skylab crewmen based on standard 6-ft posterior–anterior planar roentgenograms. Two other independent measures of heart size are also tabulated. Triggering from electrocardiographic signals provided both systolic and diastolic exposures. Differences between pre- and postflight sizes are statistically shown. (After Nicogossian et al., 1974.)

stroke volume. Return to preflight dimensions occurred between 11 and 31 days after recovery (Henry et al., 1974).

Collectively, these data strongly support a hypothesis of decreased postflight cardiac filling and stroke volume, probably directly related to decreased blood volume. An immediate consequence is decreased orthostatic tolerance long observed and now well documented. In the great majority of specific tests, crewmen have demonstrated adequate cardiovascular compensation by one or more mechanisms—especially by elevated heart rate and possibly by altered peripheral resistance.

Altered Exercise Capacity

In a somewhat counter, but further confirmatory argument, exercise capacity, quantitated by bicycle ergometry, which has almost universally been reduced postflight, never deteriorated inflight for Skylab crewmen.

On the contrary, they demonstrated progressively increased levels of exercise activities in the succeeding missions (Michel et al., 1974). It may be reasoned that, regardless of the absolute blood volume deficit induced by orbital flight, the effective resting volume was adequate for basal metabolic needs. It is also probable that, with a facilitated cardiac return postulated from headward fluid shifts and perhaps enhanced by any lower extremity activity, cardiac output satisfied inflight metabolic requirements of even high levels of work output. Apparently only during application of an orthostatic stress (LBNP or gravity by tilt or by stand, inflight or postflight) while absolute blood volume is decreased, is the net volume deficit functionally manifest.

Summary

The keystone datum in support of this hypothesis, therefore, probably involves an inverse relationship between orthostatically stressed heart rates (Hoffler et al., 1974; and Johnson et al., 1974) and blood volume (Johnson, 1975). Since both of these measurements have been made pre- and postflight on a large number of space crewmen, it is possible to express a sort of population response. Figure 16 depicts percentage changes in these

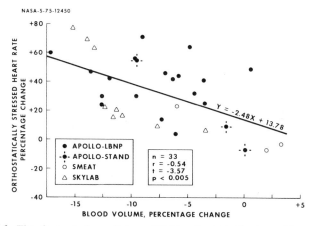

Figure 16. The change in immediate postflight orthostatically stressed heart rates (in percentage) from preflight mean reference values as a function of change in corresponding post- and preflight total blood volumes (in percentage) measured by radioisotope dilution methods. Both LBNP and passive 90° standing orthostatic stress techniques are included. The equation of the best fit linear regression through all 33 data points is given and the r value of -0.54 is statistically significant ($p < 0.005$).

data after flight for 21 Apollo, 3 Skylab Medical Experiments Altitude Test (SMEAT, *v.s.*), and 9 Skylab crewmen. The negative correlation is highly significant ($r = -0.54$, $p < 0.005$) and would seem to offer strong support for the hypothesis.

SURMISED DETERMINATIONS

If a hypothesized decrease in total absolute blood volume be granted, with central blood volume either maintained or perhaps even augmented, certain indirect evidences of these blood volume changes may have been detectable. Among these are systolic time intervals, vectorcardiographic elements, leg blood flow, and leg compliance.

Systolic Time Intervals

Systolic time intervals (STI) are temporal measurements derived from noninvasive sensors yielding important physiologic and clinical assessments of contraction characteristics of the heart. The major signals and intervals required are shown in Figure 17. Taken pre- and postflight on the last

NASA-S-74-4940 **SYSTOLIC TIME INTERVALS**

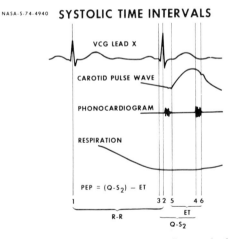

Figure 17. A composite of traces from an electrocardiogram lead, a carotid pulse wave, a phonocardiogram, and a pneumogram to show the temporal relationships from which systolic time intervals (STI) are derived. PEP, preejection period; ET, left ventricular ejection time; Q, initiation of the QRS complex; S_2, initiation of the second heart sound; and R-R, the cardiac cycle interval. All temporal values are usually expressed in milliseconds. (After Bergman et al., 1974.)

three Apollo crewmen and on all nine Skylab crewmen (Bergman, Hoffler, and Johnson, 1974) STI seem perhaps to allow some inferences regarding cardiac performance (Figure 18). It is well documented that application of LBNP causes a polling of blood in the lower part of the body, especially in the legs (Wolthuis, Bergman, and Nicogossian, 1974; Wolthuis et al., 1975). This leads to decreased central venous pressure and probably decreased right atrial filling, or preload, as evidenced by increased preejection period (PEP). In any case, left ventricular performance is diminished with decreased stroke volume and ejection time.

During preflight LBNP stress tests, the preejection period (PEP) considerably lengthened on all crewmen while left ventricular ejection time (ET) shortened. The resulting PEP/ET ratio changed markedly and is therefore a strong determinant of the degree of altered ventricular performance. During postflight evaluations, the PEP/ET ratio at supine rest was more than 20% greater than preflight recordings. Under LBNP stress, this ratio was around 30% greater postflight, and required several days to descend to preflight values.

Of course, one could as well argue that these STI data are due to depressed ventricular contractility rather than to a decreased ventricular filling, or to both factors; no direct inflight data exist to confirm or refute. It would seem rather illogical, however, that inflight exercise capacity

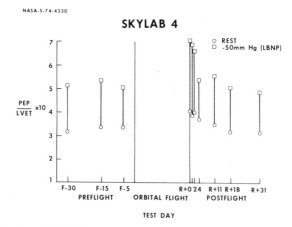

Figure 18. The ratio (unitless) of the preejection period (PEP) to the left ventricular ejection time (LVET or ET) averaged for all three crewmen of Skylab 4, under supine resting and LBNP stressed conditions, at specified pre- and postflight test dates. No inflight data for this determination have been obtained. (After Bergman et al., 1974.)

demonstrated by Skylab crewmen throughout flight even to deorbit time could be so well maintained in the presence of significant myocardial dysfunction. The immediate exercise decrements postflight must be due to some more acute process that is rapidly reversible. The fluid displacement theory fits the picture.

Vectorcardiogram

A further step using indirect data can be made with vectorcardiographic data taken pre- and postflight on the last nine Apollo crewmen and on all nine Skylab crewmen inflight as well (Hoffler et al., 1973, 1974; Smith, et al., 1974). In passing, it should be noted that no pathologic abnormalities of ultimate clinical concern have been seen, although most crewmen have demonstrated occasional ectopic and rhythm aberrations. It has been shown that certain elements of the vectorcardiogram are consistently and predictably altered upon application of LBNP (Figure 19), which, like gravity, readily displaces blood footward. Among the more sensitive respondents to LBNP is the maximal vector magnitude of the P-loop. At −50 mm Hg LBNP this maximal P-wave vector is increased in the normal adult male approximately 30%. On Apollo crewmen postflight, there was an increase of 56% during LBNP. Skylab crewmen demonstrated an astonishing 75% increase postflight, but more importantly, inflight values averaged 78% greater than the corresponding measurement at rest. A bit perplexing, however, is the fact that this P-vector at rest inflight, when one might postulate an increased intracardiac blood volume, was also greater by 24% than the preflight reference. Of course, the earliest inflight VCG was not made until the fourth mission day and the true time course of proposed fluid shifts can only be guessed.

If one allows some inference from the P-vector response during LBNP when caudad blood shifts occur, it is easy to surmise that a relatively larger effect should be assumed inflight. Without attempting an explanation of the etiology or a correlation between cardiac electrical and mechanical elements, the data stand firmly in support of a reproducible event probably related to degree of atrial filling.

Leg Blood Flow

On the opposite end of these fluid shifts are leg blood flow data derived inflight only on Skylab 4 crewmen. Using an arm blood pressure cuff from onboard medical equipment and the leg band plethysmographs from the LBNP experiment, measurements of calf blood flow were undertaken at

NASA-S-74-486b

AMPLITUDE MEASUREMENTS OF THE VECTORCARDIOGRAM

VCG MEASUREMENT	PREFLIGHT REFERENCE VALUES SUPINE, RESTING MEAN ± SD	CHANGE AFTER DESIGNATED CONDITION (%)					
		CONDITION = LBNP			CONDITION = FLIGHT		
		PREFLIGHT	IN-FLIGHT	POSTFLIGHT R + 0	IN-FLIGHT	POSTFLIGHT R + 0	
		x̄ | p	x̄ | *	x̄ | *	x̄ | p	x̄ | p
P_{MAX}MAG (mV)	0.122 ± 0.0332	+27 | <0.001	+78	+75	+24 | <0.02	+16 | NS
QRS_{MAX}MAG (mV)	1.70 ± 0.373	- 6 | <0.02	+13	+12	+12 | <0.001	+18 | <0.001
QRS-E CIRC (mV)	5.01 ± 1.027	+ 3 | NS	+24	+32	+19 | <0.005	+21 | <0.001
ST_{MAX}MAG (mV)	0.646 ± 0.206	-15 | <0.01	-32	-37	-10 | NS	- 6 | NS

* p VALUES WERE NOT COMPUTED FOR THESE COMPARISONS BECAUSE
PERCENTAGE CHANGES ARE RECKONED FROM PREFLIGHT RESTING
REFERENCES, AND COMPOUND TREATMENT EFFECTS (i.e., LBNP, SPACE
AND/OR REENTRY) ARE INVOLVED. APPROXIMATE SIGNIFICANCE
MAY BE JUDGED IN RELATION TO THE p VALUES FOR THE RELATIVELY
'PURE' TREATMENTS OF PREFLIGHT LBNP OR FLIGHT ITSELF.

Figure 19. Amplitude measurements of the vectorcardiograms from the nine Skylab crewmen. Changes (percentage) are based on the nine crewmen group mean, preflight, supine resting values as reference. Changes are given for the effect of LBNP alone in the LBNP preflight column and for the effect of space alone in the flight inflight column. Compound effects are registered in other columns due to various combinations of LBNP, the orbital state, and recovery conditions. Pmax MAG, P-wave maximum vector magnitude; QRSmax MAG, QRS complex maximum vector magnitude; QRS-E CIRC, QRS spatial eigenloop circumference; and STmax MAG, St-wave maximum vector magnitude (all in millivolts in the preflight reference column). Statistical significance is indicated under P or was not computed under columns with asterisk.

cuff occlusion pressures of 30 and 50 mm Hg. Both the initial slope and the later slope continuing for 20 sec were measured from three pressurization cycles at each of seven test periods over the 84-day mission (Thornton and Hoffler, 1974).

The initial slope more closely approximates true leg blood flow since after venous capacity is exceeded, inflow occurs against progressively increasing tissue back pressure. During three preflight reference tests, initial slopes (Figure 20) of blood flow ranged between 2 and 4 volumes percent/minute. The second slope preflight generally was ≤1 volume percent/minute. Inflight values of the initial slope varied widely, but ranged as high as 10–12 volume percent/minute and were nearly always 4 volumes percent/minute. The second slope inflight rarely exceeded 4 volumes percent/minute, but still was usually about twice preflight levels.

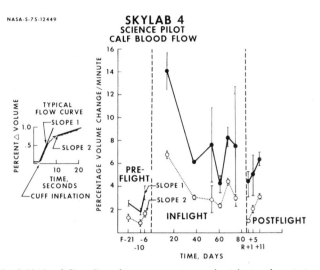

Figure 20. Calf blood flow (in volumes percent per minute) at various tests pre-, in-, and postflight for the Skylab 4 Science Pilot, based on occlusion cuff plethysmography using capacitance bands for volume determination. Slope 1 is the initial rapid volume change after inflation of the occlusion cuff; slope 2 is that after a definite hip or reduction in volume change has become evident. Bars depict ±1 SD from three successive 20-sec occlusion traces of each test. The inset at left shows one typical volume trace following cuff occlusion. Cuff occlusion pressure was 50 mm Hg.

In many cases there was no evidence of a lessening slope over the 20-sec occlusion interval, normally an indication of increasing back pressure.

Admittedly these data are crude and suffer from variation in hand inflation of the cuff, improvisation of design, and other operational discrepancies, but they point distinctly to increased inflight leg blood flow. This for the present is attributed to the decreased leg volume offering less impedance to regional arterial flow rather than to an actual increase in cardiac output as such. This, of course, needs verification.

Leg Compliance

One related datum is maximal percentage leg volume change attained during LBNP with the described plethysmograph. As already noted, in all normal subjects two distinct slopes may be described. The early and greater slope is usually attributed to the zone of free venous distensibility and the later, more shallow slope, at least in part, to stress relaxation and fluid transudation from the vascular compartment. The latter presumption is also supported by the fact that calf volume after release of LBNP almost never returns completely to prestress levels.

Apollo and Skylab data regarding maximal change in calf size during LBNP have already been described with respect to amount of blood pooled. Postflight changes have not been different from preflight, while inflight Skylab data showed almost a doubling of preflight values. Since the LBNP stressing protocol remained unchanged, it is clearly evident that an inflight compliance change must have occurred. Whether this is totally a functional phenomenon of vessels, is primarily due to altered turgor of adjacent tissue, or is some combination effect involving the whole limb, matters perhaps little. Any increased compliance of the legs would materially enhance pooling of blood out of the usable circulating compartment while a reduced absolute blood volume had already compromised cardiovascular reserves. This is the presently interpreted state of returning space crews. Not until new evidence has been made available can we more objectively understand and perhaps prevent this condition.

OUTSTANDING QUESTIONS; CONCLUSIONS

The vantage available at this juncture should allow relatively free reign in the conceptualization and design of future ground-based and inflight experiments that will further resolve and clarify principal aspects of cardiovascular function in the space environment.

Perhaps among the first basic questions should be a more refined evaluation of absolute volumes and their redistributions and time course involved in fluid shifts in space. Definitive measurements will likely necessitate multiple radioisotope or other markers for specific fluid compartments with serial quantitative determinations.

Development of techniques, preferably noninvasive, for measuring regional blood flow and perfusion are integral to volumetric evaluations. Liberal use of such devices as the gamma camera and ultrasonic probe should be encouraged. Provision must be made for continuous and/or rapidly repetitive measurements during the critical phases of flight—launch and deorbit. And, not least, there must be decision-making capability for the onboard investigator and provision for his real-time inputs into the progress and direction of researches.

Completeness requires that other organ and functional body systems be explored concurrently. Precise and definitive fluid balance studies have yet to be performed in space. Insensible water loss very likely is significant. Not only must urine output be well documented, but renal blood flow as well as neuroendocrinologic aspects accompanying hemodynamic control of urine production need unveiling. Moreover, the receptors that detect and initiate action on perceived increases or decreases in volume or pressure are in many respects hypothetical. An understanding of mechanisms is essential to intelligent and optimal therapeutic and preventative measures. Much of this is necessarily the determination and application of basic physiology.

Perhaps it can be justifiably conjectured that such enigmas as the loss of red cell mass and the space sickness syndrome of the early orbital period have etiologic foundations in circulatory disturbances. The latter condition has certain elements quite akin to hyperemesis gravidarum and to the presumed hydrops of Ménière's disease. Since the mechanisms involved in red cell production have so far escaped clinical investigators, this is a rather fertile field perhaps ready made for space researchers.

Consideration of and compensation for variations in other aspects of the space environment must be ensured. It is not yet known to what extent, if any, a hypobaric atmosphere, altered atmospheric content, maintained low humidity, or other perhaps unperceived conditions influence the subject in question. Neither can one be certain of the degree of transference permitted between so-called ground-based analogs of weightlessness and the true environment of orbital space flight.

Thus a fitting final question might be, with what may the weightlessness of space be legitimately compared? Immobilization is not the preferred analog; astronauts are entirely too active. Immersion has much to speak for it: universal buoyancy and a measure of equilibrated external forces tending to produce a centripetal shift of body mass. The diuresis accompanying water immersion perhaps has biased our thinking on what, in fact, occurs upon "space immersion." Perhaps a clear distinction should be made between the two forms of centripetal forces; the one in space is more properly cephalad in direction. Water exerts essentially equal pressure over the whole body surface. A sensation of head fullness is not appreciated. On the other hand, in weightlessness, elastic tissue forces of the lower body, always previously conditioned by the inexorable countering force of gravity, suddenly become unopposed. Tissues of the upper body are not so conditioned and experience immediately an anomalous distension, poorly opposed. And, of course, the internal organs all share equally the absence of gravitional force, which is not the case in immersion. What might be the effect, for instance, upon renal blood flow? Or upon cerebral or coronary dynamics? An intelligent guess seems not yet possible.

The last and most widely used analog for weightlessness is bed rest. Magnitude of experience, breadth of associated studies, and simplicity of performance concede to bed rest preeminence. There are also many ancillary contributions in clinical medicine dealing with fluid shifts, particularly in congestive heart failure. A slight modification recently entertained by Soviet and American investigators adds perhaps an additional degree of realism, namely, head-down tilt (Yarullin et al., 1972, and Nicogossian et al., 1975).

As of the present moment, with very few studies available, it is not possible to state categorically if head-down tilt achieves any further fidelity, or if such gain is even justified in the face of some increased subject discomfort. Nor has an optimal angle of head-down tilt been determined. But, at least subjectively, certain elements of the space syndrome are more nearly reproduced. Here is an area presently amenable to laboratory investigations. Basic physiologists and clinicians could, no doubt, contribute importantly with proposals suggested by this new ability to manipulate body fluids.

In conclusion, the cardiovascular system figures prominently in all of man's endeavors, in his sicknesses and his health, in his inner emotions and external conduct, in his exertions, failures, and achievements. It is not likely that it will preclude his frontier advances in space, for the cardiovascular system has always been adaptable. But a better understanding of its sometimes puzzling responses to the space environment will not only help lessen the cardiovascular strain from man's inquisitiveness and adventuresomeness, but also assist man in assuring optimal adaptation and function of this truly cardinal system for his overall well-being in the new environment called space.

ACKNOWLEDGMENTS

The author is grateful to the colleagues with and by whom many of these data were generated, to the flight crews who participated in each small detail of medical investigations, to many unsung supporting teams, for the extensive resources of the Johnson Space Center, and ultimately to the people of the United States for such a unique and provocative venture as is represented by this paper. He also wishes to express sincere thanks to his able and persevering secretary, Mrs. Marion Ward, who prepared the manuscript.

LITERATURE CITED

Aschoff, J., and J. Aschoff. 1969. Tagesperiodik der orthostatischen kreislaufreaktion. Pflügers Archiv 306: 146–152.

Bergman, S. A., G. W. Hoffler, and R. L. Johnson. 1974. Evaluations of the electromechanical properties of the cardiovascular system. *In* R. S. Johnston and L. F. Dietlein (Coordinators), The Proceedings of the Skylab Life Sciences Symposium, August 27–29, 1974, Lyndon B. Johnson Space Center, Houston, Texas, Vol. II, pp. 681–709, NASA TMX-58154, National Aeronautics and Space Administration, Washington, D.C.

Berry, C. A. 1973. Weightlessness. *In* James F. Parker, Jr., and Vita R. West (Managing Editors), Bioastronautics Data Book. 2nd Ed., pp. 349–411. NASA SP-3006, National Aeronautics and Space Administration, Washington, D.C.

Berry, Charles A., and Allen D. Catterson. 1967. Pre-Gemini medical predictions versus Gemini flight results. *In* Gemini Summary Conference, February 1 and 2, 1967, Manned Spacecraft Center, Houston, Texas, pp. 197–218. NASA SP-138, National Aeronautics and Space Administration, Washington, D.C.

Catterson, A. D., E. P. McCutcheon, H. A. Minners, and R. A. Pollard. 1963. Aeromedical observations. *In* Mercury Project Summary Including Results of the Fourth Manned Orbital Flight, May 15 and 16, 1963, Manned Spacecraft Center, Houston, Texas, pp. 299–326. NASA SP-45, National Aeronautics and Space Administration, Washington, D.C.

Fischer, Craig L., Philip C. Johnson, and Charles A. Berry. 1967. Red blood cell mass and plasma volume changes in manned space flight. JAMA 200: 579–583.

Gauer, O. H., and James P. Henry. 1963. Circulatory basis of fluid volume control. Physiol. Rev. 43: 423–481.

Gauer, O. H., and Hans L. Thron. 1965. Postural changes in the circulation. *In* W. F. Hamilton (Section Editor) and Philip Dow (Executive Editor), Handbook of Physiology, Section 2: Circulation, Volume III, pp. 2409–2439. American Physiological Society, Washington, D.C.

Henry, Walter L., Stephen E. Epstein, James M. Griffith, Robert E. Goldstein, and David R. Redwood. 1974. Effect of prolonged space flight on cardiac function and dimensions. *In* R. S. Johnston and L. F. Dietlein (Coordinators), The Proceedings of the Skylab Life Sciences Symposium, August 27–29, 1974, Lyndon B. Johnson Space Center, Houston, Texas, Vol. II, pp. 711–721, NASA-TMX-58154, National Aeronautics and Space Administration, Washington, D.C.

Hoffler, G. W., R. L. Johnson, R. A. Wolthuis, and D. P. Golden. 1973. Results of computer reduced vectorcardiograms from Apollo crewmembers. Preprint of the 1973 Scientific Meeting of the Aerospace Medical Association, May 7–10, Las Vegas, Nevada.

Hoffler, G. W., R. L. Johnson, A. E. Nicogossian, S. A. Bergman, Jr., and M. M. Jackson. 1974. Vectorcardiographic results from Skylab medical experiment M092: lower body negative pressure. *In* R. S. Johnston and L. F. Dietlein (Coordinators), The Proceedings of the Skylab Life Sciences Symposium, August 27–29, 1974, Lyndon B. Johnson Space Center, Houston, Texas, Vol. II, pp. 597–621, NASA-TMX-58154, National Aeronautics and Space Administration, Washington, D.C.

Hoffler, G. W., Roger A. Wolthuis, and Robert L. Johnson. 1974. Apollo space crew cardiovascular evaluations. Aerospace Med. 45: 807–820.

Johnson, Philip C. 1975. Study of the effect of space flight on red cell life span and plasma volume. NASA Contract NAS 9-7280, Final Report. Baylor College of Medicine, Houston, Texas.

Johnson, R. L., G. W. Hoffler, A. E. Nicogossian, S. A. Bergman, and M. M. Jackson. 1974. Lower body negative pressure: third manned Skylab mission. *In* R. S. Johnston and L. F. Dietlein (Coordinators), The Proceedings of the Skylab Life Sciences Symposium, August 27–29, 1974, Lyndon B. Johnson Space Center, Houston, Texas, Vol. II, pp. 545–595, NASA-TMX-59154, National Aeronautics and Space Administration, Washington, D.C.

Johnston, R. S., and L. F. Dietlein. 1974. (Coordinators) The Proceedings of the Skylab Life Sciences Symposium, August 27–29, 1974, Volumes I and II, Lyndon B. Johnson Space Center, Houston, Texas. NASA-TMX-58154, National Aeronautics and Space Administration, Washington, D.C., 862 p.

Klein, K. E., H Bruner, D. Jovy, L. Vogt, and H. M. Wegmann. 1969. Influence of stature and physical fitness on tilt table and acceleration tolerance. Aerospace Med. 40: 293–297.

Michel, E. L., J. A. Rummel, C. F. Sawin, M. C. Buderer, and J. D. Lem. 1974. Results of Skylab medical experiment M171—metabolic activity. *In* R. S. Johnston and L. F. Dietlein (Coordinators), The Proceedings of the Skylab Life Sciences Symposium, August 27–29, 1974, Lyndon B. Johnson Space Center, Houston, Texas, Vol. II, pp. 723–755, NASA-TMX-58154, National Aeronautics and Space Administration, Washington, D.C.

Nicogossian, A. E., G. W. Hoffler, R. L. Johnson, and R. J. Gowen. 1974. Determinations of cardiac size from chest roentgenograms following Skylab missions. *In* R. S. Johnston and L. F. Dietlein (Coordinators), The Proceedings of the Skylab Life Sciences Symposium, August 27–29, 1974, Lyndon B. Johnson Space Center, Houston Texas, Vol. II, pp. 785–793, NASA-TMX-58154, National Aeronautics and Space Administration, Washington, D.C.

Nicogossian, A. E., C. F. Sawin, G. W. Hoffler, and J. A. Rummel. 1975. Pulmonary functions during acute exposures to head-down tilt (possible simulation of weightless state). Preprints of the 1975 Scientific Meeting of the Aerospace Medical Association, April 28–May 1, San Francisco, California.

Shvasty, Esar. 1972. The measurement of orthostatic tolerance. Human Factors 14: 357–362.

Smith, Raphael F., Kevin Stanton, David Stoop, Donald Brown, Walter Jannsz, and Paul King. 1974. Vectorcardiographic changes during extended space flight. *In* R. S. Johnston and L. F. Dietlein (Coordinators), The Proceedings of the Skylab Life Sciences Symposium, August 27–29, 1974, Lyndon B. Johnson Space Center, Houston, Texas, Vol. II, pp. 659–679, NASA-TMX-58154, National Aeronautics and Space Administration, Washington, D.C.

Thornton, William E., and G. W. Hoffler. 1974. Hemodynamic studies of the legs under weightlessness. *In* R. S. Johnston and L. F. Dietlein (Coordinators), The Proceedings of the Skylab Life Sciences Symposium, August 27–29, 1974, Lyndon B. Johnson Space Center, Houston, Texas, Vol. II, pp. 623–635, NASA-TMX-58154, National Aeronautics and Space Administration, Washington, D.C.

Wolthuis, R. A., Stuart A. Bergman, and Arnauld E. Nicogossian. 1974. Physiological effects of locally applied reduced pressure in man. Physiol. Rev. 54: 566–595.

Wolthuis, R. A., Adrian LeBlanc, William A. Carpentier, and Stuart A. Bergman, Jr. 1975. Response of local vascular volumes to lower body negative pressure stress. Aviation Space and Environ. Med. 46: 697–702.

Yarullin, K. K., T. N. Krupina, T. D. Vasil'yeva, and N. N. Buyvolva. 1972. Changes in cerebral, pulmonary, and peripheral blood circulation. Kosmicheskaya Biol. Med. 6: 33–39.

Cardiovascular Flow Dynamics and Measurements
Edited by N. H. C. Hwang and N. A. Normann
Copyright 1977   University Park Press   Baltimore

chapter 10

CONTROL OF CARDIAC OUTPUT

Carl E. Jones

ABSTRACT

The mechanism by which cardiac output is regulated to the precise level required for adequate nutrition of the tissues of the body is described. The roles of both the heart and the peripheral circulation in this regulatory mechanism are considered, but the overall theme is that as long as the pumping ability of the heart is sufficient to pump the blood returning to it from the peripheral circulation, the peripheral vasculature determines venous return and, thereby, cardiac output. Also, a method is described by which factors affecting either cardiac or peripheral vascular function may be graphically analyzed to determine their effects on cardiac output. Using this method, the effects of such factors as autonomic nerve stimulation, oxygen insufficiency, muscular exercise, hemorrhage, opening the chest, and heart failure on cardiac output are analyzed.

INTRODUCTION

Under most physiologic conditions, the volume of blood pumped by the heart each minute is so geared to the metabolic activity of the tissues of the body that each tissue receives almost exactly the blood flow it requires for adequate nutrition. As an example, purposeful reductions of cardiac output from its normal level cause the oxygen consumption of the body to decrease significantly, but purposeful increases in cardiac output result in no substantial increase in oxygen consumption. This illustrates that under normal conditions the cardiac output is regulated at precisely that level which adequately oxygenates body tissues. This principle of cardiac output regulation is also manifest in conditions in which the metabolic rate of the tissues is altered, such as muscular exercise. The results of many studies illustrate that during muscular exercise, the increase in cardiac output is closely correlated to the increase in oxygen consumption. This correlation is illustrated in Figure 1, which is a compilation of results by Douglas and Haldane (1922), Christensen and Mitteilung (1931), Dexter et al. (1951), Donald et al. (1955), Tabakin et al. (1964), and Damato, Galante, and Smith (1966). The relationship shown in Figure 1 emphasizes the important role of adequate tissue oxygenation in the regulation of cardiac output.

It is the purpose of this chapter to present the basic mechanism by which cardiac output is regulated to ensure adequate tissue oxygenation. Both the role of the heart and the role of the peripheral circulation in the

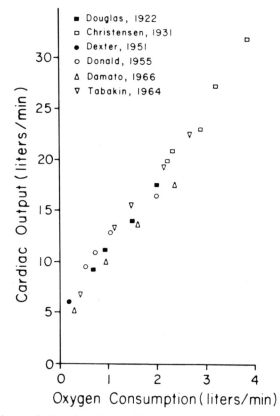

Figure 1. A compilation of results showing the relationship between cardiac output and oxygen consumption in exercise.

regulation of cardiac output are considered, but the overall theme is that as long as the cardiac pumping ability is normal, the peripheral tissues themselves regulate their own blood flows, and this regulation of local blood flows is a major factor in the regulation of total cardiac output.

NORMAL VALUES FOR CARDIAC OUTPUT

The value for normal resting cardiac output in the adult human varies with age, sex, and body size (Guyton, Jones, and Coleman, 1973). In the average young adult male, cardiac output is approximately 6 liters/min, while in the average young adult female, the value is approximately 5 liters/min. However, cardiac output decreases with age so that in the 50–60-yr-old male, cardiac output averages approximately 5 liters/min, and in the female of the same age cardiac output averages about 4 liters/min. Therefore, the value for cardiac output that is more representative of the entire adult population is approximately 5 liters/min. This is the value for normal cardiac output that will be used throughout this chapter.

REGULATION OF CARDIAC OUTPUT

The amount of blood pumped by the heart each minute is determined by two factors: first, the pumping ability of the heart, and second, the ability of blood to flow through the peripheral circulation and to return to the heart. Both of these factors and their roles in the actual regulation of cardiac output are discussed below.

Role of the Heart

Because the heart actually pumps blood through the circulation, it may at first be difficult to understand that the control of cardiac output is not normally vested in the heart itself. However, when one considers that a primary purpose of cardiac output is to supply the various tissues with nutrients, it becomes easier to see why the tissues themselves control their own blood flows and, thereby, cardiac output. This concept does not imply that the ability of the heart to pump blood is not a major factor affecting cardiac output. Rather, this concept states that so long as the pumping ability of the heart is normal, the actual adjustment of cardiac output to the precise level required by the tissues is executed by the vasculature of these tissues.

The results of a few simple experiments serve to demonstrate that the normal control of cardiac output does not lie primarily in the heart. These results are the following: (1) In resting animals and humans, increasing the heart rate by use of an electrical pacemaker fails to cause a significant increase in cardiac output (Sugimoto, Sagawa, and Guyton, 1966; Braunwald et al., 1967; Cowley and Guyton, 1971). (2) If the heart of an experimental animal is replaced by a pump that is capable of pumping blood at a much greater rate than the normal heart, the "cardiac output" cannot be made to increase significantly despite very intense activity of the pump (Guyton et al., 1957). The reason for this is that if the activity of the pump is greater than the tendency of blood to return from the peripheral circulation to the pump, the veins entering the thorax simply collapse, preventing any further increase in pump output. (3) If the pumping activity of the heart is maintained approximately constant while the resistance to blood flow through the peripheral circulation is reduced tremendously by opening a large A–V fistula, the cardiac output increases, and the change in cardiac output is approximately inversely proportional to the change in resistance (Cowley and Guyton, 1971). These experiments point out that under normal resting conditions, the factor which limits cardiac output is not the pumping ability of the heart, but is the ability of the blood to return to the heart. (4) In dogs with denervated hearts, the relationship between cardiac output and oxygen consumption during submaximal exercise is not significantly different from the relationship seen in normal dogs, despite the fact that the heart rate does not increase greatly in the denervated dogs (Donald and Shepherd, 1963). This indicates that during moderate exercise, an increase in cardiac pumping ability is not necessary to increase cardiac output to the level required by the tissues.

The discussion up to this point has centered around the theme that under normal conditions, cardiac output is regulated primarily by the peripheral vasculature. However, in any condition that reduces the pumping ability of the heart to the extent that it cannot pump even normal amounts of blood, the heart itself becomes the primary factor determining cardiac output. For example, very intense stimulation of the parasympathetic nerves to the heart, which depresses heart rate and possibly ventricular contractility, can temporarily cause cardiac output to decrease to essentially zero, regardless of the tendency of blood to return to the heart from the peripheral circulation. Other pathologic conditions that may severely depress cardiac function include myocardial infarction (Bradley,

Jenkins, and Branthwaite, 1970; Dodge and Baxley, 1968), valvular disorders (Dodge and Baxley, 1968), and myocardial inflammation (Besterman, 1954). In addition, there are conditions in which the heart can pump normal, or even two to three times normal, quantities of blood but in which the need of the tissues for blood is still greater than the ability of the heart to pump. Such a situation is seen in dogs with denervated hearts. The hearts of these dogs can pump adequate quantities of blood during moderate exercise, but cannot do so during maximal levels of exercise (Epstein et al., 1965; Donald, Ferguson, and Milburn, 1968). Under these conditions, the pumping ability of the heart is the limiting factor to cardiac output.

Thus it is evident that whenever the need for blood flow through the peripheral circulation is greater than the amount the heart is capable of pumping, the heart rather than the peripheral circulation becomes the factor that determines cardiac output. With this in mind, we can say that the heart plays a *permissive* role in cardiac output regulation.

The permissive nature of cardiac pumping may be illustrated by the cardiac function curve. Such a curve for the normal heart is illustrated in Figure 2 by the dark curve labeled "Normal," which shows the relationship between input pressure to the heart (right atrial pressure) and cardiac output. At a resting right atrial pressure of 0 mm Hg, cardiac output is 5 liters/min. If for any reason blood begins to return from the peripheral circulation to the heart more rapidly, the input pressure to the heart tends to rise, and cardiac output increases. This increase in cardiac output caused by an increase in right atrial pressure can occur when all the nerves to the heart have been cut (Herndon and Sagawa, 1969). However, there is a limit to the extent to which cardiac output can increase. Thus when right atrial pressure rises to approximately 4 mm Hg, the maximum pumping ability of the normal heart is reached, and cardiac output can increase no further. Hence the cardiac function curve simply expresses the classic law of the heart proposed by Patterson and Starling (1914) over 50 years ago, namely, that within physiologic limits the heart will pump whatever amount of blood enters the right atrium, even though the right atrial pressure increases only slightly.

It is important to note that even under normal conditions, the heart has the capacity to pump far greater quantities of blood than are required. For instance, the normal cardiac output is only 5 liters/min, even though the normal heart has the capacity to pump approximately 15 liters/min. Thus in the normal heart the permissive cardiac output is about 3 times

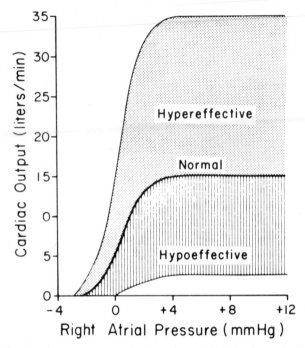

Figure 2. Cardiac function curves showing the relationship between right atrial pressure and cardiac output in the normal heart, hypereffective hearts, and hypoeffective hearts.

the actual cardiac output. It is for this reason that under normal conditions, the actual amount of blood pumped by the heart is determined primarily by the tendency of blood to return from the peripheral circulation to the heart.

There are many factors that cause the permissive level of cardiac pumping to be increased or decreased. Two conditions that have been mentioned already are intense parasympathetic stimulation of the heart and any type of cardiac damage that reduces the pumping effectiveness of the heart. Under these conditions, the cardiac function curve would lie in the area labeled "Hypoeffective" in Figure 2. Thus, if the plateau of the cardiac function curve were only 5 liters/min, the heart could pump a normal cardiac output but would not permit an increase in cardiac output above this level. Two primary factors that cause an increase in the pumping effectiveness of the heart are sympathetic stimulation of the heart (Sarnoff and Berglund, 1954; Randall, Armour, and Randall, 1971) and hypertrophy of the myocardium (Badeer, 1967). Either one of these factors would cause the permissive level of cardiac pumping to be increased such that the cardiac function curve would lie in the area labeled "hypereffective" in Figure 2. Strong sympathetic stimulation, which increases both the heart rate and the force of cardiac contraction, may increase the pumping effectiveness of the heart by approximately 60–70% such that the permissive level of cardiac pumping would be approximately 25 liters/min. Hypertrophy of the myocardium may increase the permissive level of cardiac pumping even further such that in the well-trained athlete with maximum sympathetic stimulation, the heart may be capable of pumping as much as 35 liters/min (Eckblom and Hermansen, 1968).

Fortunately, the control systems of the body operate in such a manner that the permissive level of cardiac pumping is usually maintained at a higher value than the actual blood flow required for adequate nutrition of the tissues. For instance, at the very onset of muscular exercise, an increased sympathetic stimulation of the heart along with a decreased parasympathetic inhibition greatly increases its pumping effectiveness (Rushmer and Smith, 1959; Keroes, Ecker, and Rapaport, 1969). Thus during moderate to severe exercise, the actual cardiac output can still be determined by the nutritional requirement of the tissues which, in turn, determines the rate at which blood flows through the tissues and returns to the heart.

Role of the Peripheral Circulation

In this section, the two basic mechanisms by which the peripheral vasculature determines the rate at which blood returns to the heart are presented. These are (1) the resistance to blood flow through the peripheral tissues, or the *resistance to venous return*, and (2) the filling pressure of the peripheral vasculature, termed the *mean circulatory pressure.*

Peripheral Circulatory Resistance Almost all tissues of the body have an intrinsic ability to regulate their own blood flows by changing their vascular resistances. This intrinsic regulation of local blood flows is dramatically demonstrated by two experiments as follows: (1) If perfusion pressure tending to force blood through an isolated tissue is abruptly increased, blood flow through the tissues initially increases, but over the next minute or two it returns almost to normal, despite the fact that the perfusion pressure is maintained much higher than normal. On the other hand, if the perfusion pressure is abruptly reduced, blood flow at first decreases but within the next few minutes it increases to near normal. Such an ability to maintain a constant blood flow despite changes in perfusion pressure is termed *autoregulation* and has been observed in kidney (Navar and Baer, 1970), skeletal muscle (Jones and Berne, 1965), brain (Yoshida et al., 1966), intestine (Johnson, 1964), myocardium (Berne, 1964), and liver (Brauer, 1964). (2) If an isolated skeletal muscle is stimulated, the blood flow to the muscle increases in proportion to the increased metabolic rate despite the maintenance of perfusion pressure at a constant level (Barcroft, 1964).

It is not the purpose of the present chapter to review the proposed mechanisms by which the local tissues regulate their own vascular resistances; this is discussed in detail elsewhere. However, it is important to realize that nearly all tissues possess such a mechanism and that in about 75% of the cases, this mechanism is in some way related to the balance between tissue oxygen need and transport of oxygen to the tissues (Guyton et al., 1973). Thus if the tissue oxygen requirement increases, the vascular resistance of the tissues decreases, allowing more blood flow and oxygen delivery to the tissues. On the other hand, if the tissue oxygen requirement is reduced, the vascular resistance of the tissue increases, and blood flow to the tissues is also reduced. Likewise, if the tissues become hypoxic because of a reduced concentration of oxygen in arterial blood, the vascular resistance of the tissue decreases, blood flow to the tissue increases, and the oxygen delivery to the tissues returns to approximately normal. Notable exceptions to the rule that the mechanism for local regulation of blood flows is in some way related to oxygen delivery to the tissues is found in the kidney, where the mechanism of flow regulation is probably in some way related to body fluid electrolyte balance, and in skin, where blood flow is controlled primarily by neural mechanisms related to body temperature regulation.

One can readily understand that since most tissues of the body control their own blood flows by changes in vascular resistance, the total amount of blood returning to the heart, the sum of the blood flows to all the various tissues of the body, is influenced greatly by the total resistance of the various vascular beds. The return of blood to the heart can be expressed quantitatively by the venous return curve (Guyton, Polizo, and Armstrong, 1954) as illustrated in Figure 3. In this figure, the dark curve labeled "Normal Resistance" represents the normal flow of blood into the heart, the venous return, at various right atrial pressures. When right atrial pressure is 0 mm Hg, venous return is 5 liters/min. If the pressure falls only

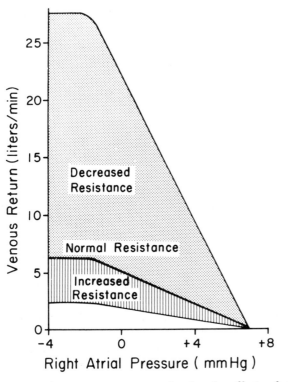

Figure 3. A family of venous return curves showing the effects of changes in resistance to venous return on the flow of blood from the peripheral circulation into the right atrium.

slightly below 0 mm Hg, venous return increases only slightly because negative right atrial pressures cause the large veins entering the thorax to collapse, preventing any additional increase in blood flow to the heart. On the other hand, if the right atrial pressure should increase above 0 mm Hg, venous return decreases rapidly, falling to 0 when right atrial pressure is increased to 7 mm Hg. The reason for this is the following: The normal mean circulatory pressure, which will be discussed in more detail later, is 7 mm Hg, and the difference between mean circulatory pressure and right atrial pressure, termed the *pressure gradient for venous return* (Guyton et al., 1957), is the driving force which tends to move the blood from the peripheral circulation to the heart. When right atrial pressure increases above zero, the pressure gradient for venous return is reduced, and when right atrial pressure reaches 7 mm Hg, there is no pressure gradient tending to force blood back to the heart. The normal curve shown in Figure 3 represents the conditions existing in the areflex animal or human. In the intact animal or human, circulatory reflexes would increase mean circulatory pressure as right atrial pressure rose and venous return tended to decrease.

If resistance to blood flow through the peripheral circulation is decreased, the entire venous return curve rotates upward or clockwise; that is, with the same pressure gradient for venous return, there is more venous return. Thus, if resistance to venous return were one-half normal, venous return at a right atrial pressure of 0 mm Hg would be 10 liters/min. On the other hand, if resistance to venous return increases, the curve rotates downward or counterclockwise. With a resistance to venous return of two times normal, venous return at a right atrial pressure of 0 mm Hg would be 2.5 liters/min.

The Mean Circulatory Pressure The mean circulatory pressure is a measure of the degree of filling of the circulation (Guyton et al., 1954; Guyton, Lindsey, and Kaufmann, 1955). It is the pressure which would be measured at all points in the circulation if all flow through the circulation were suddenly stopped, and the blood redistributed instantaneously in such a manner that all pressures were equal. Obviously, mean circulatory pressure cannot be measured clinically, but from a conceptual point of view, it is extremely important to understand its significance in cardiac output regulation.

One can readily see that if the circulation were only slightly filled with blood, the vessels would not be stretched at all, and, consequently, no pressure would develop in any of the vessels. If there were no pressure in the blood vessels, there would be no force tending to move blood from the peripheral vasculature to the heart, and cardiac output would be zero, regardless of the pumping ability of the heart. With this illustration one may see the importance of mean circulatory pressure. As explained above, the difference between mean circulatory pressure and the pressure in the right atrium, called the pressure gradient for venous return, is the driving force tending to move blood from the peripheral circulation to the heart.

There are two factors that determine the magnitude of mean circulatory pressure. From a long-term point of view, the most important factor is blood volume. A sudden increase in blood volume of 15% causes mean circulatory pressure to double immediately, and a sudden decrease in blood volume of 15% decreases mean circulatory pressure essentially to zero (Richardson, Stallings, and Guyton, 1961). However, if these changes in blood volume occur slowly, the effects on mean circulatory pressure are not nearly so great, since certain circulatory mechanisms attempt to compensate for the changes in blood volume. One form of compensation is a readjustment of blood volume; following either a decrease or an increase in blood volume, there are compensatory mechanisms that attempt to offset these changes by returning blood volume toward normal. For example, after a massive transfusion, all the pressures in the circulation, including the capillaries, rise immediately. This causes fluid to transude through the capillary walls into the interstitial spaces (Guyton et al., 1950) and through the glomeruli into the urine (Guyton et al., 1969). As a consequence, blood volume returns to near normal within 1–24 hr (Gregerson and Rawson, 1959; Prather, Taylor, and Guyton, 1969). After hemorrhage, essentially opposite effects occur. All pressures in the circulation are reduced, and the reduction in capillary pressure causes fluid to transude from the interstitial spaces into the capillaries (Gregerson and Rawson, 1959; Oberg, 1964). Also, the decrease in arterial pressure causes a reduction in the filtration of fluid into the glomeruli and, thereby, a reduction in fluid loss through the kidneys (Navar, Uther, and Baer, 1971). The rise in blood volume following hemorrhage is a slower process than the decrease in blood volume following transfusion. Nevertheless, within 24–48 hr, blood volume ordinarily returns to normal or near normal.

The second factor that determines the magnitude of mean circulatory pressure is the size, or the capacitance, of the circulatory system. One of the most important factors that affects the size of the circulatory system is the degree of sympathetic stimulation of the vessels, especially the veins (Guyton et al., 1954; Richardson, Fermoso, and Pugh, 1964). Intense sympathetic stimulation can increase mean circulatory pressure from its normal value of 7 mm Hg to approximately 18 mm Hg within 10–20 sec. On the other hand, total abrogation of the normal sympathetic impulses to the circulation decreases mean circulatory pressure to approximately 4 mm Hg. Circulatory mechanisms mediated through sympathetic reflexes help to compensate for changes in blood volume by altering the capacitance of the circulatory bed. For example, following severe hemorrhage, the very powerful central nervous system ischemic reflex (Sagawa, Ross, and Guyton, 1961; Richardson and Fermoso, 1964) causes a very intense constriction of the blood vessels that leads to a tremendous reduction in the capacitance of the circulation. This, in turn, causes the mean circulatory pressure to return toward normal. Other nervous reflexes such as the pressoreceptor reflex (Kumada and Sagawa, 1970; Chien and Billig, 1961) or reflexes originating in the pulmonary circulation, in the heart, or in the veins (Frye and Braunwald, 1960; Gupta et al., 1966) may also aid in maintaining mean circulatory pressure despite blood volume changes.

The effects of changes in mean circulatory pressure on venous return are illustrated quantitatively in Figure 4. The normal venous return is illustrated by the dark curve. If right atrial pressure remains at 0 mm Hg, and if the resistance to venous return (indicated by the slope of the venous return curve) is not altered, an increase in mean circulatory pressure to 14 mm Hg would shift the entire curve 7 mm Hg to the right and, consequently, the return of blood to the heart would double. Conversely, a decrease in mean circulatory pressure from 7 to 3.5 mm Hg would shift the curve to the left and reduce return of blood to the heart to one-half normal.

Graphical Analysis of Cardiac Output

The previous sections discussed the function of the heart in terms of the cardiac function curve and the function of the peripheral circulation in

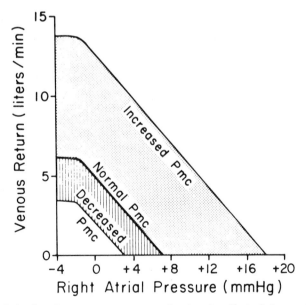

Figure 4. A family of venous return curves showing the effect of changes in mean circulatory pressure (P_{MC}) on the flow of blood into the right atrium from the peripheral circulation.

terms of the venous return curve, and showed how various factors can affect each of these curves. This section briefly illustrates how, by use of both of these curves, changes in cardiac output following changes in cardiac or peripheral vascular function may be analyzed. These analyses serve to review the roles of the heart and the peripheral circulation in the regulation of cardiac output; a thorough understanding of this type of analysis is essential for full comprehension of changes that occur during special conditions, as is presented in later sections.

Figure 5 shows several cardiac function curves and several venous

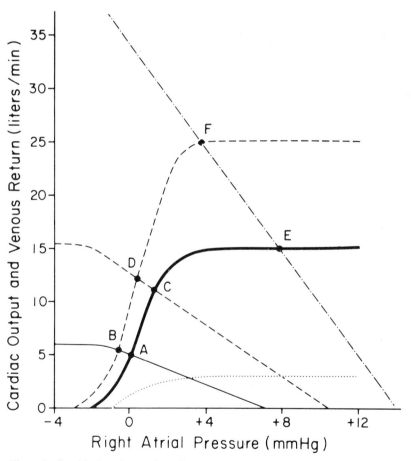

Figure 5. Graphical analyses of cardiac output showing the effects of changes in cardiac pumping ability, resistance to venous return, and mean circulatory pressure.

return curves with the normal cardiac function curve and the normal venous return curve indicated by the very dark lines. For the analyses that follow, it is important to recognize that cardiac output and venous return are always equal, except for a few heartbeats following a change in either cardiac of peripheral vascular function, and that right atrial pressure is the same for both the heart and peripheral circulation. It is obvious that for any given cardiac function and venous return curve, there is only one point that satisfies these conditions. This is the point where the two curves intersect. Thus in Figure 5 the normal cardiac output is 5 liters/min with a right atrial pressure of 0 mm Hg. This is indicated by point A.

Now let us assume that the heart becomes a much stronger pump so that the cardiac function curve is that indicated by the long-dashed line. If conditions in the peripheral circulation are not changed, the new cardiac output is represented by point B, which is only slightly higher than normal. Thus it is evident that an increase in the pumping ability of the heart alone is not sufficient to increase cardiac output. Now assume that the mean circulatory pressure is increased to 10 mm Hg and resistance to venous return is reduced to approximately one-half normal so that the venous return curve becomes that indicated by the long-dashed line. If the pumping ability of the heart is not increased from normal, the cardiac output now becomes that represented by point C, approximately 11 liters/min, with a right atrial pressure of about 1.5 mm Hg. Thus cardiac output could theoretically be increased twofold or more without increasing the pumping ability of the heart. Indeed, if the changes in the peripheral circulation just mentioned were accompanied by an increase in cardiac pumping ability, the cardiac output, point D, would still be only slightly higher than that with no alteration in the pumping ability of the heart. This emphasizes that as long as venous return is less than the permissive level of cardiac pumping, cardiac output is determined primarily by venous return.

We now examine some conditions in which the heart becomes the limiting factor to cardiac output. Assume that mean circulatory pressure is doubled, and resistance to venous return is reduced to approximately 40% of normal. These conditions are represented by the dot-dash venous return curve. If the pumping ability of the heart is not altered from normal, the cardiac output is represented by point E. Note that the heart is operating on the plateau of the cardiac function curve; it is pumping its full permissive value. Under these conditions, an increased tendency for venous return only causes a further increase in right atrial pressure. If the pumping ability of the heart is now increased as indicated by the long-dashed function curve, the new cardiac output is represented by point F, a full 10 liters/min greater than could be pumped by the normal heart (point E). This illustrates that only when the heart is the limiting factor can an increase in cardiac pumping ability cause a significant increase in cardiac output.

As a final example, assume that for some reason the pumping ability of the heart becomes very depressed such that the cardiac function curve becomes that represented by the dotted line. Here, regardless of the tendency for blood to return from the peripheral circulation, cardiac output cannot be increased even to a normal level. Under these conditions it is obvious that the pumping ability of the heart is the determinant of cardiac output.

Importance of Autonomic
Mechanisms in the Regulation of Cardiac Output

Several physiologists have proposed that cardiac output is regulated by the autonomic nervous system (Warren et al., 1945, 1948; Stead and Warren, 1947; Rushmer and Smith, 1959). However, when we recognize that the cardiac output of animals with total sympathetic block (Guyton et al., 1962), with blocked pressoreceptor reflexes (Leusen, Demeester, and Bouckaert, 1956), or with total destruction of the central nervous system (Dobbs, Prather, and Guyton, 1971) increases during muscular exercise in the same way as in normal animals, it becomes evident that a large share, if not the major share, of cardiac output regulation occurs by means of other than autonomic regulation. However, it is also true that stimulation of either the sympathetic nervous system or the parasympathetic nervous system can cause major alterations in cardiac output, under some conditions increasing output as much as double the normal value and under other conditions actually decreasing cardiac output to zero. Therefore, it is necessary to discuss the role of autonomic mechanisms in the actual regulation of cardiac output.

Autonomic Effects on the Heart   Autonomic stimulation of the heart can affect cardiac output in two very important ways: by affecting the heart rate and by affecting the strength of contraction of the heart.

Both parasympathetic and sympathetic stimulation of the heart affects heart rate; even the normal heart is constantly influenced by parasympathetic and sympathetic tone. The precise interrelationship between parasympathetic and sympathetic influences in controlling heart rate is complex, but, in general, an increase in parasympathetic tone causes a reduction in heart rate, while an increase in sympathetic tone causes an increase in heart rate. However, it is important to understand that although maximal sympathetic stimulation occurring simultaneously with parasympathetic inhibition can cause heart rate to increase to at least double the normal value (Rushmer and Smith, 1959), an increase in heart rate alone causes only a very small increase in cardiac output. If all other factors remain constant, cardiac output is affected by an increase in heart rate in approximately the following manner (Sugimoto et al., 1966; Braunwald et al., 1967; Cowley and Guyton, 1971): As the heart rate increases from normal to higher rates, cardiac output increases only a few percent, reaching a maximum at a heart rate of approximately 120–140 beats/min. As the rate rises above this level, the cardiac output progressively decreases because of decreased diastolic filling of the ventricles resulting from the greatly shortened diastolic filling time.

In contrast to the influence of heart rate on cardiac output under normal conditions, reflex changes in heart rate may be extremely important in determining cardiac output under conditions of high venous return. This was demonstrated in a study by Cowley and Guyton (1971) in which the ventricles of dogs were paced at various rates following the opening of a large aorta-venacaval fistula. With the fistula closed, increasing the heart rate from approximately 50 to 200 beats/min had very little effect on cardiac output, producing a maximum increase of only 10% at a rate of approximately 100 beats/min. However, when the fistula was opened, cardiac output increased immediately by 75%. Increasing the heart rate to 240 beats/min resulted in a further rise in cardiac output to 190% above the control value. The maximum increase in cardiac output under these conditions occurred between rates of 150 and 200 beats/min. This implies that although reflex increases in heart rate under normal conditions have very little effect on cardiac output, such increases in heart rate have a drastic effect on the permissive level of cardiac pumping. Thus, under conditions in which venous return is high, reflex increases in heart rate increase the permissive level of cardiac pumping and allow the heart to pump more effectively whatever blood returns to it.

In addition to the effect on heart rate, autonomic nervous reflexes can affect the strength of cardiac contraction. Both the parasympathetic and sympathetic nerves can affect the strength of the atrial beat, and sympathetic stimulation has a substantial effect on the strength of the ventricular beat (Sarnoff and Berglund, 1954; Carsten, Folkow, and Hamberger, 1958;

Randall, Priola, and Pace, 1967). Maximal sympathetic stimulation generally increases the strength of the ventricular beat to approximately 60–70% above normal, while complete abrogation of sympathetic impulses to the heart decreases the strength of ventricular contraction by approximately 10–20%. Recent studies indicate that parasympathetic stimulation may also affect the force of ventricular contraction, depressing the strength of ventricular contraction by approximately 5–10% (DeGeest et al., 1965; Pace and Keefe, 1970).

Here again it must be realized that although sympathetic stimulation occurring simultaneously with parasympathetic inhibition greatly increases the contractile force of the heart, in addition to increasing heart rate, the net effect is an increase in the permissive pumping of the heart as long as the tendency for venous return is not altered. Referring once again to Figure 5, we see a graphical analysis of the effects of autonomic stimulation of the heart on cardiac output. The normal cardiac function and normal venous return are represented by the dark curves, and the normal cardiac output is represented by point A. Maximum autonomic stimulation of the heart would cause the cardiac function curve to be increased to that represented by the dashed curve. Note that if the tendency for venous return is not altered, the new cardiac output is represented by point B, which is only slightly greater than that represented by point A. Note also in this figure that although cardiac output is increased only slightly, the permissive level of cardiac pumping is increased from approximately 15 liters/min to approximately 25 liters/min.

Autonomic Effects on the Peripheral Circulation   Autonomic effects on the peripheral circulation are mediated primarily through the sympathetic nervous system because of the sparsity of parasympathetic nerve fibers to the peripheral vasculature. The two major effects of sympathetic stimulation on the peripheral circulation that are of major importance in cardiac output regulation are changes in mean circulatory pressure and changes in resistance to venous return.

Total abrogation of sympathetic impulses to the circulation reduces the mean circulatory pressure from the normal value of 7 mm Hg to approximately 5 mm Hg (Guyton et al., 1954). On the other hand, maximal sympathetic stimulation, such as that caused by eliciting a maximal central nervous system ischemic reflex or by infusing a maximal amount of a sympathomimetic amine, increases the mean circulatory pressure to a level of 17–20 mm Hg (Guyton et al., 1954; Richardson and Fermoso, 1964). Since mean circulatory pressure is one of the principal determinants of the amount of blood that flows from the peripheral vasculature into the heart, this variation under the influence of autonomic impulses is a major contributor to the regulation of cardiac output.

The effect on venous return of autonomic stimulation of the peripheral circulation has been studied by many other investigators in other ways. Several workers have demonstrated that sympathetic stimulation results in constriction of the veins (Kelly and Visscher, 1956; Baum and Hosko, 1965; Zimmerman, 1966). In addition, Alexander (1954) and Mellander (1960) have shown that venous constriction produced by sympathetic stimulation increases the venous return. Eckstein and Hamilton (1957) have shown the same effect following epinephrine and norepinephrine infusion.

The effect of autonomic stimulation on the resistance to venous return is usually slight in comparison with its effect on total peripheral resistance. To understand the reason for this, one must first understand the distinction between resistance to venous return and total peripheral resistance. The resistive factors affecting total peripheral resistance are located primarily in the small arteries and arterioles. However, the resistance to venous return is a function not only of the resistance of a vessel, but also of the capacitance of the vessel (Guyton et al., 1973), and the capacitance of the venous system is much greater than the capacitance of the arterial system. Therefore, the factors affecting the resistance to venous return lie primarily in the veins. To illustrate this point, let us assume that arteriolar resistance is suddenly increased. The capacitance of the arterial system is relatively small; consequently, slight damming of blood behind the increased resistance causes the pressure in the arterial system to increase substantially. This increase in pressure in the arterial tree tends to force blood past the increased resistance. As a result, very little reduction in venous return occurs. However, if venous resistance is increased suddenly at some point along the venous tree, damming of blood behind this increased resistance causes only a very slight increase in venous pressure because of the relatively large capacitance of the venous system. Consequently, venous return is reduced substantially.

Thus the effect of sympathetic stimulation of the arteries is primarily an increase in arterial pressure with little change in venous return. However, the effect of sympathetic stimulation of the veins is primarily an increase in mean circulatory pressure with a consequent increase in venous return. The reason for this is that veins constrict along their entire length such that an increase in venous tone simply results in an increased squeezing of blood in the veins without a significant change in the diameter of the veins. As a result, mean circulatory pressure increases, but resistance to venous return does not increase appreciably.

REGULATION OF CARDIAC OUTPUT UNDER SPECIAL CONDITIONS

In the preceding section, the effects of cardiac and peripheral circulatory factors in the regulation of cardiac output have been presented, and it has been demonstrated that the effects of changes in cardiac function or peripheral circulatory function on cardiac output may be graphically analyzed by use of the cardiac function curve and the venous return curve. In the present section, such graphical analyses are used to illustrate how changes in cardiac function and peripheral circulatory function affect cardiac output in specific physiologic and pathologic states.

Effect of Oxygen Insufficiency on Cardiac Output

Oxygen insufficiency increases cardiac output in the same way that an increase in metabolism increases cardiac output. Increases in cardiac output to as much as two, or more, times normal have been observed in simple hypoxia resulting from reduced ambient oxygen concentration (Gorlin and Lewis, 1954; Vogel and Harris, 1967; Carrell and Milhorn, 1971), cyanide poisoning (Krasney, 1971), and carbon monoxide poisoning (Oberg, Richardson, and Guyton, 1961). Identical effects occur in all three types of hypoxia: cardiac output initially rises on the average to almost 100% above normal at optimal levels of hypoxia. However, when the degree of hypoxia increases further, the heart begins to fail, and the cardiac output then falls, instead of rising, as the degree of hypoxia increases still further. Figure 6 shows an analysis of the effects of oxygen insufficiency on cardiac output. The solid curves represent the normal venous return and cardiac output curves, with the equilibrium point at point A showing a cardiac output of 5 liters/min and a right atrial pressure of zero. After the effects of oxygen insufficiency have begun, the resistance to venous return decreases moderately, causing the venous return curve to rotate upward. The dashed curve illustrates the venous return curve under these conditions and shows a reduction in resistance to venous return of approximately 50%. Note also that the venous return has been shifted slightly to the right, indicating a slight increase in the mean circulatory pressure. Such a decrease in the resistance to venous return

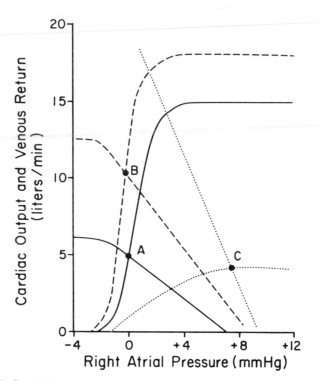

Figure 6. Graphical analyses showing effect of oxygen insufficiency on cardiac output.

with an increase in the mean circulatory pressure has been observed in hypoxic animals by Smith and Crowell (1967). The reduction in resistance to venous return is caused by dilatation of the arterioles in the various tissues of the body as explained above, and the increase in mean circulatory pressure is due to an increase in sympathetic stimulation of the veins.

The exact mechanism by which the sympathetic activity is increased during hypoxia is somewhat uncertain, but may be due to an oxygen insufficiency in the central nervous system such as occurs in the central nervous system ischemic reflex (Richardson and Fermoso, 1964). At the same time as sympathetic stimulation of the veins is increased, sympathetic stimulation of the heart causes the heart to become a more effective pump. As a result, the cardiac function curve increases to that represented by the dashed curve. Such an increase in cardiac pumping ability during the initial phases of hypoxia has been observed by Downing, Mitchell, and Wallace (1963) and Levy, Ng, and Zieske (1968). Because of this increased cardiac pumping ability, along with a reduction in resistance to venous return and an increase in mean circulatory pressure, the new cardiac output becomes that represented by point B in Figure 6. Note that under these conditions, the cardiac output is increased approximately 100%, even though right atrial pressure is not changed or may even be slightly reduced. This is precisely the observation made by Smith and Crowell (1967).

It should be pointed out that nervous reflexes involving the capacitance vessels, or the veins, play a significant role on the effects of hypoxia on cardiac output. For example, Smith and Crowell (1967) observed that when intact animals were respired with 8% oxygen, cardiac output was increased by approximately 50%; this increase in cardiac output was associated with dilatation of the peripheral resistance vessels and a 25% increase in the mean circulatory pressure. On the other hand, when the animals were given total spinal anesthesia, this same degree of hypoxia caused no significant increase in cardiac output, even though there was still a tremendous dilatation of the peripheral resistance vasculature. This failure of cardiac output to increase significantly was caused by an absence of venous constriction. Indeed, after spinal anesthesia, there was actually a drop in the mean circulatory pressure during hypoxia. Similar findings have been made by Korner and Uther (1969), Uther et al. (1970), and Banet and Guyton (1971). Thus it is apparent that in order for the reduction in resistance to venous return to be effective in increasing cardiac output, this reduction in resistance must be accompanied by a constriction of the veins, thereby maintaining, or even increasing, mean circulatory pressure. This increase in mean circulatory pressure forces blood to return to the heart, causing an increase in cardiac output, thereby maintaining arterial pressure despite the drop in peripheral resistance.

Referring once again to Figure 6, if the hypoxia becomes more severe and is sustained, the resistance to venous return is decreased even further, and mean circulatory pressure is further increased. Therefore, the venous return becomes that represented by the dotted curve. Also, severe hypoxia ultimately results in a reduction in cardiac contractility and cardiac failure (Jose and Stitt, 1969) such that the cardiac function curve becomes that represented by the dotted curve. Under these conditions, the cardiac output is reduced to that represented by point *C*, showing a cardiac output of approximately 4 liters/min and a right atrial pressure of approximately 8 mm Hg.

Effect of Muscular Exercise on Cardiac Output

Figure 7 illustrates an analysis of the sequential changes in cardiac output and right atrial pressure at different times after the onset of moderate exercise. The solid curve represents the normal resting circulation, the normal operating state being represented by point *A*. Now assume that there is a sudden onset of moderate exercise. An immediate tensing of the muscles throughout the body causes the mean circulatory pressure to rise from 7 to 10 mm Hg. Studies in areflex animals have shown that sudden tensing of the abdominal muscles and muscles of the lower leg can cause

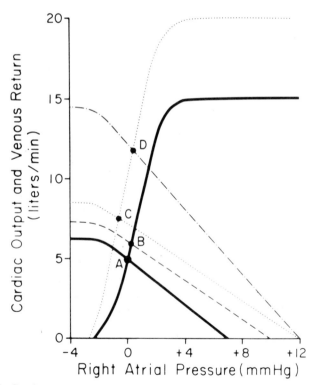

Figure 7. Graphical analyses showing effect of muscular exercise on cardiac output.

such an increase in mean circulatory pressure within 1 sec (Guyton et al., 1962). However, contraction of the muscles around the vessels, particularly of the abdominal muscles around the veins leading to the heart, simultaneously increases the resistance to venous return. Therefore, the venous return curve becomes that represented by the long dashed curve, which illustrates a mean circulatory pressure of 10 mm Hg and a slightly increased resistance to venous return, as denoted by the decreased slope. This venous return curve represents the function of the peripheral circulation during the first few seconds after the onset of moderate exercise. During this time the heart still has not increased its pumping ability, and the normal cardiac output curve is still applicable. Therefore, the instantaneous effect is an increase in cardiac output to that represented by point *B*, which shows a cardiac output of 6 liters/min and a slightly increased right atrial pressure.

During the next few seconds after the onset of exercise, sympathetic stimulation of the circulation will have developed significantly, causing major effects both on the heart and on the peripheral circulation. Sympathetic stimulation of the heart during exercise increases both heart rate (Braunwald et al., 1967; Faulkner et al., 1971) and cardiac contractility (Keroes et al., 1969). Both of these effects on the heart cause the cardiac function curve to be elevated to that represented by the dotted curve in Figure 7. Increased sympathetic stimulation of the peripheral vasculature also causes an increased constriction of the veins (Guyton et al., 1962; Bevegard and Shepherd, 1965; Shepherd, 1967). These effects of sympathetic stimulation on the peripheral circulation cause the venous return curve to be elevated and shifted to the right as represented by the dotted curve. Thus, the resulting cardiac output becomes that represented by point *C*, which shows a cardiac output of 8 liters/min and a right atrial pressure slightly less than 0 mm Hg. Moderate increases in cardiac output with no change, or even reductions, in right atrial pressure have been observed in human subjects during moderate exercise (Braunwald et al., 1963; Ekelund and Holmgren, 1967).

Within a minute or so following the onset of exercise, the arterioles in the active muscles undergo vasodilatation (Stainsby, 1962; Bevegard and Shepherd, 1967; Costin and Skinner, 1971). The precise mechanism of this vasodilatation in exercising muscle is not well defined, but it is almost certainly related to the balance between oxygen requirement by the tissue and oxygen transport to the tissue, as discussed above. For example, during exercise, the muscles utilize oxygen so rapidly that the oxygen available to the tissue is reduced. The muscle then becomes hypoxic. This muscle hypoxia in some way causes the arterioles to dilate, reducing vascular resistance, thereby allowing greater blood flow and increased oxygen transport to the active tissue. Referring once again to Figure 7, the vasodilatation reduces resistance to venous return and causes the venous return curve to rotate to the right, as represented by the dashed-dot venous return curve. This reduction in resistance to venous return causes cardiac output to increase to that represented by point D, which depicts a cardiac output of 13 liters/min and a right atrial pressure still essentially zero.

It is the vasodilatation in response to the increased requirement for oxygen of the active muscles that causes cardiac output to increase to precisely that level required by the tissues. And it is this mechanism that explains the almost linear correlation between oxygen consumption and cardiac output during muscular exercise, as illustrated in Figure 1.

In very strenous exercise, the mean circulatory pressure may increase above that shown in Figure 7. In addition, the resistance to venous return may be reduced even further. Under these conditions, the venous return curve may intersect with the cardiac function curve at a point on the plateau of the cardiac function curve. This means that during strenous exercise, the venous return may be so high that the cardiac output is equal to the maximum permissive pumping ability of the heart, and further increases in venous return would not result in further increases in cardiac output. This is demonstrated by the study of Robinson et al. (1966), who compared the effect of acute blood volume expansion on cardiac output in humans both at rest and during severe exercise. Expansion of volume by 1 liter at rest produced a small increase in right atrial pressure but a substantial increase in cardiac output. However, during exercise, the same expansion of blood volume resulted in a much greater increase in right atrial pressure but no increase in cardiac output.

Effect of Hemorrhage and Circulatory Shock on Cardiac Output

The immediate effect of acute blood loss on the circulation is a reduction in mean circulatory pressure. This reduction in mean circulatory pressure leads to several secondary effects that are graphically analyzed in Figure 8.

The dark curves depict the function of the normal circulation, with equilibrium at point A showing a cardiac output of 5 liters/min and a right atrial pressure of 0 mm Hg. If a large amount of blood is suddenly removed from the circulation, the mean circulatory pressure is suddenly

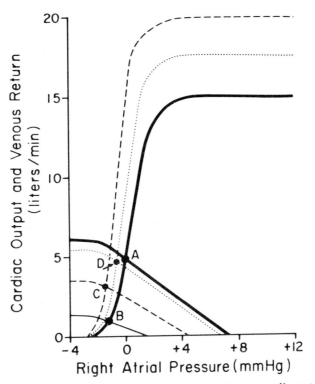

Figure 8. Graphical analyses showing effect of hemorrhage on cardiac output.

reduced, causing the venous return curve to shift to the left as shown by the light solid curve in Figure 8. If we assume that this reduction in mean circulatory pressure occurred before any compensatory factors could result, the cardiac function curve would still remain normal. The new venous return curve and the cardiac function curve would equate at point *B*, showing a cardiac output of approximately 0.6 liters/min and a right atrial pressure of −1.3 mm Hg. Within 20–40 sec after the acute blood loss, circulatory reflexes will have taken place, changing both the venous return curve and the cardiac output curve. For instance, the sympathetic reflexes cause the mean circulatory pressure to rise back toward normal; therefore, the mean circulatory pressure is shown to rise back to 4 mm Hg. This is precisely the observation made by Banet and Smith (1973). Thus the new venous return curve is now represented by the dashes. Simultaneously, reflexes to the heart make it a stronger pump so that the cardiac output curve becomes that represented by the dashes (Regan et al., 1965). These two curves equate at point C, which shows that within 20–40 sec after removal of this large amount of blood, the cardiac output has returned to 2.5 liters/min.

During the next 20–60 min, other compensatory mechanisms attempt to return blood volume to normal as discussed above. Therefore, the mean circulatory pressure increases even further and becomes that represented by the dotted curve. The increase in mean circulatory pressure causes a further increase in cardiac output; consequently, the heart becomes less stimulated by the sympathetic nervous system. As a result, the cardiac function curve now becomes that represented by the dotted curve. The new cardiac output is that represented by point D showing that cardiac output has returned almost to normal.

If the degree of blood loss were greater than that depicted in Figure 8, compensatory mechanisms may not be able to return cardiac output to near normal. The sustained reduction in cardiac output causes a sustained reduction in coronary blood flow (Jones et al., 1970). As a result, cardiac failure is a consistent finding in prolonged hemorrhagic shock (Crowell and Guyton, 1961, 1962; Regan et al., 1965; Bethea, Jones, and Crowell, 1972).

Effect of Opening the Chest on Cardiac Output

Since the heart is located in the thoracic cavity, the effective filling pressure of the heart is determined not only by the intra-atrial pressure but also by the intrapleural pressure; that is, it is determined by the *transmural pressure*, which is equal to intra-atrial pressure minus intrapleural pressure (Coleridge and Linden, 1954). Therefore, any factor that changes the intrapleural pressure also changes the entire cardiac function curve at the same time. Changing the intrapleural pressure does not alter the level or the plateau of the cardiac function curve but only shifts the curve horizontally. Thus, when the chest is opened, the intrapleural pressure immediately increases to atmospheric pressure or 0 mm Hg. As a result, the right atrial pressure must rise approximately 4 mm Hg to cause the heart to pump the same output it had been pumping before the chest was opened (Fermoso, Richardson, and Guyton, 1964).

The effect of opening the chest on cardiac output is graphically analyzed in Figure 9. Again the normal cardiac function curve and the normal venous return curve are shown by the dark curves with a normal

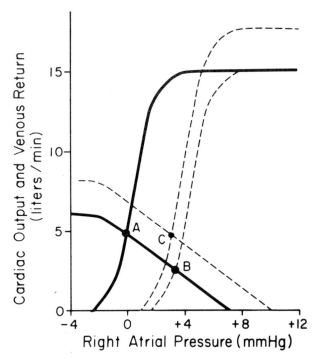

Figure 9. Graphical analyses showing the effect of opening the chest on cardiac output.

cardiac output of 5 liters/min and a right atrial pressure of 0 mm Hg. When the chest is opened, the intrapleural pressure rises from −4 mm Hg to 0 mm Hg, and the initial effect is a shift in the cardiac function curve to the right. This effect occurs before any change in peripheral circulatory function occurs so that the new cardiac output is that represented by point *B*, showing a cardiac output of approximately 2.5 liters/min and a right atrial pressure of approximately 4 mm Hg. However, compensatory effects immediately begin. During the 20–40 sec following the opening of the chest, cardiovascular reflexes cause an increase in mean circulatory pressure, thereby shifting the venous return curve upward and to the right, as illustrated by the dashed curve. Cardiovascular reflexes also enhance the pumping ability of the heart such that the cardiac function curve is increased. Thus, the cardiac output is increased to that represented by point *C*, which is only slightly less than the normal value.

The results of this graphical analysis are in accord with the results of Fermoso et al. (1964) who showed that opening the chest of dogs decreases the cardiac output only slightly.

Effect of Heart Failure on Cardiac Output

In this section the term "heart failure" is used to denote any condition in which the heart fails to pump blood as well as it does normally. Thus, whether the cause of heart failure be myocardial damage, valvular damage, toxic damage of the heart, arrhythmia, or any other cardiac abnormality, the effect on cardiac function is the same; this can be represented graphically by a depression of the cardiac function curve. When heart failure occurs, compensatory effects take place both on the heart and on the peripheral circulation, and these compensatory effects tend to offset the effects of heart failure on cardiac output. In this section the effects of heart failure and the resulting circulatory compensations on cardiac output are examined.

The solid curves of Figure 10 illustrate cardiac and peripheral circulatory function for the normal circulation with equilibrium at point A. Assume that a moderate myocardial infarction suddenly occurs such that cardiac pumping ability is abruptly reduced to approximately 25% of normal. Cardiac function would then be represented by the long dashed cardiac function curve in Figure 10. The venous return is not altered during the first few seconds after the sudden diminishment of cardiac pumping ability because the blood volume and the vasomotor tone are still the same. Therefore, the normal venous return curve is still operative in the circulation. Under these conditions, the new cardiac function curve equates with the normal venous return curve at point B, showing a cardiac output of approximately 2 liters/min and a right atrial pressure of slightly over 4 mm Hg.

Within a few seconds following the reduction of cardiac output, cardiovascular reflexes begin to develop. For instance, a cardiac output of only 2 liters/min would lead to a depressed arterial pressure, which in turn would elicit the pressoreceptor reflex. Also, the central nervous system ischemic reflex and possibly reflexes originating in the heart or lungs would be elicited. Thus increased sympathetic stimulation of both the heart and peripheral circulation would occur. As a consequence, the heart becomes a more powerful pump, as depicted by the lower dotted cardiac function curve in Figure 10. Simultaneously, the sympathetic reflexes

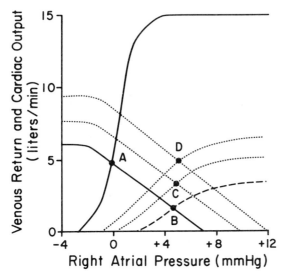

Figure 10. Graphical analyses showing effect of cardiac failure on cardiac output.

increase the vasomotor tone throughout the body, which increases the mean circulatory pressure, and, consequently, the venous return curve. This is depicted in Figure 10 by the lower, dotted venous return curve, which shows a shift in the venous return curve to the right and upward. The new cardiac output becomes that represented by point *C*, which indicates a cardiac output of approximately 3.5 liters/min and a right atrial pressure of 5 mm Hg. Thus it is obvious that within the first few seconds, the cardiovascular reflexes play a major role in returning the cardiac output back toward normal.

When cardiac output equals that represented by point *C*, a person can live quite satisfactorily as long as he lies in bed and performs no exercise. However, chronic compensations begin to occur, and these may further improve functions of both the peripheral circulations and the heart. For example, one of the principal long-term mechanisms of compensation for cardiac stress of many types is hypertrophy of the undamaged cardiac musculature (Badeer, 1964*a, b;* Dodge and Baxley, 1968). The clinical course of patients after a myocardial infarction indicates that the usual time course of the hypertrophy lasts over a period of several months, and in some patients the remaining musculature probably hypertrophies enough after a myocardial infarction to make the pump almost as strong a pump as it had been previously (Friedberg, 1956). In Figure 10, the cardiac function curve is shown to increase to that represented by the upper, dotted curve. It is assumed that this increase in cardiac function occurs over a period of weeks or months and is the result of repair of some of the myocardial damage that had been sustained by the infarction as well as to hypertrophy of undamaged portions of the heart.

Another chronic compensation is retention of fluid with a consequent increase in blood volume and mean circulatory pressure. This retention of fluid probably results in part from a decreased filtration of fluid across the glomeruli along with an increased reabsorption of fluid by the renal tubules (Davis, 1965; Baumber et al., 1970) and in part from an increased secretion of the hormone aldosterone by the adrenal cortex (Davis, 1958). Aldosterone enhances sodium reabsorption by the renal tubules and this, in turn, promotes water reabsorption from the tubules. Referring again to Figure 10, the retention of fluid increases blood volume and causes the mean circulatory pressure to increase, as indicated by a shift in the venous return curve to the right. Thus the venous return curve becomes that represented by the upper, dotted curve.

After all chronic compensations have occurred, cardiac output becomes that represented by point D, with a normal cardiac output and a right atrial pressure of between 5 and 6 mm Hg. Once the cardiac output has returned to normal, the renal retention of fluid ceases, and normal urinary output returns. However, the urinary output rises only back to normal and not above normal. Therefore, the fluid that had been accumulated in the body will remain.

When the chronic stage of compensation is in progress, even before the cardiac output has returned essentially to normal, the cardiovascular reflexes lose most of their effect on cardiac output. One of the reasons for this is that the pressoreceptors almost always adapt to the new pressure level conditions over a period of several days, and the reflex diminishes (Kubicek et al., 1953; Krieger, 1970). Furthermore, in chronic heart failure the catecholamine stores of the myocardium become almost completely depleted (Spann et al., 1965, 1967; Pool and Braunwald, 1968). Finally, as other compensatory mechanisms become active in heart failure—fluid retention to increase the mean circulatory pressure or hypertrophy of undamaged portions of the heart—the cardiac output rises, and as a result the reflexes lose their initiating stimulus.

ACKNOWLEDGMENTS

I am grateful to Mrs. Dianne Langford and Mrs. Paulette Fortenberry for their assistance in preparing this manuscript.

LITERATURE CITED

Alexander, R. S. 1954. The participation of the venomotor system in pressure reflexes. Circ. Res. 2: 405–409.

Badeer, H. S. 1964a. The stimulus to hypertrophy of the myocardium. Circulation 30: 128–136.

Badeer, H. S. 1964b. Biological significance of cardiac hypertrophy. Am. J. Cardiol. 14: 133–138.

Badeer, H. S. 1967. "Contractility" of the nonfailing hypertrophied heart. Am. Heart J. 73: 693–699.

Banet, M., and A. C. Guyton. 1971. Effect of body metabolism on cardiac output: role of the central nervous system. Am. J. Physiol. 220: 662–666.

Banet, M., and E. E. Smith. 1973. Mean circulatory pressure in hemorrhagic shock. J. Appl. Physiol. 34: 846–849.

Barcroft, H. 1964. Circulatory changes accompanying the contraction of voluntary muscle. Aust. J. Exp. Biol. Med. Sci. 42: 1–16.

Baum, R., and M. J. Hosko, Jr. 1965. Response of resistance and capacitance vessels to central nervous system stimulation. Am. J. Physiol. 209: 236–242.

Baumber, J. S., J. O. Davis, J. W. Machenzie, E. G. Schneider, J. A. Johnson, and C. A. Robb. 1970. Chronic experimental left heart failure in the dog. Am. J. Physiol. 219: 74–81.

Berne, R. M. 1964. Regulation of coronary blood flow. Physiol. Rev. 44: 1–29.

Besterman, E. M. 1954. The cardiac output in acute rheumatic carditis. Brit. Heart J. 16: 8–12.

Bethea, H. L., C. E. Jones, and J. W. Crowell. 1972. Effect of pharmacologic coronary flow augmentation on cardiac function in hypotension. Am. J. Physiol. 222: 95–100.

Bevegard, B. S., and J. T. Shepherd. 1965. Changes in tone of limb veins during supine exercise. J. Appl. Physiol. 20: 1–8.

Bevegard, B. S., and J. T. Shepherd. 1967. Regulation of the circulation during exercise in man. Physiol. Rev. 47: 178–213.

Bradley, R. D., B. S. Jenkins, and M. A. Branthwaite. 1970. The influence of atrial pressure on cardiac performance following myocardial infarction complicated by shock. Circulation 42: 827–838.

Brauer, R. W. 1964. Autoregulation of blood flow in the liver. Circ. Res. 15 (Suppl. 1): 213–221.

Braunwald, E., A. Goldblatt, D. C. Harrison, and D. T. Mason. 1963.

Studies on cardiac dimensions in intact, unanesthetized man. III. Effects of muscular exercise. Circ. Res. 13: 448–467.

Braunwald, E., E. H. Sonnenblick, J. Ross, Jr., G. Glick, and S. E. Epstein. 1967. An analysis of the cardiac response to exercise. Circ. Res. 20 (Suppl. 1): 44–58.

Carrell, D. E., and H. T. Milhorn, Jr. 1971. Dynamic respiratory and circulatory responses to hypoxia in the anesthetized dog. J. Appl. Physiol. 30: 305–312.

Carsten, A., B. Folkow, and C. A. Hamberger. 1958. Cardiovascular effects of direct vagal stimulation in man. Acta Physiol. Scand. 41: 68–76.

Chien, S., and S. Billig. 1961. Effect of hemorrhage on cardiac output of sympathectomized dogs. Am. J. Physiol. 201: 475–487.

Christensen, E. H., and U. Mitteilung. 1931. Minutenvolumen und Schlagvolumen des Herzens wahrend schwerer korperlicher Arbeit. Arbeitphysiologie 4: 470–495.

Coleridge, C. G., and R. J. Linden. 1954. The measurement of affective atrial pressure. J. Physiol. 126: 304–318.

Costin, J. C., and N. S. Skinner, Jr. 1971. Competition between vasoconstrictor and vasodilator mechanisms in skeletal muscle. Am. J. Physiol. 220: 462–466.

Cowley, A. W., and A. C. Guyton. 1971. Heart rate as a determinant of cardiac output in dogs with arteriovenous fistula. Am. J. Cardiol. 28: 321–325.

Crowell, J. W., and A. C. Guyton. 1961. Evidence favoring a cardiac mechanism in irreversible hemorrhagic shock. Am. J. Physiol. 201: 893–896.

Crowell, J. W., and A. C. Guyton. 1962. Further evidence favoring a cardiac mechanism in irreversible shock. Am. J. Physiol. 203: 248–252.

Damato, A. N., J. G. Galante, and W. M. Smith. 1966. Hemodynamic response to treadmill exercise in normal subjects. J. Appl. Physiol. 21: 959–966.

Davis, J. O., B. Kliman, N. A. Yankopoulor, and R. E. Peterson. 1958. Increased aldosterone secretion following constriction of the inferior vena cava. J. Clin. Invest. 37: 1783–1790.

Davis, J. O. 1965. Physiology of congestive heart failure. In P. Dow (ed.), Handbook of Physiology. Circulation, Vol. III, Section 2, Chapter 59, pp. 2071–2122. American Physiology Society, Washington, D.C.

DeGeest, H., M. N. Levy, H. Zieske, and R. I. Lipman. 1965. Depression of ventricular contractility by stimulation of the vagus nerves. Circ. Res. 17: 222–235.

Dexter, L., J. L. Whittenberger, F. W. Haynes, W. T. Goodale, R. Gorlin, and C. G. Sawyer. 1951. Effect of exercise on circulatory dynamics of normal individuals. J. Appl. Physiol. 3: 439–453.

Dobbs, W. A., J. W. Prather, and A. C. Guyton. 1971. Relative importance of nervous control of cardiac output and arterial pressure. Am. J. Cardiol. 27: 507–512.

Dodge, H. T., and W. A. Baxley. 1968. Hemodynamic aspects of heart failure. Am. J. Cardiol. 22: 24–34.

Donald, D. E., and J. T. Shepherd. 1963. Response to exercise in dogs after complete cardiac denervation. Am. J. Cardiol. 14: 853–859.

Donald, D. E., D. A. Ferguson, and S. E. Milburn. 1968. Effect of beta-adrenergic receptor blockade on racing performance of greyhounds with normal and with denervated hearts. Circ. Res. 22: 127–134.

Donald, K. W., J. M. Bishop, G. Cumming, and O. L. Wade. 1955. The effect of exercise on the cardiac output and circulatory dynamics of normal subjects. Clin. Sci. 14: 37–73.

Douglas, C. G., and J. S. Haldane. 1922. The regulation of the general circulation rate in man. J. Physiol. 56: 69–100.

Downing, S. E., J. H. Mitchell, and A. G. Wallace. 1963. Cardiovascular responses to ischemia, hypoxia, and hypercapnia of the central nervous system. Am. J. Physiol. 204: 881–887.

Eckblom, B., and L. Hermansen. 1968. Cardiac output in athletes. J. Appl. Physiol. 25: 619–631.

Eckstein, J. W., and W. K. Hamilton. 1957. The pressure–volume response of human forearm veins during epinephrine and norepinephrine infusion. J. Clin. Invest. 36: 1663–1671.

Ekelund, L. G., and A. Holmgren. 1967. Central hemodynamics during exercise. Circ. Res. 20 (Suppl. 1): 33–43.

Epstein, S. E., B. F. Robinson, R. L. Kahler, and E. Braunwald. 1965. Effects of Beta-adrenergic blockade on the cardiac response to maximal and submaximal exercise in man. J. Clin. Invest. 44: 1745–1753.

Faulkner, J. A., D. E. Roberts, R. L. Elk, and J. Conway. 1971. Cardiovascular responses to submaximum and maximum effort cycling and running. J. Appl. Physiol. 30: 457–461.

Fermoso, J. D., T. Q. Richardson, and A. C. Guyton. 1964. Mechanism of decrease in cardiac output caused by opening the chest. Am. J. Physiol. 207: 1112–1116.

Friedberg, C. K. 1956. Diseases of the Heart. 2nd Ed. W. B. Saunders, Philadelphia. 487 p.

Frye, R. L., and E. Braunwald. 1960. Studies of Starling's law of the heart. I. The circulatory response to acute hypervolemia and its modification by ganglionic blockade. J. Clin. Invest. 39: 1043–1050.

Gorlin, R., and B. M. Lewis. 1954. Circulatory adjustments to hypoxia in dogs. J. Appl. Physiol. 7: 180–185.

Gregerson, M. I., and R. A. Rawson. 1959. Blood volume. Physiol. Rev. 39: 307–342.

Gupta, P. D., J. P. Henry, R. Sinclair, and R. Von Baumgarten. 1966. Responses of atrial and aortic baroreceptors to nonhypotensive hemorrhage and to transfusion. Am. J. Physiol. 211: 1429–1437.

Guyton, A. C., J. E. Lindley, R. N. Touchstone, C. M. Smith, Jr., and H. M. Batson, Jr. 1950. Effects of massive transfusion and hemorrhage on blood pressure and fluid shifts. Am. J. Physiol. 163: 529–538.

Guyton, A. C., D. Polizo, and G. G. Armstrong, Jr. 1954. Mean circulatory filling pressure measured immediately after cessation of heart pumping. Am. J. Physiol. 179: 261–267.

Guyton, A. C., A. W. Lindsey, and B. Kaufmann. 1955. Effect of mean circulatory filling pressure and other peripheral circulatory factors on cardiac output. Am. J. Physiol. 180: 463–468.

Guyton, A. C., A. W. Lindsey, J. B. Abernathy, and T. Q. Richardson. 1957. Venous return at various right atrial pressures and the normal venous return curve. Am. J. Physiol. 189: 609–615.

Guyton, A. C., B. H. Douglas, J. B. Langston, and T. Q. Richardson. 1962. Instantaneous increase in mean circulatory pressure and cardiac output at onset of muscular activity. Circ. Res. 11: 431–441.

Guyton, A. C., T. G. Coleman, J. C. Fourcade, and L. G. Navar. 1969. Physiologic control of arterial pressure. Bull. N. Y. Acad. Med. 45: 811–830.

Guyton, A. C., C. E. Jones, and T. G. Coleman. 1973. Circulatory Physiology: Cardiac Output and Its Regulation. W. B. Saunders, Philadelphia. 556 p.

Herndon, C. W., and K. Sagawa. 1969. Combined effects of aortic and right atrial pressures on aortic flow. Am. J. Physiol. 217: 65–72.

Johnson, P. C. 1964. Origin, localization, and homeostatic significance of autoregulation in the intestine. Circ. Res. 15 (Suppl. 1): 225–232.

Jones, R. D., and R. M. Berne. 1965. Evidence for a metabolic mechanism in autoregulation of blood flow in skeletal muscle. Circ. Res. 17: 540–554.

Jones, C. E., H. L. Bethea, E. E. Smith, and J. W. Crowell. 1970. Effect of a coronary vasodilator on the development of irreversible hemorrhagic shock. Surgery 68: 356–362.

Jose, A. D., and F. Stitt. 1969. Effects of hypoxia and metabolic inhibitors on the intrinsic heart rate and myocardial contractility in dogs. Circ. Res. 25: 53–66.

Kelly, W. D., and M. B. Visscher. 1956. Effect of sympathetic nerve stimulation on cutaneous small vein and small artery pressures, blood flow and hindpaw volume in the dog. Am. J. Physiol. 185: 453–469.

Keroes, J., R. R. Ecker, and E. Rapaport. 1969. Ventricular function curves in the exercising dog. Circ. Res. 25: 557–568.

Korner, P. I., and J. B. Uther. 1969. Dynamic characteristics of the cardiovascular autonomic effects during severe arterial hypoxia in the unanesthetized rabbit. Circ. Res. 24: 671–687.

Krasney, J. A. 1971. Cardiovascular responses to cyanide in awake sino-aortic denervated dogs. Am. J. Physiol. 220: 1361–1366.

Krieger, E. M. 1970. Time course of baroreceptor resetting in acute hypertension. Am. J. Physiol. 218: 486–490.

Kubicek, W. G., F. J. Kottke, D. J. Laker, and M. B. Vischer. 1953. Adaptation in the pressoreceptor reflex mechanisms in experimental neurogenic hypertension. Am. J. Physiol. 175: 380–382.

Kumada, M., and K. Sagawa. 1970. Aortic nerve activity during blood volume changes. Am. J. Physiol. 218: 961–965.

Leusen, I., G. Demeester, and J. J. Bouckaert. 1956. Pressorecepteurs arteriels et de'vit cardiaque au cours de l' exercise musculaire. Arch. Intern. Physiol. 64: 564–570.

Levy, M. N., M. L. Ng, and H. Zieske. 1968. Cardiac response to cephalic ischemia. Am. J. Physiol. 215: 169–175.

Mellander, S. 1960. Comparative studies on the adrenergic neuro-hormonal control of resistance and capacitance blood vessels in the cat. Acta Physiol. Scand. 50 (Suppl. 176): 1–86.

Navar, L. G., and P. G. Baer. 1970. Renal autoregulatory and glomerular filtration responses to gradated ureteral obstruction. Nephron 7: 301–316.

Navar, L. G., J. B. Uther, and P. G. Baer. 1971. Pressure diuresis in dogs with diabetes insipidus. Nephron 8: 97–102.

Oberg, B., T. Q. Richardson, and A. C. Guyton. 1961. Effect of sodium cyanide on cardiac output. Physiologist 4: 84.

Oberg, B. 1964. Effects of cardiovascular reflexes on net capillary fluid transfer. Acta Physiol. Scand. 62 (Suppl. 229): 1–98.

Pace, J. B., and W. F. Keefe. 1970. Influence of efferent vagosympathetic nerve stimulation on right ventricular dynamics. Am. J. Physiol. 218: 811–818.

Patterson, S. W., and E. H. Starling. 1914. On the mechanical factors which determine the output of the ventricles. J. Physiol. 48: 357–379.

Pool, R. E., and E. Braunwald. 1968. Fundamental mechanisms in congestive heart failure. Am. J. Cardiol. 22: 7–21.

Prather, J. W., A. E. Taylor, and A. C. Guyton. 1969. Effect of blood volume, mean circulatory pressure, and stress relaxation on cardiac output. Am. J. Physiol. 216: 467–472.

Randall, W. C., D. V. Priola, and J. B. Pace. 1967. Responses of individual cardiac chambers to stimulation of the cervical vagosympathetic trunk in atropinized dogs. Circ. Res. 20: 534–544.

Randall, D. C., J. A. Armour, and W. C. Randall. 1971. Dynamic response to cardiac nerve stimulation in the baboon. Am. J. Physiol. 220: 526–533.

Regan, T. J., F. M. La Force, D. Teres, J. Block, and H. K. Hellems. 1965. Contribution of left ventricle and small bowel to irreversible hemorrhagic shock. Am. J. Physiol. 208: 938–844.

Richardson, T. Q., J. O. Stallings, and A. C. Guyton. 1961. Pressure volume curves in live, intact dogs. Am. J. Physiol. 201: 471–474.

Richardson, T. Q., and J. D. Fermoso. 1964. Elevation of mean circulatory pressure in dogs with cerebral ischemia-induced hypertension. J. Appl. Physiol. 19: 1133–1134.

Richardson, T. Q., J. D. Fermoso, and G. O. Pugh. 1964. Effect of acutely elevated intracranial pressure on cardiac output and other circulatory factors. J. Surg. Res. 5: 318–322.

Robinson, B. R., S. E. Epstein, R. L. Kahler, and E. Braunwald. 1966. Circulatory effects of acute expansion of blood volume: Studies during maximal exercise and at rest. Circ. Res. 19: 26–34.

Rushmer, R. F., and D. A. Smith, Jr. 1959. Cardiac control. Physiol. Rev. 39: 41–68.

Sagawa, K., J. M. Ross, and A. C. Guyton. 1961. Quantitation of the cerebral ischemic pressor response in dogs. Am. J. Physiol. 200: 1164–1168.

Sarnoff, S. J., and E. Berglund. 1954. Ventricular function. I. Starling's law of the heart studied by means of simultaneous right and left ventricular function curves in the dog. Circulation 9: 706–718.

Shepherd, J. T. 1967. Behavior of resistance and capacity vessels in human limbs during exercise. Circ. Res. 20: (Suppl. 1): 70–82.

Smith, E. E., and J. W. Crowell. 1967. Influence of hypoxia on mean circulatory pressure and cardiac output. Am. J. Physiol. 212: 1067–1069.

Spann, J., Jr., C. A. Chidsey, P. E. Pool, and E. Braunwald. 1965. Mechanism of norepinephrine depletion in experimental heart failure produced by aortic constriction in the guinea pig. Circ. Res. 17: 312–321.

Spann, J. F., Jr., F. A. Buccino, E. H. Sonnenblick, and E. Braunwald. 1967. Contractile state of cardiac muscle obtained from cats with experimentally produced ventricular hypertrophy and heart failure. Circ. Res. 21: 341–354.

Stainsby, W. N. 1962. Autoregulation of blood flow in skeletal muscle during increased metabolic activity. Am. J. Physiol. 202: 273–276.

Stead, E. A., Jr., and J. V. Warren. 1947. Cardiac output in man; analysis of mechanisms varying cardiac output based on recent clinical studies. Arch. Intern. Med. 80: 237–248.

Sugimoto, T., K. Sagawa, and A. C. Guyton. 1966. Effect of tachycardia on cardiac output during normal and increased venous return. Am. J. Physiol. 211: 288–292.

Tabakin, B. S., J. S. Hanson, T. W. Merriam, Jr., and E. J. Caldwell. 1964. Hemodynamic response of normal men to graded treadmill exercise. J. Appl. Physiol. 19: 457–464.

Uther, J. B., S. N. Hunyor, J. Shaw, and P. I. Korner. 1970. Bulbar and suprabulbar control of the cardiovascular effects during arterial hypoxia in the rabbit. Circ. Res. 26: 491–506.

Vogel, J. A., and C. W. Harris. 1967. Cardiopulmonary responses of resting man during early exposure to high altitude. J. Appl. Physiol. 22: 1124–1139.

Warren, J. V., E. S. Brannon, E. A. Stead, Jr., and A. J. Merrill. 1945. The effect of venesection and the pooling of blood in the extremities on the atrial pressure and cardiac output in normal subjects with observation on acute circulatory collapse in three instances. J. Clin. Invest. 24: 337–344.

Warren, J. V., E. S. Brannon, H. S. Weens, and E. A. Stead, Jr. 1948. Effect of increasing blood volume and right atrial pressure on circulation of normal subjects by intravenous infusions. Am. J. Med. 4: 193–200.

Yoshida, K., J. S. Meyer, K. Sakamoto, and J. Handa. 1966. Autoregulation of cerebral blood flow: Electromagnetic flow measurements during acute hypertension in the monkey. Circ. Res. 19: 726–738.

Zimmerman, B. G. 1966. Separation of responses of arteries and veins to sympathetic stimulation. Circ. Res. 18: 429–436.

Cardiovascular Flow Dynamics and Measurements
Edited by N. H. C. Hwang and N. A. Normann
Copyright 1977   University Park Press   Baltimore

chapter 11

QUANTITATIVE ANALYSIS OF THE ARTERIAL SYSTEM AND HEART BY MEANS OF PRESSURE-FLOW RELATIONS

N. Westerhof,
G. Elzinga, P. Sipkema, and G. C. van den Bos

ABSTRACT

An overview of the basis of arterial models is given. A segment of artery is described by two pressure–flow relations (longitudinal and transverse impedances); an entire arterial tree is then considered as the proper geometric combination of many segments. Each segment has its own parameters such as size and elasticity. The behavior of the entire arterial system, in terms of pressure–flow relations, is explained from its reflective characteristics and its length. The understanding of the pressure–flow relation of the whole arterial tree leads to a lumped model: the three-element windkessel. This windkessel is used in an attempt to derive aortic flow from aortic pressure; it is also used, in its hydraulic representation, as a load for the pumping heart. Cat hearts loaded with the model can be studied in terms of pressure and flow. It is shown that graphs relating mean left ventricular pressure with mean aortic flow describe the heart as a pump. Since these graphs are straight, they can be given in terms of slope (source resistance) and intercept with the pressure axis (hydromotive pressure, HMP). A time-changing compliance model is used to gain a better understanding of the pumping characteristics of the heart.

403

INTRODUCTION

The function of the arterial system is transport of blood from heart to periphery. Because the large arteries are distensible, they act as an elastic reservoir that stores a time-varying amount of blood. One of the results of this reservoir function is that pressure oscillations in the arterial system are much smaller than in the heart. The transport system is a regulated and controlled system. Flow distribution is regulated by local or overall demand, and mean pressure is usually controlled at fixed levels. To complicate analysis, the system, like most living systems, is nonlinear. An example of this nonlinearity is the pressure–volume relationship of a segment of artery: experimental results show that the relationship is not a straight line (Bergel, 1961a).

Models of the arterial tree are an abstraction and simplification of the real system. The development of a model is started with what one considers to be the most essential characteristics of the arterial tree. If the model is based on the simplifying assumptions of linearity and steady state, the result of the model should be tested against the real system. The test indicates how far the assumptions are correct.

Here we start with a model of a segment of artery based on linear theory for steady-state conditions. Models of the entire arterial system are then considered as geometrically determined combinations of such segments. Results of these models have shown a satisfactory comparison with the real system and it is therefore thought that the linear approach is sufficient for the understanding of the basic characteristics of the arterial tree.

Blood flow is intimately related to the transport function of the arterial system. It was therefore desirable to measure blood flow long before it was technically possible. To get information on transport, several investigators tried to derive flow from pressure. These attempts are of interest from the theoretic point of view, and they are discussed together with a new approach to the problem.

On the basis of the described theory a simplified hydraulic model of the arterial system can be constructed. This hydraulic model is chosen to be linear and can be used as the load for an ejecting heart.

Analysis of the heart (left ventricle) is more complicated than that of the arterial system because of its time-dependent parameters and nonlinear characteristics. This may be the reason why quantitative analysis of the heart, although initiated almost simultaneously with the quantitative analysis of the arterial system, proceeded less rapidly (Frank, 1899). Until now the heart was usually described by considering left ventricular pressure and its time derivative rather than by pressure and flow. To avoid the effect of the periphery on left ventricular pressure, only the isovolumic part of the pressure rise is analyzed. An attempt to analyze the heart as a pump in terms of pressure–flow relations is discussed. If the heart's pumping action is given in terms of slope and intercept of mean left ventricular pressure and mean outflow plots, the nonlinear characteristics of the aortic valve can be avoided.

ARTERIAL SYSTEM

Historical Remarks and Outline

Arterial models of the systemic and of the pulmonary arterial tree have a fairly long history. The oldest models were of the windkessel type (Frank, 1899). Models that included the traveling waves of pressure and flow emerged later. Although Frank (1905) already discussed wave transmission, descriptions of models that specifically included the traveling waves apparently had to wait until the frequency-domain approach was introduced in cardiac physiology. The windkessel models were almost exclusively based on time-domain considerations: the (total) arterial compliance (C) was charged during systole and during diastole [where inflow is zero and part of the volume (V) stored in the large arteries $(V = CP)$ leaves the arterial system via the peripheral resistance R_p, i.e., $F = P/R_p$] the decay of the pressure (P) could be calculated from

$$C \frac{dP}{dt} + \frac{P}{R_p} = 0 \qquad (1)$$

The solution of Eq. 1 is

$$P(t) = P_0 e^{-t/R_p C}, \qquad (2)$$

where P_0 is a reference pressure.

After the introduction of Fourier analysis of cardiovascular signals, assuming that the cardiovascular system is in a steady state of oscillation and no transients are present (Apéria, 1940; Porjé, 1946), pressure and flow waves were written as a sum of sine waves and each sine wave was considered separately (linear system). The system is thus approached in the frequency domain. Only slightly later, studies on elastic tubes were carried out (Taylor, 1957) and the arterial system was then approached from elastic-tube theory and the relations were described in the frequency domain (McDonald and Taylor, 1959). The windkessel was from then on almost completely neglected. We will show that both types of models (tube models and windkessel models) are useful and not contradictory, but rather two descriptions with emphasis on different aspects. Our description is, however, based on the frequency domain rather than on the time-domain approach.

The main purpose of the construction of arterial models is to obtain a better insight into the behavior of the arterial tree in terms of pressure–flow relations (impedance) and pressure–pressure relations (reflection). Indeed, animal experiments and work on arterial models have both contributed to a good understanding of the behavior of the arterial tree in these terms. Although a discussion that starts with the description of the windkessel would be logical from the standpoint of history, we prefer to start with principal notions on pressure and flow in a segment of artery. Summation of many of these segments leads to a distributed model that imitates the input impedance as well as wave travel in the arterial tree. From these distributed models we return to the windkessel model that only describes the input impedance of the arterial tree.

Knowledge of the characteristics of the arterial tree and arterial models can provide a basis for the computation of aortic flow from aortic pressure. A new method for the derivation of flow from pressure is discussed. Finally the obtained knowledge will make it possible to construct a load for the isolated pumping heart.

Pressure–Flow Relations in a Segment of Artery

Longitudinal and Transverse Impedances The simplest model of a segment of artery is a hollow, cylindrical distensible tube. Extensive linear theory is now available to describe oscillatory pressure–flow relations in such a segment (Womersley, 1957; Noordergraaf, 1969; McDonald, 1974).

The pressure and flow waves as functions of time can be individually written as a sum of sine waves by means of Fourier analysis (Attinger, Anné, and McDonald, 1966a; Malindzak, 1970); each sine wave is now treated separately. The theory predicts flow velocity profiles and pressure–flow relations for a rigid segment of tube. Pressure–volume relations are obtained from the continuity equation for a distensible segment.

The approach is now as follows. The longitudinal impedance is derived for a rigid segment of artery, neglecting all aspects of distensibility. The transverse impedance is given for a compliant segment. The solution for the general case is given in the literature (Womersley, 1957; Jager, 1965; Cox, 1968, 1969). The longitudinal and transverse impedances for the general case turn out to be much more complex than for the case of the simplifying assumptions mentioned above. If it is assumed that the tube is strongly tethered, then the results turn out to be equal to those of the simplified approach (Jager, 1965; McDonald, 1974). Because the assumption of longitudinal constraint is a reasonable one (McDonald, 1974), the results of the simpler approach are accurate enough for us here. The results of importance can be given in two equations that relate pressure drop ($\partial P/\partial z$) to flow, and flow drop ($\partial F/\partial z$) to pressure (Jager, Westerhof, and Noordergraaf, 1965),

$$\frac{\partial P}{\partial z} = F \cdot Z_l' \tag{3a}$$

$$\frac{\partial F}{\partial z} = \frac{P}{Z_t'} \tag{3b}$$

where P is pressure, F is (volume) flow, z is the longitudinal coordinate, and Z_l' and Z_t' are the so-called longitudinal and transverse impedances per length. The derivation of Eq. 3a is given by Womersley (1957) and can also be found in McDonald (1974). The Z_l' is a complex quantity in the mathematical sense, and can be written as a function (a quotient of Bessel functions) of a dimensionless parameter (α). The parameter α was introduced by Womersley (1957) and is $\alpha^2 = r_0^2 \, \omega/\nu$, where r_0 is the (internal) radius of the tube, ν is the kinematic viscosity of blood ($\nu = \mu/\rho$ where μ is viscosity and ρ is density), and $\omega = 2\pi f$ where f is the frequency. Tables are available that give Z_l' as a function of α (Womersley, 1957). For steady flow or very small radii ($\alpha \cong 0$)

$$Z_l' \simeq 8\mu/\pi r_0^4 = R' \tag{4}$$

In other words, Poiseuille's law is obtained: a viscous relationship, the oscillatory pressure gradient and flow are in phase. For very high frequencies or large radii (as observed in the aorta, $\alpha > 10$) the longitudinal impedance becomes

$$Z_l' \simeq j\omega\rho/\pi r_0^2 = j\omega L', \tag{5}$$

which specifies that for large arteries the longitudinal impedance reduces to an inertial relationship, the flow lags the pressure gradient by $90°$. For the general case where α is neither large nor small, Z_l' can be represented by a combination of resistances and inertances (Jager, Westerhof, and Noordergraaf, 1965) as shown in Figure 1.

The transverse impedance is directly related to the compliance per length of the tube. Compliance is defined as $C' = dS/dP$ where $S = \pi r_0^2$. The relation is

$$Z_t' = 1/j\omega C' \qquad (6)$$

The compliance per unit length can be computed from the radius, wall thickness, and modulus of elasticity (E) of the tube (Love, 1927; Bergel, 1961a):

$$C' = \frac{3\pi r_0^3 (1 + h/r_0)^2}{E(\omega)\cdot 2h(1+h/2r_0)} \simeq \frac{3\pi r_0^3}{2E(\omega)h} \qquad (7)$$

where h is wall thickness. The last approximation holds for a thin-walled tube ($h \ll r_0$). The Young modulus $E(\omega)$ is a function of frequency. Extensive measurements of the Young modulus as a function of frequency were first performed by Bergel (1961b) and later by Learoyd and Taylor (1966). For large arteries the frequency dependence of the Young modulus is rather small, so that we can write $E(\omega) = E$, i.e., a purely elastic

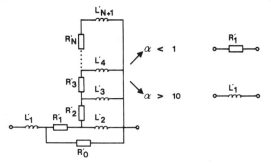

Figure 1. The longitudinal impedance of a segment of artery can be modeled by a combination of resistances and inductances. The longitudinal impedance relates pressure gradient over and flow through the segment. Primed quantities are used to indicate that they are given for a unit length. $R_m' = (8\pi\mu/S^2)m$; $L_m' = (\rho/S)[1/(2m-1)]$; $S = \pi r_0^2$; $m = 1,2,\ldots$ Explanation of symbols in text. The R_0 is the resistance for the correction of the anomalous viscosity of blood (see Jager et al., 1965). The quantity α is defined in the text. For small radii and low frequencies the network reduces to a resistor (Poiseuille's law); for large radii and high frequencies an inertial relationship between pressure and flow is found.

wall. Another (theoretic) limiting case is that of a purely viscous wall; in such a case Z_t' is a resistor. If $E(\omega)$ is known then $Z_t'(\omega)$ can be obtained. In general, Z_t' can be approximated by a series arrangement of capacitors and resistors. For the purely elastic wall a single capacitor is sufficient, as shown in Figure 2 (Westerhof and Noordergraaf, 1970).

Propagation Constant; Characteristic Impedance and Reflection Coefficient We have now defined, in very general terms, pressure–flow relationships in a segment of artery. If we have a single segment of tube that is characterized by Z_l' and Z_t' we can differentiate Eq. 3 with respect to location:

$$\frac{\partial^2 P}{\partial z^2} = Z_l' \frac{\partial F}{\partial z} = \frac{Z_l'}{Z_t'} \, P = \gamma^2 P \tag{8a}$$

and

$$\frac{\partial^2 F}{\partial z^2} = \gamma^2 F \tag{8b}$$

The quantity $\gamma = \sqrt{Z_l'/Z_t'}$ is frequency dependent (Eqs. 5 and 6) and is called the propagation constant. If we take the coordinate of location zero at the end of the tube we can solve the (one-dimensional) wave equations

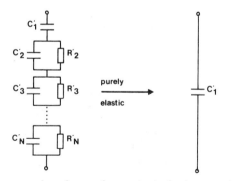

Figure 2. The transverse impedance of a segment of artery can be modeled by a combination of resistances and capacitances. The transverse impedance relates flow gradient over and pressure in a segment. Primed quantities are used to indicate that they are given for a unit length. The values of R and C are determined from the frequency characteristic of the Young modulus of elasticity (see Westerhof et al., 1970). For the case in which the artery is purely elastic, a single capacitor results (= segment compliance).

(Eq. 8). The solutions are (Karakash, 1950, p. 8)

$$P(z) = P_L [e^{\gamma z} + \Gamma e^{-\gamma z}] \tag{9a}$$

$$F(z) = P_L [e^{\gamma z} - \Gamma e^{-\gamma z}]/Z_0 \tag{9b}$$

Note the similarity and the differences in the pressure and flow equations.

The P_L is a reference pressure and the newly introduced, frequency-dependent quantity Z_0 is the characteristic impedance:

$$Z_0 = \sqrt{Z_l' Z_t'} \tag{10}$$

A special case is observed for the large arteries such as the aorta, where Z_l' = $j\omega L'$ (Eq. 5) and $Z_t' = 1/j\omega C'$ (Eq. 6). For these large arteries it holds that Z_0 is a real constant:

$$Z_0 = \sqrt{L'/C'} \tag{11}$$

The input impedance of a uniform tube without reflections is equal to its characteristic impedance. Inversely, if a segment of artery is loaded with its characteristic impedance the artery seems infinitely long and no reflections are present (Eqs. 12 and 17).

The quantity Γ is the reflection coefficient and is defined as the ratio of the backward (i.e., reflected) and forward pressure wave at the end of the tube ($z = 0$). Γ is a pressure–pressure relationship. If we define the load impedance Z_L by $P(0)/F(0)$ ($z = 0$ is at the end of the tube), then we find from Eq. 9 that

$$\Gamma = \frac{Z_L - Z_0}{Z_L + Z_0} \tag{12}$$

The reflection coefficient is a complex quantity (designated by $|\Gamma|$ and ϕ). It relates backward and forward pressure and can be written as an impedance relation. Mismatch of impedances at junctions and stenoses was studied theoretically by Womersley (1957) and experimentally by Newman and Bowden (1973) and Newman, Walesby, and Bowden (1975).

It is often more convenient to work with the propagation constant and characteristic impedance (γ and Z_0) than with the longitudinal and transverse impedances (Z_l' and Z_t'), but because there exists a direct relationship between them, either choice gives a complete description of the segment.

Pulse Wave Velocity   The propagation constant, which is the same for pressure and flow, can be written as

$$\gamma = a + jb \tag{13}$$

where a indicates the attenuation of the traveling wave and b is directly related to the so-called phase velocity (v_p) of the pressure and flow waves,

$$v_p = \omega/b. \tag{14}$$

The phase velocity in the artery can now be written in various forms if α can be assumed large and the arterial wall purely elastic as is the case in large arteries (Eq. 5–7),

$$v_p = \frac{\omega}{\sqrt{Z_l'/Z_t'}} = \frac{1}{\sqrt{L'C'}} \simeq \sqrt{\frac{2Eh}{3r_0\rho}} = \sqrt{\frac{dP}{dS}\frac{S}{\rho}} = \sqrt{\frac{X}{\rho}} \tag{15}$$

(Moens, 1878; Bramwell and Hill, 1922). X is distensibility of the tube wall. These equations (Eq. 15) were commonly used to obtain information about arterial elasticity from the pulse wave velocity. It should be stressed that the phase velocity is equal for pressure and flow waves. The velocity with which the wall displacement travels along the artery is also v_p.

Reflections affect pressure and flow and thus the apparent wave velocity of the pressure and flow waves. The apparent wave velocity (v_{app}) is measured if two transducers, separated by distance Δz, measure the time delay, Δt, of the signals: $v_{app} = \Delta z/\Delta t$. The apparent wave velocity for pressure is not equal to the phase velocity when reflections are present, but may be larger or smaller than the phase velocity depending on the reflection coefficient and on the location where it is measured (Taylor, 1957; Milnor and Nichols, 1975).

It is customary to define the apparent wave velocity in terms of pressure. There also exists an apparent wave velocity for flow. The apparent wave velocities of pressure and flow are not identical in contrast to their phase velocities, which are the same for both (Cox, 1971; Cox and Pace, 1975; Milnor and Nichols, 1975).

For the very special case that we deal with, a frictionless tube with complete reflection ($|\Gamma| = \pm 1$, open or closed end), the apparent wave velocity is infinite. If v_{app} is infinite, a standing wave is created. The estimation of arterial elasticity based on measurements of pulse wave velocity therefore can be erroneous if reflections are present. When pulse wave velocities are measured, the "foot" of the pressure or wall displacement wave is usually taken as the reference point. The relatively sharp corner of the "foot" is related to the higher harmonics in the signal, which are not much modified by reflections.

The above characterization of a segment of artery led to the notion of input impedance.

Measurements of Input Impedance and Wave Transmission   To characterize an entire arterial system or a peripheral bed, the hydraulic input impedance of that bed was introduced. Pressure drop over and flow through the system should be measured. Since venous pressure is normally negligible, it is often sufficient to measure arterial pressure only. Input impedance completely characterizes the system over which pressure difference is measured. Therefore the pump (heart) and the proximal part of the system only play a role in the generation of the pressure and flow signals, but their contribution is eliminated through the calculation of impedance. Pressure and flow are usually measured as functions of time, and Fourier analysis gives the various sine waves that should be related. We can write

$$P(t) = P_m + \sum_{n=1}^{N} P_n \cos(\omega n\, t + \phi_n), \qquad (16)$$

where m indicates mean and n is the harmonic number.

Summation is in most cases sufficient to $N = 20$; each harmonic is characterized by a modulus (P_n) and a phase (ϕ_n). The modulus of the impedance is obtained by division of corresponding pressure and flow moduli ($|Z_{in}|_n = P_n/F_n$). The phase angle of the impedance is found by subtracting the phase of a flow harmonic from the phase of the corresponding pressure harmonic. The system to be analyzed should be in a steady state; transients should not be analyzed in this way. The heart beat to be analyzed should be preceded by at least three or four identical sequences. Heart rate determines the frequencies for which the impedance values can be obtained. If heart rate is 120 beats per minute (2 Hz) then the harmonics, and thus the impedance values, are found at 0, 2, 4, ... Hz; the resolution in frequency is the inverse of the period of the heart beat. For details and limitations of the Fourier analysis method see Attinger et al. (1966a) and Malindzak (1970).

From Eq. 9 we obtain, for a tube of length l,

$$Z_{in}(\omega) = \frac{P(l,\omega)}{F(l,\omega)} = Z_0 \frac{1 + \Gamma e^{-2\gamma l}}{1 - \Gamma e^{-2\gamma l}} \qquad (17)$$

We see that the input impedance of a tube of length l is dependent on the local characteristics of the tube (Z_0) as well as on the reflection coefficient (Γ). If arterial tree were a uniform tube of infinite length, the input impedance would be equal to the characteristic impedance of the aorta, as mentioned above. As is discussed later, it turns out that for high frequencies the input impedance of the arterial system approaches the characteristic impedance, suggesting that reflections are small for these frequencies. For the special case of a tube that is closed or open at the end ($\Gamma = 1$ or $\Gamma = -1$) and where losses are negligible, there results an impedance modulus that oscillates between zero and infinity. This situation is approximated for low frequencies in the arterial system where the input impedance is grossly different from the characteristic impedance of the aorta.

Data of the modulus and phase of the input impedance of the entire arterial tree in man, dog, and cat all show the same qualitative behavior. Data reported by Patel, Austen, and Greenfield (1964), Gabe et al. (1964), Patel et al. (1965), and Mills et al. (1970) pertain to man. Data on the systemic arterial tree of the dog are reported by Randall and Stacy (1956), Attinger et al. (1966d), Taylor (1966b), O'Rourke and Taylor (1966, 1967), Noble et al. (1967), O'Rourke (1968), and Westerhof, Elzinga, and Van den Bos (1973). The input impedance of the pulmonary arterial bed is reported by Caro and McDonald (1961), Bergel and Milnor (1965), Milnor et al. (1969), and Reuben et al. (1971). Figure 3 gives the input impedance of seven dogs as measured in our laboratory. There are considerable differences between dogs; the average value of all seven dogs is given at the right-hand side of Figure 3. The input impedance of the systemic arterial tree of a cat, determined from 11 successive heart beats in a steady state, is given in Figure 4.

All impedances show the same behavior with frequency: a precipitous drop of the modulus is found at the low frequencies and thereafter it remains reasonably constant. The phase is strongly negative for low frequencies and approaches zero values for higher frequencies.

The apparent pulse wave velocity can be obtained from the simultaneous measurements of two pressures at distance Δz. After Fourier analysis of the two pressures (basic frequency f_0) the phases of corresponding harmonics (n) are related ($\Delta\psi_n$) and the apparent wave velocity is calculated from (Luchsinger et al., 1964)

$$v_{\mathrm{app},n} = 2\pi f_0 \Delta z n / \Delta\psi_n \qquad (18)$$

When the apparent wave velocity is plotted as a function of frequency, it shows characteristics similar to the modulus of the impedances. For low

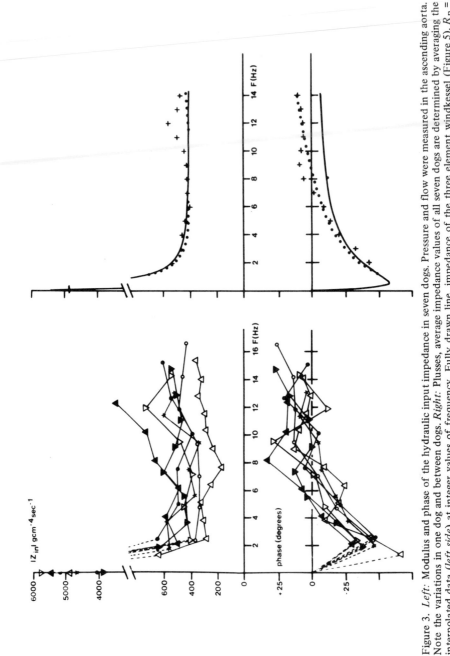

Figure 3. *Left*: Modulus and phase of the hydraulic input impedance in seven dogs. Pressure and flow were measured in the ascending aorta. Note the variations in one dog and between dogs. *Right*: Plusses, average impedance values of all seven dogs are determined by averaging the interpolated data (*left side*) at integer values of frequency. Fully drawn line, impedance of the three element windkessel (Figure 5). $R_p =$ 4450 g/(cm⁴ sec); $R_c = 420$ g/(cm⁴ sec) and $C = 240 \times 10^{-6}$ g⁻¹ cm⁴ sec². Dotted line, impedance of the same windkessel but with an inertia element (1.5 g/cm⁴) in series with the R_c

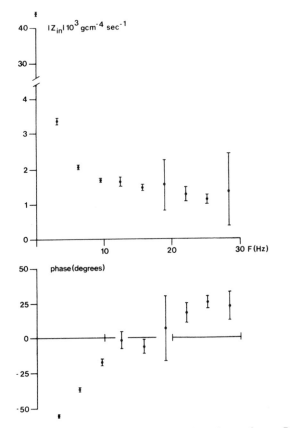

Figure 4. Modulus and phase of the hydraulic input impedance of a cat. Pressure and flow are measured in the ascending aorta. Eleven heart beats are analyzed and the results averaged. Bars give 1 S.D.

frequencies the apparent wave velocity is high; for high frequencies the apparent wave velocity is low and approximately equal to the phase velocity. The amplitudes of the pressure harmonics as a function of location (Eq. 9a) have been measured in man (Luchsinger et al., 1964) and dog (McDonald, 1974). Although it appears that most harmonics show a maximum at the inguinal ligament, this does not necessarily indicate that the arterial tree can be replaced by a single tube with a resistive load (Sipkema and Westerhof, 1975). Measurements that give more information have been reported, namely reports that give pressure–flow relations as well as pressure–pressure relations in the same animal (Gabe et al., 1964; Milnor et al., 1969; Cox and Pace, 1975).

The input impedance of the arterial tree is not the only way to characterize its hydraulic behavior. An alternative manner is to use the reflection coefficient in the ascending aorta. The reflection coefficient can be calculated from the characteristic impedance of the ascending aorta and the input impedance of the entire arterial tree (Eq. 12). The reflection coefficient, together with the characteristic impedance of the aorta, completely describes the whole systemic arterial system. The description is in other terms but it is as complete as the description by means of impedance. The modulus of the reflection coefficient decreases with frequency (somewhat as the impedance modulus) (Westerhof et al., 1972). Westerhof et al. (1972) also showed that an increase in peripheral resistance and occlusion of the aorta increase the reflection coefficient.

Arterial Hemodynamics

Models Used to Explain the Hydrodynamic Relationships in the Arterial Tree   Extensive models consisting of many segments of artery, each with its own parameters (Z'_l and Z'_t or Z_0 and γ), can be divided into mathematical and physical models. Extensive reviews are given by Noordergraaf (1969) and Beneken (1972). For all segments put in series or in parallel, the values of Z'_l and Z'_t (or γ and Z_0) must be calculated. Although mathematical models started out with single uniform tubes (Taylor, 1957, 1959), it was soon recognized that these models were too simple.

An extensive mathematical analog of the arterial tree, consisting of an assembly of uniform tubes with random lengths, was modeled by Taylor (1966a, 1966c) on a digital computer. A less extensive mathematical model, consisting of 49 segments of artery, was reported by Attinger et al. (1966a). Both models show close correspondence in their pressure–flow relationships to the behavior of the arterial tree. A simpler mathematical model consisting of two tubes in parallel ("eccentric T-tube") was recently discussed by O'Rourke (1971). Nonuniform tubes as arterial models and other approaches are reported (Taylor, 1965; Attinger et al., 1966c). Extensive hydraulic models are difficult to construct. Therefore they are mostly reduced to simple representations of the system such as the model proposed by Wetterer and Kenner (1968). The model constructed by these authors consists of two tubes, with different characteristics, in series. A more extensive hydraulic model consisting of thin-walled flexible tubing in a pressurized container has recently been constructed by Reul et al. (1974). The geometry of the large systemic arteries was closely approximated by means of plastic moldings of these arteries. The input impedance of this system is not reported and it is therefore difficult to judge to what degree it imitates the arterial tree. Since compliance results from the flexible tubes in a container that is partly filled with air, it seems that pulse wave velocities do not exist.

Extensive electrical analogs have been constructed by De Pater and Van den Berg (1964), Pollack, Reddy, and Noordergraaf (1968), and Westerhof et al. (1969). It is possible to model in electrical terms Womersley's oscillatory flow theory as shown above (Figures 1 and 2). All these models mimic input impedance and wave travel in the large arteries well. It appears that many refinements (such as viscoelasticity of the arterial wall and the introduction of Womersley's oscillatory flow theory) do not improve these models much. The basic overall behavior of the arterial models already showed the basic pressure–flow relations as observed in the arterial tree (Westerhof, 1968).

Interpretation of Arterial Impedance and Wave Travel   Arterial models as well as animal experiments led to important conclusions about the behavior of the arterial tree in terms of input impedance and wave travel. For a better understanding it is best to return for a moment to the eccentric T-tube mentioned above. Both tubes are in parallel and loaded with their own peripheral resistances. For low frequencies the two reflection sites are, compared to the wavelength of the waves under consideration, relatively close to the heart. The wave length (λ) is calculated from

$$\lambda = v_p/f \tag{19}$$

(for instance, in the large arteries v_p = 400 cm/sec; for frequencies less than 1 Hz the wave length is larger than 400 cm). Thus for the very low frequencies the waves generated by the heart are reflected at the two reflection sites and return in phase since the wave length is so long that the waves travel only a fraction of a wave length. For higher frequencies the wave length is not longer than the length of the system. Certain frequencies that are reflected at the two ends of the model may now travel over a difference in distance equal to half a wavelength; the waves return out of phase at the heart. When waves return in phase, the reflection coefficient is large; when the two reflected waves return out of phase, the reflection coefficient is small.

In the arterial system many reflection sites exist, all at different distances from the heart. For low frequencies reflection is high. As a result of the many sites, reflection is small for all high frequencies (Westerhof et al., 1972).

The shape of the input impedance as a function of frequency can now be explained on the basis of what was said of the reflection coefficient. Referring to Eq. 17 we see that for low frequencies Z_{in} deviates considerably from the characteristics impedance (Γ large) but for high frequencies Z_{in} approaches Z_0 (Γ is small). These results hold true for man, dog, and cat. In principle, one can expect that the longer the arterial system the more rapidly the impedance approaches the characteristic impedance, since the phase velocities are approximately equal in all animals.

Because apparent wave velocity deviates strongly from the phase velocity when the reflection coefficient is large (Westerhof, 1968), the apparent wave velocity is high for low frequencies. For high frequencies the apparent wave velocity approaches the phase velocity because reflections become very small.

The combination of large reflection and short system explains the increase of the pulse pressure (systolic–diastolic pressure) toward the periphery. The low harmonics increase in amplitude from heart to periphery. The high frequencies oscillate as a function of location. Since low harmonics have larger amplitudes than the high harmonics, the pulse pressure increases towards the periphery. The high frequencies mainly contribute to the details of the particular wave shapes.

The simplest model that imitates the input impedance of an arterial tree or part thereof is the modified windkessel model as suggested by Westerhof (1968). The model is shown in Figure 5. It consists of a resistor (R_c), representing the characteristic impedance of the aorta ($R_c = \sqrt{L'/C'}$, Eq. 11) in series with a parallel arrangement of a capacitor (representing total arterial compliance, C) and a peripheral resistance (R_p). The input impedance of this model (here given in electrical and hydraulic components, Figure 5) is indeed high for low frequencies and constant (equal to R_c) for high frequencies. We can now return to the original windkessel as proposed by Frank (1899). Frank was not able to measure oscillatory flow but he did measure pressure. The diastolic decay of pressure during diastole is explained by the time constant $\tau_1 = R_p C$, which is the same constant for the windkessel described by Frank (1899) and the modified windkessel. From time considerations of pressure only (flow was not known) it was not possible for Frank to infer the existence of the resistance R_c. We also see that extensive models mimic input impedance to

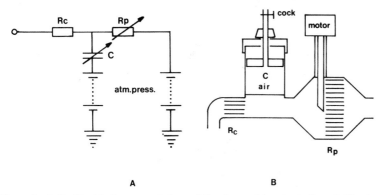

Figure 5. *Left:* Electrical representation of the three element windkessel. The two batteries are added to indicate atmospheric pressure. Batteries have zero impedance. *Right:* Hydrodynamic equivalent of the three-element windkessel. Heart is connected to cannula at left.

the same degree of correctness as the modified windkessel. Windkessel models, of course, completely disregard wave travel, while extensive models take wave travel into account.

Calculation of Flow from Pressure   If arterial models correctly predict the pressure–flow relations, then they can, in principle, be used to obtain aortic flow from aortic pressure. The methods should be simple to use and unique in their solution. Extensive models have so many parameters to adjust that they are useless for practical purposes. Simpler models like the windkessel model were used to predict flow from pressure, as originally attempted by Frank (1899). His followers improved on the approach for many years, as reviewed by Wetterer and Kenner (1968). If the decay time of the diastolic part of aortic pressure is measured and total arterial compliance is determined through measurements of pulse wave velocities, the peripheral resistance can be calculated from Eq. 2.

More recent attempts to obtain flow from aortic pressure are reviewed by Starmer et al. (1973). Some methods are intuitive and others are based on strong simplifications of the pressure–flow relationships in the ascending aorta. Some methods claim close correspondence between stroke volume and pulse pressure, while others claim a good relation between stroke volume and the area under the systolic part of the aortic pressure above the end diastolic level (Psa). Still others use a corrected Psa by taking into account heart rate and time of systole. The methods based on Psa often use the assumption that during early systole, pressure and flow are related via the characteristic impedance of the aorta only; i.e., the system is then without reflections. Westerhof et al. (1972) doubted this assumption. It seems that until now not one single method works satisfactorily under all conditions.

The approach used by Fry, Mallos, and Casper (1956), Greenfield and Fry (1962, 1965), and Greenfield, Starmer, and Walston (1971) has a firm physical basis. The method is based on the measurement of the pressure gradient in the aorta (pressure difference over a small distance in actual use) rather than a single pressure. As described above (Eq. 3a), pressure drop and flow are related by the longitudinal impedance. The longitudinal impedance is derived by Womersley and is known for a segment if the dimensions are known (together with blood density and viscosity). The longitudinal impedance was simplified and replaced by a single resistor ($1.6 \times R_1'$ of Figure 1; the correction factor is given by Fry) in series with an inertia term ($1.1 \times L_1'$ of Figure 1). Now we can write

$$\frac{\partial P(\omega)}{\partial x} = F(\omega) \cdot (j\omega L + R) \tag{20}$$

The last equation can be rewritten in the time domain as

$$\frac{\partial P(t)}{\partial x} = \frac{L \partial F}{\partial t} + RF \tag{21}$$

The last step in the simplification is the use of average velocity of blood instead of volume flow, $u = F/\pi r_0^2$ and replacement of δ by Δ, and $\rho = 1$

$$\frac{\Delta P}{\Delta x} = 1.1 \frac{du}{dt} + 1.6 \cdot (\frac{8\mu}{r_0^2})u \tag{22}$$

The viscosity of blood (μ) is known or can be determined. If the two pressures are measured and the difference taken, it is quite practical to feed this difference into an adjustable electrical analog of the simplified longitudinal impedance and calculate flow on line. The analog is adjusted such that zero flow during diastole is approximated. This last step is necessary because the radius of the aorta is not known. The method is consequently limited to aortic and pulmonary artery flow because in other arteries flow is not zero during diastole. Yet another method was tried at our laboratory. The approach is based on the idea that if the three-element windkessel (Figure 5) is a good model of the input impedance of the arterial system, flow can be derived from pressure if the parameters of the windkessel are known. Figure 3 shows the windkessel model fitted to the average impedance measured in seven dogs. The impedance of the windkessel can be written as

$$Z(\omega) = (R_p + R_c)\frac{1 + j\omega\tau_2}{1 + j\omega\tau_1} \qquad (23)$$

where

$$\tau_1 = R_p C$$

$$\tau_2 = \tau_1 R_c/(R_p + R_c)$$

The time constant, τ_1, can be estimated from the diastolic decay of aortic pressure (as suggested by Frank). A second adjustment, that of τ_2, is performed by trying to obtain zero flow during diastole. A simple analog can be constructed consisting of one high-gain amplifier with an input impedance consisting of a capacitor in series with an adjustable resistor (for time constant τ_1) and a feedback impedance of the same configuration (for time constant τ_2). Calibration is not directly possible because the individual components are not known; therefore only the wave shapes are obtained.

A result that was extremely promising is given in Figure 6. The derived and measured flows are virtually identical. However, not all attempts to derive flows were as successful as the above example. Several derived flows

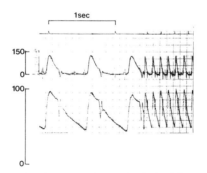

Figure 6. A good example of superposition of a derived flow and a flow measured with an electromagnetic flowmeter. The patterns are almost identical. The measured flow has more high-frequency noise superimposed. Derived flow was obtained from aortic pressure (bottom tracing). Aortic pressure was, via an amplifier, fed into the windkessel model. The windkessel was adjusted for zero flow during diastole. Pressures in mm Hg, flows in cm^3/sec.

did not compare well with flows measured simultaneously with the electromagnetic flow meter. The abnormalities often found are similar to the patterns reported by Greenfield and Fry (1962, 1965). The explanation for the findings is unknown but it seems that the modified windkessel is still too much a simplification of the input impedance of the arterial tree. Skalak (1972) mentioned that experiments on models showed better results when pressure was computed from flow than when the flow was computed from pressure.

HEART

Historical Remarks and Outline

One of the first devices used as a load for the heart that replaces the real arterial system is the Starling resistor. It consists of a thin-walled collapsible tube through which the blood flows, surrounded by a pressurized chamber. If external pressure is higher than blood pressure, the tube collapses and flow stops almost completely; a very high resistance is created. If blood pressure exceeds external pressure, the tube opens and offers almost no resistance to flow. The Starling resistor is more a valve than a resistor: it has strong nonlinear properties quite unlike those of the arterial system. Other investigators used clamps on the aorta or pressure reservoirs (Bemis et al., 1974). We have constructed a relatively simple hydraulic model as a load for the isolated cat heart. The model consists of the hydraulic equivalent of the three-element windkessel discussed above (Figure 5). The model allows changes in peripheral resistance and total arterial compliance without their interaction. For instance, an increase in peripheral resistance in the real arterial system results in an increase of mean arterial pressure and a secondary decrease of arterial compliance follows. The compliance change is a result of the nonlinear pressure–volume relationship in arteries (Bergel, 1961a). Increase in the peripheral resistance of the model does not change the compliance of the model.

Once the heart is loaded with the model, a description of the heart is not easily given. It is not possible to use aortic flow and pressure directly since these quantities are a result of the interaction of heart and arterial system (or model). It is also not possible to analyze by Fourier technique left ventricular pressure and aortic flow (Abel, 1971) and relate harmonics as is done with aortic flow and pressure. The valves are highly nonlinear and harmonics can no longer be related. The only possibility is to study left ventricular pressure before the valves open, since that part of the curve is not affected by the arterial system. However, we have chosen a new and different approach. To give a description of the heart alone, the concepts of source impedance and hydromotive pressure are introduced. With the results obtained in these terms, a suggestion is given for the explanation of source impedance. The explanation is based on the time-varying ventricular pressure–volume ratio. It is indicated below that power dissipation is related to source impedance.

Description of the Arterial Model Used as Load to the Heart

The components of the windkessel (resistors and capacitor) were constructed in our laboratory. An extensive description on their construction is given elsewhere (Westerhof, Elzinga, and Sipkema, 1971). The resistors consist of many narrow tubes of relatively large lengths. A slide provides the possibility of changing the number of open tubes and thus the value of the resistors. The capacitor is an air volume and the size of the volume determines its compliance. Input impedance of the system, as determined with a sine wave pump, is reported elsewhere (Westerhof et al., 1971). The input impedance obtained from the pressure and flow waves generated by an isolated heart pumping into the model is shown in Figure 7. The impedance is similar to the impedance of the open-thorax cat shown in Figure 5.

Description of Heart and Load in Terms of Pressure and Flow

Another comparison of the isolated heart and model with the open-thorax cat is given in Figure 8, where left ventricular pressure and aortic pressure and flow are compared for the two cases. Again one can see that the heart is actually unaware that it pumps into an artificial system instead of the real arterial tree. The preparation, the Tyrode solution with washed bovine erythrocytes used as perfusate, the filling system, and so on are described in more detail elsewhere (Elzinga and Westerhof, 1973). Left atrial filling pressure can be kept constant at any desired value. The heart is usually paced at fixed rates. It is not possible to study pressures and flows under different loading conditions. An increase in peripheral resistance (constant compliance) results in increased systolic, diastolic, and mean pressures in the aorta and a decrease in peak flow and stroke volume (and cardiac output, because heart rate is kept constant). A decrease in arterial compliance (constant peripheral resistance) slightly increased systolic pressure, greatly decreased diastolic aortic pressure, and decreased mean pressure. Mean flow also decreased, but mean aortic pressure over mean aortic flow

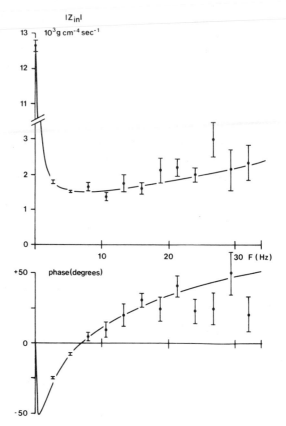

Figure 7. Hydraulic input impedance of the artificial load for the cat heart as determined from "aortic" pressure and "aortic" flow. Seven beats were analyzed and the results averaged. Bars give 1 S.D. Variation in high harmonics is, even for this ideal system, considerable. Modulus increases and phase reaches positive values as a result of the inertial effects of the input cannula (see Figure 5). The solid line gives the impedance of the system as determined with a sine wave pump.

remained constant since peripheral resistance was kept constant. Here we see that the heart keeps neither mean aortic flow constant nor mean left ventricular nor aortic pressure. The heart is thus neither a flow source (always the same flow) nor a pressure source; it is affected in its pumping action by the periphery. Wave shapes change also with changes in arterial load.

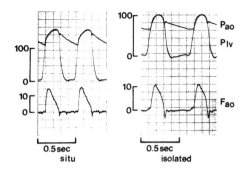

Figure 8. Left ventricular and aortic pressures and aortic flow as measured in the open thorax cat (*left*) and when an isolated cat heart pumps into the hydraulic model (*right*). Pressures in mm Hg; flows in cm³/sec.

Description of the Heart in Terms of Pumping Action

Pressure and flow are a result of the interaction between heart and arterial tree. The systemic input impedance, on the other hand, is a characterization of the arterial tree only. For this reason we have used an analysis method that characterizes the heart only; i.e., a characterization that does not include the arterial tree. The basis for this analysis is a model consisting of a pressure generator that generates a fixed oscillatory pressure under all circumstances (hydromotive pressure, HMP) and a source impedance (Z_s) that modifies the generator pressure depending on the load on the heart but is constant in time. The two unknowns (HMP and Z_s) can be obtained from two equations with left ventricular pressure and aortic flow as known variables when two different loads are used (Elzinga and Westerhof, 1973, 1974). Until now mainly the mean terms of pressures and flows were studied and thus mean HMP and source resistance (R_s) were calculated. The source resistance can be calculated from (Elzinga and Westerhof, 1974)

$$R_s = (\bar{P}_{\text{lv},1} - \bar{P}_{\text{lv},2})/(\bar{F}_{\text{ao},2} - \bar{F}_{\text{ao},1}), \qquad (24)$$

where $\bar{P}_{\text{lv}}$ and $\bar{F}_{\text{ao}}$ are mean left ventricular pressure and mean aortic flow. Aortic flow is assumed to be equal to left ventricular outflow. The indices 1 and 2 pertain to the two different situations. The nonlinearity of the aortic valves is avoided. Determination of differences may result in large errors.

To circumvent this complication we made plots of mean left ventricular pressure against mean aortic flow for a series of changes in arterial load and computed slope and intercept by linear regression. The intercept with the pressure axis is the mean value of the HMP and the slope gives the source resistance. A typical representative graph of a normal isolated cat heart is given in Figure 9. Capacitive changes and resistive changes of the load do not change the relationship, indicating that source resistance characterizes the heart and not the arterial system. In most isolated hearts the relationships between mean left ventricular pressure and mean flow turn out to be linear (Elzinga and Westerhof, 1974), so that slope and intercept completely define the relationship, and thus characterize the pump.

Whether or not the relationship is straight from such graphs we can predict mean left ventricular pressure for a certain mean aortic flow. Inversely, given a mean left ventricular pressure aortic flow can be obtained. If the peripheral resistance is also known, then mean aortic pressure can be obtained. Oscillatory terms can be treated similarly but in this case three graphs per harmonic are needed as a result of the complex nature of the data.

It was found that the source resistance is approximately equal to the (normal value of the) peripheral resistance. A series of hearts was studied

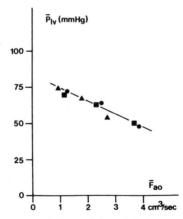

Figure 9. Source resistance graph (mean left ventricular pressure against mean aortic flow) of an isolated cat heart. Intercept with pressure axis represents HMP. Slope of graph gives source resistance. Dots, three different settings of peripheral resistance for a large arterial compliance; squares and triangles, as dots but now for medium and small arterial compliances. Note that the different types of variations all give essentially the same graph.

in this way; it turned out that an increase in left ventricular filling increased the HMP but left the source impedance unchanged (Elzinga and Westerhof, 1974). In other words, the same mean left ventricular pressure results in a larger mean flow.

Power Dissipation for Various Pumps

External power of one ventricle has been measured by several investigators (Milnor, Bergel, and Bargainer, 1966; O'Rourke, 1967; Cox, 1974) and it can be divided into three terms:

$$\dot{W}_t = \dot{W}_m + \dot{W}_0 + K_t, \tag{25}$$

where $\dot{W}_t$ is total power, $\dot{W}_m$ mean power $(\bar{P} \cdot \bar{F})$, $\dot{W}_0$ oscillatory power, and K_t the kinetic energy (McDonald, 1974). The term K_t is small and we neglect it here. The instantaneous power can be calculated from

$$\dot{W}_t = P(t) \cdot F(t) \tag{26}$$

but because some of the power, such as that stored in the arterial wall, will return to the system, it is better to calculate total power, that is, work averaged over one heart cycle:

$$\dot{W}_t = \frac{1}{T} \int_0^T P(t) \cdot F(t) \ dt \simeq \frac{1}{T} \int_0^{T_s} P(t) \cdot F(t) \ dt, \tag{27}$$

where T is the period of one heart beat and T_s is the time of systole. The integrals are the same since diastolic flow is zero. The oscillatory term $(\dot{W}_0)$ can be obtained from subtraction of the mean power from the total power. In the systemic arterial tree the oscillatory power is about 10% of total power; in the pulmonary system oscillatory power is about 25% of total power (Milnor et al., 1966). There is another way to calculate oscillatory power (Milnor et al., 1966). After Fourier analysis of pressure and flow, oscillatory power can be calculated:

$$\dot{W}_0 = \frac{1}{2} \sum_{n=1}^{N} |P_n| |F_n| \cos \phi_n, \tag{28}$$

where $|P_n|$ and $|F_n|$ are the moduli of the pressure and flow harmonics and ϕ_n is the phase angle between the pressure and flow harmonics.

For the case where aortic pressure is used, ϕ_n is the phase angle of the input impedance of the arterial system. If ventricular pressure is used to calculate oscillatory power, ϕ_n is not related to an impedance because the concept of impedance is incorrect for nonlinear systems. In Eqs. 27 and 28 both aortic pressure and left ventricular pressure may be used. Because in Eq. 27, integration over systole only is sufficient, and because during systole pressure on both sides of the valve is almost equal, we get the same total power from aortic and left ventricular pressures.

The same total power is obtained from aortic and left ventricular pressures if total power is calculated from mean power $(\bar{P} \cdot \bar{F})$ plus the oscillatory power that is calculated after Fourier analysis of pressure and flow (Eq. 28). This is so because the time-domain and the frequency-domain calculations must give the same result, and the time-domain results using either pressure were the same. However, mean left ventricular pressure and mean aortic pressure are not the same and thus the mean power terms are not the same: mean power calculated from ventricular pressure and aortic flow is the smaller one. It therefore follows that the oscillatory power calculated from left ventricular pressure and aortic flow is larger than the mean oscillatory power calculated from aortic pressure and flow. The combination of aortic valve and compliant arterial system gives a decrease in oscillatory power and an increase in mean power at the peripheral side of the valve. Separation of power into a mean and an oscillatory part is useful if the arterial system is analyzed but is difficult to interpret for the heart.

For more information on power the reader is referred to Milnor (1972), Skalak (1972), and McDonald (1974).

Contrary to input impedance and source impedance, power is a function of both the arterial tree and the heart. On the other hand, unlike the impedance, power is not restricted in its use to linear systems. Power can give us information about the heart if we determine what the power dissipation is for different loads on the heart. Because we deal with a complicated situation, we like to simplify considerably. We take the simplest case of a pump that only pumps a steady flow into the arterial system. If the pump is a flow source (it delivers the same cardiac output under all circumstances) then the source resistance graph is a vertical straight line (infinite source resistance). The power delivered by this pump is proportional to the peripheral resistance, as is indicated in Figure 10. The other extreme is a pressure source (in this situation we take aortic pressure to be fixed) and now we see that power is inversely proportional to peripheral resistance (Figure 10). A pump that is neither flow source nor pressure source acts as a flow source for extremely low peripheral resistance values $(R_p \ll R_s)$. For very high peripheral resistances the same pump seems to be pressure source $(R_p \gg R_s)$. At these extremes the power

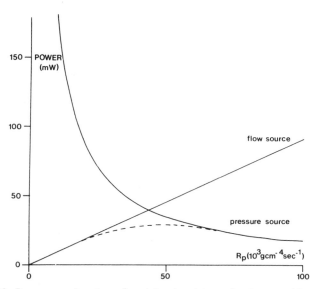

Figure 10. Power as a function of peripheral resistance for two special pumps. A flow source that always produces the same flow and a pressure source that always produces the same pressure. The broken line represents a pump with a finite source impedance. For small loads a flow source is approximated and for large loads a pressure source. Power shows a maximum.

dissipation approaches the lines given by a flow or pressure source, respectively. In the region in between, when the source resistance of the pump is of the same order as the peripheral resistance, a power maximum is observed.

For an oscillatory pump and valves the situation is more complex and is at present under study in our laboratory. Measurements on previously instrumented conscious dogs have shown that power delivered by the left ventricle decreases for very high and for very low arterial loads (Wilcken et al., 1964).

Interpretation of the Source Resistance Concept

The three elements of the modified windkessel, as discussed above, have a clear physiologic meaning. It is hard to imagine that the mean term of the source impedance, the source resistance, could be a real resistance. It is impossible to see that viscosity of the ventricular wall and of the blood could give a resistance of so large a value (same order as the peripheral resistance). One of the possible explanations of source impedance is based on the concept of a time-dependent elasticity model (Suga and Sagawa,

1972; Suga, Sagawa, and Shoukas, 1973; Suga and Sagawa, 1974). Suga et al. showed that the instantaneous pressure–volume relationships of the left ventricle are approximately straight lines with an intercept on the volume axis. During contraction the slope of these pressure–volume curves increases and subsequently decreases. The slope plotted as a function of time is almost independent of the load. A similar result (time-dependent volume stiffness) was obtained in a completely different manner. Templeton et al. (1970) introduced small volume perturbations of the left ventricle and observed a change in left ventricular stiffness in the course of an isometric contraction.

A hydraulic model that has a time-dependent compliance is shown in Figure 11. A piston powered by a strong motor moves up and down; stroke and wave shape are independent of the loading conditions. The air volume acts as a variable compliance. Two valves are incorporated in the model. One valve (the "mitral valve") connects the pump with a constant pressure head (constant "atrial pressure"), the other valve connects the pump to the arterial load ("aortic valve"). The arterial system is again modeled after the modified windkessel with variable compliance and variable peripheral resistance.

With this apparatus we can determine the pumping characteristics of the model by means of the mean left ventricular pressure–mean aortic flow graph. Figure 12 shows this source impedance graph for two different settings of the pump. It is found that the smaller the average compliance of the pump, the higher the HMP and the higher the source resistance. It can also be seen from these results that the characterization is again independent of the arterial system: peripheral resistance and arterial com-

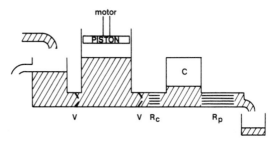

Figure 11. Pump used to gain insight into the source resistance concept. A motor drives the piston sinusoidally. The piston compresses the airvolume under it. At left is an overflow system that supplies a constant filling pressure. The two valves (V) allow flow from left to right only. The pump is loaded with the windkessel. Pressure is measured with pressure transducer; flow with beaker and stopwatch.

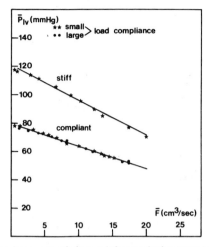

Figure 12. Source resistance graph (mean left ventricular pressure against mean flow) for the pump of Figure 11. If the airvolume of the pump is small (stiff pump) a large HMP and source resistance are found. For a large airvolume (compliant pump) HMP and source resistance are small. The bottom graph is measured with small (plusses) and large (dots) load compliance to indicate the load independence of the graph. Lines start bending close to the axes, but are straight for a large working range.

pliance changes give the same result. Figure 12 should be compared to the results obtained from the real heart.

The results indicate that a straight line is obtained over a large working range by this time-varying compliance model. The two intercepts of the source resistance plot with the pressure and flow axes can be calculated from simple thermodynamics. If, as is the case here, the piston variations are sinusoidal with volume amplitude V_1, and if the mean value of the air volume is V_0, then we find, if $V_1 \ll V_0$, that

$$\overline{HMP} \simeq kP_0 V_1/V_0 \qquad (29)$$

$$\overline{F}_0 = 2fV_1, \qquad (30)$$

where P_0 is atmospheric pressure, f is frequency, and k is a constant which is equal to 1 for an isothermic and 7/5 for an adiabatic pump (filled with a diatomic gas such as air). The slope is now

$$R_s = kP_0/2fV_0. \qquad (31)$$

The model is, of course, a simplification and the sinusoidal piston movement is not very realistic but the general features of source resistance are explained.

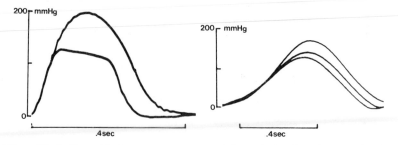

Figure 13. *Left*, ventricular pressures generated by an isolated cat heart, and *right*, by the pump (Figure 11) for different loads. Note the larger width of the pressure waves for higher loads. Pressures in mm Hg.

Another comparison between the left ventricle and the pump is given in Figure 13. Here left ventricular pressures of heart and pump are shown for different loads. Again the similarities are obvious: the smaller the load impedance, the earlier left ventricular pressure decreases. The entire curve is decreased in width.

CONCLUSION

We have given an overview of the pressure–flow relations in the arterial system and the heart. It became apparent that more is known about these relations in the arterial system than in the heart. We have spent a large proportion of this chapter on the pressure–flow relations in a segment of artery. A good understanding of these relationships is essential, because they serve as the basis for many experiments and for the construction of models. Although construction and use of models can improve the understanding of the cardiovascular system, model making should never be a goal in itself.

We have paid little attention here to nonlinear approaches of vascular dynamics since we are convinced that they are of second-order importance, i.e., they can be of use, but linear theory seems to approximate reality sufficiently. Linear theory is not adequate for the description of the coronary and venous systems. The former has time-varying properties during a heart beat, and the latter has strong nonlinear properties. Our knowledge of these systems is limited so that more work needs to be done in these fields. Research on reflections and flow profiles at and near bifurcations is still of considerable interest.

We have considered the total arterial system as a summation of many small segments for which we have defined the relation between pressure and flow. Likewise, the heart can be approached as a combination of many muscle fibers, of which the properties are defined by the theories of muscle mechanics. Some doubt has recently been cast on these theories. The extrapolation from isolated muscle to the whole heart by proper summation of individual muscles has been carried out but is extremely difficult.

Our approach to the analysis of cardiac function stems from the fact that we are familiar with pressure–flow relations in arteries. If we plot left ventricular pressure against outflow in terms of their means, then, over a working range, a linear relationship is obtained; the slope is called source resistance and the intercept with the pressure axis, as found by linear extrapolation, is the hydromotive pressure ($\overline{HMP}$). Since linear extrapolation overestimates the intercept with the pressure axis, $\overline{HMP}$ is a little higher than mean pressure in the totally isovolumic beat. Even though the concept of source resistance is not directly understood, the relationship predicts (left ventricular end-diastolic pressure kept constant) mean left ventricular pressure if ventricular outflow is given and vice versa. We have tried to relate source resistance to ventricular stiffness. Although some results indeed indicate such a relation between source resistance and ventricular stiffness, we have not yet obtained conclusive proof.

LITERATURE CITED

Abel, F. L. 1971. Fourier analysis of left ventricular performance. Evaluation of impedance matching. Circ. Res. 28: 119–135.

Apéria, A. 1940. Hemodynamical studies. Skand. Arch. Physiol. 83 (Suppl.) 16: 1–230.

Attinger, E. O., A. Anné, and D. A. McDonald. 1966a. Use of Fourier series for the analysis of biological systems. Biophys. J. 6: 291–304.

Attinger, E. O., A. Anné, T. Mikami, and H. Sugawara. 1966b. Modeling pressure–flow relations in arteries and veins. Information Exchange Group No. 3, Scientific Memo 41.

Attinger, E. O., H. Sugawara, A. Navarro, and A. Anné. 1966c. Pulsatile flow patterns in distensible tubes. Circ. Res. 18: 447–456.

Attinger, E. O., H. Sugawara, A. Navarro, A. Ricetto, and R. Martin. 1966d. Pressure–flow relations in dog arteries. Circ. Res. 19: 230–245.

Bemis, C. E., J. R. Serur, D. Borkenhagen, E. H. Sonnenblick, and C. W. Urschel. 1974. Influence of right ventricular filling pressure on left ventricular pressure and dimension. Circ. Res. 34: 498–504.

Beneken, J. E. W. 1972. Some computer models in cardiovascular research.

In D. H. Bergel (ed.), Cardiovascular Fluid Dynamics, pp. 173–224. Academic Press, London/New York.

Bergel, D. H. 1961*a*. The dynamic elastic properties of the arterial wall. J. Physiol. 156: 458–469.

Bergel, D. H. 1961*b*. The static elastic properties of the arterial wall. J. Physiol. 156: 445–457.

Bergel, D. H., and W. R. Milnor. 1965. Pulmonary vascular impedance in the dog. Circ. Res. 16: 401–415.

Bramwell, J. C., and A. V. Hill. 1922. The velocity of the pulse wave in man. Proc. Roy. Soc. London B 93: 298–306.

Caro, C. G., and D. A. McDonald. 1961. The relation of pulsatile pressure and flow in the pulmonary vascular bed. J. Physiol. 157: 426–453.

Cox, R. H. 1968. Wave propagation through a Newtonian fluid contained within a thick-walled, viscoelastic tube. Biophys. J. 8: 691–709.

Cox, R. H. 1969. Comparison of linearized wave propagation models for arterial blood flow analysis. J. Biomech. 2: 251–265.

Cox, R. H. 1970. Blood flow and pressure propagation in the canine femoral artery. J. Biomech. 3: 131–149.

Cox, R. H. 1971. Determination of the true phase velocity of arterial pressure waves in vivo. Circ. Res. 29: 407–418.

Cox, R. H. 1974. Determinants of systemic hydraulic power in unanesthetized dogs. Am. J. Physiol. 226: 579–587.

Cox, R. H., and J. B. Pace. 1975. Pressure–flow relations in the vessels of the canine aortic arch. Am. J. Physiol. 228: 1–10.

Elzinga, G., and N. Westerhof. 1973. Pressure and flow generated by the left ventricle against different impedances. Circ. Res. 32: 178–186.

Elzinga, G., and N. Westerhof. 1974. End-diastolic volume and source impedance of the heart. *In* A. Guz (ed.), The Physiological Basis of Starling's Law of the Heart, pp. 241–255. Ciba Symposium, 24. Elsevier-North Holland, Amsterdam.

Frank, O. 1899. Die Grundform des Arteriellen Puls. Z. Biol. 37: 483–526.

Frank, O. 1905. Der Puls in den Arterien. Z. Biol. 46: 441–553.

Fry, D. L., A. J. Mallos, and A. G. T. Casper. 1956. A catheter tip method for measurement of the instantaneous aortic blood velocity. Circ. Res. 4: 627–632.

Gabe, I. T., J. Karnell, I. G. Porjé, and B. Rudewald. 1964. The measurement of input impedance and apparent velocity in the human aorta. Acta Physiol. Scand. 61: 73–84.

Greenfield, J. C., and D. L. Fry. 1962. Measurement errors in estimating blood velocity by pressure gradient. J. Appl. Physiol. 17: 1013–1019.

Greenfield, J. C., and D. L. Fry. 1965. Relationship between instantaneous aortic flow and the pressure gradient. Circ. Res. 17: 340–348.

Greenfield, J. C., C. F. Starmer, and A. Walston. 1971. Measurement of aortic blood flow in man by the computed pressure derivative method. J. Appl. Physiol. 31: 792–795.

Jager, G. N. 1965. Electrical model of the human systemic arterial tree. Ph.D. Thesis, University of Utrecht.

Jager, G. N., N. Westerhof, and A. Noordergraaf. 1965. Oscillatory flow impedance in electrical analog of arterial system. Circ. Res. 16: 121–133.

Karakash, J. J. 1950. Transmission Lines and Filter Networks. Macmillan, New York. 413 p.

Learoyd, B. M., and M. G. Taylor. 1966. Alterations with age in the viscoelastic properties of human arterial walls. Circ. Res. 18: 278–292.

Love, A. E. H. 1927. A Treatise on the Mathematical Theory of Elasticity. Cambridge University Press, Cambridge. 642 p.

Luchsinger, P. C., R. E. Snell, D. J. Patel, and D. L. Fry. 1964. Instantaneous pressure distribution along the human aorta. Circ. Res. 15: 503–510.

Malindzak, G. S. 1970. Fourier analysis of cardiovascular events. Math. Biosci. 7: 273–289.

McDonald, D. A. 1974. Blood flow in arteries. Arnold, London. 496 p.

McDonald, D. A., and M. G. Taylor. 1959. The hydrodynamics of the arterial circulation. Progr. Biophys. and Biophys. Chem. 9: 105–173.

Mills, C. J., I. T. Gabe, J. H. Gault, D. T. Mason, J. Ross, E. Braunwald, and J. P. Shillingford. 1970. Pressure flow relationship and vascular impedance in man. Cardiovasc. Res. 4: 405–417.

Milnor, W. R. 1972. Pulmonary hemodynamics. In D. H. Bergel (ed.), Cardiovascular Fluid Dynamics, pp. 299–340. Academic Press, London/New York.

Milnor, W. R., D. H. Bergel, and J. D. Bargainer. 1966. Hydraulic power associated with pulmonary blood flow and its relation to heart rate. Circ. Res. 19: 467–480.

Milnor, W. R., C. R. Conti, K. B. Lewis, and M. F. O'Rourke. 1969. Pulmonary arterial pulse wave velocity and impedance in man. Circ. Res. 25: 637–648.

Milnor, W. R., and W. W. Nichols. 1975. A new method of measuring propagation coefficients and characteristic impedance in blood vessels. Circ. Res. 36: 631–639.

Moens, A. I. 1878. Die Pulskurve. Brill, Leiden.

Newman, D. L., and N. L. R. Bowden. 1973. Effect of reflection from an unmatched junction on the abdominal aortic impedance. Cardiovasc. Res. 7: 827–833.

Newman, D. L., R. K. Walesby, and N. L. R. Bowden. 1975. Hemodynamic effects of acute experimental aortic coarctation. Circ. Res. 36: 165–172.

Noble, M. I. M., I. T. Gabe, D. Trenchard, and A. Guz. 1967. Blood pressure and flow in the ascending aorta of conscious dogs. Cardiovasc. Res. 1: 9–20.

Noordergraaf, A. 1969. Hemodynamics. In H. P. Schwan (ed.), Biological Engineering, pp. 391–545. McGraw-Hill, New York.

O'Rourke, M. F. 1967. Steady and pulsatile energy losses in the systemic circulation under normal conditions and in simulated arterial disease. Cardiovasc. Res. 1: 313–326.

O'Rourke, M. F. 1968. Impact pressure, lateral pressure, and impedance in the proximal aorta and pulmonary artery. J. Appl. Physiol. 25: 533–541.

O'Rourke, M. F. 1971. The arterial pulse in health and disease. Am. Heart J. 82: 687–702.

O'Rourke, M. F., and M. G. Taylor. 1967. Input impedance of the systemic circulation. Circ. Res. 20: 365–380.

O'Rourke, M. F., and M. G. Taylor. 1966. Vascular impedance of the femoral bed. Circ. Res. 18: 126–139.

Patel, D. J., W. G. Austen, and J. C. Greenfield. 1964. Impedance of certain large blood vessels in man. Ann. N.Y. Acad. Sci. 115: 1129–1139.

Patel, D. J., J. C. Greenfield, W. G. Austen, A. G. Morrow, and D. L. Fry. 1965. Pressure–flow relationships in the ascending aorta and femoral artery of man. J. Appl. Physiol. 20: 459–463.

Pater, L. de, and J. W. van den Berg. 1964. An electrical analogue of the entire human circulatory system. Med. Elec. Biol. Eng. 2: 161–166.

Pollack, G. H., R. V. Reddy, and A. Noordergraaf. 1968. Input impedance, wave travel and reflections in the human pulmonary arterial tree: Studies using an electrical analog. IEEE Trans. Bio-Med. Eng. 15: 151–164.

Porjé, I. G. 1946. Studies of the arterial pulse wave, particularly in the aorta. Acta Physiol. Scand. 13 (Suppl.) 42: 1–68.

Randall, J. E., and R. W. Stacy. 1956. Mechanical impedance of the dog's hind leg to pulsatile blood flow. Am. J. Physiol. 187: 94–98.

Reuben, S. R., J. P. Swadling, B. J. Gersh, and G. de J. Lee. 1971. Impedance and transmission properties of the pulmonary arterial system. Cardiovasc. Res. 5: 1–9.

Reul, H., B. Tesch, J. Schoenmackers, and S. Effert. 1974. Hydromechanical simulation of systemic circulation. Med. Biol. Eng. 12: 431–436.

Sipkema, P., and N. Westerhof. 1975. Effective length of the arterial system. Ann. Biomed. Eng. 3: 296–307.

Skalak, R. 1972. Synthesis of a complete circulation. In D. H. Bergel (ed.), Cardiovascular Fluid Dynamics, pp. 341–377. Academic Press, London/New York.

Starmer, C. F., P. A. McHale, F. R. Cobb, and J. C. Greenfield. 1973. Evaluation of several methods for computing stroke volume from central aortic pressure. Circ. Res. 33: 139–148.

Suga, H., and K. Sagawa. 1974. Instantaneous pressure–volume relationships and their ratio in the excised, supported, canine left ventricle. Circ. Res. 35: 117–126.

Suga, H., and K. Sagawa. 1972. Mathematical interrelationship between instantaneous ventricular pressure-volume ratio and myocardial force–velocity relation. Ann. Biomed. Eng. 1: 160–181.

Suga, H., K. Sagawa, and A. A. Shoukas. 1973. Load independence of the instantaneous pressure-volume ratio of the canine left ventricle and effects of epinephrine and heart rate on the ratio. Circ. Res. 32: 314–322.

Taylor, M. G. 1957. An approach to an analysis of the arterial pulsewave. Phys. Med. Biol. 1: 258–269, 321–329.

Taylor, M. G. 1959. An experimental determination of the propagation of fluid oscillations in a tube with a viscoelastic wall; together with an analysis of the characteristics in an electrical analogue. Phys. Med. Biol. 4: 63–81.

Taylor, M. G. 1965. Wave travel in a non-uniform transmission line in relation to pulses in arteries. Phys. Med. Biol. 10: 539–550.

Taylor, M. G. 1966a. The input impedance of an assembly of randomly branching elastic tubes. Biphys. J. 6: 29–51.

Taylor, M. G. 1966b. Use of random excitation and spectral analysis in the study of frequency-dependent parameters of the cardiovascular system. Circ. Res. 18: 585–595.

Taylor, M. G. 1966c. Wave transmission through an assembly of randomly branching elastic tubes. Biophys. J. 6: 697–716.

Templeton, G. H., J. H. Mitchell, R. R. Ecker, and G. Blomqvist. 1970. A method for measurement of dynamic compliance of the left ventricle in dogs. J. Appl. Physiol. 29: 742–745.

Westerhof, N. 1968. Analog studies of human systemic arterial hemodynamics. Ph.D. Thesis. University of Pennsylvania. University Microfilm, Ann Arbor, Mich 69-5676.

Westerhof, N., F. Bosman, C. J. de Vries, and A. Noordergraaf. 1969. Analog studies of the human systemic arterial tree. J. Biomech. 2: 121–143.

Westerhof, N., and A. Noordergraaf. 1970. Arterial viscoelasticity: A generalized model. Effect on input impedance and wave travel in the systemic tree. J. Biomech. 3: 357–379.

Westerhof, N., G. Elzinga, and P. Sipkema. 1971. An artificial arterial system for pumping hearts. J. Appl. Physiol. 31: 776–781.

Westerhof, N., P. Sipkema, G. C. van den Bos, and G. Elzinga. 1972. Forward and backward waves in the arterial system. Cardiovasc. Res. 6: 648–656.

Westerhof, N., G. Elzinga, and G. C. van den Bos. 1973. Influence of central and peripheral changes on the hydraulic input impedance of the systemic arterial tree. Med. Biol. Eng. 11: 710–723.

Wetterer, E., and Th. Kenner. 1968. Die Dynamik des Arterien-pulses. Springer-Verlag, Berlin-Heidelberg-New York. 379 p.

Wilcken, D. E. L., A. A. Charlier, J. I. E. Hoffman, and A. Guz. 1964.

Effects of alterations in aortic impedance on the performance of the ventricles. Circ. Res. 14: 283–293.

Womersley, J. R. 1957. An elastic tube theory of pulse transmission and oscillatory flow in mammalian arteries. W.A.D.C. Techn. Report, TR56-614.

Cardiovascular Flow Dynamics and Measurements
Edited by N. H. C. Hwang and N. A. Normann
Copyright 1977   University Park Press   Baltimore

chapter 12

MECHANICAL PROPERTIES OF ARTERIES

Dali J. Patel and Ramesh N. Vaishnav[1]

ABSTRACT

Although arterial mechanics has been studied for a long time, it is only
in recent years that sophisticated techniques have been used to provide
a realistic characterization of the wall material. This is due in part to
modern technology and in part to a real need to answer a number of
practical questions that require such knowledge. For instance, any
design of vascular prosthesis or artificial organs would require detailed
knowledge of vascular architecture and rheology. Moreover, recent
researches of Fry and others have indicated that mechanical factors,
including local disturbances in flow as well as local properties of the
vessel wall, affect the permeability of the endothelial surface to various
macromolecules, which in turn could play an important role in disease
processes like atherosclerosis. Thus it is important to study, in detail,
not only the overall properties of the arterial wall but also the local
properties of the intimal surface. The importance of the latter has only
been recognized recently; therefore, very little literature exists on this
subject. The future challenge in the field of hemodynamics is to
quantify its role in disease processes like atherosclerosis through
detailed experimental studies of local flow fields and local tissue
properties in critical areas of the circulatory system.

We first consider some definitions and theoretic concepts and then
discuss the following topics: (1) motion of the arterial wall, (2) general
material properties, (3) incremental and nonlinear viscoelastic properties of the wall, and (4) local properties of the intimal surface. The
first topic is important for obtaining proper boundary conditions
assumed in fluid dynamics, and the second provides a realistic basis to

[1] Work supported by NSF Grants GK23747 and ENG 72-04259-A01 and HEW
Grant HL 15270.

make assumptions necessary in the development of a theory to describe mechanical behavior of the arterial system. Two such theories are presented. Finally, methods to study local properties of the intimal surface and associated flow fields are discussed.

INTRODUCTION

In this chapter we review the state of the art in the field of blood vessel rheology. Although, of necessity, we go through some mathematical manipulations, our primary concern is to impart an intuitive physical feel for the subject. Rather than document all factual material, which is so easily available elsewhere (Fung, 1971; Bergel, 1972; McDonald, 1974; Patel et al., 1974), we explain certain difficult physical and mathematical concepts using examples from our own work. Since students come from a wide variety of backgrounds—physiologists, clinicians, physicists, and biomedical engineers—certain areas in this chapter might appear very elementary to some yet useful to others. We hope that the material can facilitate understanding of the subject such that the interested reader can pursue independent inquiry through critical reading of the literature in the field.

Although arterial mechanics has been studied for a long time, it is only in recent years that sophisticated techniques have been used to provide a realistic characterization of the wall material (Patel and Vaishnav, 1972). This is due in part to modern technology and in part to a real need to answer a number of practical questions that require such knowledge. For instance, any design of vascular prosthesis or artificial organs requires detailed knowledge of vascular architecture and rheology. Moreover, recent researches of Fry and others (Fry, 1973; Caro, 1973; Patel et al., 1974) have indicated that mechanical factors, including local disturbances in flow as well as local properties of the vessel wall, affect the permeability of the endothelial surface to various macromolecules, which in turn could play an important role in disease processes like atherosclerosis. It is important, therefore, to study, in detail, not only the overall properties of the arterial wall but also the local properties of the intimal surface. The importance of the latter has only been recognized recently; therefore, very little literature exists on this subject (Gow and Vaishnav, 1975). It is likely that the future challenge in the field of hemodynamics will be to quantify its role in disease processes like atherosclerosis through detailed experimental studies of local flow fields and local tissue properties in critical areas of the circulatory system.

For convenience, we first consider some definitions and theoretic concepts and then follow these up with a discussion of the following selected topics: motion of the arterial wall, general material properties, incremental and nonlinear viscoelastic properties of the wall, local properties of the intimal surface, and mechanical properties of muscular arteries.

DEFINITIONS AND THEORETIC CONSIDERATIONS

When a force is applied to a material, the material deforms. When the force is removed, the deformation may or may not vanish. If the deformation vanishes, the material is said to be *elastic*. One elastic body may require a larger force to maintain a given deformation than another; the former is then said to be *stiffer* or more rigid, and the latter more *compliant*. Beyond a certain amount of deformation a body may cease to be elastic. The largest deformation it can undergo, while remaining elastic, is called the *elastic limit*. A more compliant material may have a larger or smaller elastic limit than a less compliant one. Finally, elasticity does not imply small deformations, nor does it imply force—deformation linearity.

A material is called *isotropic* when its elastic properties at a point are the same for each direction, *anisotropic* when the properties are different in different directions, and *homogeneous* when the elastic properties are the same in each direction at different points. It should be noted that the concepts of homogeneity and isotropy are basically independent. That is, it is possible for a material to be isotropic but nonhomogeneous, or to be homogeneous but anisotropic.

Elastic moduli define material properties in a unique manner and their values do not depend on the size or geometry of the material. These are calculated as stress—strain ratios, rather than force—deformation ratios, because the latter values are affected by the specimen size and geometry.

Stress is defined as force per unit area. A normal stress acts in a direction perpendicular to the surface and a shear stress acts in the plane of the surface. A typical cylindrical blood vessel segment under physiologic loading consisting of intravascular pressure and a longitudinal tethering force, develops three normal stresses. In the cylindrical coordinate system these are the circumferential, longitudinal, and radial stresses. In addition, the vascular surface adjacent to blood flow develops a shearing stress. This latter stress is small compared to the normal stresses and is therefore neglected in most rheologic considerations. However, if one were interested, for example, in transport of macromolecules across the blood–wall interface, then the shear stress would assume prime importance. This is so because the vascular endothelium is known to be delicate and susceptible to damage at relatively low values of shear stress (Fry, 1968, 1969).

Strain is defined as the ratio of increase in a particular dimension in the deformed state to that dimension in its initial undeformed state. In a cylindrical blood vessel segment under physiologic loading there are three normal strains: circumferential, longitudinal, and radial. The shearing strains, during physiologic loading, are experimentally shown to be negligible (Patel and Fry, 1969).

Next we consider the concepts of linearity and viscoelasticity, as they apply to the arterial system.

The arterial system during life operates around a mean pressure of about 90 mm Hg. There is a periodic fluctuation in this pressure of ± 20 mm Hg with each heartbeat. Although the overall elastic properties of the system are nonlinear, for many applications it is customary and reasonable to consider the behavior of the system incrementally linear around a given state of strain (Patel and Vaishnav, 1972). This approach simplifies the mathematics of system analysis considerably and has proven practical advantages. Therefore we consider next two basic properties of a linear system. First, a linear system obeys the principle of superposition. Suppose we excite such a system simultaneously with two *sinusoidal* waves of 1 and 3 Hz. Then the steady-state response of the system is a complex wave, which, when analyzed for its harmonic content, has only the two frequencies of 1 and 3 Hz. The system responds to each sinusoidal excitation discretely, changing its amplitude and phase angle but maintaining the same frequency. Second, a linear system preserves the scale factor. If the system is excited with a sinusoidal wave of amplitude e_1 and the steady-state response is a wave of amplitude w_1, then, when the system is excited with a wave of amplitude ne_1, the response is of amplitude nw_1.

Because periodic waves like the pressure and flow waves can be broken down into single sinusoidal waves by Fourier analysis, the response of the arterial system can be predicted to the extent that it behaves linearly. For instance, a sinusoidal pressure wave travels as a sinusoid of the same frequency, although its amplitude and phase angle may change. A complex pressure wave, made up of many sinusoidal waves, appears distorted downstream because the amplitude and phase angle of each sinusoid could change; however, no new harmonics are generated in the downstream wave. A sinusoidal pressure wave is associated with a sinusoidal flow wave of the same frequency.

So far, we have considered the arterial wall material to be purely elastic, whereas in reality it is viscoelastic. A viscoelastic material differs in response from a purely elastic material in three ways: (1) If we impose a step load on the material, the purely elastic material extends instantaneously and then maintains this extension as long as the load is maintained; the viscoelastic material continues to extend after the initial extension (creep). When the load is removed the elastic material instantaneously returns to its original dimensions, whereas the viscoelastic material tends to return more slowly and may or may not reach its original dimensions. (2) Under a constant strain, the elastic material immediately develops a stress that remains constant, whereas the viscoelastic material initially develops a large stress that decreases in time (stress relaxation). (3) Under sinusoidal forcing, both elastic and viscoelastic materials in the linear regime respond with a sinusoidal deformation of the same frequency. In the elastic case, there is no phase difference between force and deformation. In the viscoelastic case, deformation lags the applied force. Vascular tissue, in general, exhibits all three characteristic viscoelastic responses.

With this clarification of concepts, we now look at some of our experimental findings as they pertain to arterial mechanics.

MOTION OF THE ARTERIAL WALL

Knowledge of the geometry of the arterial system as well as its motion during a cardiac cycle provides the boundary conditions necessary for hemodynamic problems. More specifically, the solution of the Navier–Stokes equation (Ling et al., 1973) or the use of finite element methods (Davids and Cheng, 1972) to determine flow fields requires that boundary conditions be known. Because the fluid particles on the endothelial surface move with the blood vessel wall, a precise knowledge of wall motion and position could provide these boundary conditions. Mathematical solutions are not always practical, and one has to then resort to studies in physical models of the aorta and its branches. Such models, to be useful, must mimic not only the geometry but also the pressure–diameter relationships along the aorta. The value of a rigid model in these situations is limited.

Over the past few years we have acquired data on geometry and wall motion from human and dog aortas. The results from some of these studies are summarized below.

For boundary conditions it is important to know instantaneous values of four parameters, during a cardiac cycle, along the aorta: (1) the instantaneous longitudinal displacement of the aorta relative to the thoracic and abdominal cavities, (2) the pressure–length relationship, (3) the pressure–diameter relationship, and (4) the instantaneous radial displacement of the aortic wall.

The longitudinal displacement of the aortas of six dogs was measured with an electrical caliper; one leg of the caliper was fixed to the table on which the dog was lying and the other was fixed to the aorta perpendicular to the longitudinal axis (Patel, Mallos, and Fry, 1961). The results are shown in a composite diagram (Figure 1). During cardiac systole the root

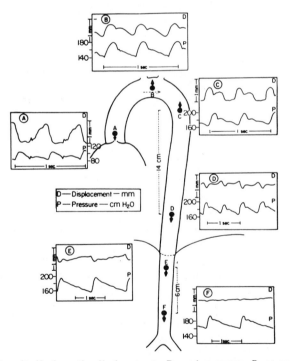

Figure 1. Longitudinal aortic displacement, D, and pressure, P, at various sites; arrows indicate main direction of displacement during cardiac systole. (From Patel et al., 1961; reproduced by permission.)

of the aorta, A, was displaced toward the heart; the highest point on the arch of the aorta, B, and the upper part of the descending thoracic aorta, C, were displaced headward; and the lower part of the descending thoracic aorta, D, was displaced toward the abdomen. Between points C and D and between points A and B in Figure 1 there was a transition zone where the motion was relatively small and difficult to characterize. The arch of the aorta, in addition to moving headward, also moved along the longitudinal axis during cardiac systole, as indicated by the dotted arrow in Figure 1B. The displacement of the abdominal aorta during cardiac systole was caudal. The absolute amount of this displacement decreased progressively with distance toward the bifurcation of the aorta (E to F). Qualitatively, therefore, the displacements follow a pattern that would be expected in a capped segment. For example, with an increase in pressure, the motion of the upper part (Figure 1C) of the descending thoracic aorta is cephalic and that of the lower part (Figure 1D) caudal. This provides a justification for treating arterial segments as capped in theoretic analysis.

The displacements shown in Figure 1 are in general small because of the longitudinal tethering that normally exists in the in vivo state between the aortic wall and the surrounding tissue in the thoracic or abdominal cavity. The significant role played by such tethering in considering the equation of dynamic equilibrium in the longitudinal direction was pointed out by Womersley (1957). We note two important aspects of the longitudinal tethering. First, it provides resistance to any longitudinal motion of the blood vessel and thus holds the blood vessel in place against the viscous drag of the blood flow within the vessel which tries to displace the vessel longitudinally. Second, it provides additional longitudinal stiffness to the blood vessel wall.

Patel and Fry (1966) carried out quantitative measurement of longitudinal tethering by isolating an aortic segment with two transverse cuts without disturbing the perivascular tissue, subjecting the segment to a known sinusoidal longitudinal displacement (0–22 Hz) and measuring the sinusoidal force required to cause this motion. They proposed a linear mechanical model[2] (Figure 2) consisting of a mass M in series with a parallel combination of an elastic element of stiffness K_1, a viscous element of viscosity C_1, and a Maxwell element that is a series combination of an elastic element of stiffness K_2 and a viscous element of viscosity

---

[2] For a description of some simple linear models used in vascular mechanics, we refer the reader to Patel and Janicki (1966).

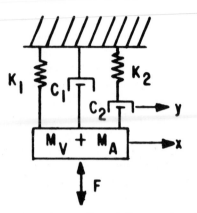

Figure 2. Model for vascular tethering. K_1 and K_2 are springs (spring constants); C_1 and C_2 are dashpots (viscosity coefficients); $M_V + M_A$ is the total mass; F is the force; x and y are the displacements.

C_2. The mass M was visualized as a sum of the vessel mass M_V and the added mass M_A of the "added" tissue consisting of short stubs of inter-costal arteries, immediately adjacent parietal pleura and some retroaortic areolar tissue. The model fits the experimental data very well over the entire frequency range. They also showed that if the response of the system for frequencies less than 1 Hz was not of interest, a simple model with $C_2 = \infty$ was equally satisfactory. In that case, the springs K_1 and K_2 would act in parallel and they can be replaced by a single spring of stiffness $K_1 + K_2$. Patel and Fry also showed that Womersley's original concept of tethering which corresponds to setting $C_1 = 0$ and $C_2 = \infty$ was accordingly limited. Any theoretic consideration of a dynamic problem wherein the longitudinal tethering enters the boundary condition must consider the viscous element as well as the elastic elements.

Another interesting aspect of tethering was also observed. The dynamic spring constant was seen to increase rapidly as one progressed along the aorta, the more peripheral vessels like the femoral artery being almost fully tethered. This longitudinal variation in tethering should also be kept in mind in quantitative modeling of circulatory dynamics.

The pressure—length and pressure—diameter relationships in the canine aorta have been studied in vivo (Patel, Greenfield, and Fry, 1964). A simultaneous recording of length, diameter, and intravascular pressure from the descending thoracic aorta is shown in Figure 3. The changes in length during a cardiac cycle were within 1% of the original length in the thoracic and abdominal aortas; a higher value of 5% was observed in the

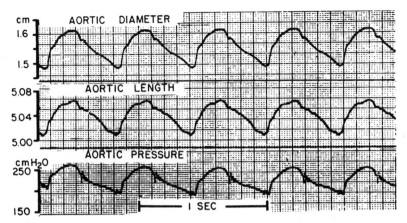

Figure 3. Simultaneous recording of length, diameter, and intravascular pressure from descending thoracic aorta. (From Patel et al., 1961; reproduced by permission.)

ascending aorta. The change in diameter during a cardiac cycle varied from 6% in the ascending aorta to approximately 1% in the iliac artery. The former value was obtained in man for a mean pressure of 95 cm H_2O and a pulse pressure of 46 cm H_2O; the latter was obtained in dog for a mean pressure of 126 cm H_2O and a pulse pressure of 34 cm H_2O. In general, as one proceeds peripherally from the ascending aorta, the vessel wall has a tendency to get stiffer.

The longitudinal and radial vessel wall velocities were calculated by taking the first derivative of the length versus time curve and of the radius versus time curve, respectively. Results from the ascending aorta of one dog are shown in Figure 4. It can be seen that the radial vessel wall velocity remains small throughout the cardiac cycle when compared to the underlying blood velocity; the longitudinal vessel wall velocity is also small except in early systole.

GENERAL MATERIAL PROPERTIES

To characterize the mechanical properties of the vascular tissue, one must first postulate a law of material behavior (or a constitutive relation), verify by actual experiments whether the postulated law is indeed applicable, and then, if the law is applicable, describe its quantitative form. The postulated law, however, must at least take into account all the experimental observations regarding material behavior unless they are specifically ruled out by some logic or deemed unimportant in a given case. Failure to do this can

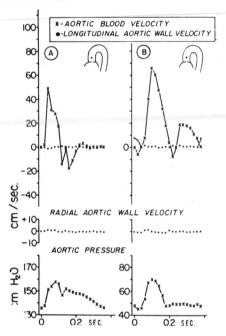

Figure 4. Relation between longitudinal aortic blood velocity, longitudinal aortic wall velocity, radial aortic wall velocity, and intravascular pressures at sites indicated. (Adapted from Patel et al., 1961; reproduced by permission.)

lead to postulation of an unjustifiably simple relation that can lead either to a merely partial description or to an erroneous one. On the other hand, failure to recognize a certain simplification can yield an unnecessarily complicated postulate that could be uneconomical or misleading. Many characteristics of tissue behavior, e.g., creep, stress relaxation, and hysteresis, can be observed simply. Numerous early papers (see McDonald, 1974) have documented such observations, many in considerable detail. However, two aspects of material behavior are not easily observable, but are nonetheless important in postulating a constitutive relation for a tissue. These are degree of tissue compressibility and degree of material symmetry. We discuss these below.

Compressibility of the Arterial Wall

An ideally incompressible material is one that undergoes no volume change when subjected to a hydrostatic stress of whatever magnitude. Identical volumes of all real material show different degrees of resistance to volume change under a given amount of hydrostatic stress; those undergoing smaller volume changes are said to have a higher bulk modulus. Steel has a higher bulk modulus ($\simeq$12.8 $\times$ 10^{11} dynes/cm^2) than water ($\simeq$2.18 $\times$ 10^{10} dynes/cm^2) and is therefore, in this sense, more incompressible than water. In practice, however, this type of incompressibility is not of importance. What is important is the relative degree of resistance that a given material offers to hydrostatic (volume-changing) stresses and deviatoric (shearing or shape-changing) stresses. Materials with a relatively high resistance to deformation under hydrostatic stresses are then said to be incompressible. Water, in this sense, is incompressible, whereas steel is compressible. Of course, for applications where the hydrostatic stress dominates, the bulk modulus, however large in comparison with the shear modulus, must be accounted for. For instance, the bulk modulus of water becomes an important quantity in the study of underwater sound propagation. With this background on the concept of incompressibility, we proceed to discuss whether arterial tissue may or may not be considered incompressible.

Various investigators have presented experimental evidence supporting the theory that the arterial tissue is either compressible or incompressible. Lawton (1954), for example, found that aortic strips preserved their volume under various degrees of stretch. Dobrin and Rovick (1967) found that canine carotid arteries were incompressible when subjected to internal pressure at a fixed length. Tickner and Sacks (1967), on the other hand, found volume changes in walls of arteries inflated with air up to pressures of 326 cm H$_2$O. The question of incompressibility of the arterial tissue was further explored by Carew, Vaishnav, and Patel (1968), who carried out experiments on various canine arterial segments, namely, the upper and lower descending thoracic aortas, abdominal aorta, and the iliac, carotid, and pulmonary arteries from 17 dogs.

Before excising the segments, the in vivo length and the mean arterial pressure were measured. At the end of each experiment, the unstretched length, radius, and tissue volume were obtained. The experiments attempted to measure the average bulk modulus k of the tissue as the ratio of the hydrostatic stress, S_h, and the volumetric strain $\Delta V/V_0$, where ΔV is the change in volume caused by the application of a state of stress with hydrostatic components S_h, and V_0 is the unstretched tissue volume. The latter is computed as the average of the three principal stresses for the state of stress in question.

To impose a known state of stress on an arterial segment, Carew et al. fixed the segment, with two hollow cylindrical plugs at its ends, into a force gauge at a length 3–10% greater than the in vivo length and inflated it with pressures greater than those in vivo (200–275 cm H_2O). The pressure p, the external radius R_0, and the extra longitudinal force F were measured. The radial, circumferential, and longitudinal stresses, S_r, S_θ, and S_z, respectively, were computed as

$$S_r = -p/2 \tag{1}$$

$$S_\theta = p(R/h - \tfrac{1}{2}) \tag{2}$$

$$S_z = p/2(R/h - 1) + F/2\pi Rh \tag{3}$$

where h is the wall thickness and R is the midwall radius. The hydrostatic component of stress, S_h, was then computed as

$$S_h = 1/3(S_r + S_\theta + S_z) \tag{4}$$

Equations 2 and 3 are obtained from simple equilibrium considerations. Equation 1 assigns a uniform value to S_r halfway between the internal and external values.

The segment was then mounted in a specially designed sealed glass flask that permitted imposition of a variable longitudinal extension and a variable internal pressure on the segment. The flask was filled with deaerated normal saline, and had a capillary side arm that could register small volume changes in the flask resulting from changes in tissue volume. These volume changes ΔV were divided by the initial volume V_0 of the tissue to give volumetric strains.

For 11 segments of the thoracic aorta, the average $\Delta V/V_0$ was 0.0006, the average S_h was 1798 g/cm^2, and the average bulk modulus K was 4.44 $\times$ 10^6 g/cm^2. Similar semiquantitative results were also obtained for other types of arterial segments.

A volumetric strain of 0.0006 clearly indicated that the arterial wall does undergo some volume change, and thus is indeed compressible in this sense. What is more important for our purposes, however, is the resistance of the wall to volume changes in comparison with its resistance to shape changes. Just as the bulk modulus k describes the former, the shear modulus G describes the latter. Thus it is the ratio k/G that provides a relative measure of incompressibility. For large deformation, it is really not permissible to talk about k and G in the same sense as in the linear theory of elasticity, but the concepts can be used for a semiquantitative analysis. If on the basis of Bergel's results (Bergel, 1960), for example, we take the value of Young's modulus, E, for the arterial tissue to be about 4.4×10^3 g/cm^2, this yields a value of $G \simeq 1.5 \times 10^3$ g/cm^2 and $k/G \simeq$ 3,000, which is very high. Thus, for states of stress such as are usually encountered in physiologic conditions, wherein the volume-changing component of stress is not dominant, the arterial tissue can be considered incompressible.

Elastic Symmetry in the Arterial Tissue

For simplicity in considering the question of elastic symmetry, we assume the artery to be linearly elastic and of cylindrical geometry. We choose a cylindrical coordinate system (r,θ,z) such that the origin is at one end, the z axis is along the vessel axis, and the r axis is directed radially outward. Because the artery is assumed to be homogeneous, a uniform state of stress in the artery also causes a uniform state of deformation. An arbitrary state of stress in a typical element could consist of up to six nonzero stresses (or the components of the stress tensor) $S_r, S_\theta, S_z, S_{\theta z} = S_{z\theta}, S_{zr} = S_{rz}$, and $S_{r\theta} = S_{\theta r}$. The first three are the normal stresses. They are directed along the axes and are perpendicular to the faces on which they act. The remaining stresses are shearing stresses and act in the planes of the faces. S_{rz}, for example, is the shearing stress acting in the z direction on a face perpendicular to the r axis. This type of stress could be generated by axial flow of blood past the inner wall of a blood vessel. An arbitrary state of strain in a typical element can likewise be described by six nonzero strains (or components of the strain tensor), say, $e_r, e_\theta, e_z, \gamma_{\theta z} = \gamma_{z\theta}, \gamma_{zr} = \gamma_{rz}, \gamma_{r\theta} = \gamma_{\theta r}$. The first three are the direct or elongating strains and the remaining ones are the shearing strains. The component e_θ, for example, describes the fractional increase in the length of a line element in the circumferential directions. The component γ_{rz} similarly describes the angle change that would accompany the deformation corresponding to the inside wall of the cylindrical segment moving axially relative to the outside wall.

In a fully anisotropic material, that is, one with no symmetry, a state of stress with only one nonzero component would be accompanied by a state of deformation wherein all strains are nonzero. If one could carry out such an experiment, six elastic constants would be obtained for a linearly elastic material. Six such experiments, one for each stress component, would give 36 elastic constants, which would then completely determine the elastic properties of this linearly elastic material. If the material is also assumed to have a strain energy density function (Patel and Vaishnav, 1972), the number of independent elastic constants needed to characterize it can be reduced to 21. However, without additional degrees of elastic symmetry, 21 is the minimum number of elastic constants. Physically, various degrees of elastic symmetry arise because of the existence of certain structural symmetries in the material composition. For example, the material might have a plane of symmetry such that the mirror image of the half reflected in that plane is identical structurally to the other half. Such symmetry would imply certain interdependence among the 36 or 21 elastic constants and the disappearance of certain others, the total number of independent constants reducing to 20 or 13. If the material exhibited further symmetry about a plane perpendicular to the first one, the number of independent elastic constants would reduce to 12 or 9. Further symmetry about a plane perpendicular to both the above planes does not further reduce the number of independent elastic constants. A material with such a degree of symmetry is called orthotropic. If the planes perpendicular to the r, θ, and z axes were the planes of symmetry, we would find that in such a material applications of S_θ, S_z, and S_r produce strains e_θ, e_z, and e_r only and $S_{r\theta}$, S_{rz}, and $S_{z\theta}$ produce only the corresponding shearing strains. A state of stress generated in an arterial segment by applying intravascular pressure and an extra longitudinal force gives rise mainly to S_θ, S_z, and S_r. If we can show that under these conditions $\gamma_{r\theta}$, γ_{rz}, and $\gamma_{r\theta}$ are negligible, we can demonstrate that an arterial segment is orthotropic. Patel and Fry (1969) carried out experiments showing that, to a first approximation, this indeed is the case. We describe these experiments briefly.

Relatively uniform segments of the middle descending thoracic aorta, abdominal aorta, and left common carotid artery were isolated and excised from dogs. A typical segment was cleaned free of loose adventitia, fitted with hollow end plugs, and hung vertically from one end. The lower end was fitted with a radial pointer that moved along the arc of a protractor. The vessel was connected to a reservoir of saline that could be raised or lowered to cause a desired pressure in the segment. As the pressure was increased, the pointer at the end rotated; the angle of rotation ϕ was measured for a series of pressures. The shearing strain $\gamma_{z\theta}$ corresponding to this rotation was obtained as

$$\gamma_{z\theta} = \frac{\phi R_0}{L}$$

where R_0 is the external radius of the vessel and L is the length of the segment.

For some vessels, a glass whisker was inserted radially through the wall from the outside, making sure that it did not pierce the diametrically opposite site in the vessel. The angular deviation of this pointer was measured as the pressure was increased through several steps to compute the shearing strain $\gamma_{r\theta}$.

In all cases it was found that the shearing strains were an order of magnitude smaller than the corresponding circumferential and longitudinal strains, the value of $\gamma_{z\theta}$ being the largest for the carotid artery. Two ancillary studies were done in vivo to corroborate the above observation. Circular imprints stamped on the thoracic aorta changed to ellipses with axes oriented circumferentially and longitudinally, indicating again that the $\gamma_{z\theta}$ was small compared to the elongating strains.

One may conclude from the above that the shearing strain $\gamma_{z\theta}$ is always small compared to the elongating strains under physiologic loading. As the other two shearing strains were also found to be small, we can conclude that the arterial tissue can be considered at least orthotropic. This reduces the number of independent elastic constants from 21 to 9. Three of these relate the shearing stresses to the shearing strains and can be ignored for a physiologic type of loading. Finally, because of incompressibility, we can reduce by three the number of independent elastic constants. The linear elastic characterization of the arterial tissue can thus be carried out in terms of only three constants which may be chosen to be the three Young's moduli in the radial, circumferential, and longitudinal directions.

OVERALL VESSEL WALL PROPERTIES

We can determine the overall vessel wall properties in two different ways. The first approach is based on the consideration that although the mechanical properties of the vascular wall are nonlinear, it is permissible to consider the mechanical response of the tissue as linear when small static or dynamic strains are superimposed on a state of large deformation. This incremental approach is motivated by the fact that pulsatile blood flow in a blood vessel causes small time-dependent strains that are superimposed on a state of large deformation of the blood vessel resulting from a mean intravascular pressure and a longitudinal tethering force. This approach is therefore a natural one because it yields data in a form that is easy to interpret and use. Much early work in vascular mechanics was ostensibly based on this approach but did not use the approach properly. Investigators often confused incremental linearity with overall linearity and neglected, in the expression for incremental stress, to account for certain terms arising from geometric changes that are significant in the incremental theory but not in the classical theory of initially unstressed linear materials. A second source of confusion arose from not realizing that the incremental properties in general depend on the state of large deformation on which the small strains are applied. The values of the incremental elastic moduli, for example, obtained at low values of initial strains cannot be compared with those obtained at higher values. In fact, this limitation of the incremental theory is indeed its major shortcoming. Finally, the third and most important source of confusion in the use of the incremental theory has been the failure to realize that even an isotropic nonlinear material would behave anisotropically, since the incremental properties depend on the state of large strain, generally unequal in different directions.

The second approach to characterizing the mechanical properties of the vascular tissue is the direct approach, wherein the stresses at all states of deformation are expressed in terms of the history of deformation. Once the tissue is characterized this way, anisotropic incremental properties can be computed about any state of large deformation. This approach is therefore far more general than the incremental approach, albeit more complicated. Below we outline our work based on both of these approaches (Patel et al., 1973; Vaishnav, Young, and Patel, 1975).

Dynamic Incremental Viscoelastic Properties

Consider a blood vessel in a state of initial strain characterized by extension ratios[3] λ_θ, λ_z, and λ_r in the circumferential (θ), longitudinal (z), and radial (r) directions. If e_θ, e_z, and e_r are small incremental sinusoidal strains and P_θ, P_z, and P_r are the corresponding sinusoidal incremental stresses, we can write the following incremental stress–strain relations:

$$e_\theta = C_{\theta\theta}P_\theta - C_{\theta z}P_z - C_{\theta r}P_r \qquad (5)$$

$$e_z = -C_{z\theta}P_\theta + C_{zz}P_z - C_{zr}P_r \qquad (6)$$

$$e_r = -C_{r\theta}P_\theta - C_{rz}P_z + C_{rr}P_r \qquad (7)$$

Equation 5, for example, states that the incremental strain in the θ direction depends linearly on all three incremental stresses. The equations as written provide for incremental orthotropy because we do not require,

---

[3] Extension ratio (or stretch) denotes the ratio of the lengths of a line segment in the deformed and undeformed states. It exceeds the engineering strain by unity and is another way of quantifying deformation.

for example, that $C_{\theta\theta}$, C_{zz}, and C_{rr} be equal. The way in which e_θ and P_θ are related can thus be different from the way in which e_z and P_z are related. In Eqs. 5–7, all quantities are complex, having real and imaginary parts.[4] This permits the incremental stresses and strains to be out of phase, as is generally the case because of tissue viscoelasticity. The negative sign in front of some of the coefficients C_{ij} is for convenience and reflects the observation that in a uniaxial test, the longitudinal extension is accompanied by transverse contractions. For a complete statement of incremental properties of the vascular tissue, three more equations relating incremental shearing stresses to shearing strains should be appended to Eqs. 5–7, but for the physiologic loading considered here, these equations are not pertinent.

There are nine complex coefficients in Eqs. 5–7. They can be reduced to six by assuming that $C_{\theta z} = C_{z\theta}$, $C_{r\theta} = C_{\theta r}$, and $C_{z\theta} = C_{\theta z}$. Implicit in this assumption is the existence of incremental strain energy density and dissipation functions that are quadratic forms of the incremental strains and strain rates, respectively (Biot, 1965).

By virtue of incompressibility, the incremental strains should sum to zero. Imposing this on Eqs. 5–7 gives three relations in C_{ij}:

$$C_{zr} = \tfrac{1}{2}(C_{zz} + C_{rr} - C_{\theta\theta}) \qquad (8)$$

$$C_{r\theta} = \tfrac{1}{2}(C_{rr} + C_{\theta\theta} - C_{zz}) \qquad (9)$$

$$C_{\theta z} = \tfrac{1}{2}(C_{\theta\theta} + C_{zz} - C_{rr}) \qquad (10)$$

These equations can be used to eliminate all but the three coefficients C_{rr}, $C_{\theta\theta}$, and C_{zz} from Eqs. 5–7, which can then be rewritten as

$$e_\theta = (P_\theta - \tfrac{1}{2}P_z - \tfrac{1}{2}P_r)C_{\theta\theta} + \tfrac{1}{2}(P_r - P_z)C_{zz} + \tfrac{1}{2}(P_z - P_r)C_{rr} \qquad (11)$$

$$e_z = \tfrac{1}{2}(P_r - P_\theta)C_{\theta\theta} + (P_z - \tfrac{1}{2}P_\theta - \tfrac{1}{2}P_r)C_{zz} + \tfrac{1}{2}(P_\theta - P_r)C_{rr} \qquad (12)$$

$$e_r = \tfrac{1}{2}(P_z - P_\theta)C_{\theta\theta} + \tfrac{1}{2}(P_\theta - P_z)C_{zz} + (P_r - \tfrac{1}{2}P_\theta - \tfrac{1}{2}P_z)C_{rr} \qquad (13)$$

These equations are available to compute the three complex unknowns or the six real unknowns, namely, the real and imaginary parts of C_{rr}, $C_{\theta\theta}$, and C_{zz}. However, these equations are linearly dependent and therefore reduce to only two equations in three unknowns for a specific state of incremental strain and the corresponding state of incremental stress. A simple multiple of these states would not provide anything new. What

---

[4] For a complex-number representation of sinusoidal events, see Patel and Vaishnav (1972).

would be required is a completely different state of strain for which the strains are in proportions different than in the first case. The two states of strain together would then give four complex equations in three complex unknowns. This overdetermined system can be solved by the method of least squares for the three complex coefficients. The remaining coefficients can then be obtained using Eqs. 8–10. This procedure can be repeated for any other state of initial strain and for any other value of the circular frequency ω of the sinusoidal strains.

Equations 5–7 can be rewritten as

$$e_\theta = \frac{1}{E_\theta} P_\theta - \frac{\sigma_{\theta z}}{E_z} P_z - \frac{\sigma_{\theta r}}{E_r} P_r \tag{14}$$

$$e_z = -\frac{\sigma_{z\theta}}{E_\theta} P_\theta + \frac{1}{E_z} P_z - \frac{\sigma_{zr}}{E_r} P_r \tag{15}$$

$$e_r = -\frac{\sigma_{r\theta}}{E_\theta} P_\theta - \frac{\sigma_{rz}}{E_z} P_z - \frac{1}{E_r} P_r \tag{16}$$

where E_θ, E_z, and E_r are the complex elastic moduli similar to Young's moduli and the σ's are the complex Poisson ratios. Comparison of Eqs. 5–7 with Eqs. 14–16 gives the following relations among these coefficients:

$$E_\theta = \frac{1}{C_{\theta\theta}} ; \quad E_z = \frac{1}{C_{zz}} ; \quad E_r = \frac{1}{C_{rr}}$$

$$\sigma_{\theta z} = \frac{C_{\theta z}}{C_{zz}} ; \quad \sigma_{zr} = \frac{C_{zr}}{C_{rr}} ; \quad \sigma_{r\theta} = \frac{C_{r\theta}}{C_{\theta\theta}}$$

$$\sigma_{z\theta} = \frac{C_{z\theta}}{C_{\theta\theta}} ; \quad \sigma_{rz} = \frac{C_{rz}}{C_{zz}} ; \quad \sigma_{\theta r} = \frac{C_{\theta r}}{C_{rr}} \tag{17}$$

We also observe that the Poisson ratios obey the relations

$$\sigma_{z\theta} + \sigma_{r\theta} = \sigma_{\theta z} + \sigma_{rz} = \sigma_{\theta r} + \sigma_{zr} = 1, \tag{18}$$

which are the counterpart of the well-known condition of Poisson's ratio being one-half for an isotropic linearly elastic incompressible material.

We carried out in vivo experiments to evaluate these incremental coefficients for the middle descending thoracic aorta in open-chested dogs at various frequencies and at various levels of initial strain (Patel et al., 1973). Each experiment was carried out in two phases. In the first phase, a constant blood volume was trapped in the vessel segment and the segment length varied sinusoidally. In the second phase, the segment length was kept constant, but the lumen volume was varied by means of a syringe driven by a sinusoidal pump. Figure 5 shows the experimental set-up used.

Ten dogs were studied. In five of them the aortic segment was studied around three mean pressures. In six dogs, the experiment was performed in vivo and in vitro. The lumen was kept filled with oxygenated blood at $26-27°C$. The pressure, external radius, longitudinal force, and segment length were measured continuously as functions of time. The pressure was measured with a Statham P23Db transducer and the radius with an electrical caliper; length and forces were measured by means of a specially designed force gauge (Plowman, Young, and Janicki, 1974).

At the end of the experiment the segment was slit open longitudinally

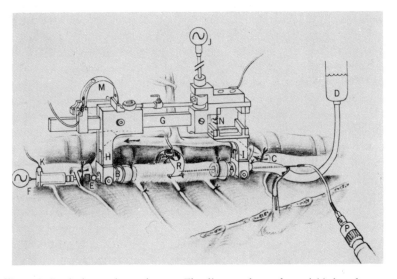

Figure 5. Typical experimental setup. The diagram shows the variable-length gauge, G, for measuring force and changes in length, attached to a segment of the middle descending thoracic aorta. The gauge has the following components: force transducer, N; length-change transducer, M; sinusoidal driver, J; movable leg, H; and fixed leg, I. The fluid displacement device, F, consists of a sinusoidal driver attached to the piston of a syringe. The volume gauge, K, senses the relative displacements of the piston and the cylinder of the syringe. R is the radius-sensing gauge, P is the pressure gauge, D is a reservoir containing blood, C is the descending thoracic aorta with bypass, and E is a Luer-lock fitting. A and B are the proximal and the distal plugs, respectively. (From Patel et al., 1973; reproduced by permission of the American Heart Association, Inc.)

and its mean unstressed length and circumference were measured. The wall thickness was calculated from the wall volume on the basis of tissue incompressibility.

For each frequency, the complex quantities e_θ, e_z, P_θ, P_z, and P_r were calculated for both phases of the experiment. Each phase gave two complex equations in three complex unknowns. These were solved by the method of least squares. Real and imaginary parts of all coefficients C_{ij}, as well as those of the Young's moduli and Poisson's ratios, were computed.

The data were divided into four groups according to the levels of initial strains in the circumferential and longitudinal directions. Group I included points with low λ_θ and λ_z, Group II with high λ_θ and low λ_z, Group III with low λ_θ and high λ_z, and Group IV with high λ_θ and λ_z. The results for these groups are shown in Figure 6 in which we plot the real (E') and imaginary parts (E'') of the incremental viscoelastic moduli. We note the following from this figure. (1) The storage moduli, E', in general, depend on the λ_θ and λ_z, thus indicating the nonlinear behavior of the arterial wall. We also see that E_θ' is influenced more by λ_θ and by λ_r. E_z' is influenced markedly by λ_z and for large values of λ_z it is relatively uninfluenced by λ_θ. E_r' seems to be equally influenced by λ_θ and λ_z. (2) E_z'' in Group I is the lowest. There is no other apparent pattern of dependence of the loss moduli, E'', on λ_θ or λ_z. (3) In general, $E_z' > E_\theta' > E_r'$ and $E_z'' > E_r'' > E_\theta''$. The vessel wall is thus anisotropic in the physiologic pressure range used in the study. (4) The ratios of loss moduli to the corresponding storage moduli are rather small, indicating that the viscous effect is small compared to the elastic effect. (5) The storage moduli increase from 0 to 2 Hz and then settle down to a relatively constant value. The loss moduli tend to increase slightly with frequency. (6) Comparison of the in vitro data with the in vivo data shows a marked decrease in the in vitro values of E_z' and E_z''. By using our data from vascular tethering, we have been able to account for most of this difference as being due to vascular tethering that is present in vivo but absent in the in vitro studies.

Nonlinear Viscoelastic Properties

The second approach toward characterization of the mechanical properties of the vascular tissue is the direct approach. We proceed to outline our recent work in this area (Vaishnav et al., 1975).

We draw upon the modern theory of continuum mechanics (see Truesdell and Noll, 1965, for example) and express the stress in the tissue at the present time as an arbitrary function of the history of the deforma-

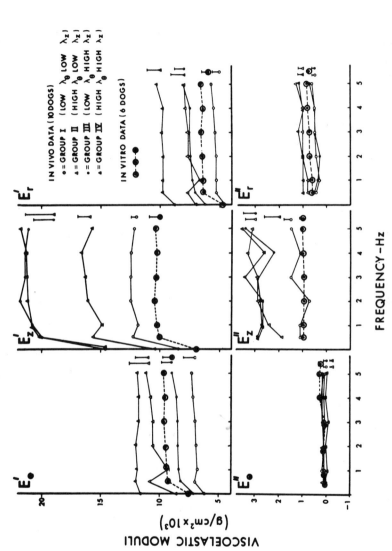

Figure 6. Incremental visoelastic moduli versus frequency. E'_θ, E'_z, and E'_r are the storage moduli in the circumferential, longitudinal, and radial directions, respectively; E''_θ, E''_z, and E''_r are the corresponding loss moduli. The vertical lines to the right represent the average SE for each curve; the symbols at the lower ends of the line segments merely identify the appropriate curves. (From Patel et al., 1973; reproduced by permission of the American Heart Association, Inc.)

tion of the tissue up to the present time. Because the history itself is a function of time, we refer to stress, more specifically, as a functional rather than a function of the history of deformation. Actually, we can restrict ourselves to the history of the deformation of the immediate neighborhood of a material particle, because such a restriction has been found to be adequate for a large class of engineering materials. We may further impose the requirement known as "the axiom of objectivity" or "the principle of material frame indifference" in modern continuum mechanics. This principle requires that the material response be invariant under changes of frames of reference or observers. With this we may express the contravariant components[5] of the stress tensor t^{kl} as

$$t^{kl}(t) = -p'g^{kl} + \frac{\partial x^k(t)}{\partial X^K}\frac{\partial x^l(t)}{\partial X^L} \underset{\tau=\infty}{\overset{0}{G}}{}^{KL}\,[E_{MN}(t-\tau)] \qquad (19)$$

where we have provided for the fact that the stress in an incompressible material can be determined only to within a hydrostatic stress p'. In Eq. 19 E_{MN} is the Green–St. Venant strain tensor of the deformation and $\partial x^k/\partial X^K$ is the deformation gradient. $\underset{\tau=\infty}{G}$ [ ] denotes a functional of the history over the stated domain of the argument function within the brackets.

The form of the functional G in Eq. 19 is too general for practical use. Following Green and Rivlin (1957), we therefore expand the functional into a series of multiple integrals. After a change of variables, we then have

$$t^{kl}(t) = -p'g^{kl} + \frac{\partial x^k(t)}{\partial X^K}\frac{\partial x^l(t)}{\partial X^L}\,[\int_{-\infty}^{t}K^{KLMN}(t-\tau)\dot{E}_{MN}(\tau)\,d\tau$$

$$+ \int_{-\infty}^{t}\int_{-\infty}^{t}K^{KLM_1N_1M_2N_2}(t-\tau_1, t-\tau_2)\dot{E}_{M_1N_1}(\tau_1)\dot{E}_{M_2N_2}(\tau_2)\,d\tau_1\,d\tau_2 +$$

$$\cdots + \int_{-\infty}^{t}\cdots\int_{-\infty}^{t}K^{KLM_1N_1\cdots M_nN_n}(t-\tau_1, \ldots, t-\tau_n)\dot{E}_{M_1N_1}(\tau_1)$$

$$\cdots \dot{E}_{M_nN_n}d\tau_1\cdots d\tau_n] \qquad (20)$$

In Eq. 20 a superior dot stands for differentiation with respect to time t. The K functions in Eq. 20 are called kernel functions; specification of material response requires specification of the form of all the pertinent kernel functions. Here we restrict ourselves only to terms involving no higher than double integrals.

For application to an orthotropic tissue, we must require that histories

---

[5] In this section we use the notation of Eringen (1962, 1967) as far as possible.

of only the invariants of E_{KL} relative to orthotropic symmetry appear as arguments. As shown by Adkins (1958), these invariants are

$$E_{11}, \ E_{22}, \ E_{33}, \ E_{23}^2, \ E_{13}^2, \ E_{12}^2, \ E_{23}E_{13}E_{12} \tag{21}$$

where E_{KL} are the components of strain referred to the local axes of symmetry.

For a cylindrical segment of a homogeneous blood vessel under a physiologic loading consisting of only an inflating pressure and an extending force, the shearing strains E_{23}, E_{13}, and E_{12} vanish. Furthermore, E_{11}, E_{22}, E_{33} are interrelated by the requirement of incompressibility. Thus histories of only E_{22} and E_{33} are pertinent here. Furthermore, recognizing that

$$p' = -\tfrac{1}{3}(t^{(1)(1)} + t^{(2)(2)} + t^{(3)(3)}), \tag{22}$$

we can eliminate p' from Eq. 20. In Eq. 22, $t^{(1)(1)}$, etc., are the physical components of t^{kl}, that is, components referred to local cartesian axes.

After simplifying and introducing new kernel functions, we have the following two equations for two stress differences:

$$t^{(2)(2)} - t^{(1)(1)} = \left(\frac{\partial x^{(2)}}{\partial X^{(2)}}\right)^2 [\int_{-\infty}^t \bar{K}^{2222}(t-\tau)\dot{E}_{22}(\tau)\,d\tau + \int_{-\infty}^t \bar{K}^{2233}(t-\tau)\dot{E}_{33}(\tau)$$

$$d\tau + \int_{-\infty}^t \int_{-\infty}^t \bar{K}^{222222}(t-\tau_1, t-\tau_2)\dot{E}_{22}(\tau_1)\dot{E}_{22}(\tau_2)\,d\tau_1\,d\tau_2 + \int_{-\infty}^t \int_{-\infty}^t \bar{K}^{222233}(t$$

$$-\tau_1, t-\tau_2)\dot{E}_{22}(\tau_1)\dot{E}_{33}(\tau_2)\,d\tau_1\,d\tau_2 + \int_{-\infty}^t \int_{-\infty}^t \bar{K}^{223333}(t-\tau_1, t-\tau_2)\dot{E}_{33}(\tau_1)$$

$$\dot{E}_{33}(\tau_2)\,d\tau_1\,d\tau_2] \tag{23}$$

$$t^{(3)(3)} - t^{(1)(1)} = \left(\frac{\partial x^{(3)}}{\partial X^{(3)}}\right)^2 [\int_{-\infty}^t \bar{K}^{3322}(t-\tau)\dot{E}_{22}(\tau)\,d\tau + \int_{-\infty}^t \bar{K}^{3333}(t-\tau)\dot{E}_{33}(\tau)$$

$$d\tau + \int_{-\infty}^t \int_{-\infty}^t \bar{K}^{332222}(t-\tau_1, t-\tau_2)\dot{E}_{22}(\tau_1)\dot{E}_{22}(\tau_2)\,d\tau_1\,d\tau_2$$

$$+ \int_{-\infty}^t \int_{-\infty}^t \bar{K}^{332233}(t-\tau_1, t-\tau_2)\dot{E}_{22}(\tau_1)\dot{E}_{33}(\tau_2)\,d\tau_1\,d\tau_2$$

$$+ \int_{-\infty}^t \int_{-\infty}^t \bar{K}^{333333}(t-\tau_1, t-\tau_2)\dot{E}_{33}(\tau_1)\dot{E}_{33}(\tau_2)\,d\tau_1\,d\tau_2] \tag{24}$$

Let us now consider a cylindrical arterial segment subjected to a sudden deformation at zero time such that, at a generic location in the deformed segment, the circumferential stretch is λ_θ and the longitudinal stretch is λ_z at time $t = 0+$ onward. The circumferential and longitudinal Green–St. Venant strains are related to λ_θ and λ_z as

$$E_{(2)(2)} = \tfrac{1}{2}(\lambda_\theta^2 - 1), \qquad E_{(3)(3)} = \tfrac{1}{2}(\lambda_z^2 - 1) \tag{25}$$

We permit E_{22} to vary through the thickness of the artery but assume E_{33} to be constant throughout. The strain history corresponding to above deformation, which is the usual type of deformation one imposes when studying the relaxation response of a viscoelastic material, can be expressed as

$$E_{(2)(2)}(t) = aH(t) \tag{26}$$

$$E_{(3)(3)}(t) = bH(t) \tag{27}$$

where a and b are constants and $H(t)$ is the Heavyside step function defined as

$$H(t) = 0, \quad t < 0$$
$$= 1, \quad t > 0 \tag{28}$$

For such a history, Eqs. 23 and 24 simplify greatly. In fact, the integrals vanish completely and we have the relations

$$S_\theta - S_r = (1 + 2a)[\bar{K}^{2222}(t)a + \bar{K}^{2233}(t)b + \bar{K}^{222222}(t,t)a^2$$
$$+ \bar{K}^{222233}(t,t)ab + \bar{K}^{223333}(t,t)b^2] \tag{29}$$

$$S_z - S_r = (1 + 2b)[\bar{K}^{3322}(t)a + \bar{K}^{3333}(t)b + \bar{K}^{332222}(t,t)a^2$$
$$+ \bar{K}^{333322}(t,t)ab + \bar{K}^{222222}(t,t)b^2] \tag{30}$$

where we have renamed the stresses $t^{(1)(1)}$, $t^{(2)(2)}$, $t^{(3)(3)}$ as S_r, S_θ, and S_z, respectively.

Equations 29 and 30 can be used to evaluate the 10 unknown kernel functions experimentally by imposing properly spaced steps a and b in strains for which the corresponding stresses are known. These kernel functions can then be used in Eqs. 23 and 24 to evaluate stresses for any other history of strain.

For convenience, we rewrite Eqs. 29 and 30 as follows:

$$S_\theta - S_r = C_2^2(t)(2a + 4a^2) + C_3^2(t)(b + 2ab) + C_{22}^2(t,t)(3a^2 + 6a^3)$$
$$+ C_{23}^2(t,t)(2ab + 4a^2 b) + C_{33}^2(t,t)(b^2 + 2ab^2) \tag{31}$$

$$S_z - S_r = C_2^3(t)(a + 2ab) + C_3^3(t)(2b + 4b^2) + C_{22}^3(t,t)(a^2 + 2a^2 b)$$
$$+ C_{23}^3(t,t)(2ab + 4ab^2) + C_{33}^3(t,t)(3b^2 + 6b^3) \tag{32}$$

where the kernel functions have been renamed and terms rearranged.

If in Eqs. 23 and 24 only the first-order integrals are retained, a simpler method with only four relaxation kernel functions follows and Eqs. 31 and 32 take the form

$$S_\theta - S_r = C_2^2(t)(2a + 4a^2) + C_3^2(t)(b + 2ab) \tag{33}$$

$$S_z - S_r = C_2^3(t)(a + 2ab) + C_3^3(t)(2b + 4b^2) \tag{34}$$

If the viscous effects are negligible, the kernel functions become constants and elastic theories follow. The stress–strain equations for 10-constant and 4-constant elastic theories are then obtained from Eqs. 31 and 32 and 33 and 34, respectively.

In our previous work (Vaishnav et al., 1972, 1973) we proposed elastic theories at three levels, involving 12, 7, and 3 constants and showed that the 7-constant theory in general sufficed for an adequate representation of the elastic behavior of the aortic tissue. The development of these was based on assuming the existence of a strain energy density function from which the expressions for stress differences were derived. There, as here, we assumed the material to be incompressible and orthotropic. The 7- and 3-constant theories are the counterparts of the 10- and 4-constant theories resulting from the present formulation. Working backwards then, we postulate, in addition to the 10- and 4-function theories, two more corresponding theories involving 7 and 3 functions, respectively. Theoretically, such a transition implies existence of a strain energy density function at each instant of time for the viscoelastic case. The exact significance of this is unclear to us at present. The theories, however, forcefully present themselves as extensions of their elastic counterparts and we conditionally accept them at present. The formulations for the 7- and 3-function theories, are then,

$$\begin{aligned}S_\theta - S_r = {}& A(t)(2a + 4a^2) + B(t)(b + 2ab) + D(t,t)(3a^2 + 6a^3) \\ & + E(t,t)(2ab + 4a^2 b) + F(t,t)(b^2 + 2ab^2)\end{aligned} \tag{35}$$

$$\begin{aligned}S_z - S_r = {}& B(t)(a + 2ab) + C(t)(2b + 4b^2) + E(t,t)(a^2 + 2a^2 b) \\ & + F(t,t)(2ab + 4ab^2) + G(t,t)(3b^2 + 6b^3)\end{aligned} \tag{36}$$

and

$$S_\theta - S_r = A(t)(2a + 4a^2) + B(t)(b + 2ab) \tag{37}$$

$$S_z - S_r = B(t)(a + 2ab) + C(t)(2b + 4b^2). \tag{38}$$

Experiments were performed to test the four different theories on aortic tissue. Segments of middle descending aorta were excised from seven dogs. A typical segment was subjected to 38 steps in circumferential and longitudinal strains by sudden injection of a known volume of blood simultaneously with a specified increase in length of each segment. The pressure and longitudinal force required to maintain the imposed steps were recorded continuously. Most of the decay occurred within the first 100 sec.

The experimental range covered in λ_θ was 1.17 to 1.72 and in λ_z from 1.28 to 1.61. The average maximum value for the intravascular pressure was 222 cm H_2O.

From the data, relaxation kernel functions for the 3-, 4-, 7-, and 10-function theories were computed. Most of the functions decayed with time as would be expected in a viscoelastic material. From an analysis of the degree of applicability of the four theories we concluded that both the 7- and 10-function theories adequately describe the nonlinear viscoelastic behavior of the aortic tissue and either may be used in critical application; for less critical applications, even the 3- and 4-function theories can be used.

From the general theory we have also arrived at formulations for incremental storage and loss moduli at any state of large initial strain and for any frequency of sinusoidal excitation. The numerical application of these formulations is in progress.

Thus we have what we consider to be a fairly general theory of nonlinear viscoelastic behavior of the vascular tissue treated as incompressible and orthotropic. The theory has been successfully applied to the aortic tissue and will, hopefully, find successful application to other tissues.

LOCAL MECHANICAL PROPERTIES OF THE INTIMAL SURFACE

As mentioned before, study of the rheology of the intimal surface has recently assumed increased importance. For example, Fry (1968) developed a method to study the shear strength of the vascular endothelium of the ventral aspect of the descending thoracic aorta. This method, however, does not yield the discrete information required to study atherosclerosis. The atherosclerotic process is a discrete process and therefore it is important to develop discrete methods that characterize rheologic properties at sites where the disease is known to occur. In our laboratory, we have therefore begun looking at methods to characterize discrete rheologic properties of the intimal surface. Two such methods are described below.

The first method (Gow and Vaishnav, 1975) was designed to study the local compliance of the vascular intima using a microindentor. To this end, a segment of canine middle descending thoracic aorta was excised, slit longitudinally, and stretched to in vivo dimensions in a stretch rack. The vessel was supported on the adventitial side by a plaster-of-paris slurry that was allowed to harden. Small forces (120 mg typically) were then applied to various locations on the intimal surface using a modified analytical balance, one pan of which was replaced by a metal rod with a prodder tip 0.19 mm in diameter. The displacement due to indentation caused by the tip was measured as a function of time by means of a differential transformer. The indentation at the end of 30 sec (δ_{30}) was considered to be indicative of the local compliance of the intima and its substructure. A considerable number of segments was tested using this method at various sites on the intima including the regions adjacent to intercostal orifices. These were found to be less compliant than the regions far away from the orifices. This is consistent with the histologic finding of collagen-rich intimal pads near the orifice regions.

The second method (Patel et al., 1975) was designed to study the strength of the endothelium using saline jets. An instrument was designed to apply jets at specific sites on the endothelium by modifying a microscope with turret-mounted objectives, one of which was replaced by a jet nozzle (diameter, 0.4 mm). A carefully handled aortic segment was stretched as above in a stretch rack and backed by a piece of Lucite. Controlled jets of saline were then applied to the endothelium for various durations and the resulting lesions made visible by staining the tissue subsequently with Evans blue dye. From a study of the lesions created by saline jets it was noted that the endothelium could resist high normal stress but was susceptible to damage by relatively low shear stress. This was evident from the fact that an intermediate jet strength gave rise to an annular lesion consisting of an undamaged core where the jet hit directly and a ring of damaged endothelium where the shearing stress due to jet efflux exceeded the endothelial yield strength. Experiments are underway to refine the method and to quantify the endothelial yield strength using this method.

The importance of these methods can be appreciated from the following. Hemodynamic shear stress, for example, can alter the permeability of the endothelium to the macromolecules in the blood. The jet studies should provide valuable information on the strength of the endothelial surface and its permeability to macromolecules. Likewise, it has been observed that regions of the vascular intima subjected to chronic high undirectional stresses appear to develop densely oriented collagen in the subendothelial region that seems to protect them from subsequent lipid deposition. The microindentor studies on local compliance of the vascular intima reported above are significant in that they provide a rheologic counterpart to the histologic finding stated above.

MECHANICAL PROPERTIES OF MUSCULAR ARTERIES

Although in recent years we have learned a great deal about large arteries, like the aorta, no precise model exists to date to predict the mechanical behavior of relatively smaller muscular arteries and the arterioles. The difficulty arises because these arteries, in addition to having passive visco-elastic properties, possess an active control mechanism mediated through the smooth muscle in the wall. Most of the studies on these arteries essentially fall into two categories. In one case, the response to various vasoactive agents is studied in excised arterial segments (Bohr and Uchida, 1969; Dobrin and Doyle, 1970; Gow, 1972) and in the other, the resistance to flow of a given vascular bed is studied under control conditions and following administration of vasoactive drugs (Folkow et al., 1973; Patel, Mallos, and DeFreitas, 1961). The latter method gives some idea of the caliber of arterioles in the vascular bed because the resistance is inversely proportional to the fourth power of the radius; an increase in resistance would indicate narrowing of the vascular bed and vice versa. Because the caliber of these vessels is also influenced passively by the transmural pressure (i.e., intravascular pressure minus the pressure acting on the outer surface), one must be careful to separate the passive effects from active contraction in a vascular bed. A valid comparison between any two states can only be made at identical transmural pressures.

The vasoconstriction in a vascular bed can also be demonstrated anatomically by injecting a casting material at a chosen pressure head into a vascular bed under control and test conditions and then examining the casts under a microscope after digesting the soft tissue. Patel and Burton (1957) used this semiquantitative technique in vivo in rabbits; their results are seen in Figures 7 and 8. Figure 7 is a photograph of lung casts from one animal following administration of Privine, a long-acting vasoconstrictor drug, into the left pulmonary artery. The marked vasoconstriction in the left lung is obvious. Microscopic photographs of similar casts obtained in the control state as well as following administration of norepi-

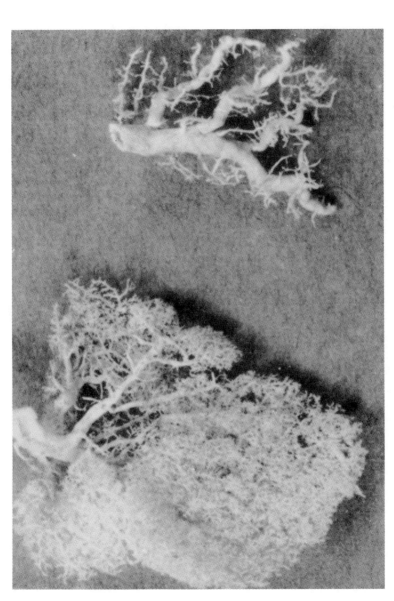

Figure 7. Photograph of lung cast. *Left*, control lung; *right*, after Privine. (From Patel and Burton, 1957; reproduced by permission of the American Heart Association, Inc.)

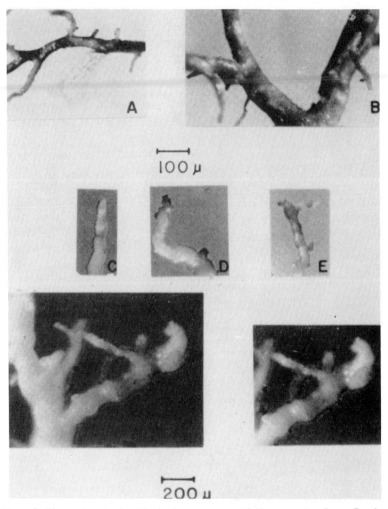

Figure 8. Photomicrographs of plastic casts. *A* and *B,* controls; *C* to *G,* after norepinephrine. (From Patel and Burton, 1957; reproduced by permission of the American Heart Association, Inc.)

nephrine (NE) are seen in Figure 8. The vasoconstriction following NE administration is apparent.

Although the above methods provide useful quantitative data, a precise mathematical model of the muscular arteries and arterioles still eludes the physiologist and presents a formidable challenge. Recent attempts to measure, in vivo, the pressure, diameter, and velocity of blood flow in the microvasculature of various animals (Intaglietta and Zweifach, 1974) should prove useful in this regard. A detailed description of such microvascular techniques is beyond the scope of this paper.

CONCLUDING REMARKS

In this chapter, we have attempted to review the state of the art in the field of blood vessel rheology. Throughout the chapter the tutorial approach is maintained. Rather than review all the recent work in this area, we have emphasized certain important concepts used in this field. For convenience, we have used our own data to illustrate these concepts. Where appropriate, other pertinent studies are also mentioned directly or through books or review articles. We hope this material will provide the reader with some basic understanding of the subject and encourage independent future studies in important but yet unexplored areas of blood vessel rheology to resolve basic mechanisms of disease processes.

ACKNOWLEDGMENTS

We are thankful to Dr. D. L. Fry for critically reviewing the manuscript and Dr. J. Kamal for her help in the preparation of the manuscript. We also thank the American Heart Association, Inc. and the American Physiological Society for permission to reproduce illustrations from previous publications.

LITERATURE CITED

Adkins, J. E. 1958. Dynamic properties of resilient materials: Constitutive equations. Phil. Trans. Roy. Soc. London (A) 250: 519–541.
Bergel, D. H. 1960. The visco-elastic properties of the arterial wall. Ph.D. Thesis, University of London.
Bergel, D. H. 1972. Cardiovascular Fluid Dynamics. Vols. I and II. Academic Press, New York. 365 p. (Vol. I), 398 p. (Vol. II).
Biot, M. A. 1965. Mechanics of Incremental Deformations. John Wiley and Sons, New York. 504 p.

Bohr, D. F., and E. Uchida. 1969. Activation of vascular smooth muscle. *In* A. P. Fishman and H. H. Hecht (eds.), The Pulmonary Circulation and Interstitial Space, pp. 143–146. The University of Chicago Press, Chicago.

Carew, T. E., R. N. Vaishnav, and D. J. Patel. 1968. Compressibility of the arterial wall. Circ. Res. 23: 61–68.

Caro, C. G. 1973. Transport of material between blood and wall in arteries. *In* Ciba Foundation Symposium, Atherogenesis: Initiating Factors. Vol. 12, pp. 127–164. Associated Science Publishers, Amsterdam.

Davids, N., and R. C. Cheng. 1972. Transient laminar flow in ducts of arbitrary cross-section by finite element methods. J. Biomech. 5: 485–499.

Dobrin, P. V., and A. A. Rovick. 1967. Static elastic properties of the dog carotid arterial wall. Fed. Proc. 26: 1021.

Dobrin, P. V., and J. M. Doyle. 1970. Vascular smooth muscle and the anisotropy of dog carotid artery. Cir. Res. 27: 105–119.

Eringen, A. C. 1962. Nonlinear Theory of Continuous Media. McGraw-Hill, New York. 477 p.

Eringen, A. C. 1967. Mechanics of Continua. John Wiley and Sons, New York. 502 p.

Folkow, B., M. Hallback, Y. Lundgren, R. Sivertsson, and L. Weiss. 1973. Importance of adaptive changes in vascular design for establishment of primary hypertension studied in man and in spontaneously hypertensive rats. Circ. Res. 32: (Suppl. 1) 2–16.

Fry, D. L. 1968. Acute vascular endothelial changes associated with increased blood velocity gradients. Circ. Res. 22: 165–197.

Fry, D. L. 1969. Certain histological and chemical responses of the vascular interface to acutely induced mechanical stress in the aorta of the dog. Circ. Res. 24: 93–108.

Fry, D. L. 1973. Responses of the arterial wall to certain physical factors. *In* Ciba Foundation Symposium, Atherogenesis: Initiating Factors. Vol. 12, pp. 92–125. Associated Science Publishers, Amsterdam.

Fung, Y. C. 1971. Biomechanics: A survey of the blood flow problem. Adv. Appl. Mech. 11: 65–130.

Gow, B. S. 1972. The influence of vascular smooth muscle on the viscoelastic properties of blood vessels. *In* D. H. Bergel (ed.), Cardiovascular Fluid Dynamics. Vol. II, pp. 65–110. Academic Press, New York.

Gow, B. S., and R. N. Vaishnav. 1975. A microindentation technique to measure rheological properties of the vascular intima. J. Appl. Physiol. 38: 344–350.

Green, A. E., and R. S. Rivlin. 1957. The mechanics of nonlinear materials with memory, Part I. Arch. Rational Mech. Anal. 1: 1–21.

Intaglietta, M., and B. W. Zweifach. 1974. Microcirculatory basis of fluid exchange. Adv. Biol. Med. Phys. 15: 111–159.

Lawton, R. W. 1954. The thermoelastic behavior of isolated aortic strips of the dog. Circ. Res. 2: 344–353.

Ling, S. C., H. B. Atabek, W. G. Letzing, and D. J. Patel. 1973. Nonlinear analysis of aortic flow in living dogs. Circ. Res. 33: 198−212.

McDonald, D. A. 1974. Blood Flow in Arteries. Williams and Wilkins, Baltimore. 328 p.

Patel, D. J., and A. C. Burton. 1957. Active constriction of small pulmonary arteries in rabbit. Circ. Res. 5: 620−628.

Patel, D. J., A. J. Mallos, and D. L. Fry. 1961. Aortic mechanics in the living dog. J. Appl. Physiol. 16: 293−299.

Patel, D. J., A. J. Mallos, and F. M. DeFreitas. 1961. Importance of transmural pressure and lung volume in evaluating drug effect on pulmonary vascular tone. Circ. Res. 9: 1217−1222.

Patel, D. J., J. C. Greenfield, Jr., and D. L. Fry. 1964. In vivo pressure-length-radius relationship of certain blood vessels in man and dog. In E. O. Attinger (ed.), Pulsatile Blood Flow, pp. 293−306. McGraw-Hill, New York.

Patel, D. J., and D. L. Fry. 1966. Longitudinal tethering of arteries in dogs. Circ. Res. 19: 1011−1021.

Patel, D. J., and J. S. Janicki. 1966. Catalogue of some dynamic analogies used in pulmonary and vascular mechanics. Med. Res. Eng. 5: 30−33.

Patel, D. J., and D. L. Fry. 1969. The elastic symmetry of arterial segments in dogs. Circ. Res. 24: 1−8.

Patel, D. J., and R. N. Vaishnav. 1972. The rheology of large blood vessels. In D. H. Bergel (ed.), Cardiovascular Fluid Dynamics, Vol. II, pp. 1−64. Academic Press, New York.

Patel, D. J., J. S. Janicki, R. N. Vaishnav, and J. T. Young. 1973. Dynamic anisotropic viscoelastic properties of the aorta in living dogs. Circ. Res. 32: 93−107.

Patel, D. J., R. N. Vaishnav, B. S. Gow, and P. A. Kot. 1974. Hemodynamics. Ann. Rev. Physiol. 36: 125−154.

Patel, D. J., R. N. Vaishnav, H. B. Atabek, and F. Plowman. 1975. Measurement of endothelial strength using saline jets. Proceedings of the World Congress for Microcirculation. Toronto, Canada.

Plowman, F., J. T. Young, and J. S. Janicki. 1974. An instrument for dynamic measurement of longitudinal stresses and strains in a blood vessel in situ. Biorheology 12: 21−25.

Tickner, E. G., and A. H. Sacks. 1967. A theory for the static elastic behavior of blood vessels. Biorheology 4: 151−168.

Truesdell, C., and W. Noll. 1965. The nonlinear field theories of mechanics. In S. Flügge (ed.), Encyclopedia of Physics, Vol. III. Springer-Verlag, Berlin.

Vaishnav, R. N., J. T. Young, J. S. Janicki, and D. J. Patel. 1972. Nonlinear anisotropic elastic properties of the canine aorta. Biophys. J. 12: 1008−1027.

Vaishnav, R. N., J. T. Young, and D. J. Patel. 1973. Distribution of stresses and of strain-energy density through the wall thickness in a canine aortic segment. Circ. Res. 32: 577−583.

Vaishnav, R. N., J. T. Young, and D. J. Patel. 1975. Nonlinear viscoelastic theory for large blood vessels. Proceeding of the International Congress on Cardiovascular System Dynamics. Valley Forge, Pennsylvania. (In press.)

Womersley, J. R. 1957. An elastic tube theory of pulse transmission and oscillatory flow in mammalian arteries. WADC Technical Report TR 56-614, p. 29.

Cardiovascular Flow Dynamics and Measurements
Edited by N. H. C. Hwang and N. A. Normann
Copyright 1977   University Park Press   Baltimore

chapter 13

MECHANICAL FACTORS IN ATHEROGENESIS

Colin G. Caro

ABSTRACT

There is substantial evidence that both spontaneous atheroma and that which can be experimentally induced by feeding a high cholesterol diet occur patchily in the circulation. A brief description is given of these processes, with some mention of theories of atherogenesis. Because mass transport between the blood and the arterial wall must play an important role in atherogenesis, current knowledge of it is reviewed; this transport has attracted a considerably increased attention of late, following recognition of the fact that it can be enhanced by mechanical disturbance of the artery wall. Such a susceptibility might in part account for the patchy occurrence of atheroma.

SPONTANEOUS ATHEROMA

Atheroma occurring spontaneously in man and animals generally affects the major central arteries rather than the peripheral circulation. It is not normally seen in the smaller intraparenchymal arteries (Anitschkow, 1933) or in arterioles or capillaries (Gofman and Young, 1963). Additional evidence that there is diminishing involvement proceeding peripherally in the arteries is provided by Mitchell and Schwartz (1965, p. 54). However, within individual arteries specific patterns of occurrence are generally seen. In the aorta the abdominal segment is affected more severely than the arch or the thoracic segment (Clarkson, 1963; Zemplenyi, Lojda, and Mrhova, 1963), and there tends to be sparing, in terms of early lesions, downstream of intercostal ostia (Caro, Fitz-Gerald, and Schroter, 1971). Again, in the carotids there tends to be progressively severe involvement proceeding distally, with especially severe involvement of the carotid sinus, while immediately downstream of the carotid sinus there is relative sparing (Solberg and Eggen, 1971).

473

Some of the theories advanced to account for this localization of atheroma that involves arterial blood mechanics have been summarized in Caro et al. (1971). For example, Rindfleisch (1872, p. 250) hypothesized that atheroma develops at sites in arteries which experience the full stress and impact of the blood. Again, Fry (1968, 1969), who had shown that acute severe elevation of shear on the aortic wall in dogs results in endothelial damage and increased permeability to lipid, postulated that the arterial wall shear stress is contributory to the development of atheroma; in more recent reports, Fry (1973) appears to consider that a high wall shear stress actually protects against atheroma, possibly by stimulating structural changes in the artery wall. The converse point of view was taken by Caro et al. (1969, 1971). In light of inevitably crude analyses of arterial fluid mechanics and observations (including those mentioned above) they made on the detailed sites of occurrence of certain early atheromotous lesions, they argued that atheroma tends to occur in regions where the wall shear is relatively low and that wall shear is one of the fundamental controlling mechanisms in atherogenesis. To account for this distribution of atheroma, they postulated an egress-controlled, shear-dependent mass-transport process, with biochemical activity in the artery wall. No evidence has emerged since then that calls for total rejection of that hypothesis, although, as shown below under discussion of blood-wall transport, it now seems likely that this transport is susceptible to non-steady as well as steady stresses and to normal as well as shearing stresses, so that the theory needs appropriate refinement.

ATHEROMA INDUCED BY A HIGH CHOLESTEROL DIET

Following sudden marked elevation of the blood cholesterol level, or the introduction of radioactively labeled materials (cholesterol, albumin, oleic acid) into the circulation of animals, their concentration is initially higher in the intima than in the media (Anitschkow, 1933; Duncan and Buck, 1959; Adams, Bayliss, and Ibrahim, 1962; Day and Wahlquist, 1968). In these transient-type studies (Caro et al., 1971) where concentrations of cholesterol (or other administered material) in arterial walls are changing relatively rapidly, the distribution of the material is quite different to that described under spontaneous atheroma above (termed a quasi-steady state by Caro et al., 1971). Thus, as noted by several workers (Clarkson, 1963; Keys, 1963; Weiss, 1959), there is, at least initially, greater accumulation in the aortic arch than the abdominal aorta and on flow dividers at junctions, which tend to be spared in spontaneous atheroma. Moreover, there is accumulation of material in the small intraparenchymal arteries and in the vessels of the microcirculation. This pattern, it must be said, is modified if, for example, a low dose of cholesterol is fed for a prolonged period, or an animal has alternating periods of a cholesterol-enriched and a normal diet (Constantinides, 1965). The accumulation then more closely resembles that in spontaneous atheroma.

One longer-term study of this general type is that of Duncan and Buck (1960). They raised the blood cholesterol level in dogs from a control value of about 60 to about 800 mg/100 ml by giving thiouracil-cholesterol. They found after 1 mo that the most rapid rise of intimal cholesterol had occurred, as expected, in the ascending aorta and arch and that the least rapid rise was in the abdominal aorta. However, after 5 mo, intimal cholesterol concentration had increased faster in the lower descending thoracic and abdominal aorta, with a distribution resembling that in spontaneous atheroma. This crossover was explained by Caro et al. (1971) in terms of the wall approaching a new elevated quasi-equilibrium, with operation of wall metabolism (for example, esterification of cholesterol) and shear-dependent efflux. Although the chemical changes could not alter the fluid mechanics, it has not been established that they did not significantly influence the local wall permeability or wall metabolism.

THE TRANSPORT OF MATTER
BETWEEN THE BLOOD AND THE ARTERIAL WALL

Matter is transported between the blood and the wall of an artery via both the luminal surface of the vessel and the vasa vasorum. There are reported to be lymphatics in the arteries, but their role in mass transport has not been established. The processes that account for this transport (and inevitably interact to some extent) are bulk (pressure-driven) flow, molecular diffusion, active transport, and pinocytosis; it is shown later that pinocytosis (micropinocytosis) in arteries apparently is primarily a passive process. Attention here is confined to short-term transient studies in which labeled, essentially nondegradable materials are used because of their greater simplicity. More emphasis is placed on the behavior of macromolecules than smaller species because more is known about them.

Bulk Flow

Because the hydrostatic pressure is higher in the lumen of an artery than at its outer surface, or presumably within the vasa vasorum and lymphatics, there tends to be bulk flow across the wall, the extent of which depends on the size of the pressure difference and the resistance offered by the intervening material. Osmotic pressure combines with the hydrostatic pressure in ways that have been described.

There have been several studies designed to assess the effect of hydrostatic pressure on the transport of matter across the artery wall. Wilens (1951) pressurized serum-filled, human postmortem arteries and observed a flow of liquid through the wall, typically $0.014 \, ml/cm^2/hr$ at a pressure of 120 mm Hg. He termed this ultrafiltration because the concentration of cholesterol (cholesterol is associated with lipoprotein in serum) was much lower in the filtrate than in the retained serum, while the concentration of chloride was the same. However, the arteries were studied as long as 24 hr after the death of the subject, and there might have been deterioration of the wall, including the endothelium of the lumen and vasa vasorum. Furthermore, there might have been leakage through the vasa vasorum, which would have been cut during excision of the vessels.

In more recent studies (Duncan and Buck, 1961; Duncan, Cornfield, and Buck, 1962; Duncan, Buck, and Lynch, 1965) the effect of transmural pressure was tested on the uptake of radioactively labeled albumin by the dog aorta, both in vivo and in vitro; discussion of the latter studies is omitted because there seemed to be leakage of label, possibly through divided vasa vasorum. The concentration of the label was determined in the inner, middle, and outer layers of the vessel at different stations and related to plasma label concentration.

In the in vivo studies the average value of the ratio tissue: plasma label concentration for the inner layer at 10 min was, in control animals (blood pressure 120 mm Hg), 0.025 for the aortic arch and 0.013 for the abdominal aorta; there was a progressive decrease in the value of the ratio proceeding distally along the aorta. In animals made acutely hypertensive (blood pressure 240 mm Hg), the corresponding values were 0.08 and 0.013. Thus the spatial gradient of uptake persists, but whereas uptake by the aortic arch is increased by increase of pressure, uptake by the abdominal aorta is not. The tissue concentration of label in these studies was related to the relaxed surface area of the specimens, whereas it is appropriate to relate it to the surface area of the vessel when exposed to the label. When an appropriate correction is made, the respective average values for the tissue:plasma ratio are 0.013 and 0.01 for the controls, and 0.024 and 0.008 for the hypertensive dogs. Thus, hypertension actually increases uptake by the arch by a factor of 1.85 rather than 3.2, and does not increase uptake by the abdominal aorta; the surface area of the arch was doubled by the hypertension while that of the abdominal aorta was increased by a factor of 1.35.

Because an increase of the transmural pressure of an artery could influence its mass transport by causing both stretching and bulk flow, vessels have been mounted, in other experiments, so that their mass transport could be studied while they were stretched at constant transmural pressure, or subjected to different transmural pressures at constant surface area, by supporting them against a screen (Duncan et al., 1965). In the former experiments the uptake of labeled albumin was found to vary almost directly as the surface area exposed to the label, that is, uptake per unit area was essentially unaffected by stretch, while in the latter experiments, increase of transmural pressure caused no increase of label uptake. Fry (1973) carried out similar studies but found a slight increase of permeability[1] in the former experiment; a 40% static increase of the surface area of a relaxed artery to its in vivo dimensions increased permeability about 12%. In the latter experiment he confirmed that an increase of transmural pressure did not increase the uptake of label, whether the endothelium was intact or damaged. It is possible, however, that the artery wall tissue becomes compacted in this last experiment so that there is interference with bulk flow (Yamartino, 1974). No study is known of the effect of transmural pressure on the transport of small molecules across the artery wall, other than that by Wilens (1951), in which the vessels were probably abnormal.

The only studies that can be used to assess bulk flow are those in which it is isolated from the other means of transport (mass diffusion, pinocytosis, active transport). The finding that an increase of pressure, which does not stretch a vessel, has little effect on the uptake of a label implies that bulk flow is not a dominant mechanism for arterial mass transport. Further support for that view comes from studies of mass diffusion reported below.

Mass Diffusion

Consideration must be given to three steps: (1) diffusion in the blood adjacent to the wall, (2) the uptake process at the blood–wall interface, and (3) transport in the substance of the wall. As before, it must be recognized that transport can occur across the endothelium of the lumen and the vasa vasorum.

Diffusion in the Blood Isolated arteries were perfused with serum in

---

[1] Uptake per unit area of vessel and time and driving concentration gradient.

such a way that the flow was laminar and fully developed, and a concentration boundary layer for labeled cholesterol in the serum grew from the upstream end of the segment (Caro and Nerem, 1973). From a knowledge of the wall shear rate and the concentration of label in the serum, using an assumed value for the diffusion coefficient of the label in serum (where it is associated with lipoprotein), it is possible to predict the flux to the wall for short times. The observed flux was less by a factor of about 1,000 than that predicted and there was no spatial dependence of wall uptake; both results imply that the resistance offered by (1) is very small compared to that offered by (2) or (3).

Uptake Process at the Blood–Wall Interface   There is little doubt that (2) rather than (1) or (3) provides the dominant resistance in the short-term uptake of macromolecules by the artery wall. The basis for that statement is that the rate of transport is appreciably increased by mechanical disturbances that primarily influence the interface region (Fry, 1969, 1973; Caro, 1974; Nerem et al., 1974; Siflinger, Caro, and Parker, 1975). These studies also shed light on the location and nature of the rate-limiting uptake process; in particular, they show that it is influenced by mechanical disturbances that do not damage the wall and can be classified as physiologic; in addition, it is influenced by wall damage.

Fry (1969) found erosion of endothelial cells on experimentally elevating aortic shear stress above 1000 dynes/cm^2 and endothelial cell damage when it exceeded 400 dynes/cm^2. Moreover, there was increased uptake of labeled albumin by the wall and this was found with a shear stress as low as 140 dynes/cm^2, which is insufficient to damage the endothelium. It appeared, furthermore, that turbulent fluctuations in themselves increased label uptake. Caro (1974) found that an essentially steady shear stress increased the uptake of labeled cholesterol associated with lipoprotein by excised segments of artery, with wall permeability roughly proportional to the cube root of wall shear stress at about 10 dynes/cm^2 and to the square root of shear stress at about 100 dynes/cm^2. Nerem et al. (1974) found arterial permeability to labeled albumin dependent on oscillatory shearing stresses in the frequency range 1–5 Hz, with peak shear stresses of about 140 dynes/cm^2 (rms value 100). Fry (1973) observed that touching the endothelium with a brush enhanced the uptake of labeled albumin, and Siflinger et al. (1975) found that this procedure removes the endothelial cells and increases albumin uptake about fourfold, which implies that the rate-limiting step in the total transport is associated with these cells. Ultrastructural studies using tracer molecules reveal two routes of entry into the artery wall: pinocytic vesicles and endothelial intercellular clefts. Larger molecules, including ferritin (diameter 110 Å) (Florey and Sheppard, 1970) and lactoperoxidase (m.w.~82,000) (Stein and Stein, 1973) do not seem to enter the clefts but seem instead to be transported exclusively by the vesicles. Smaller species, including horseradish peroxidase (m.w.~40,000, diameter 40–60 Å) enter the wall both via the vesicles and through the clefts. There is no direct evidence concerning the route for lipoprotein, although radioautographs suggest that this also enters via the vesicles (Stein and Stein, 1973). Evidence obtained in quantitative studies with ^{125}I albumin (m.w. 69,000) is inconsistent with its being transported primarily in the intercell clefts (Siflinger et al., 1975); its rate of uptake by an artery was increased fourfold when the endothelial cells were removed, while that of the smaller species, sodium acetate, expected to be transported principally via the clefts, was unchanged.

Whether, in the case of macromolecules, pinocytosis is the rate-determining transport process remains to be established. In particular, the significance of the glycosaminoglycans layer at the surface of the arterial endothelial cells (Stein and Stein, 1973) has not been determined. Hyaluronidase had no effect on the uptake of labeled albumin by excised artery (Siflinger et al., 1975), but the composition of the layer is not precisely known. It would seem (see below) that there would be a negligible dependence of the uptake of molecules on their size (in an appropriate size range) if pinocytosis is the rate-determining step, and that the converse would hold if the glycocalyx were rate limiting. In fact, however, the diffusion of macromolecules through the glycocalyx is, because it is only about 100 Å thick, a membrane process rather than free diffusion; not enough is known to decide between the two mechanisms. After appropriate correction of data (Okishio, 1961; Duncan et al., 1962; Duncan, Buck, and Lynch, 1963; Bell, Adamson, and Schwartz, 1974; Bell, Gallus, and Schwartz, 1974), it is found that the smaller a diffusing species is, the higher the relative permeability of the artery wall; lack of information precludes determination of the actual permeability coefficient. On the other hand, the molecules employed were probably sufficiently large to experience some molecular sieving during the loading and unloading of the pinocytic vesicles (see below).

The kinetics of the arterial uptake of macromolecules have not been studied extensively. For short times ($\frac{1}{2}$–1 hr), uptake by the dog carotid artery is essentially constant and varies directly with plasma concentration of label. The uptake is strongly dependent on temperature and has for labeled albumin an effective activation energy of about 13 kcal/mole (Siflinger et al., 1975). Thus an increase of temperature from 20 to 37°C caused a fourfold increase in the uptake of the label by arteries incubated at zero transmural pressure. Because this increase is much greater than that seen on doubling transmural pressure in vivo (studies of Duncan et al.), it is suggested that mass diffusion, rather than pressure-driven flow, plays the dominant role in the transport of macromolecules into the artery wall.

The few quantitative studies that have been undertaken with metabolic inhibitors (Newman and Zilversmit, 1962; Siflinger et al., 1975) mainly indicate that these have no significant effect on macromolecule uptake; this is consistent with the process being primarily passive over short periods of time. It is also reported that metabolic inhibitors have no significant effect on pinocytosis, studied directly, although such studies are necessarily only semiquantitative (Jennings and Florey, 1967; Allison and Davies, 1974). There is disagreement about the effect of temperature on pinocytosis. Jennings and Florey (1967) and Casley-Smith (1969) report that cooling from 37°C to 0–4°C had little effect on pinocytosis, while the phagocytosis of larger (0.2–1.0 μ) particles was markedly inhibited. Contrary to this, Kaye et al. (1962) report that such cooling markedly inhibits the pinocytic uptake of colloidal thorium dioxide (approximately 200 Å diameter). It is important that this conflict be resolved, particularly in view of the steep temperature dependence of the uptake of macromolecules (Caro, 1973; Siflinger et al., 1975).

It is useful to devote some attention to the details of endothelial cell pinocytosis and to consider what is known of its mechanics. High-magnification electron micrographs (Bruns and Palade, 1968) suggest that the vesicles and their stalks (when they are attached to the plasmalemma) are bounded by a membrane identical to the plasmalemma. The endothelial cells vary in thickness from 0.3 to 0.9 μ. In capillaries some 30% of the non-nuclear volume of the endothelial cell consists of vesicles (Casley-Smith, 1969). When free in the cytoplasm, the vesicles are believed to be mainly solitary, spherical bodies, only infrequently interconnected. It has been suggested that when free the vesicles undergo Brownian motion (Casley-Smith, 1964; Shea and Karnovsky, 1966), and there is some confirmatory experimental evidence for this. The average size of the vesicles (6–800 Å) has been established, and it might be thought that their Brownian diffusion could be estimated. There are, however, two major difficulties: first, the viscosity of the cytoplasm in which they are suspended is not reliably known, and second, because of their small size and the size of the endothelial cells, they can be expected to experience a considerably increased cytoplasmic viscosity as the plasmalemma is approached (Green and Casley-Smith, 1972; Weinbaum, Caro, and Lewis, 1974). As a result, it has been necessary to adopt other approaches to elucidate the mechanics of pinocytosis.

Because vesicles are seldom seen attaching to, or detaching from, the plasmalemma, it can be presumed that these processes occur rapidly, but little is known about them. In most studies of attachment, the plasmalemma has been regarded as an imperfectly absorbing barrier, i.e., there is a low probability that a vesicle which collides with it will attach (Casley-Smith and Chin, 1971; Shea and Bossert, 1973). Electron micrographs (Palade and Bruns, 1968) suggest that as a vesicle approaches the plasmalemma, the latter deforms, either dimpling toward the vesicle or in some cases wrapping itself partially around it. Eventually, there is fusion between the two membranes with the formation of a diaphragm, which ultimately disappears. It appears that detachment may involve the formation of a neck in the vesicle stalk and a "pinching off" process. The fact that vesicles are attached by necks, and hence released at some distance from the plasmalemma, means that energy is not needed to prevent them from immediately reattaching.

A preliminary, hydrodynamic interaction model of these processes has recently been formulated, taking account also of London van der Waals' forces (Weinbaum et al., 1974). According to the model, a typical free vesicle is accelerated by thermal collision to a velocity of about 30 cm/sec, but it is decelerated by Stokes frictional forces, having traveled only about one thousandth of its diameter.[2] It has been suggested that thermal collision ruptures the stalks of the vesicles (Green and Casley-Smith, 1972). Weinbaum's calculations indicate that vesicle displacements are small, but repeated high-frequency, small-amplitude, impulsive loading might fracture the stalk. Experimental studies with a labeled tracer (Casley-Smith and Chin, 1971) suggest that the average time of transit of vesicles is at least 3–5 sec, and the average time of their attachment at the plasmalemma 2–3 sec. Predictions by Weinbaum et al. (1974), which are based on the assumption of an effective range for the London Van der Waals forces, match these results reasonably well.

The neck of the vesicle has a mean diameter of about 200 Å; therefore,

---

[2] There is currently uncertainty about this value; the distance traveled may be one or two orders of magnitude larger (Weinbaum and Caro, 1976).

the loading—unloading process is by no means free diffusion for the larger macromolecules of interest, including fibrinogen HDL, LDL. The ultra-structural studies suggest that the diaphragm which is formed during the attachment process influences the resistance to diffusional loading—unloading. A recent preliminary observation in frog capillaries (Loudon, Michel, and White, 1975) indicates that the loading process for ferritin exhibits a strong dependence on temperature.

This discussion has been concerned with undisturbed endothelial cells. Electron micrographs (Buck, 1958; Weinbaum et al., 1974) indicate that the morphology of the cells from a relaxed nonpressurized artery differs markedly from that of the cells from an artery held at in vivo length and exposed to a physiologic transmural pressure—supporting the view that the cells undergo some deformation as a result of the physiologic arterial pressure pulse, or possibly the steady and nonsteady shearing stresses affecting the vessel. Such deformation could be a means whereby mechanical disturbance of the artery wall influences its macromolecule transport. Thus there would be alteration of the tension in the plasmalemma, which might affect the attachment—detachment processes of vesicles. Moreover, deformation of a cell could set up intracellular fluid currents, which, if these were nonreversible (e.g., because of thixotropy of the cell contents), could influence vesicle diffusion. The details of these have not been worked out. Preliminary experiments (Caro, Lewis, and Weinbaum, 1975) indicate that very small (approximately 4%) periodic reductions in the length of an excised artery from its in vivo length can, at an appropriate frequency, significantly enhance its uptake of labeled albumin. There is no evidence to suggest that these disturbances widened the intercell clefts, which are apparently very strong (Constantinides, 1965).

Transport in the Substance of the Wall   The concentration profile of a labeled macromolecule across the artery wall as a function of time has been obtained in in vivo studies by several investigators (Adams, 1973; Colton et al., 1974; Bell, Adamson, and Schwartz, 1974; Bell, Gallus, and Schwartz, 1974) by sectioning arteries. There is appreciable entry of label both from the intima and the adventitia, with, at later times, a fall of wall concentration near the boundaries, indicative of efflux commencing. There has been a gradual development of theory relevant to the uptake of label by the wall. Initially the wall was viewed, for the sake of simplicity, as a semi-infinite homogeneous slab (Caro and Nerem, 1973), but it must now be regarded as a two-phase structure, consisting of a small interstitial space with a relatively high diffusion coefficient and a large dispersed intracellular space with a relatively low diffusion coefficient (Weinbaum and Caro, 1976). Studies of the uptake of albumin by normal arteries and by those with damaged endothelia provide results from which it is possible to calculate the diffusion time of vesicles across the endothelial cells (Weinbaum et al., 1974).

There is, as mentioned earlier, spatial variation of the permeability of the artery wall to macromolecules in vivo (McGill, Geer, and Holman, 1957; Duncan et al., 1965; Caro et al., 1971; Bell et al., 1974), and a similar finding has been obtained in terminally ill patients (Scott and Hurley, 1970). It is not yet established with certainty whether this is the result of local variations of the mechanical stresses acting on the wall, or of spatial variation of the intrinsic permeability of the wall. Spatial variation of the ultrastructure of the wall has been observed. There is, for example, a lining up of the endothelial cells in the direction of flow over them (Fry, 1973) and a local variation of the turnover rate of endothelial cells and of the thickness of the glycosaminoclycans layer (Schwartz et al., 1974). The significance of these findings in terms of local mass transport is not known, however.

LITERATURE CITED

Adams, C. W. M. 1973. Tissue changes and lipid entry in developing atheroma. *In* Atherogenesis: Initiating Factors, Ciba Foundation Symposium, Vol. 12, pp. 5−37. Associated Scientific Publishers, Amsterdam.

Adams, C. W. M., O. B. Bayliss, and M. Z. Ibrahim. 1962. A hypothesis to explain the accumulation of cholesterol in atherosclerosis. Lancet 1: 890.

Allison, A. C., and P. Davies. 1974. Mechanisms of endocytosis and exocytosis. *In* M. A. Sleigh and D. H. Lemmings, Society for Experimental Biology Symposium, vol. 28: Transport at the Cellular Level, pp. 419−446. Cambridge University Press, London.

Anitschkow, N. 1933. Experimental arteriosclerosis in animals. *In* E. V. Cowdry (ed.), Arteriosclerosis. Macmillan, New York.

Bell F. P., I. L. Adamson, and C. J. Schwartz. 1974. Aortic endothelial permeability to albumin: focal and regional patterns of uptake and transmural distribution of [131] I-albumin in the young pig. Exp. Mol. Pathol. 20: 57−68.

Bell, F. P., A. S. Gallus, and C. J. Schwartz. 1974. Focal and regional patterns of uptake and transmural distribution of [131] I-fibrinogen in the pig aorta in vivo. Exp. Mol. Pathol. 20: 281−292.

Bruns, R. R., and G. E. Palade. 1968. Studies on blood capillaries. J. Cell Biol. 37: 277–299.

Buck, R. C. 1958. The fine structure of endothelium of large arteries. J. Biophys. Biochem. Cytol. 4: 187–190.

Caro, C. G., J. M. Fitz-Gerald, and R. C. Schroter. 1969. Arterial wall shear and distribution of early atheroma in man. Nature 223: 1159.

Caro, C. G., J. M. Fitz-Gerald, and R. C. Schroter. 1971. Atheroma and arterial wall shear. Observation, correlation and proposal of a shear dependent mass transfer mechanism for atherogenesis. Proc. Roy. Soc. London B 177: 109–159.

Caro, C. G. 1973. Transport of ^{14}C-4 cholesterol between intraluminal serum and artery wall in isolated dog common carotid artery. J. Physiol. 233: 37–38.

Caro, C. G., and R. M. Nerem, 1973. Transport of ^{14}C-4 cholesterol between serum and wall in perfused dog common carotid artery. Circ. Res. 32: 187–205.

Caro, C. G. 1974. Transport of ^{14}C-4 cholesterol between perfusing serum and dog common carotid artery: a shear dependent process. Cardiovasc. Res. 8: 194–203.

Caro, C. G., C. T. Lewis, and S. Weinbaum. 1975. A mechanism by which mechanical disturbances can increase the uptake of macromolecules by the artery wall. J. Physiol. 246: 71–73.

Casley-Smith, J. R. 1964. The Brownian movement of pinocytic vesicles. J. Roy. Microscopy Soc. 82: 257–261.

Casley-Smith, J. R. 1969. Endocytosis: the different energy requirements for the uptake of particles by small and large vesicles into peritoneal macrophages. J. Microscopy 90: 15–30.

Casley-Smith, J. R., and J. C. Chin. 1971. The passage of cytoplasmic vesicles across endothelial and mesothelial cells. J. Microscopy 93: 167–189.

Clarkson, T. B. 1963. Atherosclerosis—spontaneous and induced. In R. Paoletti and D. Kritchevsky (eds.), Advances in Lipid Research. Academic Press, New York.

Colton, C. K., R. L. Bratzler, K. A. Smith, G. M. Chisolm, R. S. Lees, and D. B. Zilversmit. 1974. Transport of albumin and low density lipoproteins in the arterial wall. In National Science Foundation Specialists' Meeting on Fluid Dynamic Aspects of Arterial Disease, Columbus, Ohio, pp. 51–54.

Constantinides, P. 1965. Experimental Atherosclerosis. Elsevier, Amsterdam.

Day, A. J., and M. L. Wahlquist. 1968. Uptake and metabolism of ^{14}C-labelled oleic acid by atherosclerotic lesions in rabbit aorta. Circ. Rec. 23: 779.

Duncan, L. E., and K. Buck. 1959. Passage of labelled cholesterol into the aortic wall of the normal dog. Circ. Res. Res. 7: 765.

Duncan, L. E., and K. Buck. 1960. Quantitative analysis of the development of experimental atherosclerosis in the dog. Circ. Res. 8: 1023.

Duncan, L. E., and K. Buck. 1961. Passage of labeled albumin into canine aortic wall in vivo and in vitro. Am. J. Physiol. 200: 622–624.

Duncan, L. E., J. Cornfield, and K. Buck. 1962. The effect of blood pressure on the passage of labeled plasma albumin into canine aortic wall. J. Clin. Invest. 41: 1537–1545.

Duncan, L. E., K. Buck, and A. Lynch. 1963. Lipoprotein movement through canine aortic wall. Science 142: 972–973.

Duncan, L. E., K. Buck, and A. Lynch. 1965. The effect of pressure and stretching on the passage of labeled albumin into canine aortic wall. J. Atheroscl. Res. 5: 69–79.

Florey, Lord, and B. L. Sheppard. 1970. The permeability of arterial endothelium to horseradish peroxidase. Proc. Roy. Soc. London B, 174: 435–443.

Fry, D. L. 1968. Acute vascular endothelial changes associated with increased blood velocity gradients. Circ. Res. 22: 165.

Fry, D. L. 1969. Certain chronological considerations regarding the blood vascular interface with particular reference to coronary artery disease. Circulation 40 (Suppl. 4): 38.

Fry, D. L. 1973. Responses of the arterial wall to certain physical factors. *In* Atherogenesis: Initiating Factors, Ciba Foundation Symposium, Vol. 12, pp. 93–125. Associated Scientific Publishers, Amsterdam.

Gofman, J. W., and W. Young. 1963. The filtration concept of atherosclerosis and serum lipids in the diagnosis of atherosclerosis. *In* M. Sandler and G. H. Bourne (eds.), Atherosclerosis and Its Origin. Academic Press, New York and London.

Green, H. S., and J. R. Casley-Smith. 1972. Calculation on the passage of small vesicles across endothelial cells by Brownian motion. J. Theor. Biol. 35: 103–111.

Jennings, M. A., and Lord Florey. 1967. An investigation of some properties of endothelium related to capillary permeability. Proc. Roy. Soc. London B 167: 39–63.

Kaye, G. I., G. D. Pappas, A. Donn, and N. Mallett. 1962. The uptake and transport of colloidal particles by the living rabbit cornea in vitro. J. Cell Biol. 12: 481–501.

Keys, A. 1963. The role of the diet in human atherosclerosis and its complications. *In* M. Sandler and G. H. Bourne (eds.), Atherosclerosis and Its Origin. Academic Press, New York and London.

Loudon, M. F., C. C. Michel, and I. F. White. 1975. Some observations upon the rate of labelling of endothelial vesicles by ferritin in frog mesenteric capillaries. Proc. Phys. Soc. July: 85–86P.

McGill, H. C., J. C. Geer, and R. L. Holman. 1957. Sites of vascular vulnerability in dogs demonstrated by Evans Blue. A.M.A. Arch. Pathol. 64: 303–311.

Mitchell, R. A., and C. J. Schwartz. 1965. Arterial Disease. Blackwell, Oxford.

Nerem, R. M., A. T. Mosberg, J. S. Polsley, and W. E. Carey. 1974. Transport of ^{131}I-Albumin between blood and the arterial wall. *In*

77th National Meeting American Institute Chemical Engineers, Pittsburgh, Pennsylvania.

Newman, H. A. I., and D. B. Zilversmit. 1962. Quantitative aspects of cholesterol flux in rabbit atheromatous lesions. J. Biol. Chem. 237: 2078–2084.

Okishio, T. 1961. Studies on the transfer of I^{131} labeled serum lipoproteins into the aorta of rabbits with experimental atherosclerosis. Med. J. Osaka Univ. 11: 367–381.

Palade, G. E., and R. R. Bruns. 1968. Structural modulations of plasmalemmal vesicles. J. Cell. Biol. 37: 633–649.

Rindfleisch, E. 1872. A manual of pathological histology. Vol. I. New Sydenham Society, London.

Schwartz, C. J., F. P. Bell, J. B. Somer, and R. Gerrity. 1974. Focal and regional differences in aortic permeability to macromolecules. In National Science Foundation Specialists' Meeting on Fluid Dynamic Aspects of Arterial Disease, Columbus, Ohio, pp. 46–50.

Scott, P. J., and P. J. Hurley. 1970. The distribution of radio-iodinated serum albumin and low-density lipoprotein in tissues and the arterial wall. Atherosclerosis 11: 77–103.

Shea, S. M., and W. H. Bossert. 1973. Vesicular transport across endothelium; a generalized diffusion model. Microvasc. Res. 6: 305–315.

Shea, S. M., and M. J. Karnovsky. 1966. Brownian motion: a theoretical explanation for the movement of vesicles across the endothelium. Nature 212: 353–355.

Siflinger, A., K. Parker, and C. G. Caro. 1975. Uptake of ^{125}I albumin by the endothelial surface of the isolated dog common carotid artery: effect of certain physical factors and metabolic inhibitors. Cardiovasc. Res. 9: 478–489.

Solberg, L. A., and D. A. Eggen. 1971. Localization and sequence of development of atherosclerotic lesions in the carotid and vertebral arteries. Circulation 43: 711–724.

Stein, Y., and O. Stein. 1973. Lipid synthesis and degradation and lipoprotein transport in mammalian aorta. In Atherogenesis: Initiating Factors, Ciba Foundation Symposium, Vol. 12, pp. 165–183. Associated Scientific Publishers, Amsterdam.

Weinbaum, S., and C. G. Caro. 1976. A macromolecule transport model for the arterial wall and endothelium based on the ultrastructural specialization observed in electron microscopic studies. J. Fluid Mech. 74: 611–640.

Weinbaum, S., C. T. Lewis, and C. G. Caro. 1974. Theoretical models and electronmicroscopic studies on the transport of macromolecules across arterial endothelium and their uptake by the arterial wall. In National Science Foundation Specialists' Meeting on Fluid Dynamic Aspects of Arterial Disease, Columbus, Ohio, pp. 58–62.

Weiss, H. D. 1959. Variation in appearance, cholesterol concentration and weight of the chicken aorta with age and sex. J. Gerontol. 14: 19.

Wilens, S. L. 1951. The experimental production of lipid deposition in excised arteries. Science 114: 389–393.

Yamartino, E. J. 1974. Determination of the arterial filtration coefficient of the rabbit aorta. Unpublished M.Sc. thesis, MIT.

Zemplenyi, T., Z. Lojda, and O. Mrhova. 1963. Enzymes of the vascular wall in experimental atherosclerosis in the rabbit. *In* M. Sandler and G. H. Bourne (eds.), Atherosclerosis and Its Origin. Academic Press, New York.

Cardiovascular Flow Dynamics and Measurements
Edited by N. H. C. Hwang and N. A. Normann
Copyright 1977   University Park Press   Baltimore

chapter 14

THE EFFECTS OF BIFURCATIONS AND STENOSES ON ARTERIAL DISEASE

Margot R. Roach

ABSTRACT

Arterial disease is common at bifurcations, but the exact mechanism by which the two are related is unknown. Intracranial saccular aneurysms develop at the apex of bifurcations in the circle of Willis, and probably are produced by a complex interaction between the axial stream impacting at the stagnation point, and the response of the distensible artery. Once developed, the flow in these aneurysms is turbulent and the aneurysms grow progressively. Both small and large aneurysms are less distensible than arteries, probably because of elastin fragmentation.

Atherosclerosis develops at the lateral angles of Y bifurcations and on the aortic wall distal to orifices of branches. Model studies and animal studies suggest that hemodynamic factors are involved. A major problem in correlating engineering and pathologic studies is the lack of uniform terminology for different parts of the bifurcation region.

Arterial stenoses may be congenital (coarctation) or acquired (atherosclerosis or external compression). The geometry of the stenosis, the peripheral resistance, and the availability of collaterals determine the flow decrease and pressure drop produced by the stenosis. Stenoses that produce distal turbulence produce a poststenotic dilatation (PSD). The PSD is considered a type of structural fatigue produced by low-frequency wall vibrations caused by the turbulence.

INTRODUCTION

In the past 10 years, both physicians and engineers have become increasingly aware that altered arterial geometry and/or bifurcations may be associated with arterial disease. Both aneurysms and atherosclerosis have an increased incidence near bifurcations, and it has been assumed that local flow disturbances at bifurcations may be factors in the production of both diseases. Unfortunately, no hard data are available to support this assumption. While several laboratories have developed physical and mathematical models to study bifurcation flow, biologic information needed to provide exact information for these models is not available.

Two major types of bifurcations are discussed: (a) those where the branch forms a side arm from a trunk that continues, and (b) those where the flow divides completely into two branches.

Side Branches

The branches of the aorta are the main examples of branches that come off a trunk. These may be small, such as the intercostals and lumbars, or large, such as renals and coeliac. Even relatively small branches, such as the intercostals, may cause significant flow distortions distal to their orifices. This is illustrated in Figure 1, by P. D. Fawcett, the late Dr. J. C. Paterson,

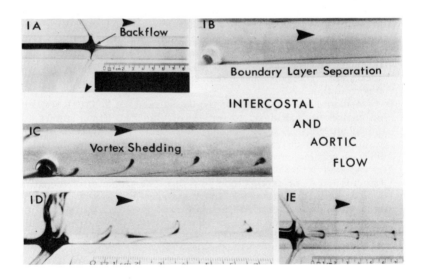

Figure 1. Model studies of intercostal flow from unpublished data of Fawcett, Paterson, and Roach. For details, see text.

and myself (unpublished data). An apparently normal aorta was obtained from a 43-yr-old female at autopsy and injected in situ with latex rubber that hardened when subjected to a pressure of 100 mm Hg. The aorta was then removed, rigidly clamped to prevent shortening, and immediately immersed in 10% formalin for 24 hr. The aorta was then slit longitudinally and the cast removed. Intercostal angles were measured by photographing the cast from above, from one side, and end-on. The image was projected onto a viewing screen where angles could be measured with a protractor. The circumferences of the intercostals and of the aorta in different places were then measured. The information was given to a glass blower, who produced a large scale model of one set of intercostals plus the aorta. The aorta and its branches were then perfused with steady flow from a large, constant-pressure reservoir and flow studied with the standard method of Evans blue dye. The branches were joined by Tygon tubing to provide a single outflow.

In this cast, the mean direction of the intercostal was $120°$ from the direction of aortic flow as demonstrated in Figure 1a. The mean intercostal diameter was 0.23 cm and the mean aortic diameter 1.93 cm. Thus the area ratio of the branch to the trunk is 1.42%. Flow into the aorta and the two paired intercostals was varied with screw clamps on the Tygon tubing attached to the outlets. The flow patterns varied with the amount of branch flow, and with the Reynolds number.

At Re = 1,000, and no branch flow, only laminar flow was seen. At 4% branch flow (Figure 1A) a sudden thinning of the boundary layer occurred, indicating new boundary-layer formation. Backflow occurred distal to the orifices as shown at the arrow. At 10% branch flow (Figure 1B) boundary-layer separation occurred downstream from the junction, and appeared at the site known to be associated with intimal cushions. At 12–16% branch flow, an unsteady boundary-layer disturbance occurred distally but was damped out 6–7 tube diameters (TD) downstream. At 14–16% branch flow, vortex shedding occurred (Figure 1C and D), and the vortices moved centrally as they passed downstream (Figure 1D and E). At branch flows above 25%, the vortices were broken up a few diameters downstream.

At higher Reynolds numbers of 1,800–2,000, the vortices seen on Figure 1D and E persisted with branch flows 10–12% rather than with the higher branch flow required at lower Reynolds numbers.

We have found that virtually all subanophilic lesions on the aortic wall of cholesterol-fed rabbits occur distal to orifices (Figure 2), and showed that these lesions could be mapped with a polar coordinate method (Cornhill and Roach, 1974). The lesions, as well as being affected by flow into the branch, are probably also affected by flow profiles in the aorta, since the lesions around the upper intercostals tend to be skewed (Figure 3) as described by Cornhill and Roach (1975).

With larger branches, such as occur in the abdominal aorta, the flow into the branch is usually great enough to alter the flow in the trunk, even at a distance, as found by Malcolm (1976) in my laboratory (Figure 4). The sudanophilic lesions that appear around these orifices are similar to those around the intercostals, but larger. In the abdominal aorta the branches originate close to each other, and so fully developed flow is unlikely near the distal branches.

The arch of the aorta must also have a significant effect on the flow distortions at the branches that leave its outer curvature. The sudanophilic lesions that occur in rabbits are complex and develop early (Figure 5).

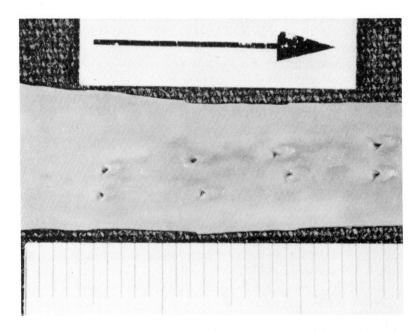

Figure 2. A rabbit aorta showing the lesions distal to the paired intercostal arteries. The arrow shows the flow direction.

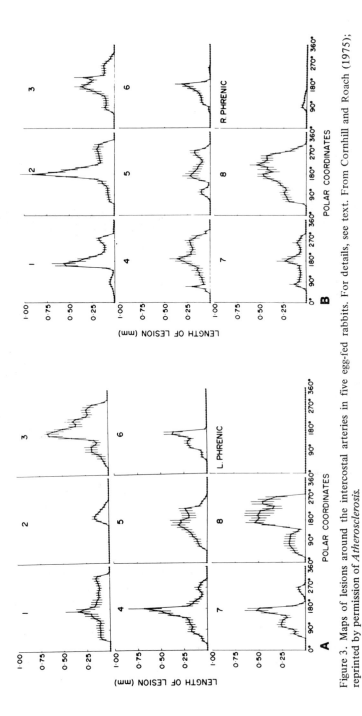

Figure 3. Maps of lesions around the intercostal arteries in five egg-fed rabbits. For details, see text. From Cornhill and Roach (1975); reprinted by permission of *Atherosclerosis*.

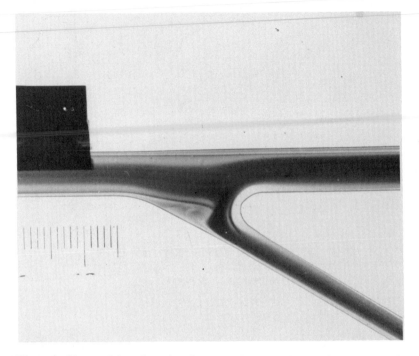

Figure 4. Glass model to show that flow into a large branch alters flow in the trunk. The branch is at 30° and β = 1.32. From Malcolm (1976) (unpublished).

Symmetric Bifurcations

In general, the distributing arteries have relatively symmetrical bifurcations, with varying angles and branch–trunk area ratios. Although these are easier to study with mathematical and physical models, they have been less thoroughly studied biologically.

Intracranial saccular aneurysms tend to occur at the apex of these bifurcations in the circle of Willis (Figure 6); they have been studied in some detail by Ferguson and Roach (1972a). They are associated with fragmentation of the single elastic membrane at the apex of these bifurcations.

Atherosclerosis also occurs at these Y bifurcations. If the vessels converge as at the vertebro-basilar junction, the lesion tends to be in the stagnant zone near the junction. By contrast, if the vessels diverge as most arteries do, the atherosclerotic lesions tend to develop at the lateral angles.

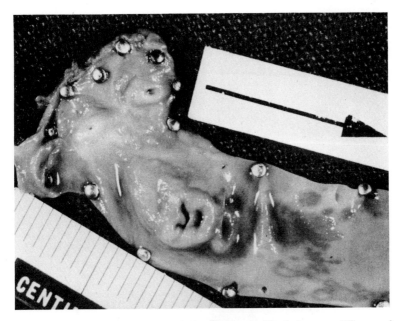

Figure 5. Sudanophilic lesions in rabbit aortic arch. The lesions are diffuse, and completely encircle the coronary arteries and the large orifices off the arch.

ANALYSIS OF FLOW IN GLASS MODEL BIFURCATIONS

There is no practical method at present to study flow profiles or velocity fluctuations at bifurcations in arteries of live animals (except perhaps large ones such as the cow or horse). Available anemometers are about 1 mm in diameter and would cause significant measurement artefacts.

In order to determine how flow differences in different parts of the bifurcation region can cause aneurysms at the apex and atherosclerosis at the lateral angles, a number of authors have used glass or plastic models to determine what type of flow profiles occur in various parts of the bifurcation.

We analyzed flow in a series of glass model bifurcations with a branch–trunk ratio of 1 and angles of 45°, 90°, 135°, and 180° (Ferguson and Roach, 1972b; Roach, Scott, and Ferguson, 1972). Both steady and pulsatile flow were used, and dye injected in thin streamlines. This study showed, as Stehbens (1959) had suggested earlier, that the critical Reynolds number, Re_{crit}, for turbulence varied with bifurcation angle (Figure

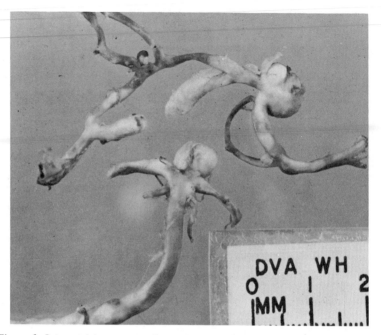

Figure 6. Intracranial aneurysms from a human circle of Willis. Note the two large and two small aneurysms present.

7A). With pulsatile flow, if the Re_{crit} was calculated from the mean flow, rather than the peak flow, then the Re_{crit} for the same bifurcations was lower than for steady flow. If "reverse flow" is put through the bifurcation (i.e., from the branches into the trunk) the curves are different, as illustrated in Figure 7B. In all of these experiments turbulence was defined by the presence of enough dye mixing that streamlines could no longer be identified. With both steady and pulsatile flow, at Re = 500, a stagnation point with reverse flow, or no flow, exists at the apex of the bifurcation in these models (Roach et al., 1972). No studies have been done, to my knowledge, on the size of the stagnation zone and on how it varies with branch–trunk ratio (β), angle (θ), and Re, with either steady or pulsatile flow. Ferguson and Roach (1972) postulated that this "battering ram" effect at the apex might be a key factor in the initiation of intracranial saccular aneurysms.

The biologic significance of studies of the stagnation zone in glass or plastic models is unclear. Recent work in my laboratory by Macfarlane

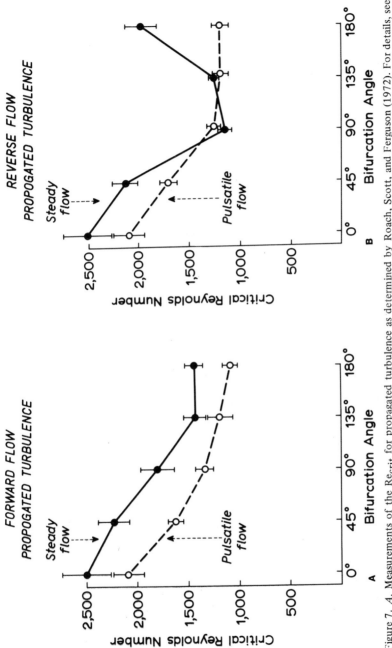

Figure 7. *A*, Measurements of the Re$_{crit}$ for propogated turbulence as determined by Roach, Scott, and Ferguson (1972). For details, see text. The reason for the differences with steady and pulsatile flow through a converging bifurcation is not obvious. Reproduced by permission of *Stroke*.

(1975) suggests that the elastic properties of the saddle region in isolated intracranial arteries are highly complex. Because the pressure and flow curves may be out of phase, we do not know whether the increase in bifurcation size with systolic pressure corresponds to the phase of accelerated systolic flow or not.

The stagnation point, or effective apex, may change as vessels are occluded. For example, Figure 8 shows flow in a glass model of the anterior cerebrals and anterior communicating artery (ACA) from the circle of Willis. Note that with both vessels open, there is virtually no flow through the anterior communicating artery (ACA) unless the pressures in the two anterior cerebral arteries are out of phase. However, if one branch is occluded, the ACA provides collateral flow to the other anterior cerebral artery and a new stagnation zone develops.

Dye studies (Roach et al., 1972) also show zones of apparent boundary-layer separation at the lateral angles of these bifurcations, and these are particularly marked if the branch comes off at an obtuse angle, as does the posterior cerebral artery. However, it should be pointed out that separation zones are best studied by plug injections of dye rather than with narrow streams. A vortex is set up in the separation zone because of the local pressure gradients and so dye both enters and leaves the separation zone slowly.

Malcolm (1976) has recently embarked on studies of the separation zone in a variety of glass models. This apparatus is basically similar to that previously described (Ferguson and Roach, 1972), except that the bifurcation is mounted in a tank filled with glycerol in order to eliminate reflections from the outer wall of the glass tubes. Because glycerol and glass have the same index of refraction, better pictures can be obtained. Flows are measured in the parent trunk and in one of the daughter branches with cannulated-type electromagnetic flowmeters made by Carolina Medical Electronics Inc. The perfusate is 0.5 normal saline, and is recirculated with a Littla Giant 2E-NT pump to a constant-pressure reservoir. Screw clamps applied to the outflows from the branches allow the branch resistance and flow (Q_{BT}) to be modified. Temperature is monitored to calculate viscosity.

A few experiments were done with pulsatile flow created with a Harvard type 1421 piston pump, with pulse rates of 18 and 12 cpm (based on the principle of dynamic similarity). The results were comparable to those with steady flow, but have not been analyzed completely.

Malcolm studied symmetric bifurcations with area ratios of 0.78, 1.03,

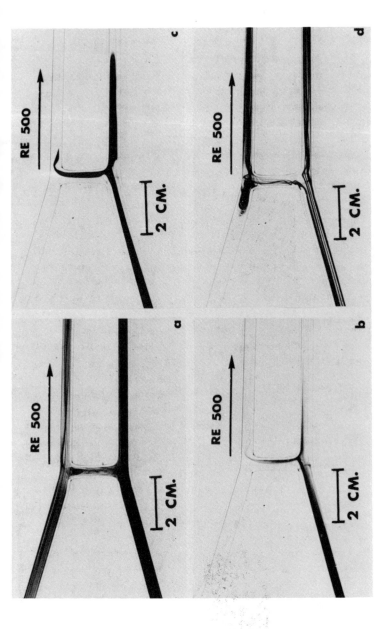

Figure 8. Flow studies in glass models of the anterior communicating artery (ACA). In (A), both anterior cerebrals (AA) are open. Dye fills the anterior communicating artery only by diffusion or if a pressure difference develops between the two trunks. The others have no flow in the top branch. Note in (B) that a stagnation point has developed at the junction of the ACA and low AA. In (C), flow is seen in the distal part of the occluded branch. There is also a zone of boundary-layer separation. In (D), some backflow is seen in the occluded trunk. From Roach et al. (1972); reproduced by permission of *Stroke*.

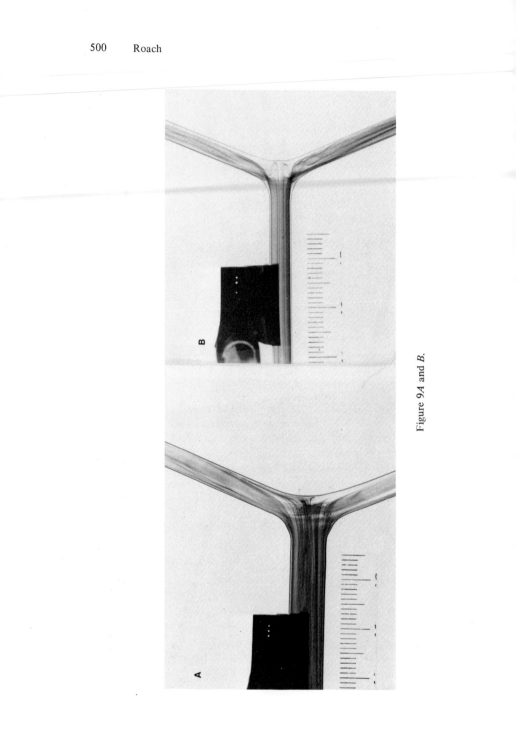

Figure 9*A* and *B*.

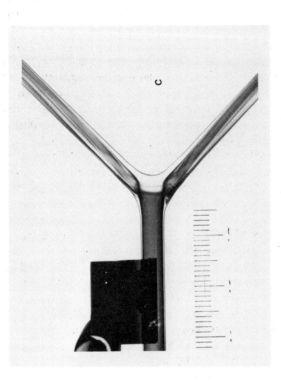
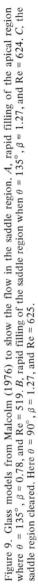

Figure 9. Glass models from Malcolm (1976) to show the flow in the saddle region. *A*, rapid filling of the apical region where $\theta = 135°$, $\beta = 0.78$, and Re = 519. *B*, rapid filling of the saddle region when $\theta = 135°$, $\beta = 1.27$, and Re = 624. *C*, the saddle region cleared. Here $\theta = 90°$, $\beta = 1.27$, and Re = 625.

and 1.27, branching angles of 45°, 90°, 135°, and 180°, and Reynolds numbers of 300–1600.

The apex was defined as the point of minimum radius of curvature facing the oncoming flow. This zone filled quickly from trunk core flow (Figure 9A), and then cleared rapidly as the axial and periaxial dye was deflected into the daughter branches (Figure 9B). Helical patterns often developed in the daughter branches from these deflected streamlines. Presumably this apical region is a zone of high shear. With time, the whole of the saddle region cleared (Figure 9B) while residual dye remained in the trunk and daughters. This pattern appeared independent of β and θ. The whole of the saddle region appeared to be swept continuously by central incident and peripheral reflected streamlines. Thus the saddle region (Figure 9C) was defined as the zone demarcated proximally by the interface between the dyed trunk boundary-layer fluid and the nondyed swept area. The correlation between this zone and the geometric saddle zone of arteries defined by two mutually perpendicular radii of curvature, as defined by Macfarlane (1975) and by the multiple muscle layer described by Walmsley and Canham (1973), remains to be determined.

These bifurcations, if viewed from above, also show separated zones at the lateral angles. These were most prominent in bifurcations with area ratios of 1.27, and in the 180° bifurcations (Figure 10). The separated region in the lateral angles was always swept vigorously with core fluid reflected from the apex. Thus these zones are not really stagnant zones, and may have high shear rates. Occasionally, a wedge of slowly recirculating fluid was seen beneath the separated boundary layer streamline, e.g., in the 45° bifurcations with $\beta = 1.03$ and 1.27 (Figure 10) and in the 135° bifurcation with $\beta = 1.03$. These wedges were fed by streamlines turned back from the medial wall of the daughter branches a short distance downstream from the apex. The part of the wedge adjacent to the lateral angle (i.e., in the expansion) contained dye moving slowly backward (with reference to the direction of bulk flow), and thus created a stationary vortex (Figure 10). These separated zones increased with both β and θ.

If one of the daughter branches was narrowed, two distinct flow phenomena developed. First, as shown in Figure 11, the streamlines entering the other branch were brought closer to the lateral angle of the parent tube as flow had to accelerate into the branch. As before, the lateral angle was swept by dye streams reflected off the apex from the core flow in the trunk. Second, as shown in Figure 11, the narrowed branch

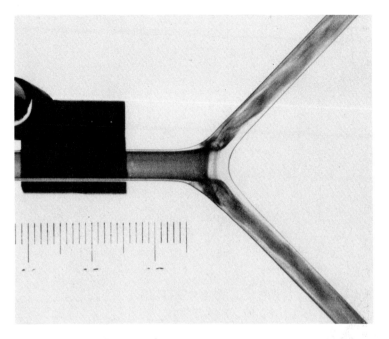

Figure 10. A glass model of a 90° bifurcation with β = 1.27 and Re = 1063 to show separation zones and a stationary vortex. From Malcolm (1976).

developed an increasingly prominent wedge-like formation in the lateral angle. These wedges occurred in the 45° bifurcations with balanced flow with high area ratios, but developed in all bifurcations with unbalanced flow.

Malcolm (1976) has also done a few studies with asymmetric glass model bifurcations. These were formed by attaching side arms to a glass trunk at 30°, 90°, and 150°. The area ratio thus produced was 1.16 and 1.32. In these, the geometrical apex of the distal lip acted as a flow divider (Figure 12). The dye entered and left this region quickly, probably indicating that fairly high local shear rates were present. Most of the fluid entering the branch was drawn from streamlines close to the side wall from which the branch opened (Figure 13A). On the opposite wall, a shallow region of boundary-layer separation developed (Figure 13B). In the 30° models, this zone of boundary-layer separation elongated progressively

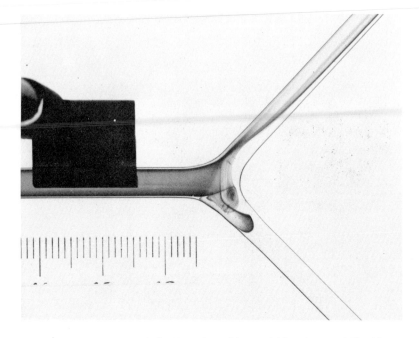

Figure 11. A symmetrical 90° bifurcation with β = 1.27 and Re = 276 with one branch partially occluded. Note that the streamlines now hug the lateral angle. A wedge-shaped zone is seen in the bottom partially occluded branch. From Malcolm (1976).

with increasing Reynolds numbers. In the 90° and 150° branch models, the streamlines associated with the separated boundary layer were never seen to reattach distally.

Wedge-shaped regions of recirculating flow were prominent in the lateral angle of the 30° models (Figure 14). Serial studies showed that these regions were swept by dyed fluid reflected from other parts of the junction.

When the branch was occluded, dyed fluid from the trunk still circulated within the proximal part of the branch for a distance of up to one tube diameter (Figure 15). Flow in the trunk was distorted, even though the branch was closed, particularly with smaller angles (Figure 15). Conversely, occlusion of the trunk caused a vigorous figure-of-eight vortex at the entrance of the occluded part, and this extended for several tube

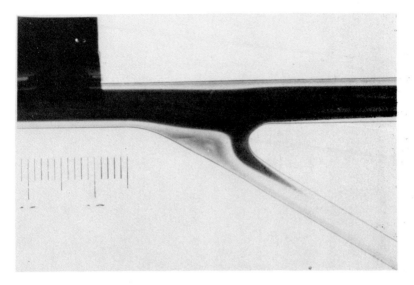

Figure 12. A glass model of a side arm at 30° form a β = 1.32 to illustrate that the distal part of the junction acts as an apex. From Malcolm (1976).

diameters distal to the side arm regardless of branch angle or Reynolds number (Figure 16). Here the streamlines adhered more closely to the lateral angle, and the wedge described previously was not seen.

Brech and Bellhouse (1973) studied two model branches with a 25.4-mm trunk and 19.0-mm branches (β = 1.12) set at an angle of 90°. One of their models had sharp lateral angles, the other smooth ones. Dye studies and measurements with hot-film probes indicated that very high shear stresses developed on the inside of the limb for about one diameter downstream, while low shears occurred on the outside of the limb. They did not investigate the effect of different β or θ, but they varied Re from 750 to 1,500 and the Strouhl number from 0.4 to 0.2 and left Womersley's α parameter at 22.

Crowe and Krovetz (1972), using flow birefringence techniques, studied steady and pulsatile flows in plastic bifurcations with angles of 30°, 60°, and 90°, and area ratios of 0.11, 0.44, and 1.0 for the side arm. They observed boundary-layer separation on the outer branch walls and Re = 20–50, and regions of locally increased shear on the inner walls at Re > 150. With pulsatile flow, these regions were approximately one diameter

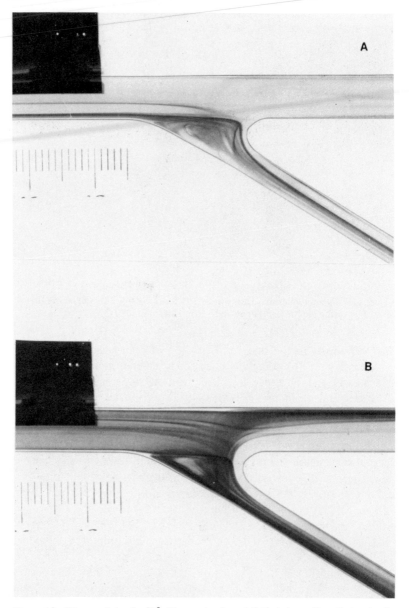

Figure 13. Glass models of a 30° side arm to show (*A*) that streamlines that enter the branch come from the part of the trunk next to the branch and (*B*) that boundary layer separation occurs on the opposite wall. From Malcolm (1976).

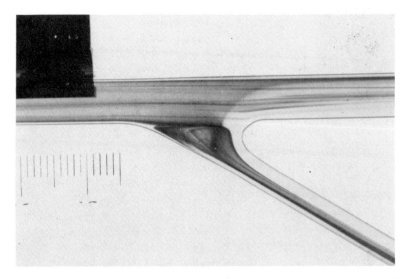

Figure 14. A glass model study to show the development of wedge-shaped regions of recirculating flow in a 30° branch. From Malcolm (1976).

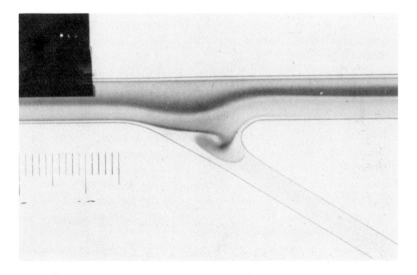

Figure 15. A glass model with the side arm closed. Note the complex dye pattern in the mouth of the occluded branch. From Malcolm (1976).

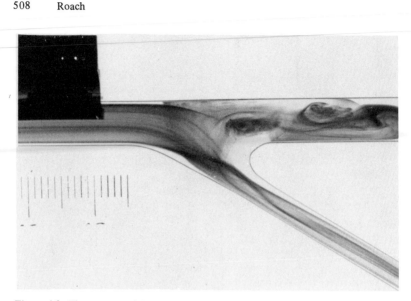

Figure 16. The same model as in Figure 15 but with the trunk occluded. Note the figure-of-eight vortex that has formed. From Malcolm (1976).

downstream from the point of bifurcation. They concluded that the area ratio was the most important parameter for determining entrance lengths and distribution of disturbed flow.

Rodkiewicz and Roussel (1973) studied 16 plastic bifurcations, and concluded that the mass flow ratio (1) decreased with entrance Reynolds number, (2) increased with diameter ratio, and (3) decreased as a function of the branching angle. They found also that interdependent separation regions occurred in each branch, with "banana-shaped" vortices from the main branch, and a double helicoidal flow in the side branch.

Schroter and Sudlow (1969) investigated air flow patterns in models of the bronchial tree with Re = 100–1,500. They found secondary motions at all flow rates, with the form depending on the direction of flow.

A number of other authors also have studied glass and plastic models simulating rigid arteries. The major problem with all of these studies is that we still do not have sound data on biologic values for the area ratio and branch angle. I believe, as discussed below, that we, as bioengineers and biophysicists, have been unable to describe these values in such a way that biologists, and particularly pathologists, who deal with arterial disease, can extrapolate our studies to what they can observe.

BIFURCATIONS AND ARTERIAL DISEASE

Bifurcations in arteries seem to be associated with a higher incidence of arterial disease than do the trunks of the arteries. Two conditions are discussed: (a) cerebral aneurysms and (b) atherosclerosis.

Cerebral Aneurysms

Cerebral aneurysms are saccular outpouchings that occur at the apex of bifurcations in the circle of Willis (Figure 6). For many years, these aneurysms were considered to be congenital in origin, because a defect was often seen in the muscle in the media of the artery near the bifurcation. However, recent investigations support the idea that these aneurysms may be produced hemodynamically. Most of this information comes from our laboratory, and was initiated by Ferguson between 1968 and 1970. We started with the premise that, because turbulence caused poststenotic dilatation (PSD), it might also cause aneurysms. Ferguson (1970a) found that aneurysms characteristically occurred at the apex of bifurcations in the circle of Willis or in its major branches. However, our model studies (see preceding section) showed that turbulence was unlikely below Reynolds numbers of 700, even with $180°$ bifurcations. Ferguson (1970b) calculated that peak Reynolds numbers in the human internal carotid artery were probably from 600 to 750, so turbulence was unlikely. However, his dye studies showed turbulence in model aneurysms at Re $\simeq$ 400. He then studied 17 patients at the time of surgery and found bruits in 10 of the 17. Because all of our patients are operated on with profound hypotension, it seems likely that turbulence is common in aneurysms but rare at normal intracranial bifurcations. Dye studies at Re = 500 in three configurations of aneurysm all showed turbulence (Roach et al., 1972). This suggests that although turbulence may be a factor in the progression of intracranial aneurysms, it is unlikely to be a factor in their initiation.

I showed previously (Roach, 1963a) that turbulence distal to an arterial stenosis altered the elastic properties of the artery so that it became more distensible. Scott, Ferguson, and Roach (1972) then showed that aneurysms were much less distensible than the cerebral arteries from which they arose (Figure 17). Analysis of the curves, using the method of Roach and Burton (1957), suggested that the major change was a loss of elastin. This supported the histologic data of Nyström (1963) and others that elastin was fragmented in the walls of these aneurysms. We then showed that the elastic properties of brain arteries could be altered to

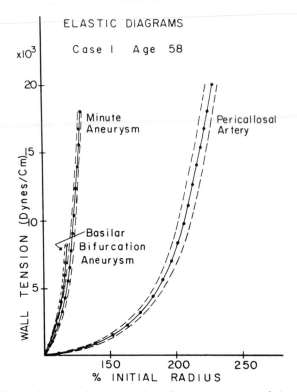

Figure 17. Elastic diagrams of a large basilar bifurcation aneurysm of about 8 mm diameter, and a minute aneurysm of 1 mm diameter and a cerebral artery from the same patient. The dotted lines show the SEM from three measurements. From Ferguson, 1972*b;* reprinted by permission.

make them like those of aneurysms by repeated exposures to pressures of ⩾200 mm Hg (Scott et al., 1972). Melton and Roach (unpublished) subsequently found that the elastin in isolated brain arteries seemed to snap at any pressure over 200 mm Hg, and this was confirmed both with elastic diagrams and histologically.

Since Ferguson (1972*a*) had demonstrated that the pressure inside human intracranial aneurysms was comparable to that in systemic arteries, Scott et al. (1972) concluded that the stress in the walls of these aneurysms could be very high. Roach (1970*a*) and Canham and Ferguson (unpublished) have since developed a method, based on conservation of wall volume, to predict when these aneurysms will rupture. This is important clinically, because these aneurysms are often multiple, and so the question of prophylactic surgery then arises if one ruptures.

Ferguson (1972b) concluded that the impacting force of the axial stream damaged the apex of intracranial bifurcations in some undetermined way, causing elastin to fragment and a minute aneurysm to develop. He suggested that turbulence might cause growth of the aneurysm, and that wall factors, coupled with transient blood pressure increases, might cause rupture. We still do not know why some patients, and some bifurcations of these patients, develop aneurysms while others do not. The answer probably lies in a better understanding of the hemodynamic forces acting at the bifurcation of these distensible vessels.

Mycotic aneurysms, or those caused by bacteria traveling in the blood stream, are quite different (Roach and Drake, 1965). They often are multiple, and tend to occur peripherally rather than in the circle (Figure 18). Their localization probably is related to stagnant flow zones where the bacteria can settle out. So little work has been done on them that no further discussion seems warranted.

Atherosclerosis

Atherosclerosis is a patchy disease that occurs in large arteries near bends and bifurcations, as illustrated in the Introduction. Recent studies in the coronary circulation (Montenegro and Eggen, 1968) and brain circulation (Solberg and Eggen, 1971) showed an increased incidence of atherosclerosis around bifurcations. Unfortunately, the bifurcation was not split into apical regions and lateral angles, so no conclusions can be drawn about what hemodynamic forces are involved.

Figures 2 and 5 illustrate the problems of mapping atherosclerotic lesions. We concluded 3 yr ago that this was impractical, for the moment, in large arteries except the aorta. However, the aorta is known to develop atherosclerosis in both man and animals, and so we embarked on a long-term project to determine how the lesions on the aortic wall were produced by flow into the branches. Thus we needed a mapping technique so we could determine how flow in the trunk or aorta was modified by flow into the branches.

Cornhill and Roach (1974) devised a polar coordinate mapping technique to achieve this. Atherosclerosis was created in rabbits by feeding a diet high in cholesterol. After variable periods, the rabbits were sacrificed and the aorta measured, removed, opened, and pinned at in situ dimensions. They were then stained with Sudan III, which stains fat red. Color

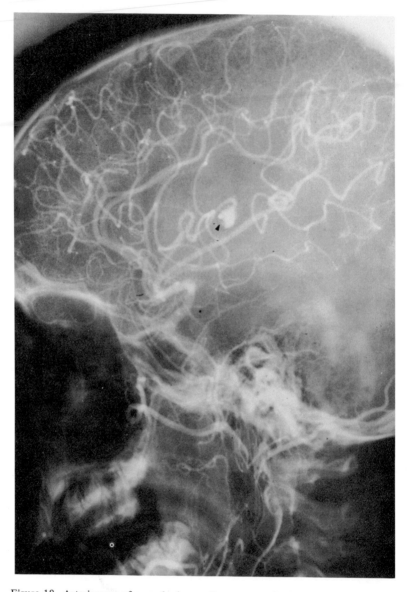

Figure 18. Arteriogram of a cerebral mycotic aneurysm (at arrow) in a young child with congenital heart disease. Note that the aneurysm has developed at the end of a vessel rather than at a bifurcation.

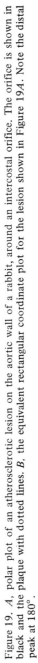

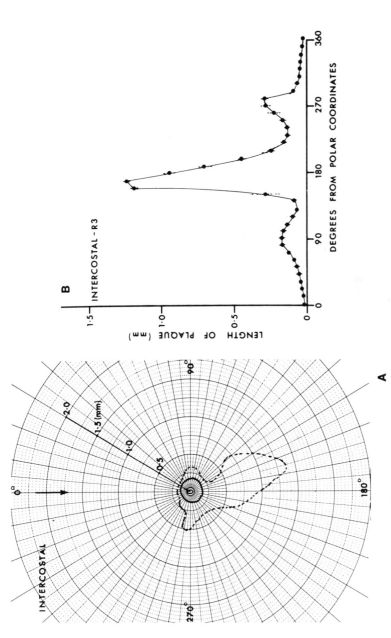

Figure 19. *A*, polar plot of an atherosclerotic lesion on the aortic wall of a rabbit, around an intercostal orifice. The orifice is shown in black and the plaque with dotted lines. *B*, the equivalent rectangular coordinate plot for the lesion shown in Figure 19*A*. Note the distal peak at 180°.

photographs were obtained and projected onto the polar coordinate grid with the orifice centered around zero, 0° proximal, 90° to the animals' left, 180° distal, and 270° to the animals' right. A typical plot is shown in Figure 19A. We then measured the length of plaque beyond the edge of the orifice at 10° intervals around the orifice, and replotted the data on rectangular coordinates (Figure 19B). Each orifice was analyzed five times, and the results were very reproducible. We found (Cornhill and Roach, 1974; Roach, 1975) that all lesions except those in the arch (Figure 5) and those around the coronaries (Figure 20) were distal to the orifices. Flow in the arch is complicated, and flow around the coronaries probably is in the form of a vortex (Bellhouse and Bellhouse, 1969).

We then studied the lesions on the aortic wall around the intercostals, coronaries, coeliac and renal orifices in detail in five rabbits (Cornhill and Roach, 1975). The intercostal lesions, as shown in Figure 3, were distal but skewed, presumably because of secondary flow set up in the arch. The size of lesions was directly proportional to the area of the associated orifice, suggesting that they might be associated with high shear stress. If

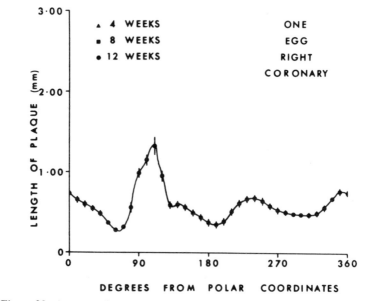

Figure 20. A rectangular coordinate plot of the lesion around the right coronary orifice after 12 wk on a one-egg diet. The lesions were present after four and eight weeks on the diet. From Fletcher, Cornhill, and Roach (unpublished).

the flow into an orifice is roughly proportional to the area of the orifice, then the reduction in thickness of the boundary layer at a branching point would increase as orifice area increased. Thus the shear stresses distal to large orifices would be greater than those distal to small ones (Figure 21).

We then found that with increased duration of feeding on the same diet, the lesions grew around each orifice, but tended to retain roughly the same shape (Figure 22) (Roach, Fletcher, and Cornhill, in press). As lesions progressed, they became elevated and often granular, so that the lesions themselves could modify the flow profile. Lesions around adjacent orifices were fused in 48% of the cases after a diet of 2% cholesterol and 6% corn oil for 10 wk. There seemed to be some correlation between the size of lesions around any one orifice (e.g., the coeliac) and the cholesterol concentration-time index, but these results were not statistically significant.

These results show clearly that fat deposits occur preferentially near orifices. However, they do not show whether this is a direct or indirect effect of hemodynamic forces. Structurally, as is discussed below, the

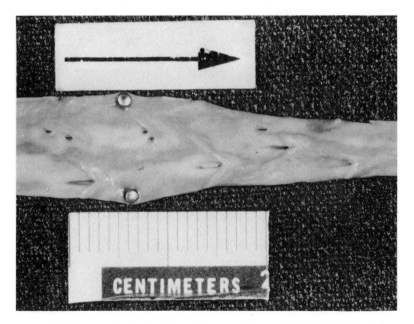

Figure 21. Photograph of the abdominal aorta of a rabbit. Note that the lesions around large orifices are large, while those around small orifices are small.

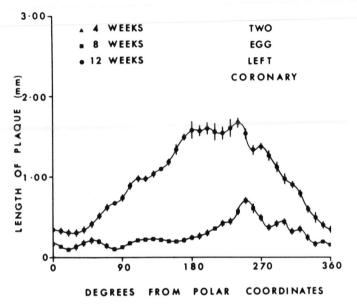

Figure 22. The development of lesions around the left coronary artery of rabbits fed a two-egg diet. Note that the shape stays the same as the lesion grows.

composition of bifurcations is complex. Thus we altered the flow around the renal orifices by doing unilateral nephrectomies, leaving a blind stump of renal artery (Roach and Fletcher, in press). Lesions now developed proximally as well as distally (Figure 23A). Removal of the right kidney (which is proximal) altered the shape of the lesion around the left renal orifice (Figure 23B), but removal of the left kidney had no effect on the lesion around the right renal orifice (Figure 23C). In addition, it should be noted in Figure 23 that sham operation is essential, because the operation alone (without flow distortion) modifies the lesions, particularly distally. Whether this is the result of altered tethering or some other factor remains to be determined.

Several other laboratories have also investigated the role of hemo-dynamic forces in creation of the early lesions of atherosclerosis. Fry (1968, 1969a, 1969b) showed with in vivo dog experiments that high shear damaged the endothelium and increased transport of both choles-terol and albumin into the arterial wall. He then proposed that high shear could be a factor in early atherosclerosis. About the same time, Caro, Fitz-Gerald, and Schroter (1971) proposed that low shear caused atherosclerosis by decreasing the mass transfer of lipid out of the wall in certain regions. These conclusions were based on the flow studies of Schroter and Sudlow (1969), coupled with mapping of atherosclerotic lesions in human aortas.

Mapping of endothelial cells around bifurcations by Flaherty et al. (1972) indicates that these cells are very sensitive to shear forces acting on them, and that the orientation of the cells is different near bifurcations. There is no evidence concerning whether the fiber distribution and geometry of bifurcations are also flow dependent.

An obvious way to resolve this controversy would be to measure shear forces around bifurcations in vivo. Unfortunately, this is impractical at present because of the large size of the probes. Thus we must get the answers with indirect methods.

BIOLOGIC STUDIES ON BIFURCATIONS

Glass model studies have indicated that flow profiles at bifurcations are complex and depend on branch—trunk ratios and the angle of the bifurcation, as well as on the Reynolds number, and presumably on the flow pattern in the parent vessel (developed or nondeveloped flow). The model studies are hard to interpret biologically because there has been no systematic study of the geometry of biologic bifurcations.

Measurement artifacts are a major problem. Most casting materials shrink, and in addition are very viscous, so that they may not fill vessels adequately. Figure 24 shows the best cast that Fletcher (unpublished) has obtained on a rabbit aorta, using Louiscraft clear casting resin. From this cast, branch—trunk ratios and angles can be measured, but radii of curvature cannot. Both values vary widely, and no sound data are available on a large enough series to draw definite conclusions.

Some information is available from arteriograms. These give valid branch—trunk diameter ratios as long as the vessels are circular in cross section. However, even minor degrees of rotation may give incorrect values for the angle. Beales and Steiner (1972) measured area ratios from diameters at arteriography in a series of patients under general anesthesia. They found the following values: normal aorta, 0.77 ± 0.04; abnormal aorta, 0.75 ± 0.04; second-generation renal artery, 1.15 ± 0.04; second-generation superior mesenteric, 1.12 ± 0.04; digital arteries, 1.25 ± 0.03.

Caro et al. (1971) found, from arteriograms, area ratios at the aortic bifurcation of 0.52–1.08; at the common iliac of 0.81–1.15; and at the

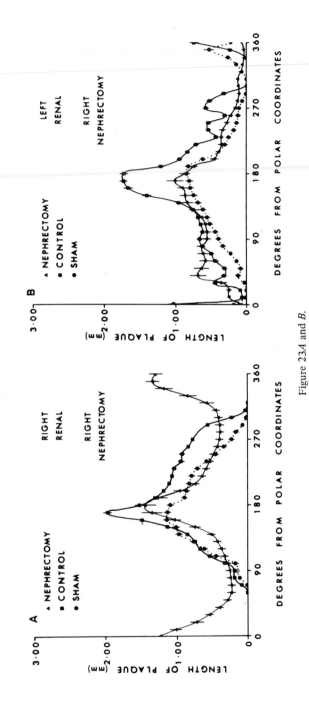

Figure 23.A and B.

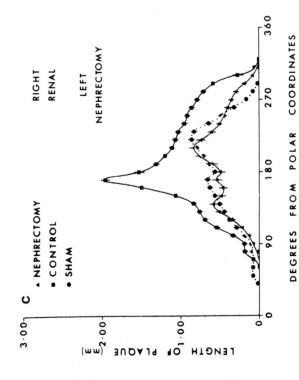

Figure 23. *A*, Sudanophilic lesions around the right renal orifice in cholesterol-fed rabbits. Note that after nephrectomy with a blind stump, the lesion becomes proximal as well as distal. *B*, Lesions around the left renal artery after right nephrectomy in cholesterol-fed rabbits. Note that the lesion has become skewed to the animal's left (i.e., 45°–75°) after removal of flow into the proximal right renal artery. *C*, Lesions around the right renal orifice after left nephrectomy in cholesterol-fed rabbits. Note that there is no difference between the sham-operated and operated groups but a marked difference from controls. The mechanism for this change from the controls to the operated groups is not clear.

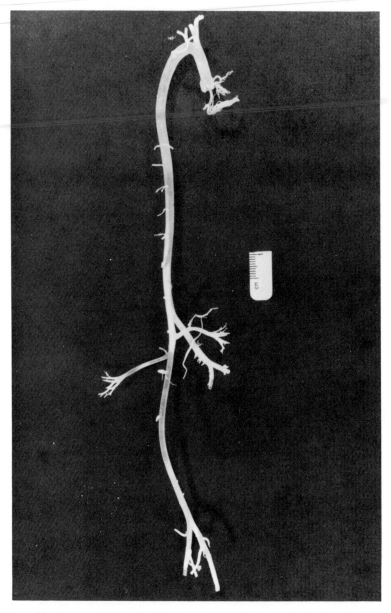

Figure 24. Cast of rabbit aorta (Fletcher and Roach, unpublished). Note the variation in vessel size and angles.

intrarenal bifurcations of 0.84–1.39. Many of their patients were hypertensive.

Gosling and his group (Gosling et al., 1971) predicted theoretically that the reflection of pressure waves depended on the area ratio, and was a minimum for an equibifurcation at 1.15 and for an equitrifurcation at 1.25. They found that in cockerels with atherosclerosis, the area ratio at the abdominal aortic junction fell well below 1.0 (Newman, Gosling, and Bowden, 1971). Lallemand, Brown, and Boulter (1972) found that five out of six women with hypoplastic abdominal aortas and thrombosis at the bifurcations had low area ratios of 0.4–0.7. The sixth patient had an area ratio of 1.0. This was lower than the age-related values measured by Gosling et al. (1971) from human aortograms. This group (Lallemand, Gosling, and Newman, 1972) then predicted that abnormal reflections of incident pressure pulse waves at bifurcations (in particular, the abdominal aortic bifurcation) could cause medial damage. They were unable to decide if this defect was present from birth, or if it developed later in life.

The histologic structure of bifurcations of arteries has only recently been investigated. Berry (1973), in a study of cerebral arteries, noted that two patterns of elastic tissue developed late in intra-uterine life, probably based on the tension in the wall. He found no evidence of selective growth of bifurcations, but proposed that medial defects were due to widening of the angles resulting from growth of the hemispheres. Our own studies (unpublished) suggest that the pattern is even more complex than proposed by Berry.

Stehbens (1974) studied the lower half of the aorta in 17 rabbits. After fixation at physiological pressure, he found area ratios of 131–219% with a symmetric and eccentric enlargement. He found the greatest area increase was 1–2 mm proximal to the apex of the bifurcation, and was due to divergence of the lateral walls while the facial and dorsal surfaces approximated only slightly. In dogs, the area ratio was 1.32; the lumen expanded laterally by 74.5% and diminished vertically by only 20%. He found expansions at most forks, but the dilatation was greatest with wide angles.

In our lab, Canham, Walmsley, and Smith (1975) have developed a detailed stereologic technique to investigate the orientation of fibers in cerebral arteries, and cerebral artery bifurcations. Their methods allow exact measurement of artifacts, so that within the next few years they should be able to provide a detailed analysis of the exact orientation of different types of fibers in the bifurcation.

OPTIMALITY PRINCIPLES IN BIFURCATIONS

Gosling et al. (1971) suggested that if the aortic bifurcation is optimally matched to minimize the reflection coefficient, atherosclerosis will not occur there. Other authors have suggested that other physical factors should be "optimized" at bifurcations. For example, Murray (1926a, 1926b) and Rosen (1967) concluded that, with the exception of the aorta and its branches, bifurcation geometry appeared to be designed to maintain a state of minimum work. Kamiya and Togawa (1972) suggest that at the capillary level volume flow is minimized. Zamir (in press) recently suggested that branch angles and area ratios might be designed to minimize shear. He then did an ingenious analysis combining the four hypotheses of minimum surface area, minimum total volume, minimum work or power, and minimum drag (Zamir, 1976). He found a small region of overlap with $\beta = 1.1-1.4$ and $\theta = 75°-100°$. It is interesting that most bifurcations (other than those with the aorta) fall within these values. The next logical question is whether bifurcations outside the values are more or less susceptible to disease.

MAJOR UNSOLVED PROBLEMS
ABOUT THE ROLE OF BIFURCATIONS IN ARTERIAL DISEASE

The major problem that must be solved before further work is how to define the component parts of a bifurcation. This is particularly important if we hope to get pathologists to map lesions.

To stimulate argument, and in the hope of obtaining more suitable definitions, I suggest we adhere to the following definitions.

1. *Bifurcation region* could be defined as that region from the first part of the trunk when either the walls are not parallel, or the flow is divided by the apex (whichever provides the greater trunk length) to the first part of each branch where the walls are parallel. One might argue that this region should be extended one tube diameter (T.D.) on each side of this. Rather than do this, I have chosen to call these zones the *entrance zone* and *exit zone.*

2. *Lateral angles* could be defined in a variety of ways, and will be very dependent on the angles involved. For the present, let us consider the lateral angle as that part of the bifurcation region bounded by the central axis of each daughter branch, and extending to meet lines drawn parallel to the axis of the trunk and roughly the same width as the part in the

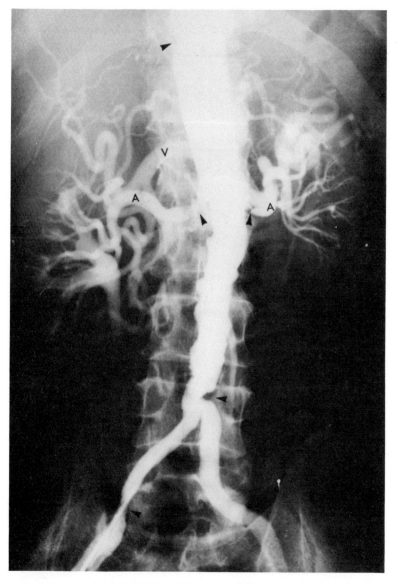

Figure 25. Aorta with diffuse atherosclerosis at arrows. Some of the major vessels are totally occluded. Both renal arteries (A) have tight stenoses. The right renal vein (V) is seen, while the left is not.

daughters. If $\beta > 1$, then there will be an undefined region in the center of the trunk in the entrance zone. If $\beta < 1$, then the axes of the branches will intersect, and their point of intersection could be used to drop an axis parallel to the trunk walls.

3. The *saddle region* will be considered the part of the bifurcation region not included by the lateral angles. Two parts of the saddle may be of particular importance: (a) the *stagnation zone* is the part near the apex of the saddle where flow direction reverses or where flow is zero. The dimensions of this zone, which may be related to aneurysm formation, should be defined; (b) the *medial angles* are the parts of the daughter branches that exist beyond the internal radius of curvature of the bifurcation. In some bifurcations it may be impractical to separate the medial angles from the saddle region.

These zones may bear no relationship to either the flow patterns, or the anatomic peculiarities of the bifurcation. However, they provide some place to start.

Figure 25 shows a high-quality aortagram on which we can attempt to

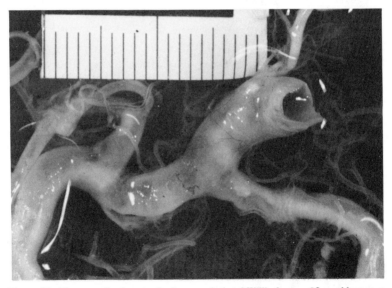

Figure 26. Photograph of part of a human circle of Willis from a 58-yr-old woman. The vessels are translucent except where atherosclerotic lesions occur, i.e., largely at bends and bifurcations.

apply these definitions. Area ratios can be obtained readily, but angles (unless clearly in the right plane) are inaccurate. This two-dimensional view cannot allow a good definition of anything but the bifurcation region and the entrance and exit zones. The arrow at the bottom right points to a filling defect that is probably an atherosclerotic plaque at the lateral angle in the main trunk. However, the diffuse aortic disease (marked irregularity) makes even defining the trunk difficult.

Figure 26, which is part of an isolated circle of Willis, shows several zones of atherosclerosis. Qualitative descriptions can be made, but quanti-

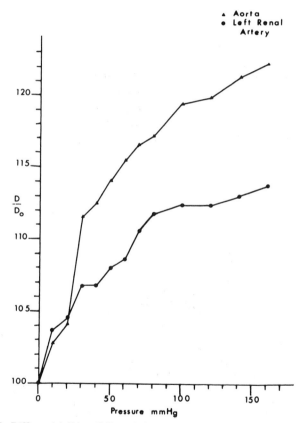

Figure 27. Differential distensibility of the abdominal aorta and renal artery of a cat, both normalized with respect to their values at zero pressure. From Reuber (unpublished).

tative ones are probably useless because the arteries are not under their normal distending pressure.

Figure 27 shows diameter—pressure curves obtained by Reuber and Roach (unpublished data) from the aorta and renal arteries of a cat. Note that, because of the different distensibility of different parts of the arterial tree, the branch—trunk ratios almost certainly change in response to pressure. Our data indicate that, in vitro, the angles also change in response to pressure. No in vivo data at different pressures are available to my knowledge.

An alternative approach is that of Schroter and Sudlow (1969), who divided the artery into quadrants. This probably is simpler than our method for the lateral angle, but less useful for the saddle region, which they treat only as a simple flow divider.

In the saddle region, there are two radii of curvature, as indicated in Figure 28. Because these are in opposite directions, an infinite force could develop at the apex. The light-pipe technique used by Macfarlane (1975), illustrated in Figure 29, seems the best way to study the internal radius of curvature. These are not feasible for clinical studies at present.

In the lateral angles there also are two radii of curvature, one around the vessel and one along the outside of the branch—trunk junction. Perhaps

$$\Delta P = \frac{T_1}{R_1} - \frac{T_2}{R_2}$$

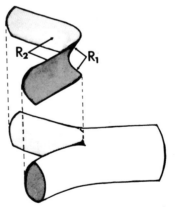

Figure 28. Schematic diagram of a bifurcation to show the two radii of curvature. From Macfarlane (1975); reproduced by permission.

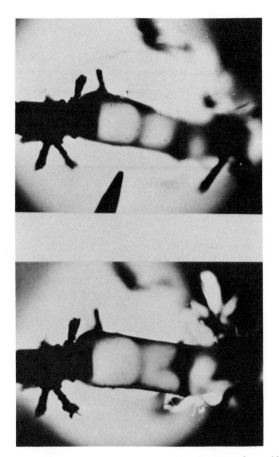

Figure 29. Photograph of the internal radius of curvature of a middle cerebral bifurcation from a 54-yr-old male. A light pipe was used to show the curvature and the two photographs are at 5 and 165 mm Hg transmural pressure. Note the change in curvature. From Macfarlane, 1975; reproduced by permission.

the difference in volume between the latter and the projected sides of these vessels may prove useful for describing the expansion that occurs before the daughter branches are fully developed.

FLOW IN THE ARCH OF THE AORTA

Atherosclerosis is common in both the arch of the aorta (Figure 5) and in the major vessels arising from it. Flow measurements are inaccurate here

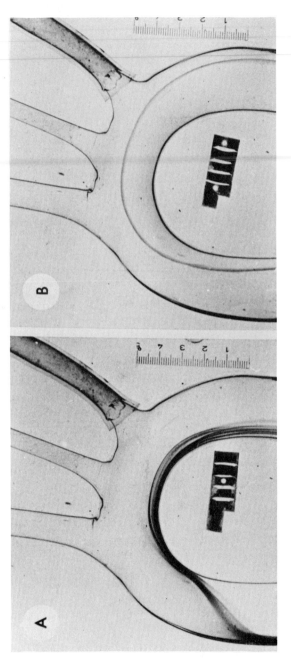

Figure 30A and B.

528

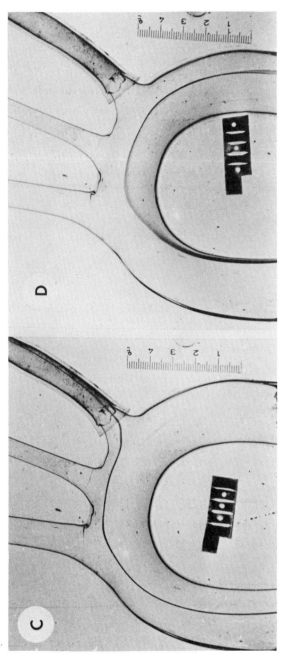
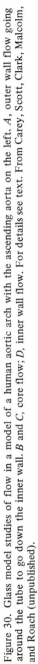

Figure 30. Glass model studies of flow in a model of a human aortic arch with the ascending aorta on the left. *A*, outer wall flow going around the tube to go down the inner wall. *B* and *C*, core flow; *D*, inner wall flow. For details see text. From Carey, Scott, Clark, Malcolm, and Roach (unpublished).

because the asymmetry distorts flow signals with electromagnetic flow-meters, and secondary flows may distort flow profiles with anemometers or ultrasound flowmeters. Scott, Carey, Clark, Malcolm, and Roach (un-published) have recently investigated this in glass models. Figure 30A shows a typical flow pattern with dye injected on the outer wall travelling helically around the circumference to reach the inner wall of the arch, and finally the inner wall of the descending aorta.

Core flow tended to remain in the core and then be diverted up one or more branches. Preliminary experiments suggested there was some prefer-ential streaming into certain branches from different parts of the core (Figure 30B and C).

Flow on the inner wall was slower moving, and tended to fan out as it reached the arch (Figure 30D). With higher Reynolds numbers, secondary motions developed. The relationship of these results to the in vivo situa-tion remains to be determined.

ARTERIAL STENOSES AND POSTSTENOTIC DILATATION

Arterial stenosis, or narrowing, is most often due to atherosclerosis (Figure 31) with or without thrombosis, and frequently occurs near bifurcations. In many cases a poststenotic dilatation (PSD) is present as shown here. Some stenoses are congenital, such as the coarctation shown in Figure 32. Others are produced by external compression of the artery by a cervical rib or fibrous band (Figure 33). The geometry of the stenosis and its location both determine the associated decrease in pressure and flow.

Some of these stenoses increase progressively (e.g., by growth of the plaque), while others increase and then stop, e.g., a coarctation that gets more severe until the surrounding aorta stops growing. Other stenoses, particularly those in the coronary tree, may increase after bypass surgery decreases the flow through the constricted segment. Other circulations may also have unique time courses as discussed previously (Roach, in press).

A number of authors (Mann et al., 1900; Shipley and Gregg, 1944; May, DeWeese, and Rob, 1963; May et al., 1963; Vonruden et al., 1964; Christophersen et al., 1965; Killen and Oh, 1968; Kindt and Youmans, 1969; Kreuzer and Schenk, 1971) have studied the effects of experimental stenoses on flow and pressure beyond the stenosis, and occasionally on turbulence production. Most authors agree that fairly tight stenoses ($\geqslant$ 60% area decrease) are required to alter flow significantly. One of the technical problems is how to estimate the degree of stenosis, and to assess whether it is constant throughout the cardiac cycle (Roach, in press).

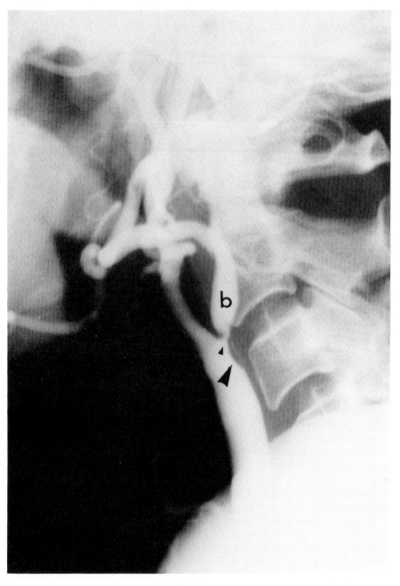

Figure 31. Arteriogram of a carotid stenosis. Note that there is a large plaque in the trunk (at the large arrow), a tight stenosis in the artery (small arrow), and a poststenotic dilatation (Roach et al., 1972).

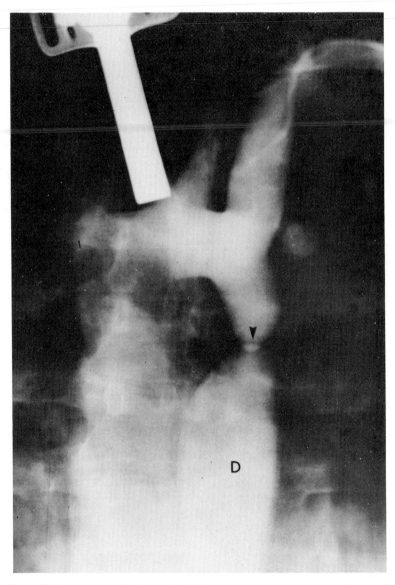

Figure 32. Aortogram of a 14-yr-old child to show a tight coarctation of the aorta (at arrow) and a large poststenotic dilatation (D).

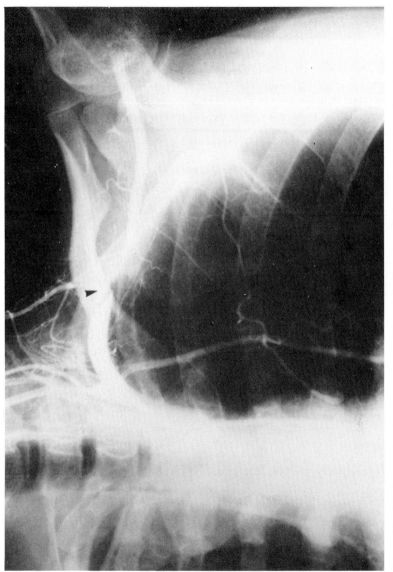

Figure 33. Arteriogram showing compressing of the subclavian artery at the level of the thoracic outlet (see arrow).

Stenoses may cause arterial disease either locally, because the rough wall tends to induce thrombus formation and progression of the stenosis, or by giving rise to emboli that are trapped in small vessels distal to the stenosis.

Stenoses are often associated with poststenotic dilatation, an interesting paradox (Roach, 1963*b*; Zamir, 1976). I showed that this phenomenon occurred in vivo (Roach, 1963*c*) and in vitro (Roach and Harvey, 1964) only if the stenosis created distal turbulence as indicated by the presence of a thrill and bruit. In the regions exposed to turbulence, the vessel became

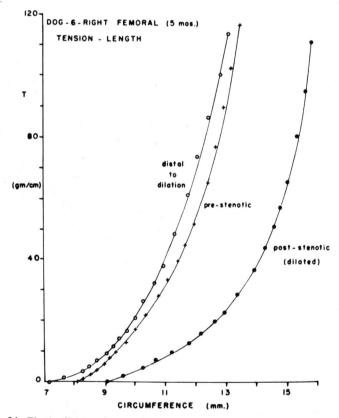

Figure 34. Elastic diagram from a dog artery. Note the marked increase in distensibility in the dilated segments. From Roach (1963*a*); reproduced by permission of Amer. J. Cardiol.

more distensible (Roach, 1963a), as shown in Figure 34. This change was primarily in the elastin and in the intercollagen links.

Boughner and Roach (1971a) subsequently showed that certain frequencies seemed more effective than others in causing this dilatation. Foreman and Hutchison (1970) and Hutchison (1974) suggested this could be due to resonance, and Sinclair (1974) subsequently showed theoretically and experimentally what factors would modify the resonance. Boughner and Roach (1971b) subsequently showed that turbulence from high flow (e.g., in the pulmonary artery in patients with atrial septal defects) also caused the same change in the elastic properties of arteries.

This evidence shows that PSD is a type of structural fatigue induced by resonant vibrations in the wall secondary to the turbulent vibrations in the fluid distal to the stenosis. The exact molecular changes are unknown, and my observation that the process is reversible if the stenosis is removed (Roach, 1970b) makes speculation even more difficult.

We found also (Roach and MacDonald, 1970) that the length of the dilatation tended to be inversely proportional to the diameter of the stenosis. Stockley (1971) and Valin and Roach (unpublished) found the length of the jet distal to the stenosis was also inversely related to the diameter of the stenosis. Thus the length of the PSD gives a better estimate of the degree of stenosis than does the diameter of the PSD.

SUMMARY

Information presented here clearly shows that bifurcations and stenoses probably produce arterial disease. The evidence for how stenoses cause a poststenotic dilatation is well developed. Hemodynamic studies on how bifurcations cause aneurysms and atherosclerosis still are rudimentary. We urgently need a way to define the parts of a bifurcation so that flow studies and pathologic studies can be correlated.

ACKNOWLEDGMENTS

I would like to thank my students and colleagues for allowing me to present these unpublished data, particularly Dr. Alasdair Malcolm and Dr. Colin Clark, and Joan Fletcher, J. F. Cornhill, Mark Carey, Sheila Scott, Barbara Reuber, Christine Melton, and T. W. R. Macfarlane. The work of many other students is quoted also, but has been published. Dr. R. E. Gold and Dr. John Allcock provided the x rays and Dr. Bruce Warren some of the pathologic slides. Mrs. Dorothy Elston provided technical help for all of us.

LITERATURE CITED

Beales, J. S. M., and R. E. Steiner. 1972. Radiological assessment of arterial branching coefficients. Cardiovasc. Res. 6: 181–186.

Bellhouse, B. J., and F. H. Bellhouse. 1969. Fluid mechanics of model normal and stenosed aortic valves. Circ. Res. 25: 693–704.

Berry, C. L. 1973. The establishment of the elastic structure of arterial bifurcation and branches. Atherosclerosis 18: 117–127.

Boughner, D. R., and M. R. Roach. 1971a. Effect of low frequency vibration on the arterial wall. Circ. Res. 29: 136–144.

Boughner, D. R., and M. R. Roach. 1971b. Etiology of pulmonary artery dilatation and hilar dance in atrial septal defect. Circ. Res. 28: 415–425.

Brech, R., and B. J. Bellhouse. 1973. Flow in branching vessels. Cardiovasc. Res. 7: 593–600.

Canham, P. B., J. G. Walmsley, and J. F. H. Smith. 1976. The morphometry and sterology of cerebral arterial bifurcations, pp. 415–418. Fourth International Congress for Sterology. National Bureau of Standards Special Publication 431. U.S. Government Printing Office, Washington, D.C.

Caro, C. G., J. M. Fitz-Gerald, and R. C. Schroter. 1971. Atheroma and arterial wall shear. Observation, correlation and proposal of a shear dependent mass transfer mechanism for atherogenesis. Proc. Roy. Soc. (Biol.) 177: 109–159.

Christophersen, E. B., A. G. May, J. A. DeWeese, and C. G. Rob. 1965. Hemodynamic alterations in arteries with critical stenosis during acute hemorrhage. Surg. Gyn. Obstet. 121: 832–836.

Cornhill, J. F., and M. R. Roach. 1974. Quantitative method for evaluation of atherosclerotic lesions. Atherosclerosis 20: 131–136.

Cornhill, J. F., and M. R. Roach. 1975. A quantitative study of the localization of atherosclerotic lesions in the rabbit aorta. Atherosclerosis (in press).

Crowe, W. J., Jr., and L. J. Krovetz. 1972. Studies of arterial branching in models using flow birefringence. Med. Biol. Eng. 10: 415–426.

Ferguson, G. G. 1970a. Physical factors in the initiation, growth, and rupture of human intracranial saccular aneurysms. Ph. D. Thesis, University of Western Ontario.

Ferguson, G. G. 1970b. Turbulence in human intracranial saccular aneurysms. J. Neurosurg. 33: 485–497.

Ferguson, G. G. 1972a. Direct measurement of mean and pulsatile blood pressure at operation in human intracranial saccular aneurysms. J. Neurosurg. 36: 560–563.

Ferguson, G. G. 1972b. Physical factors in the initiation, growth, and rupture of human intracranial saccular aneurysms. J. Neurosurg. 37: 666–677.

Ferguson, G. G., and M. R. Roach. 1972a. Physical factors in the initiation, growth, and rupture of human intracranial saccular aneurysms. J. Neurosurg. 37: 666–677.

Ferguson, G. G., and M. R. Roach. 1972*b*. Flow conditions at bifurcations as determined in glass models, with reference to the focal distribution of vascular lesions. *In* D. H. Bergel (ed.), Cardiovascular Fluid Dynamics. Vol. 2, pp. 141–156. Academic Press, London and New York.

Flaherty, J. T., J. E. Pierce, V. J. Ferrans, D. J. Patel, W. K. Tucher, and D. L. Fry. 1972. Endothelial nuclear patterns in the canine arterial tree with particular reference to hemodynamic events. Circ. Res. 30: 23–33.

Foreman, J. E. K., and K. J. Hutchison. 1970. Arterial wall vibration distal to stenoses in isolated arteries of dog and man. Circ. Res. 26: 583–590.

Fry, D. L. 1968. Acute vascular endothelial changes associated with increased blood velocity gradients. Circ. Res. 22: 165–197.

Fry, D. L. 1969*a*. Certain chemorheological considerations regarding the blood saccular interface with particular reference to coronary artery disease. Circulation. 39(Suppl.): 38–59.

Fry, D. L. 1969*b*. Certain histological and chemical responses of the vascular interface to acutely induced mechanical stress in the aorta of the dog. Circ. Res. 24: 93–108.

Gosling, R. G., D. L. Newman, N. L. R. Bowden, and K. W. Twinn. 1971. The area ratio of normal aortic junctions. Brit. J. Radiol. 44: 850–853.

Hutchison, K. J. 1974. Effect of variation of transmural pressure on the frequency response of isolated segments of canine carotid arteries. Circ. Res. 35: 742–751.

Kamiya, A., and T. Togawa. 1972. Optimal branching structure of the vascular tree. Bull. Math. Biophys. 34: 431–438.

Killen, D. A., and S. U. Oh. 1968. Quantitation of the severity of arterial stenosis by pressure gradient measurement. Am. Surg. 34: 341–349.

Kindt, G. W., and J. K. Youmans. 1969. The effect of stricture length on critical arterial stenosis. Surg. Gyn. Obstet. 128: 729–734.

Kreuzer, W., and W. G. Schenk. 1971. Hemodynamic effects of vasodilatation in "critical" arterial stenosis. Arch. Surg. 103: 277–282.

Lallemand, R. C., K. G. E. Brown, and P. S. Boulter. 1972. Vessel dimensions in premature atheromatous disease of the aortic bifurcation. Brit. Med. J. 2: 255–256.

Lallemand, R. C., R. G. Gosling, and D. L. Newman. 1972. Role of the bifurcation in atheromatosis of the abdominal aorta. Surg. Gyn. Obstet. 137: 987–990.

Macfarlane, T. W. R. 1975. The geometry of cerebral arterial bifurcations and its modification with static distending pressure. M. Sc. Thesis, University of Western Ontario.

Malcolm, A. D. 1976. Flow phenomena at bifurcations and branches in relation to atherogenesis. M. Sc. Thesis. University of Western Ontario.

Mann, F. C., J. F. Herrick, H. E. Essex, and E. J. Baldes. 1900. The effect on the blood flow of decreasing the lumen of a blood vessel. Surgery 4: 249–252.

May, A. G., L. Van den Berg, J. A. DeWeese, and C. G. Rob. 1963. Critical arterial stenosis. Surgery 54: 250–259.

May, A. G., J. A. DeWeese, and C. G. Rob. 1963. Critical arterial stenosis. Surgery 54: 250–259.

Montenegro, M. R., and Eggen, D. A. 1968. Topography of atherosclerosis in the coronary arteries. Lab. Invest. 18: 586–593.

Murray, C. D. 1926a. The physiological principle of minimum work. I. The vascular system and the cost of blood volume. Proc. Nat. Acad. Sci. U.S. 12: 207–214.

Murray, C. D. 1926b. The physiological principle of minimum work. II. Oxygen exchange in capillaries. Proc. Nat. Acad. Sci. U.S. 12: 299–304.

Newman, D. L., R. G. Gosling, and N. L. R. Bowden. 1971. Changes in aortic distensibility and area ratio with the development of atherosclerosis. Atherosclerosis 14: 231–240.

Nyström, S. H. M. 1963. Development of intracranial aneurysms as revealed by electron microscopy. J. Neurosurg. 20: 329–337.

Roach, M. R. 1963a. Changes in arterial distensibility as a cause of poststenotic dilatation. Am. J. Cardiol. 12: 802–815.

Roach, M. R. 1963b. Poststenotic dilatation in arteries. In D. H. Bergel (ed.), Cardiovascular Fluid Dynamics. Vol. 2, pp. 111–139. Academic Press, London and New York.

Roach, M. R. 1963c. An experimental study of the production and time course of poststenotic dilatation in the femoral and carotid arteries of adult dogs. Circ. Res. 13: 537–551.

Roach, M. R. 1970a. Role of vascular wall elastic tissue in hemostasis. Thromb. et Diathesis Haemorrh. 40(Suppl.): 59–77.

Roach, M. R. 1970b. Reversibility of poststenotic dilatation in the femoral arteries of dogs. Circ. Res. 27: 985–993.

Roach, M. R. 1975. Flow separation: possible effects on the vessel wall. In J. Hirsh (ed.), Platelets, Drugs, and Thrombosis, pp. 70–77. S. Karger, Basel.

Roach, M. R. Hemodynamic factors in arterial stenosis and post-stenotic dilatation. In W. E. Stehbens (ed.), Hemodynamics in Pathology. Charles C Thomas, Springfield, Ill. In press.

Roach, M. R., and A. C. Burton. 1957. The reason for the shape of the distensibility curves of arteries. Can. J. Biochem. Physiol. 35: 681–690.

Roach, M. R., and C. G. Drake. 1965. Ruptured cerebral aneurysms caused by micro-organisms. N. Engl. J. Med. 273: 240–244.

Roach, M. R., and J. Fletcher. Altered renal flow in the localization of sudanophilic lesions in rabbit aortas. In G. W. Manning and M. D. Haust (eds.), Atherosclerosis. Plenum, New York. In press.

Roach, M. R., J. Fletcher, and J. F. Cornhill. The effect of the duration of cholesterol feeding in the development of atherosclerotic lesions in the rabbit aorta. Atherosclerosis. In press.

Roach, M. R., and K. Harvey. 1964. Experimental investigation of post-stenotic dilatation in isolated arteries. Can. J. Physiol. Pharm. 42: 53–63.

Roach, M. R., and A. C. MacDonald. 1970. Poststenotic dilatation in renal arteries. Invest. Radiol. 5: 311–315.

Roach, M. R., S. Scott, and G. G. Ferguson. 1972. The hemodynamic importance of the geometry of bifurcations in the circle of Willis (Glass Model Studies). Stroke 3: 255–267.

Rodkiewicz, C. M., and C. L. Roussel. 1973. Fluid mechanics in a large arterial bifurcation. J. Fluids Eng. 95: 108–112.

Rosen, R. 1967. Optimality Principles in Biology. Butterworths, London, Chap. 3, pp. 41–60. 198 p.

Schroter, R. C., and M. F. Sudlow. 1969. Flow patterns in models of the human bronchial airways. Resp. Physiol. 7: 341–355.

Scott, S., G. G. Ferguson, and M. R. Roach. 1972. Comparison of the elastic properties of human intracranial arteries and aneurysms. Can. J. Physiol. Pharm. 50: 328–332.

Shipley, R. E., and D. E. Gregg. 1944. The effect of external constriction of a blood vessel on blood vessel on blood flow. Am. J. Physiol. 141: 289–296.

Sinclair, A. S. 1974. The dynamic response of a cylindrical elastic vessel to disturbed flow: A case for arterial resonance. Ph. D. Thesis, University of Western Ontario.

Solberg, L. A., and Eggen, D. A. 1971. Localization and sequence of development of atherosclerotic lesions in the carotid and vertebral arteries. Circulation 43: 711–724.

Stehbens, W. E. 1959. Turbulence of blood flow. Quart. J. Exp. Physiol. 44: 110–117.

Stehbens, W. E. 1974. Changes in the cross-sectional area of the arterial fork. Angiology 25: 561–575.

Stockley, D. F. 1971. The effect of stenosis diameter and length on the distribution, spectrum, and energy of poststenotic arterial wall vibrations. M. Sc. Thesis, University of Western Ontario.

Vonruden, W. J., F. W. Blaisdell, A. D. Hall, and A. N. Thomas. 1964. Multiple arterial stenoses: Effect on blood flow. Arch. Surg. 89: 307–315.

Walmsley, J. G., and P. B. Canham. 1973. The orientation of smooth muscle at the middle cerebral artery bifurcation. Proc. Can. Fed. Biol. Soc. 6:17.

Zamir, M. 1976. The role of shear forces in arterial branching. J. Gen. Physiol. 67: 213–222.

Zamir, M. Optimality principles in vascular branching. J. Theor. Biol. In press.

Cardiovascular Flow Dynamics and Measurements
Edited by N. H. C. Hwang and N. A. Normann
Copyright 1977   University Park Press   Baltimore

chapter 15

MECHANICS OF PULSATILE FLOWS OF RELEVANCE TO THE CARDIOVASCULAR SYSTEM

A. K. M. Fazle Hussain

ABSTRACT

Following a brief survey of the flow characteristics of the cardiovascular system, the governing equations and the boundary-layer phenomena are reviewed. The diffusion of vorticity and the layered phase lag of motion in unsteady viscous layers are discussed. Then different methods for analyzing time-dependent boundary-layer flows are summarized. Some general observations regarding transition, hydrodynamic stability, and the characteristics of turbulent shear flows are then made. The role of viscosity and pulsation in transition to turbulent flow and various interpretations of the Reynolds number are discussed.

Unsteady turbulent flows are complex to analyze; periodic turbulent flows are a simple class of unsteady turbulent flows. The concept of periodic ensemble average, namely, *phase average*, introduced by Hussain in 1969, is necessary for separating a flow variable into its mean, periodic, and (random) fluctuating components. The governing equations for the three components and the interplay between them are discussed as a way of understanding the mechanics of pulsatile turbulent flows. Some recent experiments involving periodic turbulent

Preparation of the manuscript was made possible through the financial support of the U.S. National Science Foundation under Grant ENG75-15226 and of the U.S. Office of Naval Research under Grant N00014-76-C-0128 and partially through the National Institute of Health under Grant HM-1330-06 awarded by the Baylor College of Medicine.

541

flows are reviewed and the effect of controlled flow pulsation on vortex shedding and vortex pairing is discussed briefly.

Finally, two experiments of possible direct significance to cardiovascular flows are presented. In the first case, the effects of controlled pulsation on the circular jet–orifice flow and the role of organized vortex rings are discussed; this study may be of relevance to the flow through arterial and valvular stenoses including coarctations. In the second case, in vitro measurements behind a natural human mitral valve are presented. Signals from an X hot-film probe are analyzed digitally to obtain the phase-averaged, longitudinal and lateral periodic velocities, turbulent intensities, and Reynolds stress at different instants of the diastolic and systolic phases. From these data, profiles of these phase-averaged quantities at different instants of the cardiac cycle are derived. The large values of Reynolds stress and correlation coefficient during the diastolic phase indicate that flow in the ventricle is turbulent.

1 INTRODUCTION

1.1 Purpose

The purpose of this chapter is to provide an introduction to fluid dynamics and the mechanics of pulsatile flows with emphasis on those aspects that may be of relevance to cardiovascular flow systems; it is addressed primarily to physiologic and bioengineering researchers. While fluid mechanics cannot be treated well without mathematics, the loss of rigor due to intentional underplay of mathematics has been offset by an overindulgence in the discussion of mechanics. The minimal mathematics involved in this chapter, however, is necessary to provide some understanding of the basic fluid dynamical considerations. Even to those without any familiarity with the mathematical notations used, reading through the text without serious attention to the equations may prove rewarding.

1.2 The System

The human body provides the fluid dynamicist with a very versatile flow laboratory: it involves flows of blood, air, lymph, urine, lubrication fluids,[1] and a variety of convective and diffusive transports of foods and nutrients, and various other chemicals. Although it is limited by the noninclusion of extremely high Reynolds numbers of aerodynamic, geo-

---

[1] This chapter is limited to blood flows only.

physical, and galactic consequence, the Reynolds numbers involved do cover a wide range (up to 15,000). For concise surveys of physiologic fluid dynamics see Lighthill (1972, 1975), and for a general introduction see Carlson, Johnson, and Calvert (1965), Jones (1969), and Rushmer (1970). Figure 1 represents a simplistic hydraulic analog of the vertebrate cardio-vascular tree. Note that typically the length of each of the millions of capillaries is short; together, they hold only about 6% of the total blood; they have the total largest flow cross section and lowest average velocity. In the arteries, the pressure oscillates between 80 and 120 mm Hg; the arteries are much thicker than the veins, which support the low-pressure (0–10 mm Hg) return flow. For limited aspects of venous flows see Holt (1969), Katz, Chen, and Moreno (1969), Snyder and Rideout (1969), and Brower and Noordergraaf (1973). Our discussion relates to the blood flow through heart and arteries only; for reviews of capillary flows see Fitz-

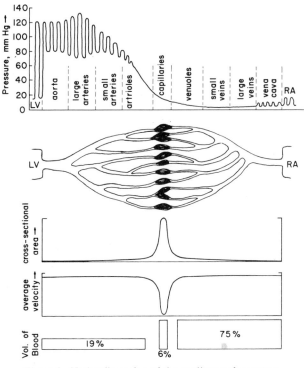

Figure 1. Hydraulic analog of the cardiovascular system.

Gerald (1972), Skalak (1972), and Charm and Kurland (1974). Flow in the arteries is pulsatile at the rate of 70–80 beats per minute; typically 0.3 sec systole and 0.5 sec diastole. Spectral analysis of pressure and velocity pulses shows that the oscillations include first 4–6 harmonics of the heart rate; at locations where the flow is turbulent or highly disturbed, however, a larger spectral bandwidth is present.

Before launching into the classical fluid dynamical aspects of the cardiovascular system, it is desirable to be aware of the limitations of the system. The characteristics of both the fluid (material) and the configuration involved in the cardiovascular system are quite different from those encountered in classical hydro-aerodynamics.

1.3 Material Characteristics

Blood is a viscous, living fluid suspension; typically 1/13th the weight of the body and 40–50% of its volume consist of suspended small-sized, deformable particles called the *formed elements;* the remaining 50–60% is liquid medium, called *plasma.* The formed elements consist primarily of highly flexible,[2] biconcave, discoid red blood cells or erythrocytes (about 8 μ in diameter and 2 μ wide); the less numerous, semitransparent white blood cells (leukocytes); and the roughly disk-shaped platelets (or thrombocytes). Typically there are 5×10^6 erythrocytes, 10^4 leukocytes, and 3 $\times 10^5$ thrombocytes in each cubic millimeter of blood. The plasma contains colloidal (macromolecular) proteins, 7–9% by volume, dissolved in 90% water plus traces of salt, sugar, foods, hormones, carbon dioxide, wastes, etc. The formed elements are slightly heavier (sp.gr. 1.09) than plasma (sp.gr. 1.03); this difference as well as the particle sizes are small enough to maintain a homogeneous state when in motion. (The Reynolds number of the formed elements is small so that they faithfully track the fluid.) Since we do not concern ourselves here with microcirculation, we can regard blood as a continuum of a single homogeneous substance of specific gravity 1.06. Even when blood flow is turbulent, the smallest scales (eddies) are many times the size of the erythrocytes so that blood flow in the arteries is indeed a *continuum.* The continuum hypothesis is obviously invalid at the plasma wall layer (see below).

Viscosity is a measure of the resistance to the flow of a fluid and is

---

[2] The flexible constitution of the erythrocytes is crucial for their passage through capillaries (which are relatively nondistensible and noncontractile; Zweifach, 1972) and alveoli (Weibel, 1972). Inside its deformable but essentially unstretchable membrane it contains the nearly Newtonian hemoglobin solution.

responsible for maintaining arterial pressure; for a given tube the pressure drop is higher with a fluid of higher viscosity. The (absolute) shear viscosity[3] μ of a fluid is the ratio of shear stress τ to shear rate $\partial u/\partial y$; when it is constant at all shear rates the fluid is called Newtonian; otherwise it is non-Newtonian. For the latter case μ, being a function of shear rate, is called the effective (or apparent) viscosity. Usually, ν (defined as μ/ρ, where ρ is the fluid density) rather than μ becomes the material property of interest; because its units $[L^2/T]$ do not contain mass or force units, it is called kinematic viscosity.

The viscosity of plasma is primarily due to proteins; plasma is nearly Newtonian; at body temperature the value of plasma viscosity ν is about 1.5 mm^2/sec. Values of viscosities of both plasma and whole blood vary somewhat between results reported by different investigators.

The viscosity of whole blood is a function of hematocrit. Particles in suspension in a fluid increase viscous (dissipation) loss due to the disturbance velocity field shear rates induced by the particles. The net effect is that of an equivalent fluid with higher shear viscosity. This shows that for a given heart power, the benefit of higher hematocrit in carrying more oxygen is offset by a corresponding decrease in flow, due to higher viscosity, so that there is an optimum hematocrit that maximizes oxygen transport (or, say, hemoglobin flow). This optimum hematocrit is 27% for camels, 32% for sheep, and 47% for man (Burton, 1972). In view of the shape of the erythrocyte, the maximum hematocrit possible without cell deformation is 63%. (Hematocrit can exceed this limit when one is afflicted with polycythemia and in children.) With increasing hematocrits, the blood kinematic viscosity increases nonlinearly (i.e., concave upwards), increasing nearly linearly up to about 4.5 mm^2/sec at the normal hematocrits of 40–50% and then increasing rapidly; at 80% hematocrit the kinematic viscosity is about 8 times that of plasma. Blood viscosity increases 2.2 times when the temperature is decreased from 37 to 0°C.

Blood is basically a non-Newtonian fluid; the application of viscometry shows that with decreasing shear rates its apparent viscosity increases substantially. This effect is increasingly pronounced with increasing hematocrits, as expected. Normal human blood viscosity is constant for shear rates above 100 sec^{-1} and can be represented by the Newtonian equation $\tau^{1/2} = \mu^{1/2}\gamma^{1/2}$. Merrill and Pelletier (1967) have shown that below the shear rate of 20 sec^{-1} the stress–strain rate relation is of the

---

[3] This contrasts the bulk viscosity which is not of concern here.

type proposed by Casson (1959) for shear thinning fluid like printer's ink; i.e.,

$$\tau^{1/2} = \mu^{1/2}\gamma^{1/2} + Y^{1/2}$$

where Y is the yield shear stress, i.e., the stress that must be exceeded before flow occurs (the yield stress is independent of temperature, increases with hematocrit, and is a strong function of proteins; Cokelet, 1972). The transition from the Casson to the Newtonian region occurs in the shear rate range $16-100$ sec^{-1}; it is interesting to note that the slope of the $\tau^{1/2}$ versus $\gamma^{1/2}$ curve in the Casson range is that of the Newtonian range. Merrill et al. (1966) have shown that the yield stress is due to reversible aggregation of erythrocytes; it is zero in suspensions containing no fibrinogen; it increases with higher concentration of fibrinogen; it is greater in suspension of erythrocytes in their original plasma than in fractionated fibrinogen; and plasma proteins other than fibrinogen have no effect in the absence of fibrinogen. Merrill and Pelletier (1967) suggest that above the shear rate of 20 sec^{-1} the erythrocyte contact time is too small for the development of aggregation. However, the in vivo study of Frasher, Wayland, and Meiselman (1968) indicates that factors other than fibrinogen may also be involved. For further discussion on yield stress see Chien et al. (1970) and Charm and Kurland (1972).

One peculiarity of blood flow is that its apparent viscosity drops with decreasing tube internal diameter below 1 mm; in a 20-μ-diameter tube, the asymptotic viscosity is 50% of its value in a large tube (see Burton, 1972; McDonald, 1974). This effect is named after Fahraeus and Lindquist, who in 1931 first observed it; their observation also resulted in the recognition of the presence of a cell-free zone near the wall, i.e., the plasma wall layer (Phibbs, 1968; Sevilla-Larra, 1968; Barbee and Cokelet, 1971; Hyman, 1973). This effect, explained variously and investigated extensively through both theoretical and experimental efforts, would be important only when the layer thickness (about 5 μ) is comparable to the lumen size. Interesting consequences of this "pinch" effect are that the erythrocytes travel with a higher average velocity than plasma and that the viscosity is lowest near the wall. Thus the velocity gradient near the wall must be higher than that of the Poiseuille flow at the same axial pressure gradient; this suggests a flatter velocity profile at the tube center, which has been confirmed by experiments.

One important fluid mechanical aspect is blood trauma or hemolysis; the threshold value of the shear stress for causing cell damage decreases with increasing exposure time. An examination of the literature reveals no study of the effect of time-dependent stress on hemolysis. It seems that for time-dependent flows, the quantity $\gamma + \sqrt{\gamma'^2}$ should be the primary variable; here γ is the mean shear rate and $\sqrt{\gamma'^2}$ is the rms shear rate. This should be especially important for turbulent flows where the damage may be mostly due to turbulent shear rather than fluctuating pressure; it seems that, contrary to the claim of Blackshear (1972), in-bulk hemolysis is possible, at least in turbulent flows. In a turbulent flow, because the cells track the fluid, the average Reynolds stress $-\rho \overline{u'v'}$ is not the stress the cell is exposed to. However, because Lagrangian measurement[4] following the cell is impractical, local Eulerian rms strain rate, which can be measured with hot-film (possibly laser) anemometry, may provide an adequate measure of mechanical forces responsible for cell damage.

Note that, owing to an exceedingly thin boundary layer, wall shear stress in the entry region is much higher than in fully developed Poiseuille flow. Thus wall shear stress can be as high as 10^4 dynes/cm^2 in some arteries, while 1,500 dynes/cm^2 is the claimed long-duration threshold for cell damage (the stress threshold for platelet damage is much lower, about 10^2 dynes/cm^2). Although this may tend to suggest high wall shear as the cause of atherosclerosis prevalent in entry regions, these locations in branchings are also associated with separation, i.e., low shear.

Flow pulsation modifies the velocity profile in a fully developed tube flow of a Newtonian fluid. In a non-Newtonian fluid, the viscosity itself is modified through its dependence on the time-dependent strain rate of the pulsatile flow. For the cardiovascular system the non-Newtonian effect can be considered negligible (Kunz and Coulter, 1967).

When the flow is turbulent, the presence of erythrocytes seems to have

---

[4] Eulerian specification describes properties, e.g., velocity and pressure as a function of position in space (x) and time (t). These properties are associated with different fluid particles (elements) occupying x at different times t. Lagrangian specification, on the other hand, provides the time history of properties associated with an identifiable (material) fluid particle: the initial position X_0 (at time $t = 0$, say) of a particle (i.e., centroid of a fluid element) can be used to identify that particle; particle X_0 will be at different locations in the flow field at different times t. Thus $u(X_0, t)$, $p(X_0, t)$ are the velocity and pressure of that particle at time t: these are Lagrangian descriptions. For any location x in the laboratory coordinates $u(x,t)$, $p(x,t)$ are the Eulerian velocity and pressure at that location at any time t. Eulerian measurements are taken with a probe fixed with the flow boundary. Lagrangian information has to be obtained with a probe attached to a flowing fluid particle. Lagrangian description is unavoidable in particle dynamics. In fluid mechanics, we are usually interested in Eulerian description.

some influence on turbulence (Blick, Sabbah, and Stein, 1975); on the other hand, turbulence has been found to induce thrombus formation (Stein and Sabbah, 1974; Smith et al., 1972).

1.4 Configuration Characteristics

The characteristics of the configuration as well as boundary conditions put constraints on the flow. The configuration characteristics of the cardiovascular flow system include the distensibility of the tube walls, the frequent branchings, vascular taper and curvature, and non-fully developed nature of flow; the pathologic lesions of the vessel walls present yet additional peculiarities.

Note that, for pulsatile flows, similarity requires that both Reynolds number (UD/ν) and Strouhal number (nD/U) must be preserved between a prototype and its model. Thus both of these are important nondimensional parameters for pulsatile flows; the square root of the product of these two, which equals the ratio of arterial caliber to Stokes layer thickness, is an important parameter for periodic boundary layers (see Section 2.4).

1.4.1 Distensibility The flow vessels are distensible; their elasticity is due to the outermost elastic connective tissue. The distensibility of the arteries is essential in maintaining the forward flow of blood away from the heart even during diastole and in transferring the intermittent pumping of the heart to the steady continuous perfusion of blood through the capillaries so that steady, efficient exchange of materials between blood and tissues can occur. The distensibility is complicated by viscoelastic behavior, which is responsible for attenuation of the traveling pulse wave from the heart, and by nonlinear response in resisting different degrees of arterial distension. Loss of vessel distensibility results in various types of circulatory complications such as arteriosclerosis, hypertension, stroke, etc.

The aortic wall is elastic; with successive branching of the arterial tree the wall structure alters, becoming less distensible and more muscular. The transition from elastic aorta to muscular artery is gradual. Elasticity of a dog's aorta has been found to change from 3×10^6 dynes/cm^2 in the ascending part to 12×10^6 dynes/cm^2 in the abdomen—a fourfold increase. The change in arterial cross section during the cardiac cycle depends on location: for a dog it is 0.5% in the iliac artery and 16% in the pulmonary artery (Bergel, 1961). (For mechanical properties of arterial walls see Bergel, 1972, and Patel and Vaishnav, 1972.)

Unlike arteries, veins respond nonlinearly to stress; the elastic modulus of a dog's vena cava was found to increase 18 times as the pressure was increased from 0 to 20 mm Hg (Green, 1944).

1.4.2 Branched Network The cardiovascular (like the bronchial) system is a complex branched network whereby blood from the aorta passes through probably 20–30 successive branchings before reaching the millions of capillaries. The branching may be to a side and may be small such as the intercostals or large such as the renals; symmetric branching such as aortic-iliac also occurs. At each branching, the ratio β (called the branching coefficient) of cross-sectional area of the branches to that of the parent vessel is an important parameter; data show that β is typically in the range 1.1–1.4 in arterial bifurcations. For a 13-kg dog the total capillary cross section has been found to be 625 cm^2 while the aorta has a cross section of 0.8 cm^2 (Rushmer, 1970). The precise area increase in man is not known, but it is at least 3 orders of magnitude. The mean blood velocity has been found to decrease from about 50 cm/sec in the aorta to about 0.07 cm/sec in the capillary. At early stages, β should be small in order to prevent separation and transition; at later stages, large β can be tolerated because the Reynolds numbers are low. Branchings have been found to lower the Reynolds number at which transition in a tube sets in; flow pulsation and reversal further decrease transition Reynolds numbers (Ferguson and Roach, 1972).

It seems that atherosclerosis is mostly associated with locations of arterial bifurcations, bends, and ostia, and locations of turbulent flow (Schwartz and Mitchell, 1962; Brech and Bellhouse, 1973); the pulsatility of the flow further aggravates atherogenesis at branchings (Friedman, O'Brien, and Ehrlich, 1975): either the high-shear or the low-shear interpretation of atherogenesis may still hold because both occur near branchings (Friedman and Ehrlich, 1975) and pulsation introduces large excursions of both over their steady flow values. In arterial branchings, it is not uncommon to have atherosclerotic lesion depositions of the kinds shown in Figures 2A–D. (The mechanics of arteriosclerotic plaque formation is far from being understood; it is clear that a combination of hemodynamic and biochemical factors plays the central role.) The plaque deposition may result in stenosis and eventually occlusion. The flow through a stenosis may produce discrete vortex lumps, the frequency of

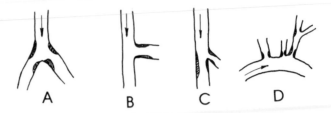

Figure 2. Some examples of atherosclerotic plaque formation at branches.

which may set the wall distal to the stenosis into resonance and thus introduce fatigue and poststenotic dilatation. These organized vortex lumps may also be the cause of systolic murmurs.

Distal to the ostium of a branch is also the beginning of the arterial wall boundary layer so that in addition to keeping a low length–diameter ratio of flow in arteries, branchings maintain the arterial flows in a state of entry flow. Symmetric branchings may also introduce aneurysms as at the bifurcations in cerebral arteries; aneurysms seem to be the result of wall rupture due to pulsatile flow impact rather than turbulence (Ferguson, 1970). The flow at branching may also roll up and shed periodic vortices (Stehbens, 1975), which is probably what Ferguson (1970) recorded as musical murmurs. This may be related to the secondary flows observed by Schroter and Sudlow (1969) in bifurcations. Although the latter study was concerned primarily with bronchial airways, the Reynolds number range is relevant to the arterial flows. They found that two vortices were formed in the daughter tube when flow entered the branches, but four vortices were formed in the parent tube when the flow was from the bifurcations to the parent tube.

The anastomotic angles of bypass grafts are of interest from the point of view of fluid mechanics. It is clear that a small angle with the branch artery would reduce separation and vortex formation at the junction (unlike the situation shown in Figure 2B, for example). However, this kind of isolated junctions does not pose any major problem, because the additional pressure drop due to local turbulent losses is insignificant; autoregulation and collateral circulation, however, would tend to mask this loss.

1.4.3 Entry Flow and Curvature   Because a long length is required for the flow in a pipe to be fully developed, flows in all the large arteries are entry region flows. Thus the Poiseuille relation for pipe flow is not applicable[5] and the wall shear stress is higher than that given by the Poiseuille equation. The pressure drop in the entry region is large because the free stream has to be accelerated from the initial velocity U_0 to a maximum velocity of $2U_0$ so that increase in kinetic energy is $\frac{1}{2}\rho U_0^2$. Taking into account the extra wall shear stress due to the thin boundary layer in the entry region, the correction is about $0.7\rho U_0^2$. In view of the numerous subsequent branchings, the total additional pressure drop is indeed substantial.

The curvature of a streamline produces a radial pressure gradient $\rho u^2/r$ (u is the axial velocity and r is the radius of curvature), so that a curved tube with potential flow has a higher velocity nearer the inner wall. The analyses of Singh (1974) and Yao and Berger (1975) indicate that the boundary-layer effect moves the peak toward the outer wall. The latter study shows that the entry length is shortened by tube bend; this still cannot explain nearly fully developed flow in man and dog found by Schultz (1972).

In a curved pipe flow the higher-velocity central fluid has a higher inertia than the boundary-layer fluid at the same radius of curvature. This causes the core fluid to move outward with respect to tube center and return, for continuity, toward the inner wall through the boundary, and thus produce a "secondary flow" normal to the "primary flow." The cross-sectional view of the pipe shows two counterrotating vortical motions (Dean, 1927, 1928) so that net axial vorticity is zero. Dye filament pictures by Scarton (1975), however, show the presence of four vortices. Secondary flow, while enhancing lateral mixing (Caro, 1966), also

---

[5] The precise determination of the entrance length in a pipe is difficult because the flow asymptotically becomes fully developed at infinite length. However, the length x_L where the centerline velocity reaches within 1% of the asymptotic velocity may be denoted as the entrance length. The entrance length in a pipe depends on the upstream condition and the pipe Reynolds number Re; for a pipe with a flat entrance profile the entrance length is given as $x_L/D = 0.08$ Re $+ 0.7$; the constant 0.7 is to account for the limiting case of creeping flow (White, 1974). For a peak Reynolds number of 8,000, this length is about 640. For man the length from aortic valve to lower thoracic aorta divided by the average diameter of aorta is 10–15. The corresponding length/diameter for a dog is about 20. It is surprising that measurements by Schultz (1972) indicate that the velocity profiles at the lower thoracic aorta in a dog and in a man are nearly fully developed. It is to be recognized that the entrance length in a pulsatile flow will also oscillate with time. On the other hand, Poiseuille flow will never be established if the period of oscillation is small compared to the flow development time R^2/ν (see Section 2.4).

appears to suppress transition in a curved tube (Lighthill, 1975). Secondary flow is produced in turbulent flows in ducts with sharp corners, e.g., rectangular, triangular, and trapezoidal cross sections, due to imbalance in turbulent stresses at the corners.

Unsteady flow in a curved tube is complex; distensibility and the noncircularity of the tube, as well as the presence of branching and taper, further compound the complexity. Irregularity in the aortic arch flow arises from branching, from aortic valve motion, from vortices originating from the ventricle and valve leaflet, and from noncircularity of the lumen and surface roughness.

Dean's calculations for steady flow in curved rigid tubes were limited to low Dean numbers $0 \leqslant De \leqslant 96$, while aortic arch flow values can reach as high as 5,000. The Dean number De is defined as $Re \sqrt{(32R/L)}$, where R is the tube radius, and L the radius of curvature. Solutions up to $De = 5,000$ were obtained later (McConalogue and Srivastava, 1968; Greenspan, 1973); the location of peak velocity was found to move outward with increasing Dean numbers. Lyne (1970) and Zalosh and Nelson (1973) studied pulsatile flow in a curved tube. Fully developed pulsatile flow in a curved elastic tube has been studied theoretically by Chandran et al. (1974). Both Lyne and Chandran et al. show quadrihelical secondary flow, but it is different from that observed by Scarton (1975); they also show a secondary flow in the tube interior opposite to that for steady flows, which is confirmed experimentally by Lyne. Chandran et al. show that the secondary flow oscillates between quadrihelical and bihelical twice in each cycle and that the velocity maximum occurs near the inner wall.

Smith (1975) has explained the change of the secondary flow direction in the potential core. Bertelsen (1975) has experimentally verified the validity of the theoretic results of Lyne (1970) and Zalosh and Nelson (1973) for high Reynolds numbers.

1.4.4 Atheroma Depositions of fatty substances (atheroma) cause hardening of the arteries (atherosclerosis) and thus decrease the distensibility and retard the ability of the arteries to transport blood. There appear to be two distinct, somewhat contradictory, possible causes of incipient atheroma (see Fry 1968, 1973; Caro, Fitz-Gerald, and Schroter, 1971; Gessner, 1973). It is generally agreed that hemodynamic factors are significant in the pathogenesis of atherosclerosis (Patel et al., 1974; Taylor, 1972; Lighthill, 1975).

Keeping in mind the above peculiarities of the cardiovascular flow system, we now proceed formally to review the governing equations and some pulsatile laminar and turbulent flows of relevance to the cardio-vascular system.

2 GOVERNING EQUATIONS AND UNSTEADY LAMINAR FLOWS

2.1 Mass Conservation

In the cardiovascular system the material velocities encountered are low enough that relativistic effects are absent. Thus the mass of an identified collection of matter must be constant.

Mass balance for the control volume V 'Figure 3) of a fluid element gives[6]

$$\int_V \left[\frac{\partial}{\partial x_j} (\rho u_j) + \frac{\partial}{\partial t} \rho \right] dV = 0$$

Because this relation is valid for any ...bitrarily small volume V, the integrand must be identically equal to zero everywhere, i.e.,[7]

$$\frac{1}{\rho} \frac{D\rho}{Dt} + \frac{\partial u_j}{\partial x_j} = 0 \tag{1}$$

This is the *mass conservation or continuity equation*. The volume of a given material element can change only through movement of its material surface, i.e.,

$$\frac{DV}{Dt} = \oint_S \mathbf{u} \cdot \mathbf{n} \, dS = \int_V \nabla \cdot \mathbf{u} \, dV$$

Hence the local rate of change of volume of a fluid element is

$$\lim_{V \to 0} \frac{1}{V} \frac{DV}{Dt} = \nabla \cdot \mathbf{u} = \frac{\partial u_j}{\partial x_j} \tag{2}$$

---

[6] The Cartesian tensor notation and repeated index summation convention are followed.

[7] The derivative Df/Dt represents the rate of change of a property f at (x,t) associated with a particle which is at $\mathbf{x}$, at time t, and is thus identical with the conventional derivative df/dt. It is not the Lagrangian derivative, but the Eulerian derivative "following the motion of the fluid"; engineers use the upper case symbol and call it substantial or material derivative to emphasize its distinction from the partial derivative $\partial f/\partial t$.

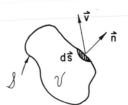

Figure 3. Mass balance in a control volume.

This is the local rate of change of volume per unit volume or *dilatation*. For a fluid element to be incompressible,

$$\nabla \cdot \mathbf{u} = 0 \tag{3a}$$

$$\therefore \quad \frac{D\rho}{Dt} = 0 \tag{3b}$$

and the corresponding fluid motion is called *isochoric* and the velocity vector field *solenoidal*. Thus, even though no fluid is truly incompressible, i.e., density is not independent of pressure, for cardiovascular flows the fluid may be regarded as incompressible provided that Eq. 3a and hence Eq. 3b is nearly satisfied. Note that Eq. 3b represents an incompressible flow rather than fluid as change of density with time and space is permitted as long as these two changes cancel each other.

The conditions (Batchelor, 1970, Section 3.6) under which a flow can be regarded as nearly incompressible are

$$
\begin{array}{lll}
\text{(i)} & U^2/c^2 \ll 1 & \\
\text{(ii)} & \omega^2 L^2/c^2 \ll 1 & \\
\text{(iii)} & \rho g L/\gamma p \ll 1 & \qquad (4) \\
\text{(iv)} & \dfrac{\beta U \nu}{c_p L} \ll 1 & \\
\text{(v)} & \dfrac{k}{\rho c_p} \dfrac{\beta \theta}{LU} \ll 1 &
\end{array}
$$

where U is the characteristic velocity, L the characteristic length, c the speed of sound, ρ the density of fluid, ν the kinematic viscosity, k the thermal conductivity, c_p the specific heat at constant pressure, β the thermal expansion coefficient, θ the temperature difference, γ the specific heat ratio, ω the circular frequency, p the pressure, and g the acceleration due to gravity.

The first condition requires that the Mach number be much smaller than one, the third requires the scale height in the gravity field to be much larger than the flow length scale, the fourth requires that viscous dissipation be not exceedingly high and the fifth requires that large amounts of heat conduction not be involved. In the cardiovascular system, as in most engineering systems, these four conditions are seldom violated. Only the second condition is important in unsteady flows and can be violated in ultrasonics but not in the cardiovascular system. Thus cardiovascular flows can indeed be regarded incompressible.

2.2 Momentum Balance

The most important fluid dynamical equation is that of the balance of momentum,

$$\rho \frac{Du_i}{Dt} = \rho b_i + \frac{\partial \sigma_{ij}}{\partial x_j} \tag{5}$$

where b_i is the body force per unit mass and σ_{ij} the stress tensor. For a Newtonian fluid under Stokes assumptions,

$$\sigma_{ij} = -p\delta_{ij} + 2\mu[e_{ij} - \tfrac{1}{3}(\nabla \cdot \mathbf{u})\delta_{ij}] \tag{6}$$

so that the balance of momentum equation becomes

$$\rho \frac{Du_i}{Dt} = \rho b_i - \frac{\partial p}{\partial x_i} + 2\mu \frac{\partial}{\partial x_j} \left[e_{ij} - \frac{1}{3} \left(\frac{\partial u_\kappa}{\partial x_\kappa} \right) \delta_{ij} \right]$$

where e_{ij} is the deformation tensor and δ_{ij} is the Kronecker delta. This is the celebrated Navier–Stokes equation; it was derived independently by Navier in 1822, Poisson in 1829, Saint-Venant in 1843, and Stokes in 1845.

For incompressible flow and in the gravitational field, the Navier–Stokes equation takes the form

$$\rho \frac{D\mathbf{u}}{Dt} = \rho \mathbf{g} - \nabla p + \mu \nabla^2 \mathbf{u} \tag{7a}$$

Taking p to represent pressure in excess of hydrostatic pressure, we get

$$\frac{D\mathbf{u}}{Dt} = -\frac{1}{\rho} \nabla p + \nu \nabla^2 \mathbf{u} \tag{7b}$$

Taking a curl of this equation we get the equation for vorticity, $\boldsymbol{\zeta} \equiv \nabla \times \mathbf{u}$,

$$\frac{D\boldsymbol{\zeta}}{Dt} = (\boldsymbol{\zeta} \cdot \nabla)\mathbf{u} + \nu \nabla^2 \boldsymbol{\zeta} \tag{8}$$

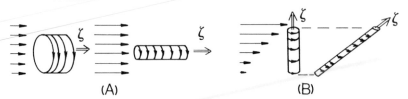

Figure 4. Physical interpretations of $\zeta \cdot \nabla u$; (*A*) vortex stretching, (*B*) vortex tilting.

Locally, vorticity is twice the angular velocity. Central to viscous fluid flows is the vorticity whose dynamics in an incompressible fluid (in a conservative body force field such as gravity) is given by Eq. 8. This equation shows that a fluid element without vorticity can obtain vorticity only through viscous diffusion due to the gradient of vorticity (the second term on the right-hand side).

The first term on the right-hand side represents both vortex stretching and tilting. The former occurs in the presence of a longitudinal velocity gradient (Figure 4A) so that as a longitudinal vortex filament is stretched, its angular velocity, i.e., vorticity, increases due to conservation of angular momentum (a principle taken advantage of by ice skating dancers). A vortex element aligned with a transverse velocity gradient will be tilted and thus stretched to produce vorticity (Figure 4B). As we will see later, turbulent flow is a field of three-dimensional random vorticity which is constantly generated through vortex stretching.

Equations 3a and 7 represent four scalar equations for the four unknowns $u(t)$, $v(t)$, $w(t)$, and $p(t)$; they thus constitute a well-posed problem that should have solutions for given initial and boundary conditions. Unfortunately, because of the nonlinearity (hidden in D/Dt) of the partial differential equation 7, it has no general solution. Consequently, solutions have been obtained for cases where the troublesome nonlinear terms identically disappear. These fall into two groups: the steady flow cases like fully developed flow in a pipe or a channel, and the periodic flow like that near an oscillating plate (see Section 2.4). In addition, approximate solutions have been obtained both analytically and numerically by applying the *Prandtl boundary-layer hypothesis*.

In the following we discuss some pulsatile flows of possible relevance to the cardiovascular system. The minimal amount of mathematics used is necessary to illustrate the physics of the flow.

2.2.1   *Oscillating Manometer*   The effect of oscillation of a fluid in a U-tube manometer is of interest for understanding manometer response;

the manometer is a very simple apparatus used for vascular pressure measurements. If the flow is laminar and inviscid the liquid oscillates with a simple harmonic motion with a circular frequency of $\sqrt{(2g/L)}$ where L is the length of the liquid column along the tube. Viscous effect obviously cannot be neglected; one must also take into consideration the entry length effect. If one assumes fully developed Poiseuille flow, one obtains the damped spring-mass oscillator type equation: the disturbance will decay or oscillate while decaying depending on tube diameter, length of liquid, and viscosity. If the flow is turbulent, an assumption of constant friction factor (valid at large Reynolds numbers) permits numerical solution. For further details see Streeter and Wylie (1975) and McDonald (1974).

2.3 Viscosity and Boundary-Layer Phenomena

Except for superfluid helium (below $-270.96°C$) all fluids have viscosity. However, there are regions of flow, e.g., core flow of pipe entrance region and flows around aerodynamic shapes, where the effects of viscosity are not brought into play so that the fluid behavior is inviscid. In spite of the inability of theoretical fluid dynamicists until the nineteenth century to recognize the role of viscosity (d'Alembert's paradox[8] being an example), a great deal of the mathematicians' preoccupation with the simple, ideal-fluid theory has not been in vain; the ideal-fluid theory can still be applied to some regions of flows of viscous fluids. A fluid adjacent to the wall experiences a drag at the wall due to viscosity so that the no-slip condition is satisfied, except at low Reynolds numbers and high Mach numbers

---

[8] The result that the drag of a rigid body moving with uniform velocity in an inviscid fluid of infinite extent and with irrotational motion everywhere is *zero* is called *d'Alembert's paradox*, because in real fluids the body will experience a drag consisting of *form drag* and *skin friction drag;* these two are respectively due to pressure and shear stress distributions on the surface of the body. The drag will be large in the case of a bluff body due to increased form drag caused by flow separation, which is again due to viscosity. For a streamlined body the drag is mainly due to skin friction. For two bodies with identical cross sections, a streamline body will have a much lower drag than a bluff body provided that the Reynolds number is not low; if the Reynolds number is very low, just the opposite will happen. If the boundary layer is turbulent, the drag of the bluff body will be decreased due to delayed separation while that of the streamline body will increase due to increased skin friction. Golf balls have dimples for inducing turbulence in the boundary layer so that their drag is reduced through decreased form drag.

It must be recognized that when a body is moving near a free surface or with supersonic speed the body experiences a different kind of drag (*wave drag*) for which the d'Alembert's paradox does not arise.

(these exceptions do not apply in liquid flows); here we assume the no-slip condition to hold.

When a fluid moves over a solid (or flexible) wall, especially at high Reynolds numbers, the effect of viscosity is felt only over a thin region adjacent to the boundary; the flow outside this region can be treated as inviscid. This thin region adjacent to the boundary is the *boundary layer;* it is this region where the adjustment of the fluid velocity from free-stream to the wall velocity takes place. It is characterized by the presence of vorticity which is generated at the wall and continually diffused away from the wall by the action of viscosity (this diffusion is analogous to heat conduction and is denoted by the second term on the right-hand side of Eq. 8). However, vorticity of a fluid element as it is convected downstream is also affected by rotation (tilting) and stretching of the vortex lines, this effect being represented by the first term on the right-hand side of Eq. 8. The boundary is a source of vorticity but a sink for momentum (Figure 5), the wall shear stress accounting for the loss of momentum.

It is interesting to note that mathematicians and theoretical hydro-dynamicists until the beginning of the twentieth century did not recognize that even though the boundary layer would continue to shrink as the viscosity is reduced to zero, the ideal-fluid behavior permitting fluid slip over a boundary is not a limiting case of the viscous flow because the no-slip condition must always be satisfied even in the presence of an extremely small viscosity.[9] The wide discrepancy between theoretical pre-dictions based on ideal-fluid theory and experimental results remained unexplained because the role of viscosity in producing large drag through separation and transition was not recognized for a long time.[10] It was only in 1904 that Prandtl first bridged the gap by proposing that viscosity effects were large and comparable in magnitude to the inertia effects in layers adjacent to solid boundaries and in other (e.g., free-shear) layers, the thickness of which decreases with increasing Reynolds numbers. It was

---

[9] The condition of zero relative velocity of the fluid at a solid surface was shown as early as 1851 by Stokes to be the only tenable boundary condition for the equations of motion in a viscous fluid. This assumption was confirmed by his wide range of experiments as well as by the capillary-tube resistance experiments of Poiseuille in 1840 and Hagen in 1839. Some writers then suggested that the no-slip condition was valid only for slow motion and that in fast motion a stagnant fluid layer adjacent to the wall will provide a cushion. But there was no mention of the continuous variation of velocity in the layer due to viscosity nor was there any mention of the values of pressure in this layer.

[10] Many sophisticated ideal-fluid analyses included flows near walls with enormous adverse pressure gradients or with sharp corners which would in reality cause flow separation and large increases in drag.

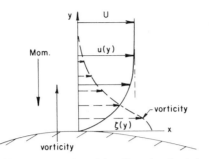

Figure 5. Momentum and vorticity fluxes in a boundary layer.

now possible to reconcile that the irrotational flows predicted by ideal-fluid theory applied to viscous fluids outside the boundary layer. While no general mathematical proof of the boundary-layer hypothesis exists, its validity has been proven in a large number of flows. For "streamlined" bodies the drag coefficient has been found to be very small—close to the zero value predicted by ideal-fluid theory. The flow separation in a diverging channel and behind a bluff body provides a useful warning that the boundary-layer hypothesis does not apply to all flow systems and that the ideal-fluid prediction does not approximate all flow situations, even away from the wall. Although a precise statement of the class of flow field to which the hypothesis does apply cannot be given, situations where the hypothesis does not apply can be identified through a review of the approximations involved. Situations where the boundary-layer hypothesis would not apply include large streamwise radius of curvature, low Reynolds number, near separation, etc.

The primary condition for the boundary-layer hypothesis is that the boundary layer be thin; this in turn states that the pressure gradient transverse to the wall is negligible so that the external pressure is *impressed* on the boundary layer flow. Under these conditions the governing momentum and continuity equations for a two-dimensional boundary layer become, respectively,

$$\frac{\partial u}{\partial t} + u \frac{\partial u}{\partial x} + v \frac{\partial u}{\partial y} = -\frac{1}{\rho}\frac{dp}{dx} + \nu \frac{\partial^2 u}{\partial y^2} \tag{9a}$$

$$\frac{\partial u}{\partial x} + \frac{\partial v}{\partial y} = 0 \tag{9b}$$

where dp/dx is specified by the irrotational flow outside the boundary layer. These two are the *Prandtl boundary-layer equations.*

Rigidity of the boundary is not required for the existence of a boundary layer, although most applications involve a rigid boundary. The no-slip condition requires that fluid velocity at the boundary be that of the boundary.

In general, a boundary layer will exist near any boundary whenever the conditions required at the boundary are not exactly satisfied by the inviscid-fluid solution. At the free surface of a liquid where the tangential stress must be zero, a boundary layer must exist. The shear layer between two parallel streams of irrotational flows of different speeds is a boundary layer. At sufficiently high Reynolds numbers, jets and wakes have boundary-layer behavior.

2.3.1 Blasius Layer   The simplest example of the boundary layer is the flow over a flat plate of no thickness, of length L and much larger width placed in a steady uniform flow of velocity U parallel to the plate and normal to its leading edge. This flow does not occur in reality (although it is approximated by flow over a wing, in the entry region of a tube, or in an artery downstream from a branch) but serves as a flow standard for understanding boundary-layer behavior and streamwise variation of skin friction. For the flow of an inviscid fluid the flat plate produces no disturbance, while in a real fluid the no-slip condition introduces at the leading edge a thin vorticity layer whose thickness increases in the downstream direction because of viscous diffusion. The streamlines both inside and outside the boundary layer are deflected laterally as if the plate were now endowed with a thickness increasing with the downstream direction; this displacement effect causes a decrease in the effective flow cross section in the entrance flow in a tube, resulting in a corresponding flow acceleration and thus increased pressure drop.

The boundary-layer thickness is small if the Reynolds number is large, i.e., $UL/\nu \gg 1$. Consequently, the free-stream velocity U is constant in x and the first term in the right-hand side of Eq. 9a is approximately zero, i.e., $dp/dx \cong 0$. Solution of Eqs. 9 with $dp/dx = 0$ (*Blasius Soln.*) shows that the boundary-layer thickness δ increases with increasing x as $\delta \sim \sqrt{(\nu x/U)}$. This result can be intuitively derived as follows. At any distance x downstream from the leading edge, the time taken for a particle to travel from the leading edge is of order x/U, which must equal the time for diffusion of vorticity from the wall to the outer edge of the boundary layer, i.e., δ^2/ν. Thus $x/U \sim \delta^2/\nu$ so that $\delta \sim \sqrt{(x\nu/U)}$. This parabolic growth of the boundary-layer thickness has been well confirmed by experiments. Two other characteristic length scales in a boundary layer are the displacement thickness $\delta^* \equiv \int_0^\infty (1 - u/U)\ dy$ and the momentum thickness $\theta \equiv \int_0^\infty (u/U)(1 - u/U)\ dy;$ their ratio, i.e., the shape factor $H \equiv \delta^*/\theta$, is an important parameter that indicates whether the boundary layer is laminar or turbulent; its value is 2.59 for laminar flow and 1.4 for turbulent flow. For a boundary layer the point where the velocity is 99% of the free-stream velocity is taken as the thickness; this quantity cannot be determined unambiguously from data. Because they are integral quantities, both δ^* and θ have low uncertainties and thus are better length scales of the boundary layer.

Note that the condition for the existence of a boundary layer, i.e., $UL/v \gg 1$, is satisfied in a boundary layer except near the leading edge (a singular point) where $Ux/v \sim 1$.

So far, we have considered laminar flow over a flat plate only. If the values of $U\delta^*/v$ exceed about 600, the flow becomes unstable and acts as a bandpass filter so that natural disturbances within the unstable band are amplified through flow instability and, finally, transition introduces the random, three-dimensional, vortical, turbulent structure. Even for a turbulent boundary layer, the boundary-layer hypothesis is valid for the average quantities. The wall shear stress in the turbulent boundary layer is significantly higher than in the laminar boundary layer, the transport of momentum from free-stream to the wall being enhanced by the turbulence.

The transition Reynolds number R_x based on the length x from the leading edge varies over the range $10^5 \leqslant R_x \leqslant 4 \times 10^6$, the value decreasing with increasing free-stream turbulence intensity. The lower value corresponds to a length of 12 cm, in a water flow of speed 1 m/sec, of a flat plate, for example.

2.4 Unsteady Viscous Layers

This section emphasizes the mechanism of vorticity diffusion and the boundary-layer behavior in unsteady and periodic flows. The case of periodic flows is different because flow oscillation generates opposite vorticities during the phases when the motions are in opposite directions. Vorticity cancels out during a complete period so that there is no net diffusion of vorticity far away from the wall. Although the boundary-layer concept was introduced at the beginning of the twentieth century, the following first two boundary-layer problems were solved in an earlier epoch. These are examples where the governing equations become linear because the velocity vector has the same direction everywhere and is independent of the distance in the flow direction; the nonlinear convective terms thus vanish identically, permitting an exact solution.

2.4.1 The Rayleigh Layer   Consider a semi-infinite region of stationary fluid bounded by a rigid wall (at $y = 0$) that is suddenly given a velocity U in its own plane at $t = 0$ and maintained constant thereafter. Because of parallel motion (Figure 6a),

$$v = 0, \quad w = 0, \quad \therefore \partial p/\partial z = 0, \quad \partial p/\partial y = 0$$

$$\therefore p = f(x); \quad \text{but away from the wall, } p = \text{const.}$$

$$\therefore \ \frac{\partial p}{\partial x} = 0$$

Thus the governing equation merely represents a balance between local acceleration and the viscous term, i.e.,

$$\frac{\partial u}{\partial t} = \nu \frac{\partial^2 u}{\partial y^2} \tag{10a}$$

and the boundary conditions are

$$u(y,t) = 0, \qquad t \leqslant 0 \tag{10b}$$

$$\left. \begin{aligned} u(0,t) &= U \\ u(\infty,t) &= 0 \end{aligned} \right\}, t > 0 \tag{10c} \tag{10d}$$

Equation 10a along with the boundary conditions is identical to the (parabolic) heat conduction equation and is thus also known as the

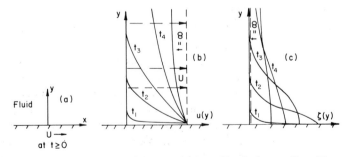

Figure 6. The Rayleigh layer; (A) flow condition, (B) velocity profiles, (C) vorticity profiles.

diffusion equation. Because the problem has no characteristic dimension, we can assume a *similarity solution* where the similarity variable is $\eta = y/L$, L being an appropriate length scale. Since the only variable other than y and t that $F \ (\equiv u/U)$ can depend on is ν, clearly from dimensional grounds $L = 2\sqrt{(\nu t)}$, the factor 2 is added for convenience. Substituting these and using the boundary conditions one can show that the solution of Eq. 10 is the *errorr function*, i.e.,

$$\frac{u}{U} = 1 - \mathrm{erf}\,(\eta) \qquad (11a)$$

where

$$\eta = y/2\sqrt{(\nu t)} \qquad (11b)$$

and vorticity is

$$-\frac{\partial u}{\partial y} = \frac{U}{\sqrt{(\nu \pi t)}}\, e^{-\eta^2}, \qquad (11c)$$

wall shear stress is

$$\tau_w = \mu \left.\frac{\partial u}{\partial y}\right|_0 = -\frac{U\rho}{\sqrt{\pi}}\sqrt{\left(\frac{\nu}{t}\right)} \qquad (11d)$$

and drag coefficient is

$$\frac{\tau_w}{\frac{1}{2}\rho U^2} = -\frac{2}{U\sqrt{\pi}}\sqrt{\left(\frac{\nu}{t}\right)} \qquad (11e)$$

At time $t = 0$, because of the no-slip condition, the velocity is U at the wall and zero everywhere and vorticity is a *delta function* at $y = 0$. With increasing time, the vorticity diffuses away from the flat plate so that at infinite time the velocity is uniform and vorticity zero, everywhere. The velocity and vorticity profiles with increasing times are shown in Figure 6. Note that if the fluid is suddenly accelerated, rather than the plate, the solution 11a takes the form

$$u/U = \mathrm{erf}\,(\eta)$$

This example illustrates the central character of viscous boundary-layer flows. The jump in the plate velocity at $t = 0$ produces a concentrated vorticity at the wall. The vorticity is then essentially spread in a thin layer adjacent to the wall of thickness $\sqrt{(\nu t)}$. The gradual diffusion or spreading away of the velocity variation (vorticity) across streamlines from the wall is due to the tangential viscous force exerted across planes normal to the y axis. The thickness $\delta_R = \sqrt{(\nu t)}$ or diffusion length which increases both with time and with increasing viscosity is called Rayleigh layer thickness; even though Stokes first introduced it in 1851, Rayleigh's name is attached to remove confusion with the Stokes layer discussed in the next section. The distance at which the velocity is 99% of free-stream velocity is about $4\delta_R$. The rate of penetration of the velocity variation decreases as t increases because the velocity gradients (and thus the momentum transfer rate) decrease with time; so with decreasing viscosity. The wall shear stress and the drag coefficient decrease with time because of the weakening of the velocity slope near the wall.

Two important points to notice are that in spite of the fact that the vorticity at a point away from the wall increases with time, it is not a wave phenomenon because the effect of the wall movement is felt everywhere at $t > 0$ (a characteristic of the parabolic equation) and that the velocity distribution shape is independent of the initial form of velocity transition.

2.4.2 Stokes Layer The effect of flow periodicity on the viscous diffusion of vorticity is discussed in this section. Consider in this case, however, that the bounding rigid plane of the previous example moves in its own plane with a simple harmonic motion with frequency ω (Figure 7A). In this case the governing equation and the boundary conditions remain the same as in the previous case except that the boundary condition 10c will be $u(0,t) = U \cos(\omega t)$.

If the motion is set up from rest, the velocity field will consist of "transients" before becoming a harmonic function of t. It is clear that the time scale is ω^{-1} so that, ν being the only other parameter, the length scale is $\sqrt{(\nu/\omega)}$. The solution to the problem (obtained by separation of variables) is

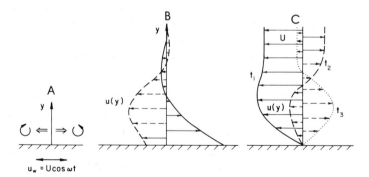

Figure 7. The Stokes layer; (A) flow condition, (B) velocity profiles, (C) velocity profiles with stationary wall.

$$\frac{u}{U} = e^{-\eta} \cos (\omega t - \eta) \qquad (12a)$$

where

$$\eta = \frac{y}{\sqrt{(2\nu/\omega)}} \qquad (12b)$$

The factor 2 in η makes the solution look simpler. Thus the velocity profile (Eq. 12) can be described as that due to a shear "wave" of wavelength $2\pi(2\nu/\omega)^{1/2}$ "propagating"[11] in the y direction with phase velocity $\sqrt{(2\nu\omega)}$, the damping in the y direction being such that the velocity falls off as $e^{-\eta}$. This being the solution of a diffusion equation, the phenomenon is not truly a wave phenomenon. The decay in velocity over one wavelength is $e^{-2\pi} \cong 0.002$ so that the motion is effectively confined to a layer near the wall of thickness $\sqrt{(\nu/\omega)}$, called the *Stokes layer thickness* δ_s (Figure 7B); this layer progressively becomes thinner with increasing frequency as less time is permitted for the vorticity to diffuse out before being canceled by opposite vorticity created by reversed motion of the plate. Thus very little vorticity is diffused away from the plate.

Instead of the plate, if the free-stream is oscillating over a fixed plate the solution 12a becomes $u/U = \cos \omega t - e^{-\eta} \cos(\omega t - \eta)$; the corresponding velocity profile is shown in Figure 7C. One can see that the wall friction *leads* the free stream by $45°$.

Since the differential equation and the boundary conditions are linear, response to any arbitrary, periodic function can thus be analyzed in this fashion.

Notice that the peak velocities at two y locations differ from each other in time, i.e., the phase of the motion changes from layer to layer; the motions at two y locations separated by a distance $\pi\sqrt{(2\nu/\omega)}$ are $180°$ out of phase. Notice that this layered motion is purely a consequence of viscosity. This layered phase lag plays an important role in unsteady viscous flows.

In both the above problems there is no outflow of fluid material away from the unsteady boundary layers; there is outflow if the outer flow depends on x, i.e., if $dp/dx \neq 0$; steady streaming is an example that is discussed later.

---

[11] In Figure 8, $y = f(x - ct)$ is obtained by shifting $f(x)$ by $x = ct$ to the right. Thus the value of $f(x)$ at $x = 0$ at time t_1 is the same as that at $x = ct$ at time $t + t_1$. This means that the pattern moves to the right by a distance $x = ct$ in time t, i.e., with speed c. Thus $y = f(x - ct)$ represents a wave traveling to the right with speed c.

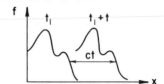

Figure 8. Wave traveling to the right.

2.4.3 Heisenberg–Tollmien Layer   This unsteady layer occurs when a vorticity wave travels in a shear flow with a mean velocity profile $\bar{u}(y)$; it occupies the location where the wave phase velocity c equals the local mean velocity u_c. This layer is also called the *critical layer* because it is critical in the instability of viscous shear flows (e.g., boundary layer and channel flows) whose noninflexional profiles are stable according to the inviscid theory (see Section 3.3). The equation for this layer is obtained in terms of vorticity fluctuations $\zeta(x,y,t)$ from Eq. 8 after linearization, i.e.,

$$\frac{\partial \zeta}{\partial t} + \bar{u}\frac{\partial \zeta}{\partial x} - v'\frac{d^2 \bar{u}}{dy^2} = \nu \frac{\partial^2 \zeta}{\partial y^2} \tag{13}$$

An important characteristic of this layer, like the x-dependent Stokes layer case, is that it promotes a phase difference between the orthogonal velocity fluctuations u' and v' such that it is different from the usual 90°, and thus produces a wave Reynolds stress $-\rho\overline{u'v'}$; thus the disturbances associated with the vorticity wave can extract kinetic energy from the mean field and thus possibly destabilize the flow. This additional phase shift is brought about by viscosity, from which comes the name "viscous instability." The Orr–Sommerfeld theory is thus a study of the Heisenberg–Tollmien layer also. In a boundary layer of thickness δ this layer is embedded within the boundary layer and has a thickness of the order $(1/\delta)[cv/\omega\overline{\zeta}_c]^{1/3}$ where ω is the wave frequency and $\overline{\zeta}_c$ the mean vorticity at the location of the Heisenberg–Tollmien layer.

The above three problems all have some relevance to the cardiovascular system. The flow in larger arteries is pulsatile, with flow reversals existing in many peripheral arteries, so that the flow oscillation problem is relevant for understanding not only the boundary-layer growth but also its possible transition to turbulent flow. Pulsation introduces acceleration and deceleration in the flow. If the frequency is large the Stokes layer dominates the flow. For low frequencies, one can treat the accelerating and decelerating phases separately. When the pulsation period is very large, the flow can be regarded as quasi-steady i.e., the boundary-layer profile remains undistorted but adjusts itself to match the instantaneous free-stream velocity.

Transition of pulsatile flows is discussed later (see Section 3.3.2).

2.5 Unsteady Boundary-Layer Analyses

The boundary layers on the walls of the arteries are examples of boundary layers in the presence of time-dependent free-stream velocity $U(t)$. Even though arterial flow often reverses, we assume that there is a time-dependent unidirectional flow. In order to determine the boundary-layer characteristics, the unsteady boundary-layer equations 9 must be solved, using the free-stream condition,

$$-\frac{1}{\rho}\frac{\partial p}{\partial x} = \frac{\partial U}{\partial t} + U\frac{\partial U}{\partial x} \tag{14a}$$

The question that must be answered is, Under what situations are the Prandtl boundary-layer equations still valid for unsteady flows? We need to discuss (1) boundary layers starting from rest and (2) boundary layers in periodic flows (Stuart, 1963b).

In the case of boundary layers for start of motion from rest, only two limiting cases permit identification of physical nondimensional parameters: small times and large times. Consider time-dependent flow with L as the characteristic length scale. For small times t, Eqs. 9 and 14a represent boundary-layer flow if

$$L^2/\nu t \gg 1 \quad \text{and} \quad UL/\nu \gg 1 \tag{14b}$$

The first equation is equivalent to stating that the velocity gradient normal to the wall is instantaneously much higher than along the wall. The second equation states that the instantaneous Reynolds numbers must be large or convection (by U) is much faster than viscous diffusion. For large times t after start, the same two conditions 14b apply. In that case, $L^2/\nu t \gg 1$ states that the streamwise diffusion rate is small compared to the rate of change of motion. The meaning of $UL/\nu \gg 1$ is the same.

In the case of a periodic boundary layer if it is oscillating (i.e., zero mean), $u = U_\omega \cos \omega t$, the boundary-layer approximation can be applied if $\omega L^2/\nu \gg 1$, i.e., $\delta(t) \ll L$. If $\delta \sim L$, a solution can still be obtained if $\omega L/U_\omega \gg 1$. If the mean is nonzero and the fluctuating velocity amplitude is small, then the important parameters are the mean Reynolds number $U_0 L/\nu$ and the frequency parameter $\alpha = \sqrt{(\omega\delta^2/\nu)} =$ (boundary layer thickness/Stokes layer thickness). If α is large, i.e., if the frequency is high, the Stokes layer is thin enough that it exists independently as a secondary boundary layer embedded in the main boundary layer. If $\alpha \sim 1$ the Stokes layer is comparable to the mean flow boundary layer and is subject to interaction with the boundary layer. When the oscillation amplitude is large clearly both the Reynolds numbers, $U_0 L/\nu$ and $U_\omega L/\nu$, and α will be important parameters (see Section 3.3.2).

In the following we briefly outline some techniques for analyzing unsteady flows.

2.5.1 Successive Approximation for Starting Flow

In this method the convective acceleration terms are considered very small compared to $\partial u/\partial t$, which then balances the viscous term $\nu \, \partial u^2/\partial y^2$ and only $\partial U/\partial t$ is assumed to be the major contributor to pressure gradient in the free-stream (Eq. 14a). These are certainly valid assumptions at the start of motion. Then the equation for the first approximation u_0 of the velocity in the boundary layer is

$$\frac{\partial u_0}{\partial t} - \nu \frac{\partial^2 u_0}{\partial y^2} = \frac{\partial U}{\partial t} \tag{15a}$$

This "heat-conduction" equation can be solved for a given $U(t)$ and then v_0 can be determined from continuity equation, Eq. 9b. The equation for the second approximation u_1 is then written with the convective terms based on u_0, v_0 only, i.e.,

$$\frac{\partial u_1}{\partial t} - \nu \frac{\partial^2 u_1}{\partial y^2} = U \frac{\partial U}{\partial x} - u_0 \frac{\partial u_0}{\partial x} - v_0 \frac{\partial u_0}{\partial y} \quad , \tag{15b}$$

which is again a linear equation and can be solved for u_1 and so on. It is apparent that the complexity of this method increases for higher-order approximations u_2, u_3, etc.

2.5.2 Unsteady Reynolds Decomposition

This method is valid for a free stream with a mean and a periodic or random fluctuation and follows the Reynolds turbulence decomposition approach. The total free-stream as well as the boundary-layer velocities and pressures can be decomposed into time-independent and time-dependent components,

$$U(x,t) = \bar{U}(x) + U_1(x,t) \tag{16a}$$

$$u(x,y,t) = \bar{u}(x,y) + u_1(x,y,t) \tag{16b}$$

$$v(x,y,t) = \bar{v}(x,y) + v_1(x,y,t) \tag{16c}$$

$$p(x,t) = \bar{p}(x) + p_1(x,t) \tag{16d}$$

where the overbar indicates *time average* (see Section 3.8), so that

$$\bar{U}_1 = \bar{u}_1 = \bar{v}_1 = \bar{p}_1 = 0 \tag{17}$$

Notice that the mean and fluctuating components separately satisfy the continuity equation, i.e.,

$$\frac{\partial \bar{u}}{\partial x} + \frac{\partial \bar{v}}{\partial y} = 0, \tag{18a}$$

$$\frac{\partial u_1}{\partial x} + \frac{\partial v_1}{\partial y} = 0 \tag{18b}$$

Substituting expressions 16 into Eq. 14 and taking the time average yields

$$\bar{U}\frac{d\bar{U}}{dx} + \overline{U_1 \frac{\partial U_1}{\partial x}} = -\frac{1}{\rho}\frac{\partial \bar{p}}{\partial x} \tag{18c}$$

A similar operation on Eq. 9a, which can then be combined with Eq. 18a, gives

$$\bar{u}\frac{\partial \bar{u}}{\partial x} + \bar{v}\frac{\partial \bar{u}}{\partial y} = \bar{U}\frac{d\bar{U}}{dx} + \bar{v}\frac{\partial \bar{u}}{\partial y} + \bar{G}(x,y) \tag{19a}$$

where

$$\bar{G}(x,y) = \overline{U_1 \frac{\partial U_1}{\partial x}} - \overline{u_1 \frac{\partial u_1}{\partial x}} - \overline{v_1 \frac{\partial u_1}{\partial y}} \tag{19b}$$

The corresponding equation for u_1 is rather long. However, if the Stokes layer thickness δ_s $(\equiv\sqrt{v/\omega})$ is small compared to the boundary-layer thickness δ corresponding to the mean free-stream flow $\bar{U}(x)$—a restriction certainly valid for high-frequency variation of $U(x,t)$—the equation of u_1 then simplifies to

$$\frac{\partial u_1}{\partial t} = \frac{\partial U_1}{\partial t} + v\frac{\partial^2 u_1}{\partial y^2}, \tag{19c}$$

which likewise (Eq. 15a) can be solved for u_1; then v_1 can be derived from Eq. 18b. Notice that the equation for the mean flow in the boundary layer, i.e., Eq. 19a, is equivalent to that for steady laminar flow except for the source or body force term $\bar{G}(x,y)$ arising from products of purely time-dependent fluctuations (with zero mean). Unlike the typical body force term $U(dU/dx)$ in steady flow, $\bar{G}(x,y)$ is not impressed by the external flow. It is clear that if U_1, u_1, v_1 are terms like $\cos \omega t$, then

$G(x,y)$ will have terms like cos $2\omega t$, sin $2\omega t$ and some constant terms; the latter will survive time averaging and will contribute to the mean velocity field. These steady motions arising from the interaction of velocity fluctuations relative to the solid boundary are called *steady streaming;* it arises purely from the nonlinear convective terms in the Navier–Stokes equation. The steady streaming can occur either if the amplitude is a function of x (standing type) or if the phase is a function of x (progressive type) or both.

2.5.3 Harmonic Oscillations When the flow at a large Reynolds number is sinusoidal, e.g., $U(x,t) = U_0(x)$ cos ωt, the governing equation can be linearized only if the convective acceleration is small compared to local acceleration, i.e.,

$$|\mathbf{u} \cdot \nabla \mathbf{u}| \ll \left|\frac{\partial \mathbf{u}}{\partial t}\right| \tag{20a}$$

If the velocity varies with amplitude U_0 and frequency ω, and if L is the characteristic length of the flow, then the left side is of order U_0^2/L and right side of order $U_0\omega$; then from Eq. 20a

$$U_0/\omega L \ll 1 \tag{20b}$$

In cases when periodic variation of u is due to a solid body oscillation of amplitude a, then $U_0 \sim a\omega$ so that

$$a/L \ll 1 \tag{20c}$$

Thus the solution obtained by linearization is valid only when the amplitude of oscillation is small compared to the characteristic length of the body. Once again a steady "streaming" motion is induced because of viscous effect. For the details of the solution see Schlichting (1968) and Batchelor (1970).

2.5.4 An Explanation for Streaming The fact that simple sinusoidal oscillation of a rigid body or of flow produces a steady velocity far away from the body is intriguing and is of some practical interest (Longet-Higgins, 1970). If the fluid were inviscid, the periodic oscillation of the body would generate orthogonal velocity components $u(t)$, $v(t)$ that would be $\pi/2$ out of phase; the average of their product (i.e., Reynolds stress) would be zero so that no net transfer of x momentum across a surface with normal in the y direction would occur during one cycle. However, because of the fluid viscosity, there will be a Stokes layer where the amplitude and phase of the u component will depend on the distance y

from the wall (see Section 2.4). Viscosity alters the phase difference between u and v from $\pi/2$ (Lin, 1955; Stuart, 1967) so that the average of their product $\overline{uv}$ is nonzero; because of transport of x momentum across the y plane there is an effective stress (Reynolds stress) at each y plane. (We will see later that similar phase shift introduced by viscosity at the Heisenberg–Tollmien layer is the mechanism responsible for viscous instability.) Because of the large u variation with y in the Stokes layer, this stress varies across the layer so that each fluid element experiences an unbalanced force that induces steady fluid motion; the consequence of this is the steady motion outside the Stokes layer. The flow outside the Stokes layer cannot be strictly irrotational; there is a slow transfer of vorticity away from the wall layer due to streaming so that after sufficient time there is second-order vorticity throughout the fluid field.

Because of vascular taper and traveling wave pulses, streaming should be of concern in the arterial flows. I know of no analysis addressed to this aspect. The secondary flow in the interior of a curved tube as observed by Lyne (1970) and Chandran et al. (1974) is an example of steady streaming; this explains why the potential region secondary flow is from the outside to the inside of the tube.

2.5.5 Harmonic Modulation For harmonic oscillations superimposed on a stream, Lin (1957) developed a theory that essentially follows Section 2.5.2. If the external flow is represented as

$$U(x,t) = \overline{U}(x) + U_1(x) \sin \omega t, \qquad (21a)$$

where ω is the frequency of oscillation, then from Eq. 19c the solution for the oscillating components u_1 of the velocity in the boundary layer can be shown to be

$$u_1(x,y,t) = U_1(x)[\sin \omega t - e^{-\xi}] \ [\sin(\omega t - \xi)], \qquad (21b)$$

where $\xi = y/\delta_s\sqrt{2}$, and $\delta_s \ (=\sqrt{(\nu/\omega)})$ is the Stokes layer thickness due to $U_1(x) \sin \omega t$. The first bracket gives the y dependence of the amplitude of u_1 while the second gives the phase variation in y of u_1 with respect to the free-stream motion. The transverse component v_1 can be obtained from the continuity equation. One can thus obtain the body force term $\overline{G}(x,y)$ from Eq. 19b and show it to be

$$\overline{G}(x,y) = \tfrac{1}{2} U_1 \frac{dU_1}{dx} \overline{G}_1(\xi) \qquad (21c)$$

where $\overline{G}_1(\xi) = [(2 + \xi)\cos \xi - (1 - \xi)\sin \xi - e^{-2\xi}]e^{-\xi}$.

Equation 21c shows that the modification of the true mean velocity $\bar{u}$ in the boundary layer by the nonlinear term $\bar{G}(x,y)$ depends on the amplitude U_1 of free-stream oscillation and its streamwise gradient dU_1/dx. Thus large oscillations in the free stream produce no change in the boundary-layer profile if the amplitude U_1 is constant in x, i.e., $dU_1/dx = 0$.

In view of the lowest inertia of the fluid particles adjacent to the wall, these particles undergo the greatest changes under free-stream oscillation. That is, the same axial pressure gradient causing the flow acceleration produces a greater relative effect on the slow-moving fluid near the wall than on the main stream flow; this causes the outer flow to lag behind the fluid particles adjacent to the wall, i.e., the wall shear stress *leads* the outer fluid. On the other hand, because of thermal inertia, heat transfer from a heated wall lags behind the free-stream (see Lighthill, 1954).

2.5.6   Oscillating Flow Through a Pipe   The case of oscillating flow through a pipe can be of relevance to flows in some arteries and arterioles. We consider a long pipe of circular cross section with radius R under the influence of periodic pressure gradient necessary to cause the flow oscillation, i.e.,

$$-\frac{1}{\rho}\frac{\partial p}{\partial x} = K\,\cos(\omega t) \tag{22a}$$

The governing equation for the pipe flow is

$$\frac{\partial u}{\partial t} - \nu\left(\frac{\partial^2 u}{\partial r^2} + \frac{1}{r}\frac{\partial u}{\partial r}\right) = K\,\cos(\omega t) \tag{22b}$$

where r is the radial coordinate from the pipe center.

Notice that this equation, unlike Eq. 19a, is linear and thus we do not expect either higher harmonic or steady streaming in this case. The solution to this problem was worked out by Sexl and Uchida and can be found in Schlichting (1968). The solution is in terms of ω; only the limiting cases of large and small ω can be discussed for physical interpretation.

For very low frequencies the velocity distribution is parabolic and oscillates in phase with the driving pressure gradient. At very large frequencies the Stokes layer behavior discussed earlier is manifested; the pipe core fluid moves as if it were frictionless while the motion in the vicinity of the wall is phase dependent as a function of distance from the wall. In

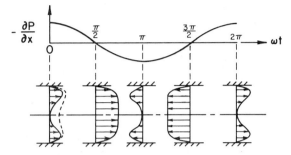

Figure 9. Pipe flow with oscillating pressure gradient.

Figure 9 the velocity distribution is shown for a complete cycle of the pressure gradient at an intermediate value of $R\sqrt{(\omega/\nu)} = 5$ so that the effect of oscillation on the flow across the entire pipe cross section can be observed. Notice that the flow on the pipe center follows the pressure gradient but lags behind the layers near the wall, as explained in Section 2.5.5. It can also be seen that the velocity amplitude has its maximum not at the pipe center but somewhere near the wall.

With increasing frequency, the Stokes layer becomes thinner, the core region becomes flatter, and the amplitude becomes smaller; for a detailed discussion see McDonald (1974).

Significant advances have been made in recent years in the development of predictive methods by retaining the nonlinear convective terms of Eq. 7 and the realistic characteristics of arterial wall; see, for example, Anliker (1972), Ling and Atabek (1972), Wemple and Mockros (1972), and Ling et al. (1973).

3 TRANSITION, TURBULENCE, AND PULSATION

3.1 The Turbulence Closure Problem

Nearly all naturally and technologically occurring flows are turbulent; these include galactic, atmospheric, and oceanic flows, motion in the earth's core, flows in pipe lines, compressors, boilers, and over trains, airplanes, ships, and submarines, etc. One can legitimately say that turbulent flow is the natural state of fluid motion and laminar flow is an exception. However, because it is a random function of position and time and because of its wideband spectrum and nonlinear nature, very little progress has been made in obtaining an adequate understanding of the turbulent flow, except for the very simple case of isotropic turbulent flow.

Some laminar flows, on the other hand, have been successfully predicted because of their relative simplicity compared to turbulent flows. It must be recognized that even for laminar flows the governing nonlinear partial differential (Navier–Stokes) equations do not produce solutions in general nor is there a general uniqueness and existence theorem of the initial valve problem (see Ladyzhenskaya, 1975). The Navier–Stokes equation does represent the evolution of a Stokesian fluid with given initial and boundary conditions. Even if the equation can be solved as a function of time t for each location x in the turbulent flow domain, such information is unmanageably voluminous and requires essentially infinite space for storage. This information could not be utilized and one has thus to look for statistical averages, e.g., a time average as a function of x.

However, as a consequence of the time averaging, the nonlinearity of the governing equations introduces new unknown moments, viz., the Reynolds stresses. This poses the *closure problem*, i.e., the unknowns now exceed the number of equations. It is natural to seek closure through equations for Reynolds stresses but these will contain third-order unknown moments. This approach is futile because the number of unknowns always exceeds the number of equations and the difference between unknown moments and equations increases progressively with the increasing order of the moment equation. This is the typical problem in nonlinear statistical mechanics.

An alternative approach is to seek closure by relating the unknown moments (e.g., Reynolds stresses) to the mean velocity field through some hypothesis like a phenomenologic theory. The gradient transport hypotheses, viz., mixing length and eddy viscosity theories, are the two most popularly applied examples. However, apart from the objections to the gradient transport hypotheses on conceptual grounds alone, these have been found to be inapplicable universally, even on an approximate basis.

Another approach to find closure has been either to neglect higher-order moments or to express them in terms of lower moments; these steps include unjustifiable and often incorrect assumptions.

To summarize, the theory of turbulent flow is far from complete. This situation has put a high demand on experimental exploration of turbulent flows and, in fact, some significant advances have been made through experimental efforts in recent years. Nevertheless, turbulent flow continues to remain elusive and may remain so for some time.

In spite of its apparent random nature, turbulent flow has a remarkable organization that is masked from the observer unless viewed through sophisticated techniques. There seem to be two independent interpretations of turbulent shear flows: the "large eddy" concept (Townsend, 1956) and the "wave" interpretation (Landahl, 1967; Lighthill, 1968; Moffatt, 1968; Hussain, 1969; Reynolds and Hussain, 1972). Since wavelike phenomena produce turbulent flow through instability of laminar flow, it is not unreasonable to expect that the resulting turbulent flow will have a wavelike behavior. Because of this, an understanding of flow instability is likely to provide further insight into the nature of turbulent shear flows. Hydrodynamic stability, however, is a fascinating subject in its own right.

In the following we give a purely nonmathematical description of the mechanics of transition and turbulent flows. As we will see later, flow in the cardiovascular system may be unstable and indeed become turbulent.

3.2 Transition

Turbulence is caused by the transition from a laminar flow. Transition represents a hierarchy of motions: growth of two-dimensional infinitesimal disturbances to finite amplitudes, three-dimensionality of the flow, and a maze of complex nonlinear interactions among the large-amplitude, three-dimensional modes resulting in a final, usually stochastically steady but instantaneously random, motion called turbulent flow (see later for discussion on turbulence). The initiation of the growth of disturbances is called instability. It precedes the manifestation of the occurrence of turbulence (spots) called transition. In an entrance region like the flow in the leading edge of a pipe, the appropriate Reynolds number is based on the distance from the leading edge. Thus the critical Reynolds number Re_{cr} representing the location of instability is lower than the transition Reynolds number Re_{tr}; the difference $Re_{tr} - Re_{cr}$ decreases with increasing free-stream turbulence intensity and with decreasing free-stream acceleration. Free-stream deceleration decreases the difference further (see Schlichting, 1968).

The solution of a governing equation with appropriate boundary conditions can occur in reality only if the solution is stable to small perturbations (the mean velocity profiles predicted by theory for a channel flow at $Re > 7700$ would not be realized because, unlike what the solution suggests, the flow is turbulent). Hydrodynamic stability predicts instability of certain basic flow states and is a testimony to the mathematicians' success in predicting some real flow behavior, their early endeavor having been mostly devoted to inviscid fluid flows; for detailed coverage of hydrodynamic stability see Lin (1955), Stuart (1963a), Yih (1969).

3.3 Hydrodynamic Stability

A basic state is a state that satisfies the governing equations and boundary conditions of the system. A basic state can be a stationary state, a laminar flow, or even a turbulent flow. When a disturbance is introduced to the system, its amplitude can grow, remain constant, or decrease in time; correspondingly, the basic state is said to be *unstable, neutrally stable*, or *stable* to the disturbance (Figure 10); the instability is called *temporal* instability in contrast with *spatial* instability. The response of a system depends on the frequency (or wavenumber) of the disturbance; typically it is unstable to a band of frequencies but stable to the others. Thus the system essentially behaves as a bandpass amplifier. A major effort of hydrodynamic stability theory is to predict the unstable bandwidth for each flow configuration.

Three approaches to stability study have been followed: *linear* (*inviscid* and *viscous*), *nonlinear*, and *energy* theories. In the linear theory the growth of infinitesimal disturbances is studied; their frequencies and wavenumbers (or phase velocities) identify them. Because disturbances are always present in a real system and any arbitrary disturbance can be Fourier decomposed into component frequencies, the instability at any frequency is sufficient for the system to be unstable. (In the cardiovascular flow system, disturbances are introduced by the motions of the heart, the valves, and the arterial wall as well as by abnormalities).

The primary advantage of the linear theory is that the nonlinear governing partial differential equations, Eqs. 7, are rendered linear (and the choice of a simple configuration, e.g., parallel flow, permits convenient

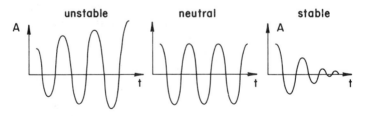

Figure 10. Unstable, neutrally stable, and stable disturbances; A is disturbance amplitude.

simple forms, i.e., normal modes of the disturbance) so that the solution to the problem can be derived analytically or numerically for each mode at a time. The linearity of the equation thus permits superposition of different modes. (The nonparallel aspect of some flows like the boundary layer can be accounted for through streamwise perturbation expansions.) Even for the simplest configurations for which solutions can be obtained, the linear theory can only predict initial growth of a disturbance but not its eventual evolution; if unstable, the theory predicts exponential growth without limit. After the disturbance has grown to finite amplitudes, however, the linear theory and thus its predictions are rendered invalid; the finite amplitude and intermodal interactions must be taken into account. This is the pursuit of the nonlinear theory. The energy theory, on the other hand, ignores the detailed characteristics of the disturbance and merely provides a sufficient condition for the stability of a state to all kinematically admissable (though not possible) disturbances; the prediction is based on a variational formulation of the integral of the disturbance energy equation and provides the global criterion under which the total kinetic energy of the disturbance will *not* increase with time. The energy theory, therefore, typically predicts highly conservative values of the critical stability parameter (e.g., critical Reynolds number) below which stability is guaranteed, and thus, until recently, has received very little attention.

Because instability centers around growth of disturbances, only those disturbances to which the system is unstable are important. The nonlinear theory thus centers around the unstable modes of the linear theory as a series expansion of the unstable mode amplitude.[12]

There are various kinds of instability, some of these attributed to outstanding researchers, viz., Benard, Rayleigh, Taylor, Marangoni, Kelvin–Helmholtz, Tollmien–Schlichting, etc. Typically, each case of instability results from lack of balance between two counterbalancing forces acting on a fluid element, one force trying to destabilize the basic state and the other restore it; instability (growth of disturbances) results when a destabilizing force overpowers a stabilizing force. In each case a critical nondimensional number is defined as the ratio (stability parameter)

---

[12] Some instabilities have been shown to be dependent on the amplitude of the disturbance; the critical Reynolds number for a channel flow has been found to decrease with increasing disturbance amplitude. It is likely that pipe flow will be found to be unstable by an appropriate nonlinear theory; this nonlinear theory obviously cannot be built on a linear theory.

of the destabilizing to stabilizing forces; exceeding this number at any point in the fluid domain indicates instability. For example, the Beñard instability results when the destabilizing buoyancy force due to heating exceeds the stabilizing viscous force; Marangoni instability sets in when the destabilizing force due to surface tension gradients exceeds the opposing viscous force; in Taylor instability the destabilizing centrifugal force exceeds the stabilizing viscous force, etc.

Instability may imply that of a nonmoving state also, e.g., Beñard and Marangoni instabilities. When a system is unstable, the disturbance may grow but reach another stable laminar state (the flow between two rotating cylinders undergoes a series of instabilities into successive states of stable, ordered motion before it becomes turbulent); this is the case of *supercritical equilibrium.* On the other hand, the critical Reynolds number of a flow can depend on the disturbance amplitude; the critical Reynolds number of a channel flow has been predicted to decrease with increasing disturbance amplitudes (see Reynolds and Potter, 1967; George, Hellums, and Martin, 1974). The latter is the case of *subcritical instability.*

For the cardiovascular system the viscous (Tollmien–Schlichting) instability is the most critical one. However, the Gortler instability is likely to be important in the aortic arch and the free shear layer (Kelvin–Helmohltz) instability in the flow behind the valve leaflet and arterial and valvular stenoses.

3.3.1 Inviscid and Viscous Instability   The instability of a shear layer (free as well as a boundary layer) is governed by the linearized form of the Navier–Stokes equation; in terms of the amplitudes of the normal mode forms for disturbance (normal velocity or stream function or vorticity), the equation is a fourth-order ordinary differential equation called the *Orr–Sommerfeld equation;* when the viscous terms are neglected it is called the *Rayleigh equation.* For sufficiently high Reynolds numbers, the stability study can neglect viscosity (except at the *critical layer* where the mean velocity equals disturbance-phase velocity and in the disturbance-induced Stokes layer adjacent to the wall); the instability so predicted is called *inviscid instability.* From the inviscid theory two important conclusions follow: parallel flows are inviscidly stable if the velocity profile has no inflection point (Rayleigh's theorem); and for inviscid instability to occur, the vorticity of the basic flow must have a maximum (Fjørtoft's theorem). While not a sufficient condition, Rayleigh's theorem suggests that profiles with inflection points, Figure 11A for example, are candidates for instability. However, the profile shown in Figure 11B is stable

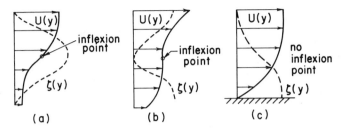

Figure 11. Linear inviscid instability of velocity profiles.

because it does not satisfy Fjørtoft's theorem. Boundary layers under adverse pressure gradients have inflection points and are known to be unstable under some circumstances. For this reason the progressive branching and associated increase in flow area in the cardiovascular system can be critical; however, the rate of increase of flow area is in general too small to induce instability. Flow downstream from some bifurcations has shown instability waves and vortex shedding; see, for example, Stehbens (1975).

The above instability criterion based on inflexion point suggests that pipe and channel flows and flat-plate boundary layers are inviscidly stable; see Figure 11C. In order to explain the instability of profiles with no point of inflection, viscosity has to be taken into account. This is done by the *viscous instability theory* initially worked out by Heisenberg, Tollmien, Schlichting, Lin, and others (see Lin, 1955). A notable distinction between inviscid and viscous instabilities is that a flow which is viscously unstable becomes stable at infinite Reynolds number; an inviscidly unstable flow is unstable even at infinite Reynolds number (Figure 12). The viscous theory has been successful in predicting transition in a channel or on a flat plate. However, the pipe flow has been theoretically found to be stable to

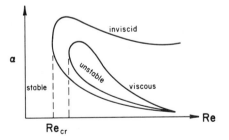

Figure 12. Linear inviscis and viscous instabilities; α, nondimensional wavenumber; Re_cr, critical value of Reynolds number Re.

infinitesimal disturbances for all Reynolds numbers. In reality, pipe flow is found to be turbulent at a Reynolds number of about 2,500, but it has been possible to maintain laminar pipe flow to a Reynolds number of 40,000 by progressively lowering the disturbance level. It is quite likely that pipe flow may be unstable to finite amplitude disturbances.

It is important to emphasize that transition in a pipe or channel is inherently different from that on a flat plate. (Consistent with Squire's theorem, it is found that the flow is unstable to two-dimensional disturbances at a lower Reynolds number than to three-dimensional disturbances. Thus it suffices to study two-dimensional disturbances, because they are more dangerous for transition. Note that for a non-Newtonian flow the three-dimensional disturbances contribute terms absent in two-dimensional flow.) The disturbances grow as two-dimensional waves and when their amplitudes are large they develop three-dimensionality; in a flat plate, transition has no effect upstream. In a pipe or a channel the disturbances grow downstream and when transition occurs the resulting higher skin friction requires a larger pressure drop so that the entire flow slows down. The Reynolds number than becomes subcritical and thus the formed turbulent slug is followed by a laminar region. When either a part or all of the turbulent region is washed out or the length of laminar flow is long enough, the reduction of required pressure drop increases the flow rate, which again precipitates transition. Thus the transitional pipe flow, of necessity, contains alternate regions of laminar and turbulent slugs (Wygnanski and Champagne, 1973). This also suggests that transitional pipe flow is inherently time dependent.

It is worthwhile to note that transition on a boundary layer is affected by flow oscillation, pressure gradient, free-stream turbulence intensity, surface roughness, wall curvature, heating, density and viscosity stratification, compressibility, wall suction and blowing, etc. For details see Schlichting (1968) and Stuart (1963a).

Most early theories were devoted to time-dependent disturbances; however, the disturbances encountered in a shear flow are spatially dependent (i.e., they grow or decay in space downstream). While early transition studies by Sato (1960) and Schubauer and Skramstad (1947) compared their experimental data with temporal theory, Gaster (1962) showed that the conversion of a spatially dependent problem to a temporal one by convection of coordinates with the disturbance phase velocity is, indeed, restrictive. Recent experimental and analytical studies have made attempts to develop and compare spatial theory with data (Michalke, 1965; Hussain and Reynolds, 1970, 1972; Hussain and Thompson, 1975).

3.3.2 Instability of Periodic Flows When the basic state is periodic, stability definitions introduced earlier need to be modified. The periodic flow is said to be unstable if the disturbance undergoes a net growth in each period, stable if it decays continuously and transiently stable if it grows for part of the cycle before decay (Davis, 1975).

In a pulsatile flow in a pipe of diameter D we can denote the velocity field as $U_0 + U_\omega \cos \omega t$; the velocity is a function of radius but we will take it to denote the centerline value. When the mean flow is dominant, the parameters characterizing the stability are: *mean Reynolds number* $Re_0 = U_0 D/\nu$, *frequency parameter* $\alpha = D/\delta_s$, and *velocity amplitude ratio* $\Delta = U_\omega/U_0$, where $\delta_s = (\nu/\omega)^{1/2}$ is the Stokes layer thickness. When the mean flow is not significant, in place of Re_0, the important parameter is the *modulation Reynolds number* $Re_\omega = U_\omega \delta_s/\nu$, which equals $Re_0 \Delta/\alpha$. Obremski and Fejer (1967), however, identified a yet different parameter, viz., *nonsteady Reynolds number* $Re_{ns} = U_0 U_\omega/\omega\nu$, which equals Re_ω^2/Δ, as the parameter controlling transition in an oscillating boundary layer.

It appears that Re_ω is likely to be the more important parameter when Δ is large (e.g., in arterial flow). In addition, there should be another characteristic parameter, viz., time-scale ratio Υ (defined as flow time scale/modulation time scale) so that modulation is *slow* if $\Upsilon \ll 1$ and *fast* if $\Upsilon \gg 1$. When mean flow is dominant, $\Upsilon = \omega D/U_0$; however, when modulation dominates, $\Upsilon = \omega D/U_\omega$. Based on the fundamental of the heart rate, the value of α in the ascending aorta is typically 28 in man and about 22 for dog (Kenner, 1972). Δ is obviously greater than 1 for arterial flow.

In a pulsatile flow the basic state may change with time so quickly that a disturbance does not get enough time to grow to large amplitudes. An inflexional profile is created in the decelerating phase so that the flow is more likely to be unstable during the decelerating phase; any turbulence so created may not have the small-scale structure because adequate time for cascade to small scales is not available. Although distensability of the arterial wall is a factor in arterial flow instability, it is necessary to understand the effect of flow modulation in a rigid pipe first. Gilbrech and Combs (1963), Yellin (1966a), Sarpkaya (1966), Sergeev (1966), and Clarion and Pelissier (1975), among others, have studied the stability of pulsatile flow in a pipe. Yellin's (1966) data show that oscillating pipe flow is more stable than Poiseuille profile. When transition occurred, it took place only in the decelerating phase; disturbances were typically restricted to the core and were destroyed during acceleration. Sarpkaya's experiments are limited to low frequencies ($\alpha < 8$). These data show that transition Reynolds number increases from steady flow value Re_{tr} with increasing Δ until it reaches a peak value; then with further increase in Δ it even falls below Re_{tr}. For increasing α the peak value of Re_{tr} occurs at lower Δ. It appears that the instability of modulated flows at large Δ and α should be controlled by Re_{ω} (which is independent of D), rather than by Re_0. Apparently, the Stokes layer (at least at large α) is stable to small amplitude disturbances but unstable to large amplitude disturbances. It must be noted that the Stokes layer, in spite of its instantaneous inflexional profile, is a very stable flow; this is not true at low α because the disturbance growth can outweigh the change of the basic state in one period. The Stokes layer has been found to become unstable typically at $Re_{\omega} \simeq 350$ (Davis, 1975). Merkli and Thomann (1975) have experimentally studied transition in an oscillating straight pipe flow and observed, by both hot-wire and smoke visualization, that transitions occurred at Reynolds number $Re_{\omega} \simeq 280$. Turbulence occurred in the form of periodic bursts followed by relaminarization within the same cycle; no case of continuous turbulence generation was found. Sergeev (1966) found that $Re_{\omega} \simeq 350$ for $\alpha > 6$.

The interest in the stability of the aortic flow is motivated primarily by the effect that the resulting turbulence, if the flow is unstable, may have on mass transport, atherosclerosis, heart murmur, post stenotic dilatation, blood damage, etc.

3.4 Role of Viscosity in Transition

Instability and transition imply that kinetic energy in the disturbance field must grow. In a plane parallel shear layer $U(y)$, the simplest flow case, the disturbance kinetic energy can increase if "production" exceeds "dissipation." The kinetic energy equation for the longitudinal component u is

$$\frac{d}{dt}\left(\frac{\overline{u'^2}}{2}\right) = -\overline{u'v'}\frac{dU}{dy} - \epsilon_1 + \cdots$$

The last term ϵ_1 represents viscous dissipation due to longitudinal turbulence u, i.e., direct conversion of turbulent kinetic energy to internal thermal energy. The transfer of kinetic energy from the mean to the turbulent field occurs through "production" $-\overline{u'v'}\,dU/dy$, which represents work done by kinematic Reynolds stress $-\overline{u'v'}$ against mean strain rate dU/dy. Note that this transfer of energy to turbulence occurs in the longitudinal mode only, pressure being responsible for redistribution of this energy to the other two components v' and w'. Thus in order for the increase of kinetic energy of disturbance to take place on the average, not only should there be shear dU/dy but also nonzero kinematic Reynolds stress $-\overline{u'v'}$; in fact, the Reynolds stress $-\overline{u'v'}$ must be positive. In an inviscid fluid the Reynolds stress $-\overline{u'v'}$ associated with a wave disturbance is zero because $u'(t)$ and $v'(t)$ are $\pi/2$ out of phase. The presence of even a small amount of viscosity produces a phase shift between $u'(t)$ and $v'(t)$ so that their correlation is no more zero, thus producing a net positive Reynolds stress $-\overline{u'v'}$ and positive production $-\overline{u'v'}\,dU/dy$. Typically, viscosity is associated with damping out oscillations, e.g., in Benard, Marangoni, Taylor instabilities; however, it is because of viscosity, on the other hand, that a viscous flow like plane Poiseuille flow (which is inviscidly stable to all disturbances) becomes unstable and undergoes transition. This is the dual role of viscosity.

Parenthetically, it is viscosity that causes separation of a boundary layer in an adverse pressure gradient (e.g., around a cylinder or in a diffuser) because the fluid in the boundary layer retarded by viscous stresses cannot continue to overcome increasing pressures in the streamwise direction. The separated shear layer may then be unstable according to inviscid instability.

Inviscid instability can be explained without any regard to viscosity, from the consideration of vorticity alone. In a shear layer with monotonic vorticity variation, any lateral displacement of a fluid element results in its being returned to its original position; that is, the flow is stable. However, Fjørtoft's theorem states that a shear layer must have a vorticity maximum in order for it to be unstable. A transfer of a fluid element with vorticity across the vorticity maximum may generate a fluid acceleration and thus produce instability. It turns out that the inviscid instability of a shear layer is associated with its roll-up into discrete vortices, which may then undergo secondary instability and become turbulent; the discrete vortices may also pair up due to subharmonic resonance (see Section 4).

3.5 Turbulent Flow

As stated earlier, most flows encountered in natural and technologic situations are turbulent. In a turbulent flow the rates of transfer of heat, mass, and momentum are much higher (typically a few orders of magnitude) than those in a laminary flow; the higher diffusivity of these properties in a turbulent flow is primarily due to eddying convection and smearing of fluid chunks compared to that due to molecular collision and migration in laminar flows. Because of the high momentum diffusivity, the friction factor for a turbulent pipe flow is higher than that for a laminar flow at the same Reynolds number; this is obvious from the mean velocity profiles in a laminar and a turbulent tube flow (see Figure 13); the case in heat transfer is similar.

Turbulent motion is characterized by random motion in space and time; for a location fixed in space, the velocity or pressure signal in a turbulent field is a random function of time; similarly, at a particular instant, the velocity and pressure are a random function of position in the flow field. Yet randomness of the velocity and static pressure as a function of position and time is a necessary condition but *not* the sufficient condition for the flow to be regarded as turbulent.

Turbulence can be defined as fluid motion with *random, three-dimensional* fluctuating vorticity. Any violation of either of these conditions renders the flow non-turbulent. For example, (1) a very low Reynolds number pipe flow with a random axial pressure gradient $\partial p/\partial x(t)$ will have a random velocity, pressure, and even vorticity field within the pipe, but the flow is clearly not turbulent. Two other examples associated with a turbulent boundary layer can be identified: (2) because of continuity of motion, flow outside the turbulent–nonturbulent interface of a turbulent boundary layer has random velocities and pressures but zero vorticity; this irrotational random flow is clearly not turbulent; (3) the sublayer flow in a thin region adjacent to the wall is random and essentially two dimensional, and thus not really turbulent.

Turbulent flow is a tangle of random, time-dependent vortex filaments

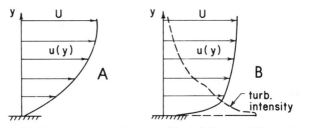

Figure 13. Boundary-layer velocity profiles; (*A*) laminar, (*B*) turbulent.

that are constantly stretched (denoted by the second term in Eq. 8) while at the same time being destroyed by the action of viscosity. A two-dimensional turbulent flow field cannot exist except in a state of decay as the vortex stretching necessary to continuously produce new vorticity will be identically equal to zero.

It is worthwhile to review some gross features of turbulent flows. Turbulent flow is highly diffusive; this is the most straightforward mechanistic test that can be employed to determine if a flow is turbulent or not. A neutrally buoyant dot of ink in a turbulent flow field of water will be obliterated much faster than if it is put in any of the three above-mentioned random flow cases that are not truly turbulent. The high diffusivity is often accounted for by an eddy viscosity which is clearly a function of position and time and not of the mean velocity field alone as usually assumed. Yet a simple eddy viscosity assumption, although conceptually incorrect, provides acceptable results for some engineering situations, involving a single length scale and a single time scale.

Turbulent flow is highly nonlinear. The primary characteristics of a nonlinear system are the creation of new frequencies and the lack of superposition of two finite-amplitude inputs. In a turbulent flow there is a continual transfer of energy between different frequency components. Figure 14 shows linear and nonlinear transfer functions.

Turbulent flow is highly dissipative. Internal thermal energy is the sink for turbulent kinetic energy: the turbulent kinetic energy from the eddies is irreversibly converted to internal thermal energy by the action of

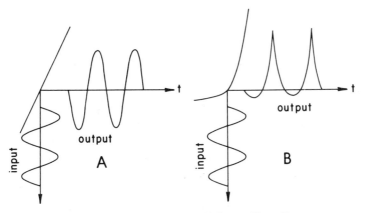

Figure 14. Transfer functions; (*A*) linear, (*B*) nonlinear.

viscosity. This transfer is called "dissipation" and is more effective with the smallest size eddies, being inversely proportional to the square of the eddy sizes. In view of this unidirectional flow of energy on the average, there is a net transfer or cascade of energy from the lower to higher frequencies (even though energy from a frequency component can transfer to both higher and lower frequencies). Most turbulent kinetic energy enters at the largest scales (or eddies) and is converted to internal thermal energy primarily at the smallest scales. Since in any flow situation there is an upper bound on dissipation, there is thus a lower bound on the size of eddies that can exist in the flow; this scale is called the *Kolmogorov scale*. The largest scale in a turbulent shear flow is of the order of the width of the shear region and is called the *integral scale*. There is an intermediate scale called the *Taylor microscale*, which was initially defined in connection with dissipation. This scale has no physical significance because most dissipation occurs in (Kolmogorov) scales much lower than this, but it is still used as a reference length scale of turbulence, presumably for historical reasons; its use is widespread in atmospheric turbulence.

Although the large eddies have preferential orientation so as to cause maximum transfer of energy from the mean field, the small-scale turbulence has no preferred orientation because their scales are typically much smaller than the integral scale, i.e., they are stochastically isotropic. This behavior of the small scales is called *local isotropy*.

Turbulent flows have other interesting characteristics. For sufficiently high Reynolds numbers the flow must be independent of viscosity and thus of Reynolds number. This Reynolds number similarity is known as *asymptotic invariance.* Turbulent flow is a high-Reynolds-number phenomenon. The Reynolds number at which the flow becomes turbulent depends on each configuration; in each case, again, appropriate velocity and length scales must be identified for forming the Reynolds number.

In spite of the presence of very small eddies, turbulent flow behavior is quite different from kinetic theory of gases. The flow still behaves as a continuum; the small length and time (Kolmogorov) scales associated with turbulent flow are many times larger than the length and time scales (i.e., mean free path and collision interval) of molecular motion. For further details on the eiementary aspects of turbulent flow see, for example, texts by Bradshaw (1971), Tennekes and Lumley (1972), and Hinze (1975).

3.5.1 Blood Turbulence Whether turbulence exists in cardiovascular blood flow or not is of interest from the point of view of mixing and transport, heart murmurs, thrombus formation, atherogenesis, etc. For general reviews see Patel et al. (1974), Robertson and Henick (1975), and

Nerem et al. (1974). Turbulence is known to occur in the aorta and behind stenoses; in Section 4 we show that flow behind the mitral valve is turbulent during the diastolic phase.

3.6 Interpretation of the Reynolds Number

The Reynolds number, Re, is the most frequently mentioned quantity in the entire field of fluid mechanics. In general, its interpretation is the ratio of inertial force term $\rho u(\partial u/\partial x) \sim \rho U^2/L$ and viscous force term $\rho\nu(\partial^2 u/\partial y^2) \sim \rho\nu U/L^2$ so that Re $= UL/\nu$. This therefore becomes the important parameter when the momentum equation is nondimensionalized. In the case of rapid velocity variation with respect to time the local acceleration is much larger than the convective acceleration so that balance is between the acceleration term $\partial u/\partial t \sim \omega U$ and the viscous term $\nu(\partial^2 u/\partial y^2) = \nu(U/L^2)$; that is, the corresponding Reynolds number is Re $= \omega L^2/\nu$. For incompressible steady flows without any free surface, the Reynolds number is the only parameter that must be maintained constant between a prototype and a geometrically and kinematically similar model for the data to be applicable to the prototype. For periodic flow, the additional important parameter is Strouhal number. In a steady-flow case, a large Reynolds number suggests that flow is unstable to disturbances and will become turbulent and that the boundary-layer thickness is small compared to the characteristic dimension of the body. In case of a pulsatile flow, large Re would indicate that the Stokes layer thickness is small compared to the body length scale.

In unsteady boundary layers, the Reynolds number $U_0 L/\nu$ signifies the ratio of convection rate by U_0 to the viscous diffusion rate, i.e., $(U_0/L)/(\nu/L^2)$ as well as the ratio of diffusion transverse to a boundary layer to that along the boundary layer, i.e., $(\nu/\delta^2)/(\nu/L^2)$. For a turbulent flow, the Reynolds number takes on newer meanings, e.g.,

$$\frac{\text{Turbulent diffusivity (eddy viscosity)}}{\text{Molecular diffusivity (viscosity)}}$$

$$\left\{\frac{\text{Length scale of a body}}{\text{Length scale of the boundary layer on it}}\right\}^2$$

For a flow with an imposed length scale (e.g., flow in a pipe) the Reynolds number can be expressed as

$$\frac{\text{Time scale for molecular diffusion}}{\text{Time scale for turbulent diffusion}}$$

For a flow with an imposed time scale, e.g., flow in the earth's atmosphere, on a rotating disk, or in periodic flow, the Reynolds number has the following significance:

$$\left\{\frac{\text{Turbulent diffusion length scale}}{\text{Molecular diffusion length scale}}\right\}^2$$

In addition to these, there are other Reynolds numbers used to characterize turbulent flows: *Kolmogorov Reynolds number,* $\eta v/\nu = 1$ for all turbulent flows where η, v are the Kolmogorov microscales of length and velocity; *turbulent Reynolds number,* $v\ell/\nu$ where v is the rms turbulent velocity and ℓ the integral scale; *Taylor microscale Reynolds number,* $R_\lambda = u\lambda/\nu$ where λ is Taylor's microscale, and the interpretation of R_λ is

$$\frac{\text{Large eddy time scale}}{\text{Strain rate fluctuation time scale}}$$

3.7 Turbulent Boundary Layer

The structure of turbulent boundary layers and the effect of the compliant wall on the structure are too complex to permit a brief review. This has been an area of vigorous research activity for the recent couple of decades, and space does not permit review of even some major publications. For some elementary aspects see Hinze (1975), Tennekes and Lumley (1972), and Zaric (1972). Willmarth (1975) has prepared an excellent summary of recent experimental studies of turbulent boundary layers. For a review of the effect of compliant wall, see Ash et al. (1975).

3.8 Time Average and Reynolds Stress

As indicated before, pressure, velocity, vorticity, temperature, concentration, etc., in a turbulent flow field are random functions of position and time. While the Navier–Stokes equations adequately represent the evolution of a given flow with adequately specified boundary and initial conditions, the nonlinearity of the governing equations precludes their solution in general. Even if the solutions to the equations were available, the values for the instantaneous pressure and velocity as a function of time at each location in the flow field would be unmanageably excessive information. One thus looks for the statistical aspects of the flow, e.g., mean velocity, rms turbulent intensity, Reynolds stress, spectra, etc. These quantities provide meaningful information if the flow is stochastically stationary,[13] i.e., its statistics are independent of time. Thus the *time average* of any random quantity f is defined as

$$\bar{f} \equiv \lim_{T \to \infty} \frac{1}{T} \int_0^T f(t)\, dt \tag{23}$$

One can thus decompose the instantaneous variables u, v, p as

$$u = \bar{u} + u' = \bar{U} + u'$$
$$v = \bar{v} + v' = \bar{V} + v' \tag{24}$$
$$p = \bar{p} + p' = \bar{P} + p'$$

so that by definition, the averages of u', v', p' are zeros (see Eq. 17) and the partial derivatives of the mean quantities, $\bar{U}$, $\bar{V}$, $\bar{P}$ are zeros. Substituting these in the momentum equation (Eq. 9) and taking its time average one gets

$$\rho \bar{U} \frac{\partial \bar{U}}{\partial x} + \rho \bar{V} \frac{\partial \bar{U}}{\partial y} = -\frac{\partial \bar{P}}{\partial x} + \frac{\partial}{\partial y} \left(\mu \frac{\partial \bar{U}}{\partial y} - \rho \overline{u'v'} \right) \tag{25}$$

Comparing this equation with the boundary layer equation, Eq. 9, we see that in addition to the convective, pressure, and viscous terms, the additional term is the gradient of the nonlinear term $\rho \overline{u'v'}$, which represents the average transverse transport of longitudinal momentum per unit mass; this appears as a pseudostress along with the viscous stress $\mu\, \partial \bar{U}/\partial y$, and is called *Reynolds stress* in honor of Osborne Reynolds, who first introduced it. This term represents the effect of the fluctuating turbulent field on the mean field that is distorted by the turbulence; this term is usually large in most turbulent shear flows. Notice that the Reynolds stress term arises from the nonlinear convective term due to the application of the time average and represents the anisotropic nature of turbulent shear flow; Reynolds stress is zero in an isotropic turbulent flow.

When a turbulent flow field changes with time, the concept of time average is not a useful concept; the concept of short time average used by some authors is not meaningful, either. One then has to use *ensemble average*. If a large number of identical experiments with identical initial and boundary conditions could be started simultaneously, then at some time later the average of any quantity over all the experiments gives the

---

[13] For general treatment of random functions see Papoulis (1965), Bendat and Piersol (1971), and Panchev (1971).

ensemble average, although individual realizations are different from one another because of the random evolution. The deviation from the ensemble average could be taken to represent the instantaneous turbulent quantity for each experiment. One can use ensemble average to determine their intensity and other turbulence measures.

Because it is unrealistic to run a large number of simultaneous identical experiments, nonstationary turbulent flows in general defy any meaningful analysis. One simplification would be to repeat the experiment a number of times and assume that the initial and boundary conditions in each case are identical. In many situations this may be prohibitively expensive.

For time-dependent turbulent flows, if the flow is periodic, each period constitutes a member of the ensemble. One can introduce a periodic ensemble average and use it to adequately characterize the flow.

3.9 Phase Average

In case of a pulsating turbulent flow the instantaneous variables consist of contributions from the mean flow, the periodic component, and the background turbulence. From the time-dependent variation of a quantity, only when the periodic component is subtracted out can one study the nature of turbulence. In the presence of a periodic perturbation, any instantaneous flow variable f at location $\mathbf{x}$ and time t can be decomposed (following Hussain, 1969) as

$$f(\mathbf{x},t) = \bar{f}(\mathbf{x}) + \tilde{f}(\mathbf{x},t) + f'(\mathbf{x},t) \qquad (26)$$

where $\bar{f}$ is the time mean value at $\mathbf{x}$, $\tilde{f}$ is the statistical contribution of the periodic disturbance at $\mathbf{x}$ and at the instant t, and f' is the background turbulence. This decomposition is clearly in the spirit of Osborne Reynolds, whose introduction of the instantaneous turbulent signal as the sum of the time mean and the random fluctuations gave rise to the appearance of Reynolds stress term in the time-averaged mean momentum equation. Clearly, presence of the periodic component will also give rise to periodic Reynolds stress.

In a stationary turbulent flow, the Reynolds decomposition requires a time average to sort out the governing equations for the mean and the turbulent fields. However, the decomposition of the total velocity into three velocity scales likewise in Eq. 26 requires introduction of another average, called the *phase average* (see Hussain, 1969), which is defined as

$$\langle f(\mathbf{x},t) \rangle = \lim_{N \to \infty} \frac{1}{N} \sum_{n=1}^{N} f(\mathbf{x}, t + n\tau) \qquad (27a)$$

where τ is the period of the pulsation. The phase average, $\langle f \rangle$, thus repeats itself in time every interval τ apart. Taking a clock synchronized with the disturbance period, the phase average at any point in space is the average at a particular phase ϕ in the cycle of the pulsation; that is, $\langle f \rangle$ can be better explained as

$$\langle f(\mathbf{x},\phi) \rangle = \lim_{N \to \infty} \frac{1}{N} \sum_{n=1}^{N} f(\mathbf{x},\phi + n\omega\tau) \tag{27b}$$

where ω is the circular frequency of the pulsation.

In a real experiment f is recorded neither over infinite time nor over an ensemble size of infinity, so that the time average $\bar{f}$ has to be determined over a finite interval T. This period is adequate if it is much larger than the integral scale or the time scale of the largest eddies in a stationary flow; a good test is to show that averages taken over intervals greater than T remain unchanged. For a periodic flow the ensemble size N that is adequate to give the phase average can be determined by ensuring that larger ensemble sizes do not affect phase average.

Definitions 27a and 27b apply to flows that are statistically periodic in time. For flows that are statistically periodic in space, such as a traveling wave, the phase average must be determined at different phases in the wavelength.

In order to understand the phase average, consider a periodic turbulent signal f with period T; suppose that the instantaneous total signal is sampled at a phase ϕ in each cycle and an average of the signal value at that phase is taken over a large number of cycles. Since background turbulence is random, it will cancel out over a large number of cycles; the average is thus the phase average of f at phase ϕ in the period T. If this averaging procedure is repeated for all phases ϕ within the period, one obtains the phase average $\langle f \rangle$ of f; any deviation of f from $\langle f \rangle$ is the background turbulence, i.e.,

$$\langle f \rangle = \bar{f} + \tilde{f}$$
$$f' = f - \langle f \rangle \tag{27c}$$

Thus given an instantaneous signal $f(t)$ at any point in a pulsatile flow field and given the period of pulsation, i.e., a reference wave with its period equal to that of pulsation, the three components of the total signal f, i.e., the time mean, the periodic component, and the background turbulence component, can be determined by the application of the time and phase averages introduced above. The statistical contribution due to the pulsation or a traveling wave can be determined by subtracting the time average from the phase average. The instantaneous deviation of the total signal from the phase average gives the contribution of the background turbulence (see Figure 15); its rms value gives the turbulence intensity.

The heart beat is the natural clock for the living body so that the cardiac cycle can be used as the most convenient reference wave for obtaining phase averages of velocity, pressure, Reynolds stress, etc., in the cardiovascular flow field. In the arteries, the periodic components of the velocity and pressure signals are large compared to their fluctuations, the period being marked by steep velocity and pressure rises during systole. This permits the use of the signal itself to define the beginning of each period (see Figure 15) and will thus render the need for another periodic signal unnecessary.

A note of warning is in order at this point; the above method of determining the pulsation-induced component and the background turbulent component is precise only if the signal is strictly periodic. However, the cardiac cycle or the velocity or pressure signal in the aorta is not always periodic; the period changes over time depending on, among other factors, the subject's consciousness or excitement level, which affects heart

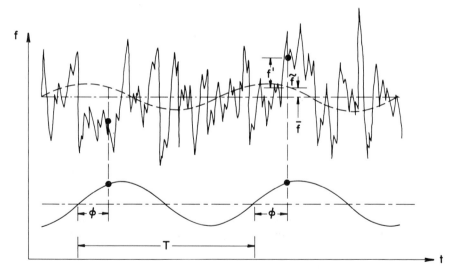

Figure 15. Time and phase averages; time average = $\overline{f}$, phase average = $\langle f \rangle = \overline{f} + \tilde{f}$.

rate. Worse yet, there is variation in the period from cycle to cycle because the heart does not repeat itself every cycle. Thus even if the signal were strictly nonturbulent, the "period jitter" would contribute to the turbulent signal, to its rms value, and to other statistical measures. For this reason turbulence analysis of periodic random signal obtained in vivo requires that the subject be maintained in a controlled state, e.g., under anesthesia, when the turbulent signal (in the heart, aorta, or arteries) is taken. In vitro data should be free from the jitter effect because the modulation period can be precisely controlled.

The phase-average technique is thus especially suited for experiments with controlled excitation; see Section 4 for some recent investigations.

3.10 Mechanics of Pulsatile Turbulent Flow[14]

In the presence of a periodic disturbance in a turbulent flow, any instantaneous quantity $f(\mathbf{x},t)$ can be represented as

$$f(\mathbf{x},t) = \langle f(\mathbf{x},t) \rangle + f'(\mathbf{x},t) \tag{28a}$$

where $\langle f \rangle$ is the property associated with the organized (i.e., periodic) field and f' the background (random) turbulent fluctuation. It follows that for two functions $f(\mathbf{x},t)$ and $g(\mathbf{x},t)$,

$$\langle f' \rangle = 0; \ \langle \langle f \rangle g \rangle = \langle f \rangle \langle g \rangle \tag{28b}$$

$$\therefore \langle f' \langle g \rangle \rangle = 0$$

We can thus represent the instantaneous velocities $u_i(\mathbf{x},t)$ and pressure $p(\mathbf{x},t)$ as

$$u_i = \langle u_i \rangle + u_i'$$

$$p = \langle p \rangle + p' \tag{28c}$$

and derive governing equations for the organized and turbulent fields. We find that each of the two fields satisfies the incompressible continuity equation, i.e.,

$$\frac{\partial \langle u_i \rangle}{\partial x_i} = \frac{\partial u_i'}{\partial x_i} = 0 \tag{28d}$$

---

[14] This section can be omitted by those not interested in the fundamental interpretations.

Substituting Eq. 28c in the Navier–Stokes equation and taking the phase average, we obtain the momentum equation for the organized field,

$$\rho \frac{\hat{D}\langle u_i \rangle}{Dt} = -\frac{\partial \langle p \rangle}{\partial x_i} + \frac{\partial}{\partial x_j}\left(\mu \frac{\partial \langle u_i \rangle}{\partial x_j} - \rho \langle u_i' u_j' \rangle \right) \qquad (28e)$$

where

$$\frac{\hat{D}}{Dt} = \frac{\partial}{\partial t} + \langle u_j \rangle \frac{\partial}{\partial x_j}$$

is the time derivative following a fluid particle moving with the organized fluid motion. $-\rho \langle u_i' u_j' \rangle$ represents the contribution of the turbulent field to the organized field; it appears in the equation along with the viscous stress $\mu(\partial \langle u_i \rangle / \partial x_j)$ of the organized field and is thus the *organized Reynolds stress*. The term $(\partial/\partial x_j)(-\rho \langle u_i' u_j' \rangle)$ denotes the net organized momentum transport by the turbulent velocity fluctuations. The momentum equation for the turbulent field is then obtained by subtracting Eq. 28e from the instantaneous equation, Eq. 7b, i.e.,

$$\rho \frac{\hat{D}u_i'}{Dt} + \rho u_j' \frac{\partial \langle u_i \rangle}{\partial x_j} = -\frac{\partial p'}{\partial x_i} + \frac{\partial}{\partial x_j}\left[\mu \frac{\partial u_i'}{\partial x_j} - \rho(u_i' u_j' - \langle u_i' u_j' \rangle) \right] \qquad (28f)$$

The effect of the organized field on the turbulence field is apparent.

Some further understanding can be obtained from the energy equations for the two fields. Multiplying Eq. 28e by $\langle u_i \rangle$ and then taking the phase average we get the kinetic energy equation for the organized field, i.e.,

$$\frac{\hat{D}}{Dt}\left(\frac{\langle u_i \rangle \langle u_i \rangle}{2} \right) = \left| \frac{\partial}{\partial x_i}\left(\frac{\langle p \rangle \langle u_i \rangle}{\rho} \right) \right.$$

$$+ \langle u_i' u_j' \rangle \frac{\partial \langle u_i \rangle}{\partial x_j} - \frac{\partial}{\partial x_j}(\langle u_i \rangle \langle u_i' u_j' \rangle)$$

$$+ \nu \frac{\partial}{\partial x_j}\left\{ \langle u_i \rangle \left(\frac{\partial \langle u_i \rangle}{\partial x_j} + \frac{\partial \langle u_j \rangle}{\partial x_i} \right) \right\}$$

$$- \frac{\nu}{2}\left\{ \frac{\partial \langle u_i \rangle}{\partial x_j} + \frac{\partial \langle u_j \rangle}{\partial x_i} \right\}\left\{ \frac{\partial \langle u_i \rangle}{\partial x_j} + \frac{\partial \langle u_j \rangle}{\partial x_i} \right\} \qquad (28g)$$

Similarly, the kinetic energy equation for the turbulence field is obtained by multiplying Eq. 28f by u_i' and then taking phase average, i.e.,

$$\frac{\hat{D}}{Dt}\left(\frac{\langle u_i' u_i' \rangle}{2}\right) = -\frac{\partial}{\partial x_j} \langle u_j'\left(\frac{p'}{\rho} + \frac{1}{2} u_i' u_i'\right)\rangle - \langle u_i' u_j'\rangle \frac{\partial \langle u_i \rangle}{\partial x_j}$$

$$+ \nu \frac{\partial}{\partial x_j} \langle u_i'\left(\frac{\partial u_i'}{\partial x_j} + \frac{\partial u_j'}{\partial x_i}\right)\rangle$$

$$- \frac{\nu}{2}\langle\left(\frac{\partial u_i'}{\partial x_j} + \frac{\partial u_j'}{\partial x_i}\right)\left(\frac{\partial u_i'}{\partial x_j} + \frac{\partial u_j'}{\partial x_i}\right)\rangle \qquad (28h)$$

In Eqs. 28g and 28h the left-hand side is the rate of change of kinetic energy per unit mass per unit time in the respective fields. The first term on the right in 28g is the convective transport of the phase-average pressure energy by the organized motion and is thus the "flow work" of the organized field. The second term represents the loss of kinetic energy of the organized flow field due to the shear work of the organized kinematic Reynolds stress $-\langle u_i' u_j'\rangle$ against the organized flow field shear $\partial\langle u_i\rangle/\partial x_j$. This is responsible for generation of turbulent kinetic energy and can be called production. Notice that this is a negative term in Eq. 28g but appears, as expected, with an opposite sign in Eq. 28h as a source term. The third term represents the energy transport due to work done by the Reynolds stresses, $-\langle u_i' u_j'\rangle$. The last two are the viscous work terms; the separation into two terms is motivated by physical reasons. The first of these is the energy transfer by viscous work and represents a redistribution of kinetic energy within the flow domain; its integration over the flow region bounded by rigid boundaries is zero. The second represents transfer of kinetic energy to thermal energy by viscosity and is called dissipation; it is a net negative quantity and represents unidirectional transfer of kinetic to thermal energy. These are, therefore, respectively the reversible and irreversible works done by the viscous stresses.

The interpretations of the corresponding terms in Eq. 28h are similar; physical interpretations are discussed below.

3.10.1 Modulated Turbulent Flows In a pulsatile turbulent flow with a non-zero mean we should be interested in the time-average quantities also; thus we need to use the decompositions

$$u_i = \bar{U}_i + \tilde{u}_i + u_i' \qquad (29a)$$

$$p = \bar{P} + \tilde{p} + p' \tag{29b}$$

and then derive the governing equations for the mean, periodic, and turbulent components.

The following consequences of time and phase averages must be recognized:

$$\langle g' \rangle = 0 \tag{30a}$$

$$\overline{g'} = 0 \tag{30b}$$

$$\overline{\tilde{g}} = 0 \tag{30c}$$

$$\overline{\tilde{g}h} = \overline{\tilde{g}}\overline{h} \tag{30d}$$

$$\langle \tilde{g}h \rangle = \tilde{g}\langle h \rangle \tag{30e}$$

$$\langle \bar{g}h \rangle = \bar{g}\langle h \rangle \tag{30f}$$

$$\overline{\langle g \rangle} = \bar{g} \tag{30g}$$

$$\langle \bar{g} \rangle = \bar{g} \tag{30h}$$

$$\overline{\tilde{g}h'} = \langle \overline{\tilde{g}h'} \rangle = 0 \tag{30i}$$

The random nature of the background turbulent signal g' is stated by the first two relations. The third states that the time average of a pulsation-induced quantity is zero. The fifth one states that the phase average of a product of a periodic quantity $\tilde{g}$ and any quantity h is the product $\tilde{g} \langle h \rangle$. The sixth emphasizes that the phase average is a linear operation. The seventh and eighth state that when both time and phase averages are applied, the result is time average. The last two relations state the key concept, i.e., the periodic and the background turbulent components are, on the average, uncorrelated.

In the following we consider all the variables to be nondimensionalized by the appropriate length scale δ (e.g., pipe diameter) velocity scale U_0 (e.g., maximum velocity) so that pressure is nondimensionalized by ρU_0^2, and $\mathrm{Re} \equiv U_0 \delta / \nu$ is the Reynolds number.

Substituting the decomposition, Eq. 29a, in the continuity equation, Eq. 3a, and first taking the phase average and then the time average, one sees that each of the components separately satisfies the continuity equation (a direct consequence of the linearity of the continuity equation and also linearity of the time and phase averaging operations), i.e.,

$$\frac{\partial \bar{U}_i}{\partial x_i} = \frac{\partial \bar{\tilde{u}}_i}{\partial x_i} = \frac{\partial u_i'}{\partial x_i} = 0 \tag{31}$$

Similarly, by substituting Eqs. 29 in the Navier–Stokes equations, Eq. 7b, we obtain Eq. A, which after phase averaging becomes Eq. B (A and B are not written here for brevity). Then, time average of B gives the equation for the mean flow in a pulsatile turbulent flow, i.e.,

$$\bar{U}_j \frac{\partial \bar{U}_i}{\partial x_j} = -\frac{\partial \bar{P}}{\partial x_i} + \frac{1}{\mathrm{Re}} \frac{\partial^2 \bar{U}_i}{\partial x_j \partial x_j} - \frac{\partial}{\partial x_j}(\overline{u_i' u_j'}) - \frac{\partial}{\partial x_j}(\overline{\tilde{u}_i \tilde{u}_j}) \tag{32}$$

Note that this equation for the mean flow differs from that of a steady laminar flow because of the last two terms; the first of these two is the familiar Reynolds stress term representing the contribution of the turbulent field to the mean field. The last term represents the modification of the mean field due to the periodic pulsation field. In a two-dimensional flow $-\rho \overline{\tilde{u}\tilde{v}}$ represents the average transverse transport of streamwise pulsation momentum by pulsation-induced velocity per unit time per unit area.

Subtraction of Eq. 32 from B gives the governing equation for the periodic pulsation velocity field:

$$\frac{\bar{D}}{Dt}\tilde{u}_i + \tilde{u}_j \frac{\partial \bar{U}_i}{\partial x_j} = -\frac{\partial \tilde{p}}{\partial x_i} + \frac{1}{\mathrm{Re}} \frac{\partial^2 \tilde{u}_i}{\partial x_j \partial x_j}$$

$$- \frac{\partial}{\partial x_j}(\tilde{u}_i \tilde{u}_j - \overline{\tilde{u}_i \tilde{u}_j}) - \frac{\partial}{\partial x_j}(\langle u_i' u_j' \rangle - \overline{u_i' u_j'}) \tag{33}$$

In addition to the typical convective, pressure gradient, and viscous terms, the equation contains the last two quadratic terms representing the contribution to the pulsation flow field by pulsation through self-interaction and by the background turbulent field because of its modulation by the periodic pulsation field. Note that $\bar{D}/Dt = \partial/\partial t + U_j \partial/\partial x_j$.

Subtraction of Eq. B from A, obviously, gives the governing equation for the background turbulent fluctuations, i.e.,

$$\frac{\bar{D}u_i'}{Dt} + \tilde{u}_j \frac{\partial u_i'}{\partial x_j} + u_j' \frac{\partial \bar{U}_i}{\partial x_j} + u_j' \frac{\partial \tilde{u}_i}{\partial x_j}$$

$$= -\frac{\partial p'}{\partial x_i} + \frac{1}{\mathrm{Re}} \frac{\partial^2 u_i'}{\partial x_j \partial x_j} + \frac{\partial}{\partial x_j}(\langle u_i' u_j' \rangle - u_i'' u_j') \tag{34}$$

The last term gives the contribution to the turbulent field due to the instantaneous turbulent momentum transport over the phase-averaged turbulent momentum transport.

Note that in each equation the quadratic terms representing momentum transport due to pulsation and turbulence arise from the nonlinear convective terms of the Navier–Stokes equation. There is a hierarchy of momentum transport involved. The average of time-dependent momentum transport by the pulsation-induced velocity fluctuations contributes to the mean momentum field; the balance of the pulsation components contributes to the pulsation momentum field only, but not to the turbulent field; the contribution of the pulsation to the turbulence field is only through modulation of the turbulence momentum transport. On the other hand, background turbulence contributes to each of the three momentum fields. The instantaneous turbulent momentum transport r_{ij} due to the turbulent field can be split into three parts:

$$-u_i'u_j' \equiv r_{ij} = \bar{r}_{ij} + \tilde{r}_{ij} + r_{ij}'$$

$$\bar{r}_{ij} = -\overline{u_i'u_j'}; \qquad \tilde{r}_{ij} = -\langle u_i'u_j' \rangle + \overline{u_i'u_j'} \qquad (35)$$

$$r_{ij}' = -u_i'u_j' + \langle u_i'u_j' \rangle$$

Thus the momentum contribution of turbulence is $\bar{r}_{ij}$ to the mean field, $\tilde{r}_{ij}$ to the pulsation field, and r_{ij}' to the turbulent field. The term $\tilde{r}_{ij}$ representing the difference of the phase and time averages of the background turbulence Reynolds stress is physically important because it represents the periodic modulation of the background Reynolds stress by the pulsation and suggests that interaction between pulsation and turbulence fields can be important.

A look at Eqs. 32–34 shows that, in spite of the success of the introduction of time and phase averages in identifying the governing equations for the mean, pulsation, and turbulent fluctuations, the three fields are indeed strongly coupled; they must be solved simultaneously and the unknowns, $\bar{r}_{ij}$, $\tilde{r}_{ij}$, r_{ij}', $\overline{u_i u_j}$, have to be expressed in terms of other variables. See Hussain (1969) for application to a simple flow (discussed briefly in Section 4.1).

The complexity of Eqs. 32–34 does not permit any direct appreciation of the three components in a pulsatile turbulent flow field. However, some further insight can be obtained from the consideration of the energetics of the flow. In a turbulent flow, there is a continual transfer (dissipation) of kinetic energy from the turbulent field to internal thermal energy by the action of viscosity. This drain, if the flow is stationary, is continually replenished by the transfer of mean flow kinetic energy by the work of the Reynolds stress against mean shear. The direct dissipation of the mean kinetic energy to thermal energy is very small owing to small strain rates of the mean flow field. In the presence of pulsations, the energetics gets complex because pulsation may add to as well as extract energy from the mean field. Because the total average energy of the flow field must be equal to the sum of the average kinetic energies of the mean, pulsation, and turbulent fields,

$$\tfrac{1}{2}\,\overline{u_i u_i} = \underset{E}{\tfrac{1}{2}\,\overline{U_i U_i}} + \underset{\mathcal{E}}{\tfrac{1}{2}\,\overline{\tilde{u}_i \tilde{u}_i}} + \underset{e}{\tfrac{1}{2}\,\overline{u_i' u_i'}} \tag{36}$$

Equations for the average kinetic energies of the mean, pulsation, and turbulence fields can be obtained by multiplying the equations for $\bar{U}_i$, $\tilde{u}_i$, and u_i', i.e., Eqs. 32, 33, and 34, by $\bar{U}_i$, $\tilde{u}_i$, and u_i', respectively, then taking first the phase average and then the time average. One can then obtain the following energy equations (see Hussain, 1969):

$$\frac{\bar{D}}{Dt}(E) = -\frac{\partial}{\partial x_i}(\bar{P}\bar{U}_i) - (-\overline{u_i' u_j'})\frac{\partial \bar{U}_i}{\partial x_j} - (-\overline{\tilde{u}_i \tilde{u}_j})\frac{\partial \bar{U}_i}{\partial x_j} \tag{37a}$$
$$+ \text{ visc. terms} + \text{triple correl.}$$

$$\frac{\bar{D}}{Dt}(\mathcal{E}) = -\frac{\partial}{\partial x_i}(\overline{\tilde{p}\tilde{u}_i}) + (-\overline{\tilde{u}_i \tilde{u}_j})\frac{\partial \bar{U}_i}{\partial x_j} - (-\overline{\langle u_i' u_j' \rangle})\frac{\partial \tilde{u}_i}{\partial x_j} \tag{37b}$$
$$+ \text{ visc. terms} + \text{triple correl.}$$

$$\frac{\bar{D}}{Dt}(e) = -\frac{\partial}{\partial x_i}(\overline{p' u_i'}) + (-\overline{u_i' u_j'})\frac{\partial \bar{U}_i}{\partial x_j} + (-\overline{\langle u_i' u_j' \rangle})\frac{\partial \tilde{u}_i}{\partial x_j} \tag{37c}$$
$$+ \text{ visc. terms} + \text{triple correl.}$$

Note the close similarity between the terms of the three equations. The term on the left of each equation denotes the increase of the average kinetic energy of the component per unit mass per unit time and the terms on the right denote the mechanics governing these changes.

Let us discuss the right-hand side. The first term represents the pressure–velocity correlation term; this term in Eq. 37c is responsible for redistribution of turbulent kinetic energy by the action of pressure fluctuation. The viscous terms in Eq. 37 have the same form and explanation as in Eq. 28g,h. The triple product of the velocity fields (last term) represents convection of kinetic energy of a component by itself; the integral of this term over the flow domain is also zero, because this represents convection of the kinetic energy. The volume integral of the pressure velocity term is also zero because this represents intercomponent transfer of kinetic energy without any net loss. See Hussain (1969) for details.

The most important terms are the second and third terms on the right-hand side, i.e., the "production" terms. The term $-\overline{u'_i u'_j}\,(\partial \bar{U}_i/\partial x_j)$ represents the production of turbulent kinetic energy by the action of the kinematic turbulent (Reynolds) stress $-\overline{u'_i u'_j}$ against the mean shear $\partial \bar{U}_i/\partial x_j$; this term thus appears as a drain term in the mean field Eq. 37a but appears with the opposite sign, i.e., as an energy source term in the turbulent kinetic energy Eq. 37c. More interestingly, the third term in Eq. 37a is the loss of mean kinetic energy to the pulsation field by the action of the pulsation-induced Reynolds stresses $-\overline{\tilde{u}_i \tilde{u}_j}$ against the mean shear. This term appears as a drain term in Eq. 37a representing a loss of mean kinetic energy and appears as an energy source term with opposite sign in the pulsation kinetic energy Eq. 37b. This term clearly shows that the pulsation can be further strengthened by the mean field. The third term on the right side in Eq. 37b is rather subtle; it represents a net transfer of kinetic energy from the periodic field to the turbulence field by the action of the oscillating Reynolds stress $\langle -u'_i u'_j \rangle$ against the pulsation-induced shear $\partial \tilde{u}_i/\partial x_j$. This oscillation is produced by the imposed flow pulsation. The same term appears as an input term (with the opposite sign) in Eq. 37c. Note that energy transfer from the pulsation-induced field to the turbulence field requires that the phase difference between the pulsation-induced periodic strain rate $\partial \tilde{u}_i/\partial x_j$ and the Reynolds stress oscillation $\langle -u'_i u'_j \rangle$ be less than $\pi/2$.

On the average, the kinetic energy of turbulence is produced by the "production" term but destroyed by the viscous "dissipation" term. The mean flow field loses energy to the periodic and turbulence fields and directly to the thermal energy through viscous dissipation. The pulsation field receives energy from the mean field but loses energy to the turbulence field and to direct viscous dissipation. This discussion, from energy considerations, once again brings out some aspects of the mechanics of interactions between the mean, pulsation, and turbulence fields.

The above discussion is more relevant when the pulsation is a traveling disturbance or it is a pulsation of an amplitude that is small compared to the mean velocity. The above formalism was applied for developing a theory for perturbations in turbulent shear flows and for predicting traveling-wave characteristics and eigenfunctions (see Hussain, 1969; Reynolds and Hussain, 1972).

4 SOME PERIODIC TURBULENT FLOWS

In the following we review some recent experiments involving pulsatile turbulent flows that may be of relevance to the cardiovascular system. The experiments in a channel flow and in a plane jet are of basic interest. The flow through a circular jet is of direct relevance to the arterial and valvular stenoses. The last one presents in vitro hot-film measurements behind a natural human mitral valve.

4.1 Channel and Plane Jet Experiments

The complexity of turbulent flows has rendered inadequate even the best theories developed so far; the search for better closures for the governing equations continues. In view of the simple mathematics of wave disturbances, the representation of a shear flow turbulence as a superposition of (vorticity) waves seems attractive. This representation is different from Fourier decomposition (transform) of the instantaneous random signal; Fourier decomposition would typically show that the phase and group velocities (ω/k, $d\omega/dk$) will take all possible values for disturbances covering the entire spectrum. On the other hand, if turbulent flow is indeed wavelike, these velocities will be essentially the same for all wavenumbers. In fact, the natural disturbances in a turbulent pipe flow have been observed to demonstrate this wavelike behavior (Morrison and Kronauer, 1970).

Based on the above motivation, Hussain (1969) studied the behavior of controlled-perturbation waves for a very simple flow geometry, viz., plane parallel flow, and theoretically predicted the traveling-wave characteristics and their eigenfunction distributions. He then carried out an experimental investigation in a turbulent air channel flow in which two thin ribbons were oscillated electromagnetically and the flow downstream was studied by hot-wire anemometry.

Central to the signal processing system were the Princeton Applied Research Waveform Eductor and the Lock-in-Amplifier. The waveform eductor performs the phase averaging defined earlier and the lock-in amplifier determines the amplitude and the phase of the fundamental of the phase-averaged signal.

Principal conclusions arrived at through this experiment are that the traveling waves in a turbulent shear flow decay essentially exponentially, the decay rate increasing with increasing frequency. The wavenumber increases with the frequency of the disturbance so that the phase velocity is essentially constant and is about 90% of maximum mean velocity. For further details see also Hussain and Reynolds (1970, 1972).

The above experiment in a fully developed turbulent channel flow showed that the wave decay increased with increasing frequencies. Thus there was an upper limit to the frequency above which data over a sufficient streamwise length could not be obtained.

It was hoped that data over a wide range in frequency could be obtained in a plane jet where the disturbances would first grow before decay. This was the motivation behind the recent experiments carried out by Hussain and Thompson (1975) in a plane turbulent jet.

The relevance of the above jet data to the cardiovascular system stems from the fact that the flows behind the aortic and the mitral valves resemble pulsatile jet flow with large pulsation amplitude. (The circular jet flow is discussed later.) The peculiarities of the constitutions and shapes of the valves must have an important effect on the flow dynamics distal to them, because we know that the near field of a jet depends also on the initial profile characteristics (see Clark and Hussain, 1975).

4.1.1 Valve Dynamics   The flow, in turn, affects the valve dynamics. The formation of organized large vortices as the flow passes through the valve leaflets seems to be critical for the effective operation of the valves. The role of the vortex formation, even though probably conjectured previously by others, was first demonstrated by Bellhouse and Bellhouse (1968, 1969a) in in vitro study. They found that the three pouches (sinuses of valsalva) in the wall behind the three cup-shaped membranes of the aortic valve were responsible for the formation of three vortices during systole; these vortices then participate in the motion of the valve leaflets themselves. The fluid rolls over each curved flexible valve leaflet and swirls into a vortex in each pouch and in the process pushes the valve leaflet back to the closed position before actual diastole of the left ventricle begins. Apart from flow visualization, they used hot-film anemometry to determine the flow velocity field and to compare the data with the predictions based on the Hill spherical vortex (Bellhouse and Talbot, 1969). Detailed in vitro study was also carried out by Bellhouse and Bellhouse (1969a, 1969b) to study the role of the vortex formation in the left ventricle in the operation of the mitral valve. (See also Taylor and Wade (1973).) When the left ventricle was allowed to fill slowly so that the vortex formation was either eliminated or sufficiently weakened, the backflow across the mitral valve due to systole was increased five times. They thus concluded that the valve leaflets rely on the vortex lump to push the leaflets back to closure and suggested that the papillary muscles and chordae tendineae serve to prevent mitral valve inversion during systole. The ventricular flow is complicated because of the papillary muscles and the chordae tendineae and the time-dependent wall distension; thus such explanations are indeed simplistic.

Another importnat role of the vortex formation in the ventricle seems to be to keep the fluid in constant motion so that essentially no area of stasis occurs in the left ventricle. Some artificial hearts as well as left ventricular bypass devices show significant areas of coagulation after some use indicating a failure to emulate the natural flow.

4.2 Vortex Shedding in the Presence of Flow Pulsation

The Tritton-Gaster controversy regarding the duality of low-Reynolds-number vortex shedding has spurred a number of investigations but the controversy still remains unresolved (Tritton, 1959, 1971; Gaster, 1969, 1971; Berger and Wille, 1972). In addition to these investigators, a number of others have speculated that the free-stream turbulence will have a noticeable influence on the vortex-shedding mechanism.

This motivated us to carry out an investigation of the effect of free-stream turbulence intensity on the vortex-shedding phenomenon. The shedding cylinder was exposed to flows with free-stream turbulence up to 8% in intensity created by different grids upstream of the cylinder. The conclusion from this study (see Hussain and Ramjee, 1975, 1976) is that turbulence of moderate intensities typical for realistic situations does not affect vortex shedding. Immediately behind the cylinder, the wake frequency is that of the low turbulence signal (see Roshko, 1954). The periodic velocity oscillation due to the vortex streets is strongest at about 5 diameters downstream. It then decays downstream because of viscous diffusion $\nu\nabla^2\zeta$ of vorticity. Sufficiently downstream, when the periodic velocity oscillation is comparable to the free-stream turbulent velocity fluctuations, the two interact nonlinearly and cause rapid decay or transition depending on the Reynolds number. For a given Reynolds number, the distance L_p behind the cylinder over which the frequency count remains constant decreases with increasing turbulence intensities, and, for a given turbulence intensity, L_p decreases with increasing Reynolds numbers. This study shows that the Kármán vortex-shedding method of measuring low velocities can be employed even for large turbulence intensities provided that the detecting hot-wire is placed 5–8 diameters behind the cylinder.

The above results prompted us to study the vortex-shedding phenomenon in the presence of controlled free-stream pulsations. Vortex shedding being a naturally occurring periodic phenomenon, this study of the interaction of a periodic phenomenon and a controlled excitation is of basic interest. The periodic streamwise excitation at controlled frequencies and amplitudes was generated in the test section of a wind tunnel with the help of a loudspeaker attached to its settling chamber.

Conclusions from this study are that for pulsation amplitudes up to 10% of the free-stream velocity, pulsation over a wide range of frequencies has no effect on the shedding frequency except that the signal is amplitude modulated at the difference frequency. Figure 16 shows hot-wire traces for the frequency of pulsation n_p in the range 60–100 Hz while the mean velocity is kept constant such that the natural shedding frequency n_s is 80 Hz. Note that in spite of the different frequencies and amplitudes of modulation, the basic "carrier" frequency is unaffected. At large amplitudes of oscillation, the typical dual frequency on the centerline disappears, suggesting that the vortex shedding is either symmetric or suppressed at large-amplitude streamwise oscillation. The smoke visualization technique that has been used for the low-amplitude pulsation study was not effective in making an exact determination of the flow situation because at these large pulsation amplitudes the smoke jet could not be kept steady or laminar.

Other aspects of this study are that the shedding frequency does not vary as the cosine of the yaw angle; it drops more rapidly at smaller angles. The shedding experiment was also carried out at mild, favorable, and adverse pressure gradients, but no effect on the shedding frequency was observed.

The vortex-shedding experiment is relevant to flow behind valves and protrusions and especially at bifurcations where vortex shedding has been reported (Stehbens, 1975). Vortex shedding in the presence of free-stream disturbances, periodic pulsation, and pressure gradient is directly relevant to the vortex shedding at bifurcations and protrusions in the cardiovascular system.

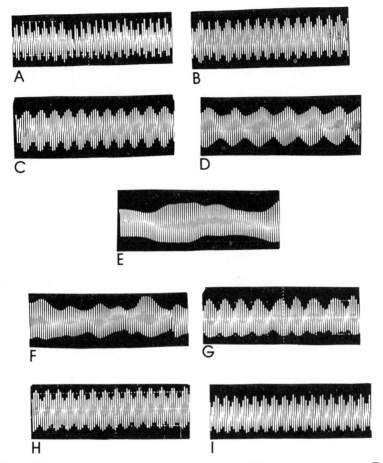

Figure 16. Hot-wire signal traces showing vortex shedding at n_s = 80 Hz, $u'_p/\overline{U}$ = 10%, at different pulsation frequencies n_p; (A) n_p = 100 Hz, (B) n_p = 95 Hz, (C) n_p = 90 Hz, (D) n_p = 85 Hz, (E) n_p = 80 Hz, (F) n_p = 75 Hz, (G) n_p = 70 Hz, (H) n_p = 65 Hz, (I) n_p = 60 Hz.

4.3 Role of Vortex Pairing

The flow behind a cylinder is related to flow behind sharp corners and bluff bodies where vortex shedding plays a critical role in generating the large-scale organized structure, in causing transition, in mixing of heat, mass, and momentum, and in unsteady loading of structures. In all these separating flows, the instability of the shear layer plays the critical role. It is conjectured that, because of the inflexional velocity profile, the shear layer becomes inviscidly unstable and becomes sinuous. A higher-velocity layer slides over the lower-velocity layer and thus eventually the shear layer rolls up into vortex trains (Figure 17A). These vortex trains then undergo transition through secondary instability and become turbulent. Any slight nonuniformity in strengths or spacing of two (or three) adjacent ones mutually induces them to roll up around each other and in the process entrain some nonturbulent fluid to which the vorticity fluctuations eventually, of course, are transferred by viscous diffusion. This is how a shear layer grows (Figure 17B).

This interpretation of mass entrainment in a free-shear layer as that due to engulfment or entrapment of nonvortical fluid slugs is consistent with recent visual studies (Brown and Roshko, 1974; Winant and Browand, 1974) but contrasts with the classical concept of entrainment as

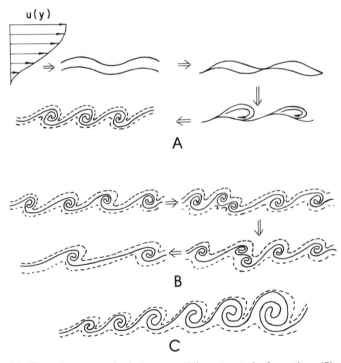

Figure 17. Shear layer organized structure; (*A*) vortex train formation, (*B*) vortex pairing, (*C*) shear layer growth.

the gradual "nibbling away" at the turbulent–nonturbulent interface (see Corrsin and Kistler, 1954; Townsend, 1956; Phillips, 1972). However, Moore and Saffman (1975) provide a mechanism of vortex pairing that agrees more with the pictures of Brown and Roshko (Figure 17C) than with those of Winant and Browand.

Our study suggests that free-stream turbulence or controlled disturbances have no influence on the primary instability of a shear layer. It seems that little is known about the influence of these factors on shear-layer instability (see Michalke, 1972). Effects of initial conditions, free-stream turbulence, and controlled excitation on the free-shear-layer structure are being studied by us. Our data show that evolution and self-preservation of a shear layer vary systematically with variations of its initial characteristics. Results of studies of the near-field shear layer may be important in the design of prosthetic devices involving blood flow, especially valves. In particular, high rates of shear caused by shear layers may cause unacceptable rates of damage of blood cells. The vortex shedding behind both normal and defective heart valves may also cause heart murmurs.

4.4 Pulsatile Flow Jet/Orifice

We have been studying the near flow field of a circular jet under controlled excitation (Hussain and Zaman, 1975); the results obtained so far are reported briefly here because of their possible relevance to the flow through a stenosis or a coarctation.

The experimental set-up is such that different nozzles can be attached at the end of the settling chamber. This study has been carried out for nozzles of three diameters, 1, 2, and 3 in., for tripped (turbulent) as well as untripped (laminar) initial boundary layers. Crow and Champagne (1971) studied limited aspects of controlled excitation of tripped jet flows over the Strouhal number range 0–0.6; the current study extends the Strouhal number range to 0–4.0. The flow through an orifice or a circular jet becomes unstable, unless the Reynolds number is very low and finally becomes turbulent; the turbulence intensity increases in the downstream direction, reaches a maximum, and then decays in the far field.

Figures 18A and 18B show downstream variation of the longitudinal turbulence intensity for 2% exit pulsation amplitude at various Strouhal numbers up to 1.0; the range is divided into two figures for better clarity. Note that the turbulence intensity reaches the peak value at $St_D = 0.3$; a local minimum occurs before a second peak. With further increase of St_D,

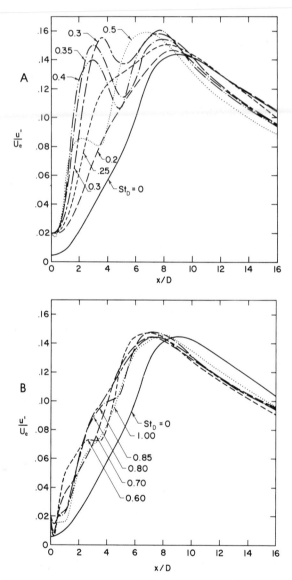

Figure 18. Variation of centerline longitudinal turbulence intensity for tripped nozzle; (A) $0 \leqslant St_D \leqslant 0.5$, (B) $0.6 \leqslant St_D \leqslant 1.0$.

the bump moves upstream. Our data in the range $0 \leqslant St_D \leqslant 0.6$ agree with the data of Crow and Champagne. Note that the far field is essentially independent of St_D. These data were taken with tripped nozzles so that the jet exit boundary layer is turbulent.

When the initial boundary layer is untripped the *preferred mode*, i.e., the Strouhal number that produces the maximum growth, is found to be 0.4 compared to 0.3 for the tripped case. We thus speculated that a subharmonic can be formed at a Strouhal number of 0.8. We were able to stabilize the subharmonic formation at this Strouhal number. The subharmonic formation is associated with laminar vortex pairing, as can be determined from the hot-wire scope traces at successive stations on the centerline of the jet (see Figures 19A–19F). All the figures have identical horizontal and vertical scales. Figure 19A shows the shear layer vortex roll up at the driving frequency. Figure 19B suggests that every alternate vortex is fusing with the next vortex which is growing in strength, finally reaching the maximum strength at $x/D \simeq 2.5$ (Figure 19D). Note that at this stage the signal period is exactly twice that of the initial signal indicated by Figure 19A and that the signal is strictly periodic. Figure 19D shows the passage of identical vortex rings passing over the probe and demonstrates that the vortex pairing is stabilized. Note that at $x/D \simeq 3$, turbulent bursts start forming at the beginning of deceleration from the maximum velocity. At $x/D \simeq 4$ the randomization has advanced significantly. We have observed the same large growth of induced oscillation at $St_D = 0.8$ for 1-, 2-, and 3-in.-diameter nozzles; we thus claim that stable, strong subharmonic formation at $St_D = 0.8$ is universal for all untripped nozzles.

The spectra of the longitudinal velocity fluctuations provide further insights. The signal at the jet exit has a peak at the driving frequency. With progressive distances downstream, first a strong subharmonic component develops; this soon dominates the fundamental. The nonlinearity is manifested by the appearance of higher harmonics. At $x/D = 2$ where the pairing is complete, there is a sudden burst of a large number of harmonics indicating nonlinear saturation and beginning of laminar flow breakdown. At $x/D = 3$, the signal has a wide spectral content. At $x/D = 4$, the randomization is essentially complete; the subharmonic, however, is still strong.

Figure 20 shows the centerline longitudinal turbulence intensity for an untripped nozzle. Note that the near-field turbulence intensity growth rate increases with St_D, reaching a maximum at $St_D = 0.8$. We have also observed vortex pairing at $St_D = 1.2$, but the subharmonic formation is

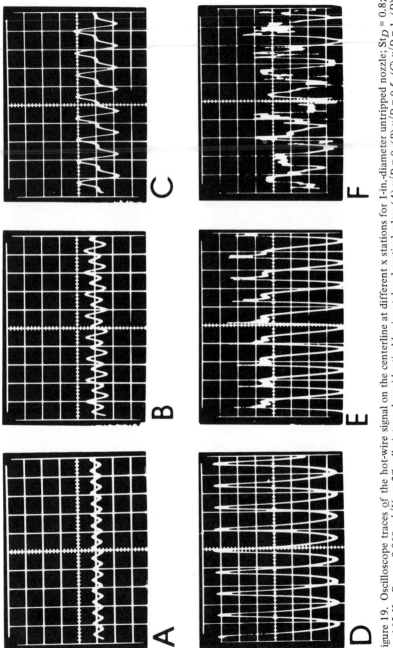
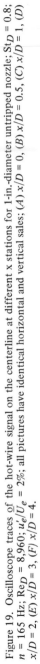

Figure 19. Oscilloscope traces of the hot-wire signal on the centerline at different x stations for 1-in.-diameter untripped nozzle; $St_D = 0.8$; $n = 165$ Hz; $Re_D = 8,960$; $u'_e/U_e = 2\%$; all pictures have identical horizontal and vertical sales; (A) $x/D = 0$, (B) $x/D = 0.5$, (C) $x/D = 1$, (D) $x/D = 2$, (E) $x/D = 3$, (F) $x/D = 4$.

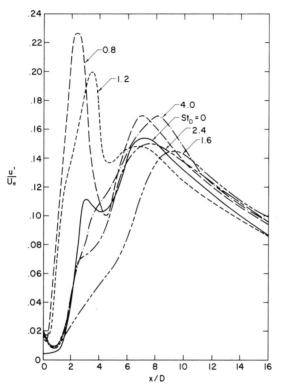

Figure 20. Variation of the centerline longitudinal turbulence intensity for 1-in.-diameter untripped nozzle for $0 \leqslant St_D \leqslant 4.0$; $u'_e/\overline{U}_e = 2\%$.

intermittent. Note that, on the other hand, there is a strong suppression of turbulence intensity at $St_D = 1.6$. With a further increase of St_D, the effect on the turbulent field decreases and becomes essentially negligible at $St_D = 4.0$.

Figure 21 shows the jet diameter corresponding to the points at which the mean velocity is half of the local maximum. Notice the large increase in the diameter immediately downstream from the exit at Strouhal numbers 0.4, 0.8, 1.2, which produce vortex pairing when two adjacent vortices must wrap around each other before merging. Notice that the far field is not significantly dependent on St_D.

We have found that the near-field mass and momentum fluxes and entrainment rate depend strongly on the Strouhal number. The large

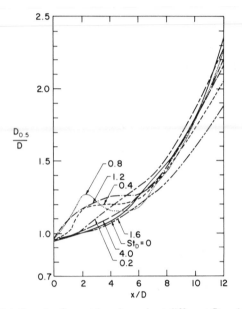

Figure 21. Jet diameter for untripped nozzle at different Strouhal numbers.

entrainment rates at St_D = 0.4, 0.8, 1.2 suggest that vortex pairing produces large fluid engulfments.

Figure 22A shows the subharmonic formation as a function of Reynolds number at a fixed pulsation level of 2%. Note that the amplification, i.e., the strength of the subharmonic, increases with decreasing Reynolds number. Although the subharmonic formation is intermittent, giving lower peak averages at higher Re, the subharmonic is stable and strong at lower Re.

Figure 22B shows the response of the jet to pulsation amplitude at a fixed Reynolds number. Notice that the longitudinal turbulence intensity increases monotonically with increasing pulsation amplitudes from 2 to 8%. The growth cannot, of course, continue to increase indefinitely with pulsation amplitude and must reach a saturation pulsation amplitude.

Shadowgraph pictures taken in the flow behind an orifice show that the orifice produces a series of vortex rings which undergo pairing (Anderson, 1956; Yellin, 1966b). Vlasov and Ginevski (1974) have observed turbulence amplification at St_D = 0.5 but suppression at St_D = 2.75 in a circular jet under acoustic excitation.

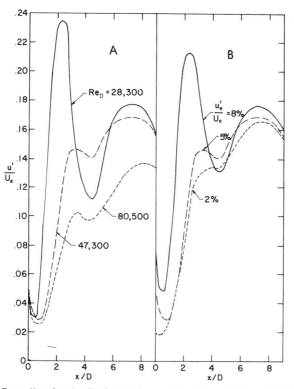

Figure 22. Centerline longitudinal turbulence intensities at $St_D = 0.8$ for an un-tripped nozzle; (A) dependence on Re_D, (B) dependence on pulsation amplitude u'_e/U_e.

These results may have some implications for arterial stenosis. For $St_D = 0.8$ if $n \sim 1$ Hz, $D \sim 0.5$ cm, then $U \sim 0.6$ cm/sec; this is a likely possibility in the cardiovascular system. A wide range in D, U, and n (changed through exercise) may combine to produce the Strouhal numbers 0.4, 0.8, and 1.2. The stenosed opening is typically noncircular; in such cases, an equivalent diameter like the hydraulic diameter can be used.

Poststenotic dilatation of arteries has been found to be related to high turbulence distal to stenosis (Roach, 1972). Boughner and Roach (1971a) showed that certain frequencies were more effective than others in causing dilatation. Hutchinson (1974) suggests that this could be related to arterial wall resonance, which can be induced by turbulence (Boughner and Roach, 1971b; Fry, 1968).

Is it quite likely that poststenotic dilatation occurs when the stenosis flow has a Strouhal number of 0.4, 0.8, or 1.2 and, simultaneously, this frequency happens to be the "resonant" frequency for the arterial wall?

4.5 Turbulent Flow Behind a Human Mitral Valve

The characteristics of pulsatile flow in the left ventricle behind the mitral valve have been determined by the application of the phase average to in vitro hot-film measurements.

Surgical replacement of diseased heart valves by prostheses has become a routine heart operation in recent years; thousands of prosthetic valves of various designs have been implanted in patients. Development of a successful prosthetic valve depends on proper characterization of the natural human valve—not only its static and dynamic characteristics, but also the mechanics of flow through it. For a moderate 5-yr duration, the valve must effectively operate approximately 2×10^8 cycles of continued operation. The flow behind the valve must be free from a stagnation region. The valve should not produce high turbulence, which might cause thrombus formation (Stein and Sabbah, 1974), or excessive shear stresses, which might cause excessive hemolysis. In view of the distensibility of the heart and the rapid and large changes of the volume of the left ventricle, in vivo study with hot-film is impractical. This provided the motivation for studying the flow behind a natural human mitral valve in vitro.

The mitral valve, situated between the left atrium and the left ventricle, consists of two cusps attached to the atrioventricular fibrous ring. The large anteromedial (aortic) cusp hangs down like a curtain and guides the flow, and the shorter posterolateral cusp joins to form a tunnel-like shape at the top. The papillary muscles exert tension simultaneously on the two cusps through the chordae tendineae. The mitral valve opens to allow blood to enter the left ventricle and closes at the end of diastole to prevent back flow into atrium during systole, thus permitting the left ventricle to impel blood into the aorta. Both cusps are extremely pliable and soft, consisting of a very thin (0.1 mm) surface tissue like the endocardial lining. They have a specific gravity nearly equal to that of blood; they provide very little inertial resistance to the flow. The motion of a mitral valve has been studied visually (Rushmer, Finlayson, and Nash, 1956), with ultrasound cardiograph (Zaky, Grabhorn, and Feigenbaum, 1967; Konecke et al., 1973; Pohost et al., 1975; Laniado et al., 1975) and with cineangiograms (Tsakiri et al., 1975).

The flow measurements reported here were performed in an ex vivo flow chamber constructed to simulate the flow configuration near the mitral valve; the ventricular wall motion is so complex that mechanical simulation is essentially impossible even though some attempts have been made. Because the change of the ventricle from mid-diastole to the presystolic period is rather small, it was decided to build a rigid chamber with a cross section to correspond this period. A normal human heart acquired at autopsy was injected with silicone rubber through the apex until the ventricular pressure reached the peak diastolic pressure. The heart tissue was then removed by chemical maceration. In order to transform this irregular shape into a chamber with smooth surface for visibility, the rubber model of the left ventricle was sliced into 2.5-mm sections parallel to the mitral valve annulus. The area of each section was then measured. These areas were then used to construct a chamber with circular cross section; the chamber looks somewhat like a Venturitube with a mitral valve located at the throat (Figure 23). The atrium and ventricle sections were fabricated from two rectangular pieces of Plexiglas that were held together with four bolts; they hold an orifice plate-like disk at the junction. A natural human mitral valve from a 32-yr-old male killed in an accident was procured at autopsy and carefully sutured to the disk, which was then mounted on the flow chamber. The flow chamber consists of straight circular sections that do not represent the ventricle. This, however, affects the vortex formation in the ventricle.

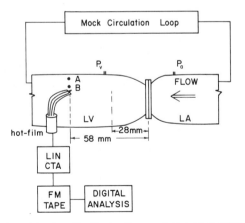

Figure 23. Experimental set-up for the in vitro measurements behind a natural mitral valve. LA, left atrium; LV, left ventricle.

The flow chamber was installed in a mock circulatory system designed to simulate the human cardiovascular system (see Wieting, Hwang, and Kennedy, 1971; Stripling, 1972). 36.7% glycerol in water at 25°C was used in the loop system as the testing fluid. The flow through the chamber was pulsated at a pulse rate of 72 beats per minute with an average flow rate of 5 liters/min. The mean atrial pressure was maintained at 5 mm Hg and the ventricular pressure at 120/0 mm Hg. A Statham P-23H differential pressure transducer was used to measure the pressure drop across the valve. A cylindrical hot-film x-probe (Thermo-Systems) oriented symmetrically with respect to the axis was used at an overheat of 1.07 to obtain the instantaneous velocity signals. The probe was calibrated in a small tow tank. The linearized hot-film signals were recorded on an FM analog tape at $7\frac{1}{2}$ in./sec through a Sandborn recorder. Velocity signals were recorded at two stations 28 and 58 mm downstream from the mitral valve, 15 points at each station for about 1 min each (about 60 cardiac cycles each); Figure 23 shows the experimental set-up.

Figure 24A shows typical scope traces of the three analog signals obtained from the experiment: the top curve shows the time-dependent pressure difference P_a-P_v across the mitral valve; the bottom two are the linearized signals from the two hot films placed 28 mm downstream from the mitral valve. These traces provide an indication of the nature of the flow during the cardiac cycle; the diastolic and systolic portions of the cardiac cycle can be identified in Figure 24B. During the diastolic phase the atrial pressure P_a is slightly higher than the ventricular pressure P_v so that the pressure difference helps to fill up the ventricle. The small positive pressure hump at the beginning of diastole would indicate atrial pressure build-up due to slower opening of the mitral valve. During systole, the pressure drop P_a-P_v is negative because of a large increase of ventricular pressure. Note the sudden pressure build-up in the ventricle at the beginning of the systolic phase. In a real heart, the pressure build-up is necessary to force open the leaflets of the aortic valve; the chordae tendineae prevents the mitral valve leaflets from being pushed into the atrium during systole even though the pressure in the atrium falls as it is being passively filled up with blood from the pulmonary vein due to suction action; the result is a continuous increase of pressure difference P_a-P_v at the start of ventricular systole. Notice also that the ratio of diastolic to systolic periods is about 2:1.5.

At the location of the x probe (i.e., position A in Fig. 23), the flow directed by the anteromedial leaflet directly impinges on the probe so that

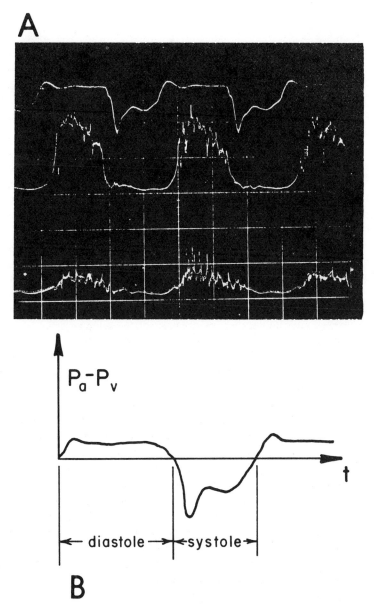

Figure 24. (A) Scope traces of analog pressure drop and linearized hot-film signals. The top trace is that of the pressure drop $P_a - P_v$ across the mitral valve. Bottom two traces are the outputs from the two hot films of an x probe. (B) Diastolic and systolic phases of the pressure trace in Figure 24(A).

the velocity is well correlated with the pressure drop. The velocity increases across the valve rapidly with the opening of the mitral valve as indicated by the start of the small pressure hump; the small delay between the velocity rise and pressure rise is due to the time required for the jet to reach the probe. The difference between the two hot-film signals arises because, at the location of the x probe, the flow impinges on one cylinder nearly normal to it but at a small angle on the second cylinder; the signal is thus larger in the former case. Note that the velocity increases rapidly; it becomes randomly oscillatory ("turbulent") during the rest of the diastolic phase when the mitral valve remains open because of the positive difference P_a-P_v. After the valve closes (because of the two vortices formed at the mitral valve leaflet) the velocity decreases and its random oscillations disappear.

The signal traces indicate that the flow is periodic; this is, of course, a consequence of the fact that the data were taken in vitro in a mock circulatory system with controlled flow periodicity. However, note that the details of the random fluctuating signal are not repeated. It is tempting to claim that the flow is "turbulent," especially during ventricular diastole. However, as indicated earlier, randomness of the velocity signal is necessary for turbulence; it is not sufficient. Nonzero Reynolds stress or random vorticity will be used to indicate the presence of turbulence. Characterization of the turbulence, namely, its intensity, Reynolds stress, etc., requires the use of phase average so that the periodic component can be subtracted out. Note that success of the phase-average technique relies on the period being repeated; if not, jitter of the period alone will contribute errors to the rms intensity of even a smooth signal. This therefore suggests that the phase-averaging technique will be more meaningful in in vitro experiments with controlled periodicity or in in vivo experiments in calm subjects, e.g., those under anesthesia.

Both the instantaneous pressure drop signal and the hot-film signals from the FM magnetic tape were digitized (in a hybrid computer at the Cullen College of Engineering, University of Houston) at a rate of 2,000 (16 bit) words per second. The Nyquest theorem, therefore, limits the upper frequency content of the hot-film signals to 1 kHz; this is an adequate upper frequency limit for turbulence in blood.

The digitized data were then processed numerically in an IBM 360/44 computer to obtain the phase average of the total velocity components $\langle U(t) \rangle$, $\langle V(t) \rangle$, phase-averaged rms turbulent intensities, $\sqrt{\langle u'(t)^2 \rangle}$, $\sqrt{\langle v'(t)^2 \rangle}$, and the phase-averaged Reynolds stress $\langle u'(t)v'(t) \rangle$ using the following digital formulas:

$$\langle U(t)\rangle = \frac{1}{N} \sum_{n=1}^{N} u(t+nT)$$

$$\langle V(t)\rangle = \frac{1}{N} \sum_{n=1}^{N} v(t+nT)$$

$$\therefore u'(t) = u(t) - \langle U(t)\rangle$$

$$v'(t) = v(t) - \langle V(t)\rangle$$

$$\sqrt{\langle v'(t)^2\rangle} = \left[\frac{1}{N} \sum_{n=1}^{N} u'(t+nT)^2\right]^{1/2}$$

$$\sqrt{\langle v'(t)^2\rangle} = \left[\frac{1}{N} \sum_{n=1}^{N} v'(t+nT)^2\right]^{1/2}$$

$$\langle u'(t)v'(t)\rangle = \frac{1}{N} \sum_{n=1}^{N} u'(t+nT)v'(t+nT)$$

where T is the period of the cardiac cycle. Since data were taken for about 1 min at each location, the number of periods (N) was 50.

Note that because the mean velocity direction was not, in general, symmetric with respect to the two cylinders of the x probe, the components $u(t)$ and $v(t)$ of the instantaneous velocity magnitude $\mathbf{u}$ were obtained from the two outputs $E_1(t)$ and $E_2(t)$ of the hot films as follows (Champagne, Sleicher, and Wehrmann, 1967; Brunn and Davies, 1972):

$$E_1(t) = \mathbf{u}(t)[\sin^2\theta + k^2\cos^2\theta]^{1/2}$$

$$E_2(t) = \mathbf{u}(t)[\sin^2(90-\theta) + k^2\cos^2(90-\theta)]^{1/2}$$

Following Champagne et. al., we use $k = 0.25$ so that

$$\mathbf{u} = [0.941\,(E_1^2 + E_2^2)]^{1/2}$$

$$\theta = \sin^{-1}\left[\frac{E_1^2 - 0.0625\,E_2^2}{0.996\mathbf{u}^2}\right]^{1/2}$$

and

$$u(t) = \mathbf{u}(t)\sin[45° + \theta(t)]$$

$$v(t) = \mathbf{u}(t)\cos[45° + \theta(t)]$$

Figures 25A–25E show $\langle U(t)\rangle$, $\langle V(t)\rangle$, $\sqrt{\langle u'(t)^2\rangle}$, $\sqrt{\langle v'(t)^2\rangle}$, $-\rho\langle u'(t)v'(t)\rangle$ at position A (see Figure 23).

The longitudinal phase average velocity $\langle U\rangle$ increases almost exponentially after the start of the diastolic phase, reaching the maximum at one-third of this phase. It drops to two-fifths of the maximum velocity at the end of the diastolic phase; the velocity continues to decrease in the systolic phase. This suggests that the vortex motion continues even though flow through the valve has stopped because of its closure. The vortex-induced motion decays, reaching a minimum velocity at the end of systole to a value of about one-tenth of the maximum velocity.

Notice from the phase-average velocity $\langle V(t)\rangle$ that the velocity at position A is nearly aligned with the probe except at the middle of the diastolic phase. Figures 25C and 25D show the turbulent intensities $\sqrt{\langle u'(t)^2\rangle}$, $\sqrt{\langle v'(t)^2\rangle}$ at position A at different instants in the cardiac cycle. Notice that both of these quantities increase rapidly along with $\langle U(t)\rangle$ remaining constant over most of the systolic phase because of the continuing vortex motion even though the mean velocity $\langle U(t)\rangle$ starts dropping; they continue to decrease during the systolic phase and reach a minimum at the end of the systolic phase.

Figure 25E shows that at location A the Reynolds stress always remains negative. The minimum values occur during the diastolic phase with a local maximum at the middle. The sign of the Reynolds stress is consistent with that of the local mean velocity gradient (see below). Figures 26A–25E show the corresponding data at location B (Figure 23).

The large Reynolds stress during the diastolic phase indicates that flow becomes unstable at the beginning of the diastolic phase and is *turbulent* for the remainder of the phase. This is confirmed by the high values of the correlation coefficient $\langle u'v'\rangle/\sqrt{\langle u'^2\rangle}\cdot\sqrt{\langle v'^2\rangle}$ during the diastolic phase (shown in Figures 25F and 26F). The turbulence can be due either to instability of the shear layer originating from the valve leaflets or to the interaction of the vortices with the wall or with each other.

The phase-average mean, turbulence, and Reynolds stress data at different stations within the flow field permit one to draw the profiles of these quantities at different periods within the cardiac cycle by cross plotting and thus enable one to analyze periodic turbulent flow at different phases of the cardiac cycle.

Figure 27A shows the phase-average mean velocity distributions at successive intervals in the diastolic phase. Figures 27B–27D show the

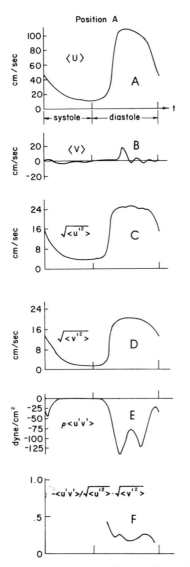

Figure 25. Phase-average measurements at position A shown in Figure 23; $(A) <U>$, $(B) <V>$, $(C) \sqrt{<u'^2>}$, $(D) \sqrt{<v'^2>}$, (E) $\rho<u'v'>$, $(F) <u'v'>/(\sqrt{<u'^2>}\sqrt{<v'^2>})$.

Position B

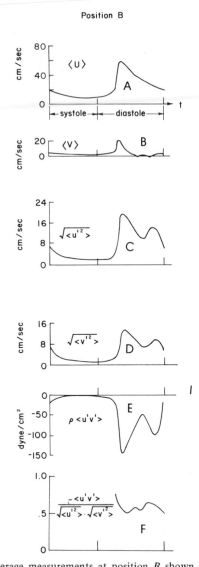

Figure 26. Phase-average measurements at position *B* shown in Figure 23. Legends (*A*)–(*F*), same as in Figure 25.

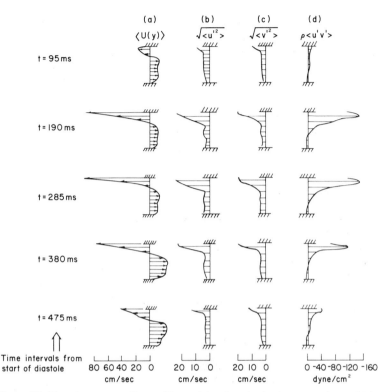

Figure 27. Phase-average profiles at 58 mm from the mitral valve across the ventricular chamber at different instants in the cardiac cycle; (A) $<U>$, (B) $\sqrt{<u'^2>}$, (C) $\sqrt{<v'^2>}$, (D) $\rho<u'v'>$.

corresponding values of $\sqrt{\langle u'^2\rangle}$, $\sqrt{\langle v'^2\rangle}$, $\langle u'v'\rangle$ at different instants within the cardiac cycle. For detailed data and discussions please see Hui (1975).

It is to be noted that the inaccuracy in the data stems from the limited number (i.e., 50) of the ensemble size and poorer resolution of the digitization from magnetic tape. The experimental set-up also has the limitation that the ventricle chamber used is cylindrical rather than of the typical closed shape, which would enable a better formation of the vortices in the ventricle.

While the data presented here are neither very accurate nor at a sufficient number of spatial locations within the flow field, they do illustrate that the phase-average concept can be applied not only to identify the nature of the mean and turbulent flow, but also to analyze the spatial distributions of these flow characteristics at different phases and instants within the cardiac cycle.

ACKNOWLEDGMENTS

The author is grateful to Drs. Ned Hwang, Dali Patel, H. Scarton, and R. K. Menon for careful reviews of the manuscript. Drs. S. H. Davis and R. Vick have reviewed portions of the text.

LITERATURE CITED

Anderson, A. B. C. 1956. Vortex-ring structure-transition in a jet emitting discrete acoustic frequencies. J. Acoust. Soc. Amer. 28: 914–921.

Anliker, M. 1972. Toward a nontraumatic study of the circulatory system. *In* Y. C. Fung et al. (eds.), Biomechanics, pp. 337–339. Prentice-Hall, Englewood Cliffs, N.J.

Ash, R. L., D. M. Bushnell, L. M. Weinstein, and R. Balasurbramanian. 1975. Compliant wall surface motion and its effect on the structure of a turbulent boundary layer. Proceedings of the Fourth Bienn. Symp. Turb. Liquids, University of Missouri-Rolla.

Barbee, J. H., and G. R. Cokelet. 1971. The fahraeus effect. Microvasc. Res. 3: 1–21.

Batchelor, G. K. 1970. An Introduction to Fluid Dynamics. Cambridge University Press, Cambridge, England.

Bellhouse, B. J., and F. H. Bellhouse. 1968. Mechanism of closure of the aortic valve. Nature 217: 86–87.

Bellhouse, B. J., and F. H. Bellhouse. 1969a. Fluid mechanics of model normal and stenosed aortic valves. Circ. Res. 25: 693–704.

Bellhouse, B. J., and F. H. Bellhouse. 1969b. Fluid mechanics of the mitral valve. Nature 224: 615–616.

Bellhouse, B. J., and L. Talbot. 1969. The fluid mechanics of the aortic valves. J. Fluid Mech. 35: 721–735.

Bendat, J. S., and A. G. Piersol. 1971. Random data: analysis and measurement procedures. Wiley-Interscience, New York.

Bergel, D. H. 1961. The static elastic properties of the arterial wall. J. Physiol. 156: 445–457.

Bergel, D. H. 1972. The properties of blood vessels. *In* Y. C. Fung et al. (eds.), Biomechanics, pp. 105–139. Prentice-Hall, Englewood Cliffs, N.J.

Berger, E., and R. Wille. 1972. Periodic flow phenomena. Ann. Rev. Fluid Mech. 4: 313–340.

Bertelsen, A. E. 1975. An experimental investigation of low Reynolds number secondary streaming effects associated with an oscillating viscous flow in a curves pipe. J. Fluid Mech. 70: 519—527.

Blackshear, P. L. 1972. Mechanical stenolysis in flowing blood. *In* Y. C. Fung et al. (eds.), Biomechanics, pp. 501—528. Prentice-Hall, Englewood Cliffs, N.J.

Blick, E., H. N. Sabbah, and P. D. Stein. 1975. Red blood cells and turbulence. Proceedings of the Fourth Bienn. Symp. Turb. Liquids, University of Missouri-Rolla.

Boughner, D. R., and M. R. Roach. 1971*a*. Etiology of pulmonary artery dilatation and hilar dance in atrial septal defect. Circ. Res. 28: 415—425.

Boughner, D. R., and M. R. Roach. 1971*b*. Effect of low frequency vibration on the arterial wall. Circ. Res. 29: 136—144.

Bradshaw, P. 1971. An Introduction to Turbulence and Its Measurement. Pergamon Press, New York.

Brech, R., and B. J. Bellhouse. 1973. Flow in branching vessels. Cardiovasc. Res. 7: 593—600.

Browand, F. K., and J. Laufer. 1975. The role of large-scale structure in the initial development of circular jets. Proc. of the Fourth Bienn. Symp. Turb. Liquids, University of Missouri-Rolla.

Brower, R. W., and A. Noordergraff. 1973. Pressure—flow characteristics of collapsible tubes: A reconciliation of seemingly contradictory results. Ann. Biomed. Eng. 1: 333—355.

Brown, G. L., and A. Roshko. 1974. On density effects and large structure in turbulent mixing layers. J. Fluid Mech. 64: 775—816.

Brunn, H. H., and P. O. A. L. Davies. 1972. Measurement of turbulent quantities by single hot-wires and X hot-wires using digital evaluation techniques. *In* Fluid Dynamic Measurements in the Industrial and Medical Environments. Leicester University Press, Leicester.

Burton, A. C. 1972. Physiology and Biophysics of the Circulation. Yearbook Medical Publishers, Chicago.

Carlson, A. J., V. Johnson, and H. M. Calvert. 1965. The Machinery of the Body. University of Chicago Press, Chicago.

Caro, C. G. 1966. The dispersion of indicator flowing through simplified models of the circulation and its relevance to velocity profile in blood vessels. J. Physiol. 185: 501—519.

Caro, C. G., J. M. Fitz-Gerald, and R. C. Schroter. 1971. Atheroma and arterial wall shear. Observation, correlation and proposal of a shear dependent mass transfer mechanism for atherogenesis. Proc. Roy. Soc. London B 177: 109—159.

Casson, N. 1959. A flow equation for the pigment-oil suspensions of the printing ink type. *In* D. C. Mill (ed.), Rheology of Disperse System, pp. 84—102. Pergamon Press, New York.

Champagne, F. H., C. A. Sleicher, and O. H. Wehrmann. 1967. Turbulence measurements with inclined hot wires. J. Fluid Mech. 28: 153—175.

Chandran, K. B., W. M. Swanson, D. N. Ghista, and H. W. Vayo. 1974.

Oscillatory flow in thin-walled curved elastic tubes. Ann. Biomed. Eng. 2: 392–412.

Charm, S. E., and G. S. Kurland. 1972. Blood rheology. *In* D. H. Bergel (ed.), Cardiovascular Fluid Mechanics, pp. 157–203. Academic Press, New York.

Charm, S. E., and G. S. Kurland. 1974. Blood flow and microcirculation. Wiley, New York.

Chien, S., S. Usami, R. J. Dellenback, and M. I. Gregersen. 1970. Shear-dependent interaction of plasma proteins with erythrocytes in blood rheology. Amer. J. Physiol. 219: 43–53.

Clarion, C., and R. Pelissier. 1975. A theoretical and experimental study of the velocity distribution and transition to turbulence in free oscillatory flow. J. Fluid Mech. 70: 59–79.

Clark, A. R., and A. K. M. F. Hussain. 1975. Effects of initial conditions on the development of a plane turbulent jet. Proceedings of the 12th Ann. Meeting of the Soc. Engr. Science, University of Texas, pp. 1149–1158.

Cokelet, G. R. 1972. The rheology of human blood. *In* Y. C. Fung et al. (eds.), Biomechanics, pp. 63–103. Prentice-Hall, Englewood Cliffs, N.J.

Corrsin, S., and A. Kistler. 1954. The free-stream boundaries of turbulent flows. NACA Technical Note 3133.

Crow, S. C., and F. H. Champagne. 1971. Orderly structure in jet turbulence. J. Fluid Mech. 48: 547–591.

Davis, S. H. 1975. The stability of time-periodic flows. Ann. Rev. Fluid Mech. 8 (in press).

Dean, W. R. 1927. Note on the motion of a fluid in a curved pipe. Phil. Mag. (7) 4: 208–233.

Dean, W. R. 1928. The streamline motion of a fluid in a curved pipe. Phil. Mag. (7) 5: 673–695.

Ferguson, G. G. 1970. Turbulence in human intracranial saccular aneurysms. J. Neurosurg. 33: 485–497.

Ferguson, G. G., and M. R. Roach. 1972. Flow conditions at bifurcations as determined in glass models, with reference to the focal distribution of vascular lesions. *In* D. H. Bergel (ed.), Cardiovascular Fluid Dynamics, Vol. 2, pp. 141–156. Academic Press, New York.

Fitz-Gerald, J. M. 1972. The mechanics of capillary blood flow. *In* D. H. Bergel (ed.), Cardiovascular Fluid Dynamics, pp. 205–239. Academic Press, New York.

Frasher, W. G., H. Wayland, and H. J. Meiselman. 1968. Viscometry of circulating blood in dogs. I. Heparin injection, II. Platelet removal. J. Appl. Physiol. 25: 751–760.

Friedman, M. H., V. O'Brien, and L. W. Ehrlich. 1975. Calculations of pulsatile flow through a branch. Circ. Res. 36: 277–285.

Friedman, M. H., and L. W. Ehrlich. 1975. Effect of spatial variations in shear on diffusion at the wall of an arterial branch. Circ. Res. 37: 446–454.

Fry, D. L. 1968. Acute vascular endothelial changes associated with increased blood velocity gradients. Cir. Res. 22: 165–197.

Fry, D. L. 1973. Response of the arterial wall to certain physical factors. *In* Atherogenesis: Initiating Factors, CIBA Foundation Symposium 12: 93–125.

Gaster, M. 1962. A note on the relation between temporally-increasing and spatially-increasing disturbances in hydrodynamic stability. J. Fluid Mech. 14: 222–224.

Gaster, M. 1969. Vortex shedding from slender cones at low Reynolds numbers. J. Fluid Mech. 38: 565–576.

Gaster, M. 1971. Vortex shedding from circular cylinders at low Reynolds numbers. J. Fluid Mech. 46: 749–756.

George, W. D., J. D. Hellums, and B. Martin. 1974. Finite-amplitude neutral disturbances in plane Poiseuille flow. J. Fluid Mech. 63: 765–771.

Gessner, F. B. 1973. Hemodynamic theories of atherogenesis. Circ. Res. 33: 259–266.

Gilbrech, D. A., and G. D. Combs. 1963. Critical Reynolds numbers for incompressible pulsating flow in tubes. *In* Developments in Theoretical and Applied Mechanics, Vol. I, pp. 292–304. Plenum Press, New York.

Goldsmith, H. L., and R. Skalak. 1975. Hemodynamics Ann. Rev. Fluid Mech. 7: 213–247.

Green, H. D. 1944. Circulatory system: Physical principles. *In* O. Glasser (ed.), Medical Physics. Yearbook Publishers, Chicago.

Greenspan, D. 1973. Secondary flow in a curved tube. J. Fluid Mech. 57: 167–176.

Hinze, J. O. 1975. Turbulence. 2d Ed. McGraw-Hill, New York.

Holt, J. P. 1969. Flow through collapsible tubes and through in situ veins. IEEE Trans. Bio-Mech. Eng. BME 16: 274–283.

Hui, P. W. 1975. Turbulent characteristics of pulsatile flow downstream from a natural human mitral valve. M.S. Thesis, University of Houston.

Hussain, A. K. M. F. 1969. The mechanics of a perturbation wave in turbulent shear flow. Ph.D. Thesis, Stanford University.

Hussain, A. K. M. F., and V. Ramjee. 1975. Vortex shedding from a circular cylinder in the presence of free-stream disturbances. Proc. Fifth Canad. Congr. Appl. Mech., pp. 485–486.

Hussain, A. K. M. F., and V. Ramjee. 1976. Periodic wake behind a circular cylinder at low Reynolds numbers. Aero. Quart. 27: 123–142.

Hussain, A. K. M. F., and W. C. Reynolds. 1970. The mechanics of an organized wave in turbulent shear flow. J. Fluid Mech. 41: 241–258.

Hussain, A. K. M. F., and W. C. Reynolds. 1972. The mechanics of an organized wave in turbulent shear flow. Part 2: Experimental Results. J. Fluid Mech. 52: 241–262.

Hussain, A. K. M. F., and C. A. Thompson. 1975. Organized motions in a plane turbulent jet under controlled excitation. Proc. 12th Ann. Meeting Soc. Engr. Sci., Univ. of Texas, pp. 741–752.

Hussain, A. K. M. F., and K. B. M. Q. Zaman. 1975. Effect of acoustic excitation on the turbulent structure of a circular jet. Proc. Third Interag. Symp. Univ. Res. Trans. Noise, Univ. of Utah, pp. 314–325.

Hutchinson, K. J. 1974. Effect of variation of transmural pressure on the frequency response of isolated segments of canine carotid arteries. Circ. Res. 35: 742–751.

Hyman, W. A. 1973. The role of slip in the rheology of blood. Biorheology 10: 57–60.

Jones, R. T. 1969. Blood flow. Ann. Rev. Fluid Mech. 1: 223–244.

Katz, A. I., Y. Chen, and A. H. Moreno. 1969. Flow through a collapsible tube. Biophys. J. 9: 1261–1279.

Kenner, T. 1972. Flow and pressure in the arteries. In Y. C. Fung et al. (eds.), Biomechanics, pp. 381–434. Prentice-Hall, Englewood Cliffs, N.J.

Konecke, L. L., H. Feigenbaum, S. Chang, B. C. Korya, and J. C. Fisher. 1973. Abnormal mitral valve motion in patients with elevated left ventricular diastolic pressures. Circulation 47: 989–996.

Kunz, A. L., and N. A. Coulter. 1967. Non-Newtonian behavior of blood in oscillatory flow. Biophys. J. 7: 25–26.

Ladyzhenskaya, O. A. 1975. Mathematical analysis of Navier–Stokes equations for incompressible liquids. Ann. Rev. Fluid Mech. 7: 249–272.

Landahl, M. T. 1967. A wave-quid model for turbulent shear flow. J. Fluid Mech. 29: 441–459.

Laniado, S., E. L. Yellin, M. Kottler, L. Levy, J. Stodler, and R. Terdiman. 1975. A study of the dynamic relations between the mitral valve echogram and phasic mitral flow. Circulation 51: 104–113.

Lighthill, M. J. 1954. The response of laminar skin friction and heat transfer to fluctuations in the stream velocity. Proc. Roy. Soc. London 224: 1–23.

Lighthill, M. J. 1968. The outlook for a wave theory of turbulent shear flows. Proceedings of the Computation of Turbulent Boundary Layers: 1968 AFOSR-1FP-Stanford Conference, Stanford Univ., pp. 511–520.

Lighthill, M. J. 1972. Physiological fluid dynamics: A survey. J. Fluid Mech. 52: 475–497.

Lighthill, M. H. 1975. Mathematical Biofluid dynamics. Society for Industrial and Applied Mathematics, Philadelphia.

Lin, C. C. 1954. Some physical aspects of the stability of parallel flows. Proc. Natl. Acad. Sci. U.S. 40: 741–747.

Lin, C. C. 1955. The Theory of Hydrodynamic Stability. Cambridge University Press, Cambridge.

Lin, C. C. 1957. Motion in the boundary layer with a rapidly oscillating external flow. Proc. 9th Intern. Congress Appl. Mech. 4, Brussels, pp. 155–167.

Ling, S. C., and H. B. Atabek. 1972. A nonlinear analysis of pulsatile flow in arteries. J. Fluid Mech. 55: 493–511.

Ling, S. C., H. B. Atabek, W. G. Letzing, and D. J. Patel. 1973. Nonlinear analysis of aortic flow in living dogs. Circ. Res. 33: 198–212.

Longuet-Higgins, M. S. 1970. Steady currents induced by oscillations round islands. J. Fluid Mech. 42: 701–720.

Lyne, W. H. 1970. Unsteady viscous flow in a curved pipe. J. Fluid Mech. 45: 12–31.

Mattingly, G. E., and W. O. Criminale. 1971. Disturbance characteristics in a plane jet. Phys. Fluids 14: 543–556.

McConalogue, D. J., and R. S. Srivastava. 1968. Motion of a fluid in a curved tube. Proc. Roy. Soc. London A. 307: 37–53.

McDonald, D. A. 1974. Blood Flow in Arteries. 2nd Ed. Williams and Wilkins, Baltimore.

Merkli, P., and H. Thomann. 1975. Transition to turbulence in oscillating pipe flow. J. Fluid Mech. 68: 567–575.

Merrill, E. W., E. R. Gilliland, T. S. Lee, and E. W. Salzman. 1966. Blood rheology: Effect of fibrinogen deduced by addition. Circ. Res. 19: 437–446.

Merrill, E. W., and G. A. Pelletier. 1967. Viscosity of human blood: Transition from Newtonian to non-Newtonian. J. Appl. Physiol. 23: 178–182.

Michalke, A. 1965. On spatially growing disturbances in an inviscid shear layer. J. Fluid Mech. 23: 521–544.

Michalke, A. 1972. The instability of free shear layers. Porg. Aero. Sci. 12: 213–239.

Moffatt, H. K. 1968. Large scale motions in a turbulent boundary layer; waves versus eddies. Proceedings of the Computation of Turbulent Boundary Layers: 1968 AFOSR-1FP-Stanford Conference; Stanford University, pp. 495–510.

Moore, D. W., and P. G. Saffman. 1975. The density of organized vortices in a turbulent mixing layer. J. Fluid Mech. 69: 465–473.

Morrison, W. R. B., and R. E. Kronauer. 1970. Structural similarity of turbulence in smooth tubes. J. Fluid Mech. 39: 117–141.

Nerem, R. M., J. A. Rumberger, D. R. Gross, R. L. Hamlin, and G. L. Geiger. 1974. Hot-film anemometer velocity measurements of arterial blood flow in horses. Circ. Res. 4: 193–203.

Obremski, H. J., and A. A. Fejer. 1967. Transition in oscillating boundary layer flows. J. Fluid Mech. 29: 93–111.

Panchev, S. 1971. Random Functions and Turbulence. Pergamon Press, New York.

Papoulis, A. 1965. Probability, Random Variables and Stochastic Processes. McGraw-Hill, New York.

Patel, D. J., and R. N. Vaishnav. 1972. The rheology of large blood vessels. In D. H. Bergel (ed.), Cardiovascular Fluid Dynamics, Vol. 2, pp. 1–64. Academic Press, New York.

Patel, D. J., R. N. Vaishnav, B. S. Gow, and P. A. Kot. 1974. Hemodynamics. Ann. Rev. Physiol. 36: 125–154.

Phibbs, R. H. 1968. Orientation and distribution of erythrocytes in blood flowing through medium-sized arteries. In A. L. Copley (ed.), Hemorheology, pp. 617–630. Pergamon Press, New York.

Phillips, O. M. 1972. The entrainment interface. J. Fluid Mech. 51: 97–118.

Pohost, G. M., R. E. Dinsmore, J. J. Rubenstein, D. D. O'Keefe, R. N. Grautham, H. E. Scully, E. A. Blarholm, J. W. Frederiksen, M. L. Weisfeldt, and W. M. Daggett. 1975. The echocardiogram of the anterior leaflet of the mitral valve: correlation with hemodynamic and cineroentgenographic studies in dogs. Circulation 51: 88–97.

Reynolds, W. C., and A. K. M. F. Hussain. 1972. The mechanics of an organized wave in turbulent shear flow. Part 3: Theoretical models and comparison with experiments. J. Fluid Mech. 52: 262–288.

Reynolds, W. C., and M. C. Potter. 1967. Finite-amplitude instability of parallel shear flows. J. Fluid Mech. 27: 465–492.

Roach, M. R. 1972. Poststenotic dilatation in arteries. In D. H. Bergel (ed.), Cardiovascular Flow Dynamics. Academic Press, New York.

Robertson, J. M., and J. F. Henick. 1975. Turbulence in blood flow. T & AM Report No 401, Dept. of Theoretical and Applied Mechanics, University of Illinois.

Roshko, A. 1954. On the development of turbulent wakes from vortex streets. NACA Report 1191.

Rushmer, R. F. 1970. Cardiovascular Dynamics. Saunders, Philadelphia.

Rushmer, R. F., B. L. Finlayson, and A. A. Nash. 1956. Movements of the mitral valve. Circ. Res. 4: 337–342.

Sarpkaya, T. 1966. Experimental determination of the critical Reynolds number for pulsating Poiseuille flow. J. Bas. Eng. 88: 589–597.

Sato, H. 1960. The stability and transition of a two-dimensional jet. J. Fluid Mech. 7: 53–80.

Scarton, H. 1975. Rensselear Polytechnic Institute, private communication.

Schlichting, H. 1968. Boundary Layer Theory. McGraw-Hill, New York.

Schroter, R. C., and M. F. Sudlow. 1969. Flow patterns in models of the human bronchial airways. Resp. Physiol. 7: 341–355.

Schubauer, G. B., and H. K. Skramstad. 1947. Laminar boundary layer oscillations and transition of a flat-plate. NBS Res. Paper RP-1772.

Schultz, D. L. 1972. Pressure and flow in large arteries. In D. H. Bergel (ed.), Cardiovascular Flow Dynamics, Vol. 2, 287–314. Academic Press, New York.

Schwartz, C. J., and J. R. A. Mitchell. 1962. Observations of localizations of arterial plaques. Circ. Res. 11: 63–73.

Sergeev, S. I. 1966. Fluid oscillations in pipes at moderate Reynolds numbers. Fluid Dyn. 1: 121–122.

Sevilla-Larra, J. F. 1968. Detailed characteristics of pulsatile blood flow in small grass capillaries. Ph.D. Thesis, Carnegie-Mellon University, Pittsburgh.

Skalak, R. 1972. Mechanics of the Microcirculation. In Y. C. Fung et al. (eds.), Biomechanics, pp. 457–499. Prentice-Hall, Englewood Cliffs, N.J.

Singh, M. P. 1974. Entry flow in a curved pipe. J. Fluid Mech. 65: 517–539.

Smith, F. T. 1975. Pulsatile flow in curved pipes. J. Fluid Mech. 71: 15–42.

Smith, R. L., E. F. Blick, J. Coulson, and P. D. Stein. 1972. Thrombus production by turbulence. J. Appl. Physiol. 32: 261–264.

Snyder, M. F., and V. C. Rideout. 1969. Computer simulation studies of the venous circulation. IEEE Trans. Bio-Med. Eng. BME 16: 325–334.

Stehbens, W. E. 1975. Flow in glass models of arterial bifurcations and berry aneurysms at low Reynolds numbers. Quart. J. Exp. Physiol. 60: 181–192.

Stein, P. D., and H. N. Sabbah. 1974. Measured turbulence and its effect on thrombus formation. Circ. Res. 35: 608–614.

Streeter, V. L., and E. B. Wylie. 1975. Fluid Mechanics. 6th Ed., McGraw-Hill, New York.

Stripling, T. S. 1972. Left ventricular flow characteristics of a healthy human heart. M.S. Thesis, University of Houston.

Stuart, J. T. 1963a. Hydrodynamic stability. In L. Rosenhead (ed.), Laminary Boundary Layers, pp. 492–579. Oxford Univ. Press, Oxford, England.

Stuart, J. T. 1963b. Unsteady boundary layers. In L. Rosenhead (ed.), Laminary Boundary Layers, pp. 349–408. Oxford Univ. Press, Oxford, England.

Stuart, J. T. 1967. Hydrodynamic stability of fluid flows. Inaugural Lecture, Imperial College, London, 14 November 1967.

Stuart, J. T. 1972. Unsteady boundary layers. In E. A. Eichelbrenner (ed.), Recent Research on Unsteady Boundary Layers. Les Presses de l'Université Laval, Quebec, Canada.

Taylor, D. E. M., and J. D. Wade. 1973. Pattern of blood flow within the heart: A stable system. Cardiovasc. Res. 7: 14–21.

Taylor, M. G. 1972. Hemodynamics. Ann. Rev. Physiol. 35: 87–116.

Tennekes, H., and J. L. Lumley. 1972. A First Course in Turbulence. MIT Press, Cambridge, Mass.

Townsend, A. A. 1956. The Structure of Turbulent Shear Flow. Camb. Univ. Press, New York.

Tritton, D. J. 1959. Experiments on the flow past a circular cylinder at low Reynolds numbers. J. Fluid Mech. 6: 547–567.

Tritton, D. J. 1971. A note on vortex streets behind circular cylinders at low Reynolds numbers. J. Fluid Mech. 45: 203–208.

Tsakiri, A. G., D. A. Gordon, Y. Mathieu, and I. Lipton. 1975. Motion of both mitral valve leaflets: A cineroentgenographic study in intact dogs. J. Appl. Physiol. 39: 359–366.

Vlasov, Y. V., and A. S. Ginevski. 1974. Generation and suppression of turbulence in an axisymmetric turbulent jet in the presence of an acoustic influence. NASA TT F-15, 721.

Weibel, E. R. 1972. Morphometric estimation of pulmonary diffusion capacity. V. Comparative morphometry of alveolar lungs. Resp. Physiol. 14: 26–43.

Wemple, R. R., and L. F. Mockros. 1972. Pressure and flow in the systemic arterial system. J. Biomech. 5: 629–641.

White, F. M. 1974. Viscous Fluid Flow. McGraw-Hill, New York.

Wieting, D. W., N. H. C. Hwang, and J. H. Kennedy. 1971. Fluid mechanics of the human mitral valve. AIAA Paper No. 71-102, New York, January 25–27.

Willmarth, W. W. 1975. Structure of turbulence in boundary layers. Advan. Appl. Mech. 15: 159–253.

Winant, C. D., and F. K. Browand. 1974. Vortex pairing: The mechanism of turbulent mixing layer growth at moderate Reynolds numbers. J. Fluid Mech. 63: 237–255.

Wygnanski, I., and F. H. Champagne. 1973. On transition in a pipe. Part 1: The origin of puffs and slugs and the flow in a turbulent slug. J. Fluid Mech. 59: 281–335.

Yao, L. S., and S. A. Berger. 1975. Entry flow in a curved pipe. J. Fluid Mech. 67: 177–196.

Yellin, E. L. 1966a. Laminar-turbulent transition process in pulsatile flow. Circ. Res. 19: 791–804.

Yellin, E. L. 1966b. Hydraulic noise in submerged and bounded liquid jets. Biomedical Fluid Mechanics Symposium, ASME, pp. 209–221.

Yih, C. S. 1969. Fluid Mechanics. McGraw-Hill, New York.

Zaky, A., L. Grabhorn, and H. Feigenbaum. 1967. Movement of the mitral ring: A study in ultrasound cardiography. Cardiovasc. Surg. 1:121.

Zalosh, R. G., and W. G. Nelson. 1973. Pulsating flow in a curved tube. J. Fluid Mech. 59: 693–705.

Zaric, Z. 1972. Wall turbulence studies. Adv. Heat Tr. 8: 285–347.

Zweifach, B. W. 1972. Biomechanics and physiology. In Y. C. Fung et al. (eds.), Biomechanics, pp. 1–13. Prentice-Hall, Englewood Cliffs, N.J.

Cardiovascular Flow Dynamics and Measurements
Edited by N. H. C. Hwang and Ñ. A. Normann
Copyright 1977   University Park Press   Baltimore

chapter 16

INSTABILITY IN ARTERIAL BLOOD FLOW

Kim H. Parker

ABSTRACT

The flow of blood in the large arteries can be disturbed, and these disturbances can have important physiological implications. The history of in vivo observations is reviewed in general and the results of one observation in the descending aorta in dogs are analyzed in detail. It is found that the disturbances occur suddenly during the deceleration phase of systole.

Understanding the origin of these disturbances requires some understanding of hydrodynamic stability theory. This theory is introduced by taking the example of steady and unsteady plane Poiseuille flow. Knowledge about this stability of flows in pipes is reviewed with particular reference to those theoretical and experimental studies that model arterial flow in some way.

Finally, some recent work on the stability of the flow in a pipe that is suddenly blocked is described. The laminar decay of blocked Hagen–Poiseuille flow is calculated. Experiments show that for low initial Reynolds numbers the flow decays as predicted, but for high initial Reynolds numbers the flow becomes disturbed.

INTRODUCTION

Blood flows through our arteries in a very complex way. Predicting how it flows is even more complex because we cannot be sure that the flow that we predict will be unique; even under identical conditions many different flows are possible. The simplest flow is a laminar flow. But there are always many other more complicated flows that are not only physically permissible but very often physically preferable to the simpler flow. Sometimes the preferred flow is a more complicated laminar flow but more often it is a far more complicated turbulent flow.

Stability is the study of which of the many possible flows is most likely to be observed. If the simplest flow is preferred it is called *stable.* If one of the more complicated flows is preferred the simpler flow is called *unstable.* The importance of studying stability is that virtually every property and characteristic of a flow depends on whether it is laminar or turbulent. And whether it is laminar or turbulent depends upon its stability.

One of the most important properties of a flow is its shear stress, or the way that momentum is transferred from place to place. In a laminar flow this transfer can only take place by molecular diffusion, that is, by viscosity. In a turbulent flow, momentum is also transported by convection, generally, a much more effective method. Thus local shear stresses in a turbulent flow can be much higher than in a laminar flow. This can be very important if we are interested in hemolysis.

Because the average shear stresses are different, the average velocity distributions are also different in laminar and turbulent flows. Knowing the radial velocity distribution in an artery can be important if we want to make accurate measurements of flow using an electromagnetic flowmeter.

Different average shear rates and velocities also cause different shear stresses at the wall of the artery. This is important if we are interested in pressure–flow waves in the artery. Also, possibly much more important, there is some suspicion that wall shear stress, or some closely allied property, may be very important in atherogenesis (Caro, Fitz-Gerald, and Schroter, 1971).

Another important difference between laminar and turbulent flows is that turbulent flows can generate sound. The mechanisms that produce murmurs are not fully understood yet, but it is clearly important to know whether the flow is laminar or turbulent. It has also been shown that extended exposure to the pressure fluctuations inherent in turbulent flows can have a profound effect on the properties of the artery walls (Roach, 1963).

What is true of momentum transfer is also true of mixing. In laminar flows mixing can only take place by molecular diffusion. In turbulent flows mixing is greatly enhanced by convection. Because different mixing can mean different distribution through the arterial tree, knowing whether a flow is laminar or turbulent can be important if we are using dilution techniques or if we are interested in regional distribution of blood.

OBSERVATIONS OF ARTERIAL DISTURBANCES

Probably the first intimation that blood flow could be disturbed is by Shakespeare, "for I have dream'd of bloody turbulence" (Troilus and

Cressida, V:3). More scientific speculation had to wait until the nineteenth century when the pioneers of auscultation tried to explain the origins of the sounds they were hearing (see McKusick, 1958, for a historical survey). Corrigan, in 1829, stated that murmurs were caused by "an alteration in the motion of the blood, instead of its equable progressive motion en masse." By 1844, Rouanet stated that the basis of murmurs was to be found in the formation of turbulence (*tourbillons*).

The first direct observation of disturbed flow in the arteries was made by MacDonald (1952), who took high-speed cinefilms of dye injected into the aorta of rabbits. He observed that during part of the cardiac cycle the dye was "seen to break up and become distributed in random threads" across the artery.

Cineradiographic studies also showed that radiopaque material is very rapidly dispersed across the arteries of dogs (see MacDonald, 1974, for the early history of observations of disturbances in the arteries). This rapid mixing indicates that the flow must be disturbed during at least part of the cycle.

The development of hot-film anemometers that could make accurate, local measurements of the instantaneous velocity in the arteries led to a more thorough investigation of arterial blood flow. Early workers (Ling et al., 1968; Schultz et al., 1969; Seed and Wood, 1971) all reported that flow in the aorta of dogs was generally undisturbed, but all reported that disturbed flows were sometimes seen, usually in smaller dogs.

Nerem and Seed (1972) studied this phenomenon systematically, again using hot-film anemometry. They discovered that in the same dog the flow in the descending aorta could be undisturbed, disturbed, or highly disturbed depending upon the heart rate and the peak velocity of the flow as shown in Figure 1. They argued that the state of the flow should depend upon two dimensionless parameters:

$$\mathrm{Re} = Ud/\nu,$$

a Reynolds number based upon the maximum velocity U, the diameter of the vessel d, and the kinematic viscosity of blood ν, and

$$\alpha = d\sqrt{\omega/\nu}$$

a frequency parameter (often called the Wormesley parameter) based upon the heart rate ω.

Nerem and Seed's observations of flow in the descending aorta of a number of dogs are shown on an R versus α plot in Figure 2. Flows on the

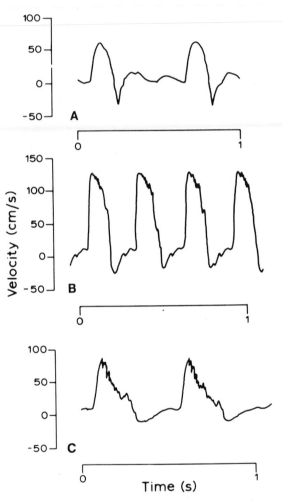

Figure 1. Velocity measured in the descending thoracic aorta of dogs. (*A*) undisturbed, (*B*) disturbed, (*C*) highly disturbed.

lower and right-hand side of the plot tend to be undisturbed while those to the top and left tend to be disturbed. The dividing line shown in the figure has some theoretical basis that will be discussed below. Nerem and Seed observed that the anesthetics used by previous workers tended to alter both heart rate and peak velocity away from those conditions for which

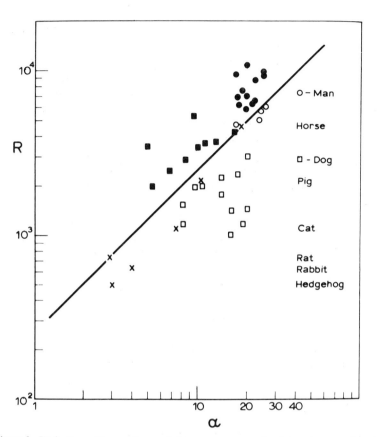

Figure 2. Peak Reynolds number and frequency parameter for various species; o, man; □, dog; x, other species. o, □, undisturbed flow; •,■, disturbed flow. The line is an empirical stability boundary.

disturbances would be expected. They concluded that disturbed flow might be common, or even prevalent, in the aorta of normal, conscious dogs.

Wondering if what was true for dogs was true for other animals, Seed (1972) collected data that enabled him to calculate R and α for the other species shown in Figure 2. The points are averages of all of the data for each species and all the data are derived from anesthetized subjects. It is striking that all of the points lie in, or very near to, the region in which disturbed flow is expected.

Finally, we must ask what happens in man. Figure 2 also contains previously unpublished data obtained by Seed from normal, conscious humans. These data were obtained by a catheter-tip hot-film anemometer placed in the ascending aorta of patients undergoing diagnostic catheterization. All of the subjects had disturbed flow. In fact, in the 40 patients in whom measurements were made (most exhibited anatomic lesions or abnormal left ventricular function and are not included in Figure 2), only one exhibited an undisturbed flow and he suffered from severe pulmonary hypertension resulting in an abnormally low cardiac output.

It is interesting to note in passing that none of the subjects included in Figure 2 exhibited any detectable murmurs in spite of having large disturbances in their ascending aortas.

Clearly, blood flow in the large arteries can be disturbed or turbulent. Disturbances have been observed in the ascending aorta of man, in the descending aorta of dogs and rabbits, and as far as the thoracic artery in horses (Nerem et al., 1974), and it seems likely that they are normally present in many different species. We are almost tempted to argue teleologically that there is some advantage (as yet unknown) in operating so that conditions in the aorta are very near to those that divide stable from unstable flows.

There is, therefore, strong justification for studying the stability of arterial blood flow. But before we can discuss that subject we must first discuss in more detail the nature of the observed disturbances and then, briefly, discuss hydrodynamic stability in general.

THE NATURE OF ARTERIAL DISTURBANCES

The data recorded by Nerem and Seed (1972) using a hot-film anemometer in the descending aorta of dogs have been reanalyzed using numerical techniques in order to study the nature of the disturbances that they measured.

The method of analysis was the basically digital technique of ensemble averaging. Records of the instantaneous velocity measured in the descending aorta over a period of about 200 heart beats were digitized at 2,000 samples per second. These digital data were then fed into a computer that first identified the start of each beat by means of the very rapid rise in velocity, as represented in Figure 3. The continuous record was thus separated into individual beats, and an ensemble average velocity was calculated by averaging the velocity at each time during the beat over all of

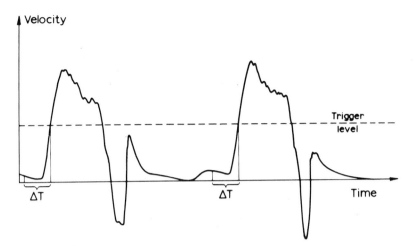

Figure 3. Velocity measured in descending aorta of a dog showing how beat starts can be identified.

the individual beats. Referring to Figure 4, this can be thought of as taking an average along the beat number axis at fixed times.

The average velocity in the descending aorta of a dog whose waveform was described as disturbed is shown as the dotted line in Figure 5A. The solid line represents the actual velocity measured for one of the beats that was included in the average. The difference between the actual velocity and the average velocity for any particular beat represents the random disturbances or turbulence during that beat. This difference, the turbulence velocity, is shown in Figure 5B for a particular beat.

The difference between the actual and the ensemble average velocity, which we have called the turbulence velocity, is not entirely due to hydrodynamic velocity fluctuations. Also included in this quantity is everything that can cause any beat-to-beat variation in the velocity, for example, respiration or variations in the length of each beat. The problem of separating fluid disturbances from other variations cannot be fully overcome, but it can be partially resolved by means of the energy spectrum discussed below.

The turbulence velocity can be calculated for each beat in the series and this turbulence velocity can be analyzed to tell us more about the nature of the disturbances that are observed. The ensemble average energy of the turbulence tells us not only the average magnitude of the distur-

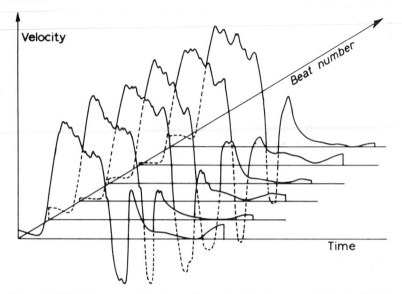

Figure 4. Velocity measured in descending aorta of a dog separated into individual beats. Ensemble averages correspond to averages taken along the beat number axis.

bances but also when in the beat they occur. The ensemble average turbulence energy is shown in Figure 5C.

For comparison with the disturbed waveform, the results of an identical analysis of the velocity data, measured in the same dog but under different stimulation so that the waveform is judged to be undisturbed, are shown in Figure 6. Note that the period of the beat is almost double that of the previous example. The average velocity and the actual velocity for an arbitrarily chosen particular beat are so similar that the two lines cannot be differentiated on the scale of this figure.

The most notable feature of the turbulence energy in the disturbed waveforms of Figure 5C is its peakedness. There is a very rapid peak in the disturbances just after the peak velocity is attained, that is, during systole but during the deceleration phase of the cycle. There is no corresponding peak in the undisturbed waveform results.

There is a second peak in the turbulence energy that occurs at the time of velocity reversal. There is a similar, although much smaller, peak in the undisturbed waveform. We attribute this peak to slight variations in the length of systole and to inaccuracies in the hot-film anenometer at the

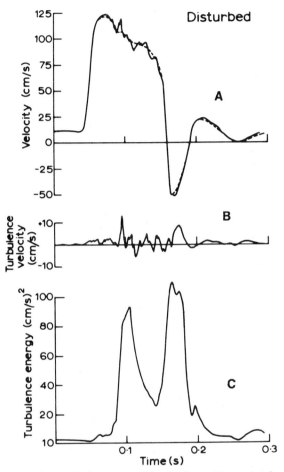

Figure 5. Analysis of the velocity measured in the descending aorta of a dog with a disturbed waveform. (A) Broken line, ensemble average velocity; solid line, velocity for a single beat. (B) Turbulent velocity for a single beat. (C) Ensemble average turbulence velocity.

time of flow reversal rather than large disturbances in the blood flow, although such disturbances cannot be ruled out. At any rate, we concentrate our attention on the disturbances that appear during the deceleration phase of systole.

We can further analyze these disturbances by calculating the development of the energy spectrum of the turbulence velocity during this part of

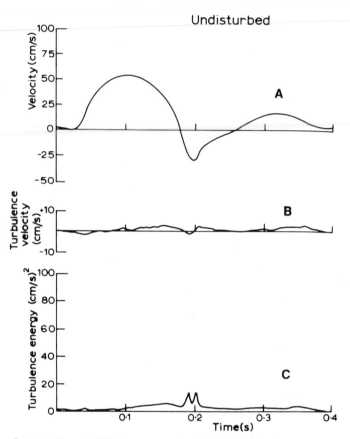

Figure 6. As in Figure 5. Velocity measured at the same location in the same dog but under conditions that resulted in an undisturbed waveform.

the beat. Numerically, this is done by taking the fast Fourier transform of the turbulence velocity at a particular time in each beat, calculating the energy spectrum, and then ensemble averaging over all of the beats to obtain the average energy spectrum of the turbulence velocity at that particular time in the beat. Physically, the energy spectrum tells us how the turbulence energy is distributed between disturbances of different wavenumbers. The energy at the lowest wavenumbers, corresponding to frequencies on the order of the heart rate, is due to beat-to-beat variations. At higher wavenumbers the energy is due to disturbances in the fluid.

By calculating the energy spectrum at different times, we can see how the turbulence develops not just in magnitude but in scale. Figure 7 shows the energy spectrum calculated for various times during the development of the first peak in turbulence energy shown in Figure 5C. We see that most of the energy appears at wavelengths similar to the diameter of the artery. The energy decreases rapidly at higher wavenumbers (i.e., shorter wavelengths) because of the increased effectiveness of viscous dissipation.

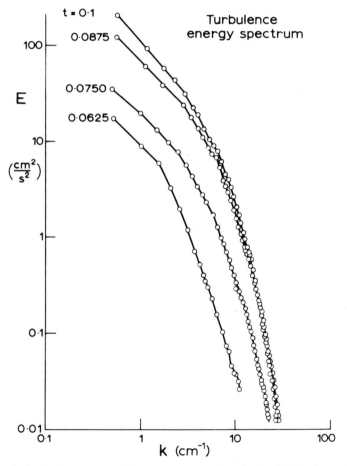

Figure 7. Ensemble average turbulence energy spectrum for the disturbed waveform in Figure 5.

Notice that this is a log-log plot and that the energy decreases over four orders of magnitude. This type of energy spectrum is typical of those measured in turbulent pipe flows (Hinze, 1959).

In conclusion, we can say that flow in the arteries of man and the larger mammals is often disturbed and there is some evidence that these disturbances are normal. There has not been much detailed analysis of these disturbances, but this analysis of data taken in the descending aorta of dogs may be typical. These disturbances appeared only during a part of the cycle. The early phase of systole, when the blood in the artery is accelerated, was completely free of disturbances. Once peak velocity was reached and the flow began to decelerate, disturbances appeared and grew very rapidly. As the flow slowed further the disturbances decreased. But as the flow actually reversed direction, there may have been another increase in the amount of disturbances in the blood. We are most concerned with the initial disturbances: where they come from, how they grow, and whether we can predict when they will appear.

STABILITY THEORY

We have seen that flow in the large arteries can be disturbed and that the disturbances can be important to the functioning of the circulation. We must now consider the origin of these disturbances.

An obvious source of disturbances in the large arteries is the heart. We know from cineangiography and hot-film anemometry that the flow in the left ventricle during filling is highly disturbed. It is very possible that these disturbances do not die down completely and are still present when the blood is ejected into the aorta.

Another source of disturbances is the aortic valve. The ridge-like valve ring could cause disturbances in the blood flowing past it. The valve flaps interact with the flow to produce vortices that assist in valve closure at the end of systole (Bellhouse and Bellhouse, 1969), but may also interact with the artery walls and with each other to produce flow disturbances. In the case of severe aortic stenosis, the jet formed by the stenosed valve certainly causes the extreme disturbances observed in this disease. Figure 8 shows the velocity measured by Seed (1972) in the ascending aorta of a patient with severe aortic stenosis and should be compared to the waveforms in Figure 1.

The qualitative nature of the flow leaving the left ventricle has been

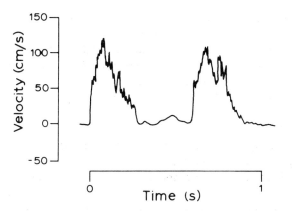

Figure 8. Velocity measured in the ascending aorta of a man with aortic stenosis.

demonstrated in model studies by Meisner and Rushmer (1963) for both normal and stenosed conditions.

All of these things can, and probably do, create disturbances. But because of the pulsatile nature of arterial blood flow, these disturbances are probably confined to the ascending aorta—to blood that has just left the heart. Because disturbances have been observed all the way down the descending aorta in blood which is three, or possibly four, beats away from the heart, there must be some source of disturbances other than the heart and aortic valve. The most likely source of these disturbances is hydrodynamic instability of the aortic blood flow.

Hydrodynamic stability is one of the most active and interesting branches of theoretical fluid mechanics. The subject is both broad and specialized, and we do not intend to review it in great detail. We do, however, need to review a few of the concepts of stability theory in order to discuss what we know about the stability of the flow in the arota.

All stability theories start from the idea that there is a known basic flow which satisfies the hydrodynamic equations and the appropriate boundary conditions. The theories then assume that there is a more complicated, as yet unknown, flow that satisfies the same equations and boundary conditions. The difference between these two flows is thought of as the disturbance flow. In theory, the theoretician solves the equations to determine how the disturbances evolve. If all possible disturbances decay then the flow is stable. If one or more of the disturbances grows in time then the basic flow is unstable and a new flow, either turbulent or a more complicated laminar flow, is predicted.

In practice, it is far too difficult to obtain a full solution for the disturbance flows. Therefore, three different methods have been developed to obtain partial solutions that can tell us something about the stability of the basic flows: linear theory, nonlinear theory, and the energy method.

Linear Theory

The linear theory of stability dates back nearly a century to the studies of Lord Rayleigh. Briefly, the theory assumes that the disturbance is very small—small enough that the nonlinear terms in the governing equations can be neglected. Because the resultant equations are linear, their solution must vary exponentially in time, $u \sim e^{\sigma t}$, where σ is a growth rate. When $\sigma < 0$, the disturbance decays exponentially in time. When this happens for all possible small disturbances the flow is stable. When, for some disturbance, $\sigma > 0$ then that particular disturbance grows in time and the basic flow is unstable. The condition $\sigma = 0$ divides stable from unstable disturbances and is often called the stability boundary.

A typical result of a linear stability analysis is sketched in Figure 9. The stability boundary divides the plane into two regions. In a flow with Reynolds number Re, a disturbance of wavenumber k decays if (k, Re) falls outside the stability boundary but grows exponentially if (k, Re) falls inside the boundary. Generally, there is a critical Reynolds number, Re_{crit}, where for Re < Re_{crit} all disturbances decay, while for Re > Re_{crit} there are some wavelengths at which disturbances grow. The wavenumber k_{crit} is often called the least stable disturbance because it is the first disturbance that can become unstable as the Reynolds number is increased.

A basic shortcoming of the linear theory is that it cannot tell us what happens to the infinitesimal disturbances once they begin to grow. As soon as they grow, the linearized equations no longer describe their behavior. Nevertheless, the linear theory has had many successes and provides the basis for most of our understanding of hydrodynamic stability.

Another shortcoming of the linear theory is that since it considers only infinitesimal disturbances, its prediction of the critical Reynolds number is a least upper bound. That is, for Re > Re_{crit} predicted by linear theory, the basic flow is unstable to the infinitesimal disturbances that are always present in a real flow. However, the finite disturbances that are often present and cannot be studied by a linear analysis may also be unstable at lower Reynolds numbers, so that a real flow can be unstable at Re <

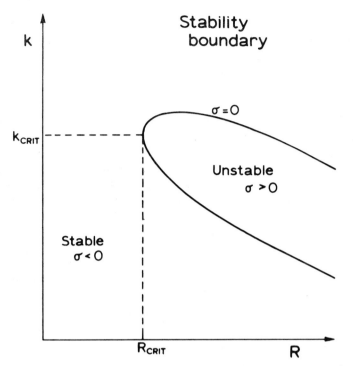

Figure 9. A typical stability boundary. Wavenumber of the disturbance and Reynolds number of the flow.

Re_{crit}. Both nonlinear theory and the energy method are attempts to study the stability of these finite disturbances.

Nonlinear Theory

Nonlinear theory of stability is a very specialized field that is impossible to discuss in general terms (see, e.g., a review by Stuart, 1971). Simply, it concerns the approximate solution of the full nonlinear equations describing the disturbance. Often this analysis takes the form of a series expansion for which the lowest-order term is the linear stability solution. Thus nonlinear theory can give more accurate predictions of critical parameters for stability. In some problems, nonlinear theory has successfully predicted the form of new, more complicated laminar flows that under certain conditions are more stable than the basic flows.

Because nonlinear theory uses full nonlinear disturbance equations, it does not suffer from the same restrictions as linear theory. The only shortcoming of the theory is the difficulty of the mathematics involved and, hence, the limitations on the types of problems to which it can be applied.

Energy Method

The energy method is, in a sense, a complement to the linear theory in that it provides a lower bound instead of an upper bound for the critical parameters. It does this by looking at the global kinetic energy equation for the disturbance formed by multiplying the momentum equation for the disturbance by the disturbance velocity and integrating over the whole flow. For some basic flows this equation can be analyzed to provide the maximum Reynolds number for which the kinetic energy for all disturbances must eventually vanish.

The energy method has not been very successful in obtaining practically useful results about stability. Its major shortcoming is that it is too comprehensive; it considers the stability of all disturbances, even those that are dynamically unrealizable. Thus the stability limits it predicts are generally unrealistically low. They are, however, rigorous and, together with results from the linear and nonlinear theories, can broaden our understanding of the problem.

STABILITY OF PLANE POISEUILLE FLOW

As an example of the methods and results of stability theory, we look at the stability of plane Poiseuille flow. This flow is qualitatively similar to flow in a pipe, but because of its two-dimensional nature it is simpler to analyze. Despite its similarity to pipe flow, as far as stability is concerned, the slight geometrical differences are significant; therefore, the results are not directly applicable to flow in arteries.

Plane Poiseuille flow refers to the two-dimensional flow between parallel plates at $y = \pm h$ under the influence of a pressure gradient, dP/dx. For a constant pressure gradient the steady solution is the parabolic profile

$$u = U(1 - (y/h)^2)$$

where h is the half-height of the channel and U is the velocity on the centerline,

$$U = -\frac{h^2}{2\mu} \frac{dP}{dx}$$

This profile is shown in Figure 10.

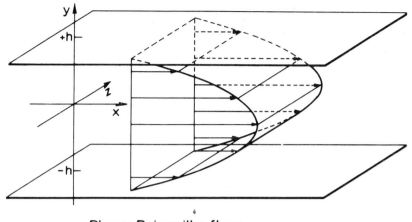

Plane Poiseuille flow

Figure 10. Steady plane Poiseuille flow.

Linear theory has been applied to this basic flow by many workers, most recently by Grosch and Salwen (1968). The result of their analysis is the neutral stability curve as shown in Figure 11. The critical parameters in this problem are the Reynolds number Re_h, based on the channel half-height, h, and k, the dimensionless wavenumber of the disturbance. These results say that for $Re_h < 5,800$ all infinitesimal disturbances decay and the basic flow is stable. For $Re_h > 5,800$, there is a range of wavenumbers at which infinitesimal disturbances grown exponentially in time.

This value for the critical Reynolds number, Re_{crit}, does not correspond very well with experimental observations. These show that disturbances occur spontaneously for Re_h as low as 1,400 (Davies and White, 1928).

The disturbance that is theoretically the least stable is a fairly complicated three-dimensional wave. Since linear theory is only valid for very small disturbances, we cannot, of course, say what happens to these waves once they grow. Neither can we predict what will happen to finite disturbances that are introduced into the flow.

To study the effect of finite disturbances on the stability of plane Poiseuille flow, we must turn to nonlinear stability theory. Stuart (1960) suggested that finite disturbances could be analyzed by an asymptotic expansion around the critical conditions found by the linear theory. This suggestion was carried out by a number of people including Pekeris and Shkoller (1969), whose results are shown in Figure 11. They found that

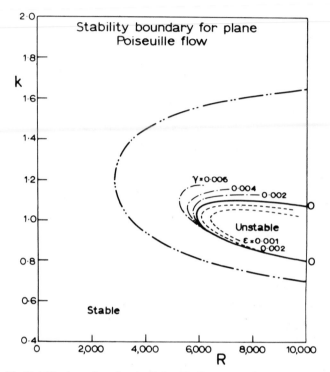

Figure 11. Stability boundary for the Poiseuille flow. —— linear theory for steady flow (Grosch and Salwen, 1968); — – – nonlinear theory for steady flow (Pekeris and Shkoller, 1969); — – – – linear theory for cellular steady flow (Zahn et al., 1974); – – – – linear theory for unsteady flow (Grosch and Salwen, 1968).

the neutral curve for finite, periodic disturbances was shifted so that Re_{crit} decreased as the amplitude of the disturbance was increased. How far this value can be shifted cannot be determined because, once again, their analysis breaks down as the amplitude of the disturbance increases.

More recent work on periodic waves by George, Hellums, and Martin (1974) has shown that a critical Reynolds number at the least stable wavelength decreases to almost half of its linear value as the amplitude of the disturbance increases.

Stewartson and Stuart (1971) broadened the scope of nonlinear analysis by considering the stability of nonlinear waves that could develop both in space and in time. This approach is particularly appealing because all experiments since Reynolds have shown that the transition from laminar to turbulent flow does not occur uniformly throughout the flow.

Instead, the turbulence appears first in localized "spots" or "bursts." These "spots" or "bursts" develop as they are convected along the tube (Wygnanski and Champagne, 1973). This approach is certainly appealing to stability theoreticians; a minor industry has developed around it. However, the results to date are of more interest to the mathematician than to the practical fluid dynamicist.

Zahn et al. (1974) used yet another nonlinear approach to demonstrate that a three-dimensional, cellular motion is possible in plane Poiseuille flow. Furthermore, they showed that this flow is less stable than the basic flow. The stability boundary they calculated for one type of possible cellular motion is included in Figure 11. The critical Reynolds number is less than half of that calculated for the basic flow.

Linear theory gives a critical Re_h that is about four times larger than the Re_h at which transition has been observed experimentally. Nonlinear theory has shown that finite disturbances are less stable than the infinitesimal disturbances of linear theory. Some finite disturbances are unstable at Re_h less than half of the critical Re_h found by linear theory. But what is the lower limit? To answer this, we must turn to the energy method that considers the stability of all disturbances. Busse (1969) has shown that plane Poiseuille flow is stable for $Re_h < 99.2$. This is a lower limit for the critical Re_h, but it may be unrealistically low because it considers dynamically unrealistic disturbances.

So far, only the stability of steady, plane Poiseuille flow has been discussed. Because we are interested in highly oscillatory flows, it is interesting to see what effects oscillations can have. There has been extensive work done on the stability of periodically modulated Poiseuille flow. Instead of being steady the pressure gradient is varied periodically in time:

$$\frac{dP}{dx} = \frac{dP_0}{dx} (1 + \epsilon \sin \omega t),$$

where ω is the frequency and ϵ is the dimensionless amplitude of the oscillation. Making the pressure gradient periodic introduces a new time scale into the problem: the period of the oscillation. This new time scale corresponds to a very important new length scale, the Stokes layer thickness,

$$\delta = \sqrt{v/\omega}$$

Physically, this is a measure of the distance that the effect of the wall can diffuse away from the wall during one period of the oscillation. Inside the

Stokes layer, viscosity and the effect of the walls are important; outside, viscosity is unimportant and the flow behaves as if it were inviscid. The basic flow for three different frequencies is shown in Figure 12. Unsurprisingly, the nature of flow inside these Stokes layers is very important to the stability of unsteady flows.

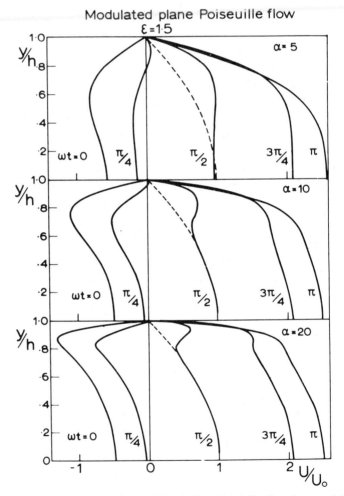

Figure 12. Velocity profiles for modulated plane Poiseuille flow for $\epsilon = 1.5$ and frequency parameter $\alpha = 5$, 10, and 20. Broken line, unmodulated profile.

If ω is large then the Stokes layer is very thin. Hall (1975) used linear theory to analyze the stability of high-frequency periodic Poiseuille flow for which $\delta/h \ll 1$. He found that Re_{crit} was less than that in steady flow. That is, the effect of high-frequency modulation of the pressure gradient is to destabilize the flow.

Grosch and Salwen (1968) used linear theory to look at another extreme of the same problem. If the amplitude of the periodic part of the pressure gradient is small, $\epsilon \ll 1$, then the basic flow is not very different from the steady flow. Some of the results of their stability analysis are shown in Figure 11. They showed that as the amplitude of the modulation increases, the flow becomes more stable. They found that this trend continues and then reverses so that, at the largest amplitudes they studied, the modulated flow was less stable than the steady flow.

For the same limit of small amplitude modulation, Herbert (1972) used the energy method to show that disturbances of a certain size must be stable. He showed that a disturbance will experience a net decay over a cycle if $\delta'/\delta \geqslant \frac{1}{2}$ where δ' is the thickness of the disturbance. Because this is a sufficient condition for stability, this is a very general result and yet it is of little practical interest since it does not tell us anything about the general stability of the flow, but only about its stability to certain size disturbances.

Finally, Davis (1975) suggests that there may be critical frequencies of oscillation at which the modulation will interact resonantly with a previously stable disturbance of the basic flow. This possibility has not been explored very far, but it could be an important type of instability.

These results of analyses of the stability of plane Poiseuille flow cannot be applied directly to flow in the aorta. They do serve, however, as an indication of the way in which more physically realistic problems may be analyzed.

STABILITY OF FLOW IN A PIPE

Our theoretical understanding of the stability of flow in pipes is not as advanced as it is in planar flows, primarily because of the additional complexity of axial-symmetric flows. There are, however, a few analyses as well as a number of experimental studies that provide some understanding of the stability of arterial flow.

The simplest possible pipe flow is steady, Hagen–Poiseuille flow in a straight, rigid pipe with circular cross section. This is the flow that

Reynolds used in his classic experiments that laid the foundation of the study of stability. Unfortunately, this is also the flow that best illustrates the failure of stability theory. Experimentally, Reynolds found that this flow is unstable for Re_d greater than about 2,000 (although with great care laminar flow has been maintained to Re_d greater than 20,000).

Linear theory predicts that this flow should be stable for all Re_d, that is, all infinitesimal disturbances decay exponentially in time under all conditions. Nonlinear theory has never yielded any results for this problem (probably because most nonlinear methods rely upon the existence of a linear solution as a starting place for their approximations). The energy method tells us only that the flow is stable for $Re_d < 81.5$ (Joseph and Carmi, 1969), that is, every imaginable disturbance must decay for $Re_d < 81.5$. For $Re_d > 81.5$ there are some disturbances that can grow.

Garg and Rouleau (1974) suggested that the discrepancy between theory and experiment might be due to the assumption of perfectly rigid walls. They therefore used linear theory to study the stability of Poiseuille flow in thin-walled, elastic pipes. They found the very interesting result that for walls with a small Youngs modulus, the flow could become unstable. The Youngs modulus below which they predict instability is somewhat larger than the Youngs modulus of the wall of a large artery. Nevertheless, their results do indicate that the flexible walls of an artery can have a destabilizing effect on the flow within it.

Two characteristics of flow in the aorta that undoubtedly have a large influence on its stability are its curvature and its pulsatility. Smith (1975) and Blennerhasset (1975) have only recently calculated the basic laminar flow for periodically modulated flow in a curved pipe. We cannot draw any definite conclusions about stability from their solutions, but with the basic solution now available, we can at least contemplate starting the stability analysis.

In the absence of a basic solution for flow in the artery, previous discussions of stability have been limited to extrapolation from the results of simpler but similar flows. There has been a great deal of work recently on the stability of pulsatile flows, including that on modulated plane Poiseuille flow discussed in the previous section. This work has been reviewed in some detail by Davis (1975).

The most important of these studies, from the point of view of flow in the arteries, is the work on the stability of Stokes layers. As mentioned above, the Stokes layer is the region near the wall in a periodic flow in which the effect of viscosity is important. It is a kind of boundary layer that gets thinner as the frequency of the oscillation increases. As the Stokes layer gets thinner in a pipe flow, it can be argued that the effects of curvature decrease and that the stability of the layer becomes approximately that of a plane Stokes layer.

This is the argument used by Nerem (1973) in his theoretical justification of the stability boundary shown in Figure 2. If $Re_\delta = K$ is the stability criterion for a plane Stokes layer where Re_δ is the Reynolds number based on the Stokes layer thickness

$$\delta = \sqrt{\nu/\omega},$$

then

$$Re_d = \frac{d}{\delta} Re_\delta = K\alpha$$

is the stability criterion for the Reynolds number based on pipe diameter, Re_d. In Figure 2, $K = 250$. Theoretical values of K range from 19 (a lower bound) for the energy method to 800 calculated for a bounded Stokes layer using linear theory (Davis, 1975). This approach does give a useful practical result. However, in view of the assumptions made, it should be treated as an empirical result rather than a theoretical one.

Apart from the in vivo measurements of disturbances in the arteries mentioned in the Introduction, there have been relatively few experiments on the stability of flows similar to those in the arteries. The earliest experiments demonstrated that in steady Poiseuille flow, blood behaves like a Newtonian fluid; transition from laminar to turbulent flow occurs at $Re_d \simeq 2,000$ (Coulter and Pappenheimer, 1949).

There have been a few experiments on the stability of purely oscillating flow in pipes, i.e., oscillatory flows with no mean velocity. Sergeev (1966) found that the critical Reynolds number based upon maximum velocity and pipe diameter varied linearly with α:

$$Re_{crit} = 700\alpha$$

Pelisier and Clarion (1975), working with oscillatory flow in a U-tube, found that disturbances occur when the Reynolds number based on maximum velocity exceeded $Re_{crit} = 190 \, \alpha^{0.8}$.

The results of experiments on the stability of oscillatory flow with a mean velocity are more difficult to summarize. It is necessary to introduce another parameter to describe these flows: a ratio of the amplitude of the velocity oscillation to the mean velocity, γ, for instance. With this extra parameter, the stability boundary is no longer a line but a surface that is only partially described by the experiments that have been reported.

Gilbrech and Combs (1963) used an optical technique to determine whether an artificially generated turbulent slug grows or decays as it is traveling along with the pulsating flow. Sarpkaya (1966) used a similar technique but detected the turbulent slug with differential pressure transducers. Fortunately, both looked at frequencies that are of interest physiologically; Gilbrech and Combs varied α from 4 to 16, Sarpkaya from 4 to 7.8. Both looked at γ, the ratio of oscillatory to mean velocity components, from 0 to 1, that is, from steady flow to when the flow just begins to reverse. For arterial flow, $\gamma > 1$.

Both experimenters defined a flow to be stable if a turbulent slug decayed as it passed down the pipe, and both report similar results. For a given α, the critical Reynolds number based on mean velocity increases as γ increases from zero, that is, small-amplitude oscillations stabilize the flow. As γ increases further, a maximum Re_{crit} is reached and thereafter Re_{crit} decreases as γ increases. The maximum Re_{crit} depends upon α; the lower the α, the larger the maximum Re_{crit}. Gilbrech and Combs and Sarpkaya found that their higher-frequency, larger-amplitude flows were less stable than the corresponding steady flow.

Yellin (1966) also looked at transition in pulsatile pipe flow over a more limited range of frequencies and amplitudes. However, he did not artificially generate turbulence. He observed naturally occurring transition and gives a good description of the transition process. His results agree, at least qualitatively, with those of previous researchers.

Minton and Clamen (1975) ingeniously obtained modulated pipe flow by oscillating their pipe rather than by generating an oscillatory pressure gradient. They studied their flow visually, using a hydrogen bubble technique, and so they were able to study the formation and nature of disturbances in much more detail than the previous researchers. They made extensive measurements of the stability of the flow over a wide range of frequencies, α up to 34, and amplitudes, γ up to 8.

Briefly, their results confirm the trends indicated by previous results. They found that for $\alpha < 10$ and $\gamma \ll 1$ the pulsating flow is more stable than the corresponding steady flow. However, for $\alpha > 10$ and $\gamma > 1$ they found the reverse: the pulsating flow is less stable than the steady flow. We emphasize that these results refer to the appearance of any disturbance rather than the grosser definition of stability used in previous studies.

All of the experiments we have mentioned were done in rigid pipes.

Olsen and Shapiro (1967) studied periodically modulated flow through elastic tubes. They measured only the variations in the diameter of the tube; they could not observe directly whether or not the flow was disturbed. However, in applying their theory to their observed results they found that under certain experimental conditions they obtained much better agreement if they used a turbulent friction relationship rather than the laminar one. From this indirect evidence, we can conclude that the flow was disturbed for certain conditions but their means of detecting turbulence was far too crude to enable us to determine any sort of stability criterion.

Another common feature of all of these experiments is that the oscillations imposed upon the flow were harmonic. Sarpkaya (1966) does report some results for periodic but nonharmonic oscillations. He found that for the same α and γ, nonharmonic flows are always less stable than harmonic flows. Arterial flow, of course, is highly nonharmonic.

We conclude this section simply by observing that, theoretically, our understanding of the stability of unsteady flow in a pipe is very poor, and, experimentally, our understanding is incomplete and qualitative, at best. We conclude the review by describing some of our experiments on the stability of another type of flow that we feel models some of the essential features of arterial flow.

STABILITY OF STOPPING FLOWS

How we define stability is a very important practical question, particularly in unsteady flows. Several definitions have been suggested and used (see Davis, 1975) but, generally, a flow is defined as stable if disturbances taken in some average sense do not grow in time. By most definitions, the disturbances measured in man (Seed, 1972), in dogs (Nerem and Seed, 1972), and in horses (Nerem et al., 1974) would be called stable because they do not grow from period to period. If we are interested in the growth of the disturbances within a period it may be convenient to take a slightly different approach to the problem.

Instead of considering the flow in the arteries as a periodic flow, consider it as a succession of completely independent beats. Each beat starts in a state of quiescence or of very slow, steady flow, is rapidly accelerated during the start of systole, decelerates as systole ends, and readjusts itself to its original state during diastole. The period of diastole need not be the same from beat to beat; we only require that it last long enough for the original state to be recovered so that each beat has the same initial conditions. This is the philosophy that underlies the ensemble averaging analysis mentioned previously.

From this point of view, the disturbances seen during the deceleration phase of the flow must be thought of as the result of the nature of the flow during that particular beat and are independent of what happens before and after that beat.

Taking this point of view, we have embarked on a study of the stability of the flow in the large arteries during a single beat. As a first step, we have made a very simple model which we feel retains many of the essential features of arterial flow. Since the flow seems to be stable during the acceleration phase, we have concentrated on decelerating flows. In particular, we have studied the simplest decelerating flow, a steady Poiseuille flow in a rigid pipe that is suddenly stopped by means of a valve.

The experimental apparatus is sketched in Figure 13. The valve is opened and steady Poiseuille flow is established. The solenoid-operated, shutter-type valve is rapidly closed and the flow is studied visually while it decelerates and eventually comes to a complete rest. The flow is made visible by the hydrogen bubble technique.

Surprisingly, the theoretical prediction of how the flow decays, assuming it remains laminar, proved to be fairly difficult (Weinbaum and Parker, 1975). Very briefly, the problem must be analyzed on three separate time scales: (1) a very short time characteristic of the passage of a pressure wave, (2) a short diffusion time during which a boundary layer grows out

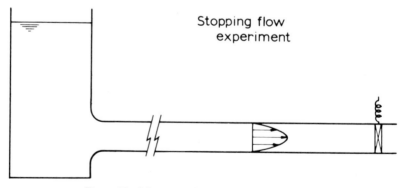

Figure 13. Schematic of stopping flow experiment.

from the wall of the pipe, and (3) a long diffusion time characteristic of the flow after the boundary layer grows to fill the entire pipe.

The short time scale characteristic of the propagation of a pressure wave is

$$\tau_1 = R/c$$

where c is the speed of sound in the fluid and R is the radius of the pipe. In a nearly incompressible fluid such as blood or water, this time is very small. During this time a pressure wave propagates through the fluid adjusting the flow to the new boundary condition of no net flux. This pressure wave acts like an impulse, giving the flow a uniform velocity equal but opposite to the mean velocity of steady Poiseuille flow. Since the mean velocity of steady Poiseuille flow is half the maximum velocity, U, the new flow after the passage of the pressure wave has the velocity profile

$$u = U(\tfrac{1}{2} - (r/R)^2)$$

The fluid in the center of the pipe continues to flow forward but at half of its initial velocity. The fluid at the wall that was originally at rest is given an equal velocity in the opposite direction. This bidirectional velocity profile is shown in Figure 14.

This profile violates the no-slip condition at the wall of the pipe because on the short, pressure-wave time scale we have neglected the effect of viscosity. The flow, which cannot ignore viscosity, adjusts by establishing a very thin boundary layer at the wall. This boundary layer is established and grows on the second time scale, a diffusion time scale

$$\tau_2 = R^2/v$$

where v is the kinematic viscosity of the fluid.

It is during this period of the growth of the boundary layer that the flow becomes difficult to analyze. The reason can be seen physically. The fluid in the boundary layer near the wall slows down as it dissipates its energy in shearing work on the wall. Since the fluid near the wall is flowing in the negative direction and the positively moving fluid in the center of the pipe is still unaffected by viscosity, there is a net flux in the positive direction. But, because the valve is shut, the continuity equation demands that the net flux at every cross section must be zero. To satisfy this condition, a pressure gradient is established that accelerates the flow in the negative direction just enough to offset the flux imbalance due to viscosity. Since the nature of the boundary layer depends on the history of

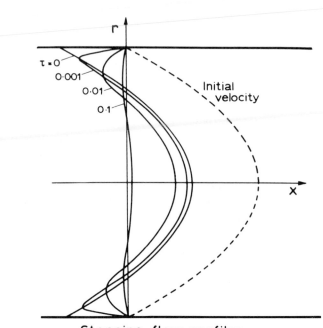

Stopping flow profiles

Figure 14. Calculated stopping flow velocity profiles. Broken line, velocity profile before the valve is shut.

the compensating pressure gradient, which in turn depends upon the history of the boundary layer, the problem becomes very complex analytically.

In the final stage, after the boundary layer grows to fill the entire pipe, the problem becomes slightly easier to analyze. However, by this time the effect of viscosity has greatly reduced the velocity throughout the fluid and the problem becomes the relatively uninteresting one of the final decay of the small residual motions. The theoretical solution for the laminar decay of a suddenly stopped Poiseuille pipe flow is shown in Figure 14.

The stability of this flow is being explored both theoretically and experimentally. Theoretically, the problem is being analyzed by making the approximation that the basic flow is quasisteady, that is, we assume that the variation in the basic flow is slow compared to the onset and development of the disturbance. This is clearly a bad assumption just after the valve is shut, but it becomes better and better as the flow begins to slow and is a reasonably good assumption during the final stages of the decay.

Experimentally, we find that the stability of the flow depends on both the velocity profile and the Reynolds number of the flow just before the valve is shut. For Poiseuille flows, and an initial Reynolds number based on maximum velocity less than about 5,000, the flow remains laminar and decays just as predicted by the laminar theory. As the initial Reynolds number is increased, a periodic disturbance appears just before the flow decays. The more the Reynolds number is increased, the earlier the periodic disturbance appears and the more it develops before it decays. Finally, at large enough Reynolds number the disturbances grow, interact, and develop into turbulence that is rapidly distributed throughout the pipe. This turbulent flow then decays much more quickly than the laminar flow because of the more effective transport of momentum in turbulent flows.

Turbulent disturbances are observed for initial Reynolds numbers greater than about 8,000. These disturbances first appear about 2 sec after the valve is shut. As the initial Reynolds number is increased, they appear earlier until at the highest Reynolds numbers the flow seems to become turbulent almost immediately after the valve is shut.

Blood flow velocity in the arteries does not have a parabolic profile, nor does it stop suddenly, so the results of this model experiment cannot be applied directly to flow in arteries. The results do, however, demonstrate that a decelerating flow can be unstable and can produce the type of disturbances that are observed in the arteries. They also demonstrate that the observed disturbances may develop during the course of a single beat and may not necessarily be the result of the periodic nature of blood flow. This may seem a trivial distinction, but it may make an important difference in the way that we approach the problem of stability in arterial flows both theoretically and experimentally.

LITERATURE CITED

Bellhouse, B. J., and F. H. Bellhouse. 1969. Fluid mechanics of model normal and stenosed aortic valves. Circ. Res. 25: 693–704.

Blennerhasset, P. 1975. Secondary motion and diffusion in unsteady flow in a curved pipe (in preparation).

Busse, F. H. 1969. Bounds on the transport of mass and momentum by turbulent flow between parallel plates. Z. Angew. Math. Phys. 20: 1–14.

Caro, C. G., J. M. Fitz-Gerald, and R. C. Schroter. 1971. Atheroma and arterial wall shear. Observations, correlation and proposal of a shear dependant mass transfer mechanism for atherogenesis. Proc. Roy. Soc. London, Series B 177: 109–159.

Coulter, N. A., and J. R. Pappenheimer. 1949. Development of turbulence in flowing blood. Amer. J. Physiol. 159: 401–408.

Davies, S. J., and C. M. White. 1928. An experimental study of the flow of water in pipes of rectangular section. Proc. Roy. Soc. London, Series A 119: 92–107.

Davis, S. H. 1975. The stability of periodic flows (in preparation).

Garg, V. K., and W. T. Rouleau. 1974. Stability of Poiseuille flow in a thin elastic tube. Phys. Fluids 17: 1103–1108.

George, W. D., J. D. Hellums, and B. Martin. 1974. Finite-amplitude neutral disturbances in plane Poiseuille flow. J. Fluid Mech. 63: 765–771.

Gilbrech, D. A., and G. D. Combs. 1963. Critical Reynolds numbers for incompressible pulsating flow in tubes. Developments in Theoretical and Applied Mechanics. Vol. I. pp. 292–304. Plenum Press, New York.

Grosch, C. E., and H. Salwen. 1968. The stability of steady and time-dependant plane Poiseuille flow. J. Fluid Mech. 34: 177–205.

Hall, P. 1975. The stability of Poiseuille flow modulated at high frequencies. Proc. Roy. Soc. London, Series A 344: 453–464.

Herbert, D. M. 1972. The energy balance in modulated plane Poiseuille flow. J. Fluid Mech. 56: 73–80.

Hinze, J. O. 1959. Turbulence: An Introduction to Its Mechanism and Theory. McGraw-Hill, New York. Section 7-9.

Joseph, D. D., and S. Carmi, 1969. Stability of Poiseuille flow in pipes, annuli, and channels. Quart. J. Appl. Math. 26: 575–599.

Ling, S. C., H. B. Atabek, D. L. Fry, D. J. Patel, and J. S. Janicki. 1968. Application of heated-film velocity and shear probes to hemodynamic studies. Circ. Res. 23: 789–801.

MacDonald, D. A. 1952. The occurrence of turbulent flow in the rabbit aorta. J. Physiol. 118: 340–347.

MacDonald, D. A. 1974. Blood Flow in Arteries. 2nd Ed. Edward Arnold, London. Chapter 4.

McKusick, V. A. 1958. Cardiovascular Sound in Health and Disease. Williams and Wilkins, Baltimore. Section 1.

Meisner, J. E., and R. F. Rushmer. 1963. Eddy formation and turbulence in flowing liquids. Circ. Res. 12: 455–463.

Minton, P., and M. Clamen. 1975. An experimental study of pulsating flow in an oscillating pipe (in preparation).

Nerem, R. M. 1973. Turbulence in blood flows. Presented at 10th Annual Meeting of the Society of Engineering Science, November 5–7, Raleigh, N. C.

Nerem, R. M., and W. A. Seed. 1972. An in vivo study of aortic flow disturbances. Cardiovasc. Res. 6: 1–14.

Nerem, R. M., J. A. Rumberger, D. R. Gross, R. L. Hamlin, and G. L.

Geiger. 1974. Hot-film anemometer velocity measurements of arterial blood flow in horses. Circ. Res. 34: 193–203.

Olsen, J. H., and A. H. Shapiro. 1967. Large-amplitude unsteady flow in liquid-filled elastic tubes. J. Fluid Mech. 29: 513–538.

Pekeris, C. L., and B. Shkoller. 1969. The neutral curves for periodic perturbations of finite amplitude of plane Poiseuille flow. J. Fluid Mech. 39: 629–639.

Pelisier, R., and C. Clarion. 1975. A theoretical and experimental study of the velocity distribution and transition to turbulence in free oscillatory flow. J. Fluid Mech. 70: 59–79.

Roach, M. R. 1963. Experimental study of the production and time-course of post stenotic dilation in the fermoral and carotoid arteries of adult dogs. Circ. Res. 13: 537–551.

Sarpkaya, T. 1966. Experimental determination of the critical Reynolds number for pulsating Poiseuille flow. J. Bas. Eng. 88: 589–598.

Schultz, D. L., D. S. Tunstall-Pedoe, G. de J. Lee, A. J. Gunning, and B. J. Bellhouse. 1969. Velocity distribution and transition in the arterial system. In G. E. W. Wolstenholme and J. Knight (eds.), Circulatory and Respiratory Mass Transport. A CIBA Foundation Symposium, pp. 172–202. Churchill, London.

Seed, W. A. 1972. Velocity profiles and turbulence in the aorta: a study by hot film anemometry. Ph.D. Thesis, Univ. of London.

Seed, W. A., and N. B. Wood. 1971. Velocity patterns in the aorta. Circ. Res. 5: 319–330.

Sergeev, S. I. 1966. Fluid oscillations in pipes at moderate Reynolds numbers. Mekh. Zh. i. Gaza, 1: 168–170 (trans. Sov. Fluid Mech. 1: 121–122).

Smith, F. T. 1975. Pulsatile flow in curved pipes. J. Fluid Mech. 71: 15–43.

Stewartson, K., and J. T. Stuart. 1971. A non-linear instability theory for a wave system in plane Poiseuille flow. J. Fluid Mech. 48: 529–545.

Stuart, J. T. 1960. On the non-linear mechanics of wave disturbances in stable and unstable parallel flows. Part 1. The basic behaviour in plane Poiseuille flow. J. Fluid Mech. 9: 353–370.

Stuart, J. T. 1971. Non-linear stability theory. In Annual Review of Fluid Mechanics, Vol. 3, p. 347. Annual Reviews, Palo Alto, Calif.

Weinbaum, S., and K. H. Parker. 1975. The laminar decay of suddenly blocked channel and pipe flows. J. Fluid Mech. 69: 729–752.

Wygnanski, I. J., and F. H. Champagne. 1973. On transition in a pipe. Part 1. The origin of puffs and slugs and the flow in a turbulent slug. J. Fluid Mech. 59: 281–335.

Yellin, E. L. 1966. Laminar-turbulent transition process in pulsatile flow. Circ. Res. 29: 791–804.

Zahn, J-P., J. Toomre, E. A. Spiegal, and D. O. Gough. 1974. Non-linear cellular motions in Poiseuille channel flow. J. Fluid Mech. 64: 319–345.

Cardiovascular Flow Dynamics and Measurements
Edited by N. H. C. Hwang and N. A. Normann
Copyright 1977   University Park Press   Baltimore

chapter 17

MECHANICS OF PULMONARY CIRCULATION

Yuan-Cheng B. Fung and Sidney S. Sobin

ABSTRACT

Pulmonary blood vessels have their particular geometry and elasticity, and blood flow in the lung has its own particular characteristics. To formulate the boundary value problems of pulmonary blood flow, we first made preliminary investigations on lung morphometry, blood rheology, vascular elasticity, and the "sluicing" or "waterfall" phenomenon. The mathematical problem is then formulated and solved. The theory can be used to analyze various physiological phenomena, such as the pressure–flow relationship, blood volume in various vessels, transit time distribution, velocity field, regional flow due to gravity, etc. The theoretical results are compared with experiments. The exchange of water between the blood vessel and the extravascular space, and the input impedance of pulsatile flow are discussed in some detail.

INTRODUCTION

The oxygenation of the mixed venous blood and the removal of the excess CO_2 by exchange between the capillaries and the alveoli is the function of the pulmonary circuit. The nutrition of the lung tissue is the function of the systemic bronchial circuit. In this chapter, we are concerned with the pulmonary circuit only. The principal distinction between the pulmonary circuit and the systemic circuit is that the former is a low-resistance system. The increase in pressure head required for an increased flow is much smaller in the lung than in the heart.

The work described in this chapter was carried out with the support of the U.S. Public Health Service, National Heart and Lung Institute, and the National Science Foundation over the past ten years.

For descriptive material concerning lung anatomy, physiology, bio-chemistry, control, radiology, etc., see the list of General References at the end of this chapter. It is a vast field with a vast literature; in this chapter we concentrate on those fluid mechanical aspects that have been subjected to a reasonably complete analysis.

A formulation of a problem is incomplete unless both the field equations and boundary conditions are well posed. Most of the descriptive material in the literature offers some data on some aspects of the lung and its function, or records some observations, but usually they are only preliminaries to a full formulation of the problem. A full theory should provide a mathematical framework capable of predicting quantitative relationship between several variables. The predictions should be con-sistent with all known facts. With this criterion, our choices are quite limited.

Of course, most work on cardiovascular dynamics applies as well to pulmonary blood vessels as to systemic blood vessels. Thus a large part of the material presented in other chapters of this book can be applied to pulmonary circulation. Of the particular theories that specifically apply to the lung, the most prominent is the mathematical analysis of pulsatile blood flow in the lung by Patel, DeFreitas, and Fry (1963), Bergel and Milnor (1965), Milnor, Bergel, and Bargainer (1966), Wiener et al. (1966), Pollack, Reddy, and Noordergraaf (1968), Milnor et al. (1969), and Milnor (1972). The principal feature of the problem is the rapid branching of the pulmonary arteries and veins. The most recent summary is given by Milnor (1975), who studied how the input impedance spectrum is affected by the distribution of physical properties with the pulmonary bed. Womersley's equation for a constrained elastic tube is used for each segment of a branching system. Taylor's method of branching analysis is applied. Milnor concluded that the significant terminal impedance of the lung is not located at the end of the veins, but in the small arteries, in a circumscribed region where the characteristic impedance matches the input impedance of the remainder of the bed. The input spectrum and the apparent termina-tion are much less sensitive to changes in the properties of the veins than to similar alterations in the arteries, but are influenced by both.

Another set of investigations is related to the special features of the pulmonary capillary blood vessels. The capillaries of the lung form a very dense network, with only a thin barrier from the air. The parenchyma of the lung (its gas-exchange portion, i.e., the capillary blood vessel network) comprises the majority (as much as 90%) of the volume of the lung,

(Weibel, 1963, p. 54). In contrast to the capillaries of the peripheral circulation, the pulmonary capillaries are distensible; in fact, very compliant. Furthermore, unlike the systemic circulation in which the pressure drop in the capillaries is minor (of the order of 10%), in pulmonary circulation a major part of the motive force (pulmonary arterial pressure − left atrium pressure) is used up in the capillaries (30−50%). The capillaries are also the site for water exchange, gas diffusion, etc., the understanding of which also requires the solution of the blood flow problem as a prerequisite. This is a problem we are familiar with; therefore, it forms the main topic of the present chapter.

1 PRELIMINARY STUDIES

To analyze pulmonary alveolar blood flow, we must know the pulmonary blood vessel geometry, the elasticity of the blood vessels, the rheology of blood in these vessels, the conditions in the pulmonary artery and left atrium, the gravitational vector, the boundary conditions, and the control mechanisms. This basic information can be pieced together with the laws of physics. From a unified treatment we should be able to deduce the pressure−flow relationship for the pulmonary circulation, the dependence of the nonlinear resistance to flow on the blood pressure, the effect of gravitation on the blood flow distribution in the lung, the distributions of stresses and strain in the parenchyma, the distribution of alveolar size, the transit time distribution, the extravascular water transport, the dynamic impedance, etc. Thus the functions of the lung can be related to the structure and the material properties of the lung.

In this section we discuss the microvascular geometry, elasticity, blood rheology, "sluicing" or "waterfall," and boundary conditions of the mammalian lung. A unified analysis of the blood flow is presented in subsequent sections.

1.1 Geometry of the Pulmonary Vessels

The hierarchy of bronchial tree and blood vessels has been studied extensively by Weibel (1963), Horsfield and Cumming (1968), and others. The smallest unit of the air space is the alveolus. The alveolus is bounded by networks of capillary blood vessels. The walls of each alveolus are shared by neighboring alveoli, and are called *interalveolar septa*. The overriding fact that determines the topology of the capillary blood vessels is that all pulmonary alveolar septa in adult mammalian lungs are similar. Each

septum contains one single sheet of capillary blood vessels, and is exposed
to air on both sides.

The dense network of the capillary blood vessels in an alveolar wall
of the frog is shown in Figure 1 (Maloney and Castle, 1969). A similar
picture of the cat's lung is shown in Figure 2, and a cross-sectional
view is shown in Figure 3. To characterize the geometry of such a network, we idealize the vascular space as a sheet of fluid flowing between
two membranes held apart by a number of more or less equally spaced

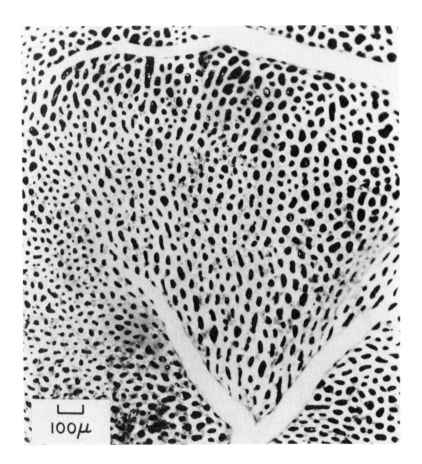

Figure 1. Photograph of a network of capillary blood vessels in the frog by Maloney
and Castle (1969). Reprinted by permission.

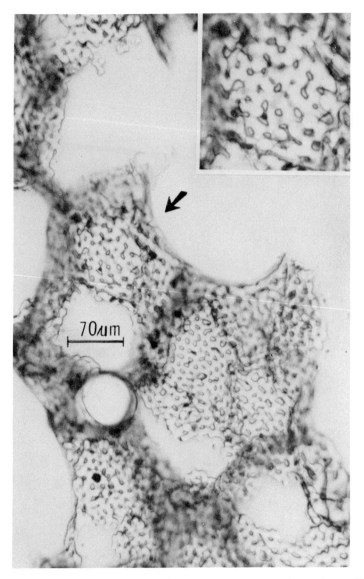

Figure 2. Cat lung. Flat view of interalveolar wall with the microvasculature filled with a silicone elastomer. This photomicrograph illustrates the tight mesh or network of the extensively filled capillary bed. The circular or elliptical enclosures are basement membrane stained with cresyl violet and are the nonvascular posts. Frozen section from gelatin-embedded tissue; glycerol-gelatin mount. The insert shows a detail from the region indicated by the arrow.

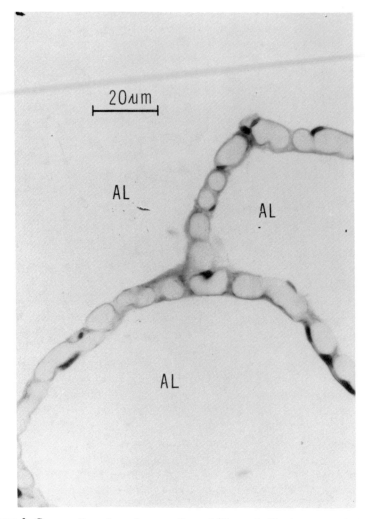

Figure 3. Cross section view of preparation of Figure 2. The intercept of three interalveolar walls and how each wall is shared by two alveoli are clearly shown. *AL*, alveolus.

"posts;" see Figure 4. In the plane view (A) this is a sheet with regularly arranged obstructions. The plane may be divided into a network of hexagons, with a circular post at the center of each hexagon. The "sheet-flow" model is therefore characterized by three parameters: L, the length of each side of the hexagon; h, the height or thickness of the sheet; ϵ, the diameter of the posts.

We shall define a "vascular-space—tissue ratio" (VSTR) as the ratio of the vascular lumen volume to a certain circumscribing volume defined below. As illustrated in Figure 4B, the circumscribing volume is that enclosed between surfaces T and B. The tissues (epithelial, interstitial, and endothelial) external to the surfaces T and B are excluded. Thus VSTR does not represent the volumetric fraction of the total interalveolar septum occupied by blood. For the sheet model, the VSTR is independent of the height h and is equal to the percentage of the area occupied by

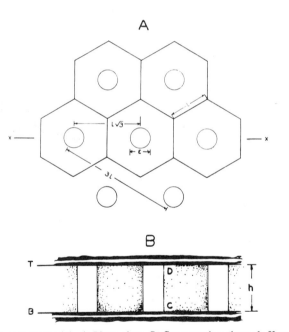

Figure 4. Sheet-flow model. *A*, Plane view. *B*, Cross section through X———X of *A*. The clear rectangular spaces are the nonvascular posts. The stippled areas indicate the flow channels. For bounding surfaces only, T, top and B, bottom. Sheet thickness, h. *C* and *D*, contact of posts with endothelial surface at T and B. From Sobin et al. (1970). Reprinted by permission.

blood in the plane cross section. From Figure 4A, we have

$$\text{The area of a hexagon} = \frac{3\sqrt{3}}{2} L^2$$

$$\text{The area of a circle} = \pi \frac{\epsilon^2}{4}$$

(1)

Hence for the sheet flow,

$$\text{VSTR} = 1 - \frac{\pi}{6\sqrt{3}} \frac{\epsilon^2}{L^2}$$

(2)

In actual practice, it is difficult to measure and evaluate L, ϵ, and h from microscopic preparations because of the random irregularities in the geometric appearance of the specimens. The VSTR, however, can be determined with greater confidence by planimetry and random sampling. The dimension of the obstructing posts (ϵ) can be calculated from Eq. 2 by determining the VSTR and measuring $3L$ as indicated in Figure 5A. Then

$$\frac{\epsilon}{L} = \sqrt{\frac{6\sqrt{3}}{\pi}(1 - \text{VSTR})}$$

(3)

The idea is illustrated in Figure 5. We choose an area that is large compared with the individual posts, and measure the area ratio of the vascular space and the circumscribing area, thus obtaining VSTR directly. ϵ/L is then calculated from Eq. 3. Let the measured average area of the posts be A_p, and that of the basic hexagon be A_s; then

$$L = \sqrt{\frac{2}{3\sqrt{3}} A_s}$$

(4a)

$$\epsilon = 2\sqrt{\frac{A_p}{\pi}}$$

(4b)

The interpost distance (the distance between post edges) is $L\sqrt{3} - \epsilon$, which is the smallest distance for free passage of the red cell in the plane of the alveolar wall.

The results for the cat lung are presented in Table 1. The VSTR for each individual lobe is not influenced by the blood pressure; the average value is 0.91. These data indicate that in the plane of the interalveolar wall, the capillary bed can occupy 91% of the area of the wall.

This high value of VSTR applies to the interalveolar septa. It does not apply to those alveoli which were noted by Miller (1947) to have capillary

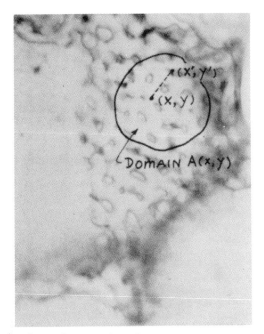

Figure 5. Domain of averaging around a point (x,y) in an alveolar sheet. From Fung and Sobin (1969). Reprinted by permission.

Table 1. Summary of data for elastomer-filled lungs of vertically positioned cats at transpulmonary pressure (alveolar–pleural pressures) of 10 cm H_2O (from Sobin et al. (1970))

Δp	VSTR (%)	Hexagon area (μ^2)	Post diameter (μ)	Interpost distance (μ)	No. fields analyzed
6.3	90.94 ± 1.94	239.51 ± 27.06	5.25 ± 0.83	10.21 ± 0.30	6
6.8	88.81 ± 2.10	275.34 ± 37.80	6.22 ± 0.66	10.34 ± 0.99	6
7.3	91.16 ± 1.50	256.53 ± 45.58	5.35 ± 0.80	10.60 ± 0.89	6
10.3	90.16 ± 1.84	202.08 ± 43.34	5.01 ± 0.82	9.15 ± 0.91	18
14.3	90.59 ± 2.12	193.25 ± 63.07	4.74 ± 1.02	8.99 ± 1.38	18
18.3	90.43 ± 2.64	203.54 ± 38.75	4.96 ± 1.11	9.24 ± 0.51	18

Values are means ± SD. Δp is the transmural pressure difference, i.e., vascular pressure minus alveolar air pressure; VSTR is vascular space–tissue ratio expressed in percent; hexogon area is planimetered sheet area divided by the number of posts in area; and interpost distance is the distance between posts edges.

beds with a "coarse" mesh, such as pleura, peribronchial, and perivascular septa, and those abutting connective tissues.

1.2 Elasticity of the Pulmonary Alveolar Sheet

As is common to most topics in science, the question of elasticity can be formulated in many different forms, varying in degree of generality and difficulty. For the blood flow problem the question of elasticity we are concerned with is this: When the pressure in the blood vessel is changed, how much does the blood volume change? In the sheet-flow model of the pulmonary alveoli, the problem is translated to the following: when the pressures of the blood and of the alveolar air change, (1) how does the thickness of the sheet change, and (2) how does the plane area of the sheet change? Note that the blood volume in an alveolar sheet is equal to

$$\text{thickness} \times \text{area} \times \text{VSTR},$$

where the VSTR is the vascular-space–tissue ratio discussed before. The morphometric data presented in Section 1.1 show that the VSTR remains constant when blood pressure changes. Hence the elasticity problem can be limited to the consideration of thickness and area.

It turns out that these questions have both a simple answer and a complicated answer. In simple terms, the thickness h varies with the pressure difference Δp (equal to the static pressure of blood minus the pressure of the alveolar air) as follows:

(1) $h = 0$ if Δp is negative, and smaller than $-\epsilon$, where ϵ is a small number about 1 cm H_2O.   (5a)

(2) $h = h_0 + \alpha \Delta p$, if Δp is positive and smaller than certain limiting value.   (5b)

(3) h tends to a limiting value h_∞ if Δp increases beyond the limiting value.   (5c)

(4) In the small range $-\epsilon < \Delta p < 0$, h increases from 0 to h_0. A rough approximation is $h = h_0 + (h_0/\epsilon)\,\Delta p$.   (5d)

Here α, h_0, h_∞, and ϵ are constants independent of Δp. The parameter h_0 is the sheet thickness at zero pressure difference when the pressure decreases from positive values. The parameter α is called the *compliance coefficient* of the pulmonary capillary bed. The thickness h is understood to be the mean value averaged over an area that is large compared with the posts, but small relative to the alveoli.

Also, in simple terms, the answer to the second question is that if A_0 represents the area of certain region on an alveolar septa when the static pressure of the blood is some physiologic value p_0, then the area of the same region A when blood pressure is changed to p is

$$A \doteq A_0 \tag{6}$$

In other words, the area is unaffected by the blood pressure.

The answers to our questions become more complex when we try to relate the constants h_0, α, h_∞, and A_0 to the airway pressure, the intrapleural pressure, the surfactants on the alveolar septa, the geometric parameters of the septa, the structure of the entire lung and the shape of the thoracic cage and the diaphragm, and whether a pathologic condition such as edema or emphysema exists. In order to unravel these relationships, we may take a two-pronged approach: we may study the problem theoretically and derive these relationships from the principles of mechanics, or we may lay out an extensive program of experiments in order to deduce empirical correlations among various parameters. It is easy to see that the required experimental program would be very large. For pragmatism one should take a combined approach: to deduce as much as possible from theoretic considerations, and to test as often as possible by experiments.

Figure 6 shows the experimental results for the cat's lung. It is seen that for positive Δp and in the linear range, the *compliance constant,* α, is quite large; $\alpha = 0.219 \ \mu m/cm \ H_2O$ when the transpulmonary pressure is 10 cm H_2O. The thickness as Δp tends to zero, h_0, is 4.28 μm. Other animals will have different h_0 and α. For the dog, we made an estimation of h_0 and α from the data of Glazier et al. (1969) and Permutt et al. (1969) and obtained the results of α equal to 0.122 $\mu m/cm \ H_2O$ at a transpulmonary pressure of 10 cm H_2O, and 0.079 $\mu m/cm \ H_2O$ at a transpulmonary pressure of 25 cm H_2O (see Fung and Sobin, 1972a and b). The lower bound of the linear range is $\Delta p = 0$. The upper bound of the linear range has not been determined. The thickness decreases rapidly; when Δp is smaller than $-\epsilon$, the thickness is practically zero.

A theoretic analysis of the sheet elasticity compliance α as a function of geometric parameters is presented by Fung and Sobin (1972a).

1.3 Apparent Viscosity of Blood in Pulmonary Alveoli

If a Newtonian fluid flows through an alveolar sheet, it encounters certain resistence. The pressure–flow relationship is influenced by the geometric parameters of the sheet. With dimensional analysis it can be shown that

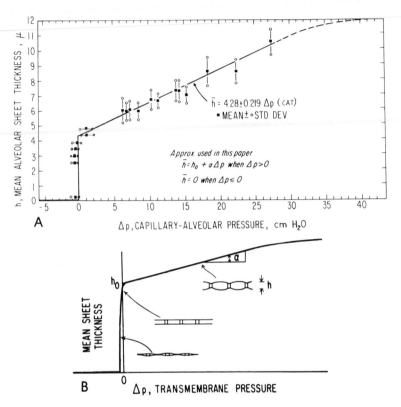

Figure 6. *A*, Sheet thickness–pressure relationship. Equations 5a–5d approximate this curve by a discontinuous curve that is composed of three line segments: a horizontal line $h = 0$ for Δp negative, which jumps to $h = h_0$ at Δp slightly greater than 0, then continues as a straight line for positive Δp until some upper limit is reached, beyond which it bends down and tends to a constant thickness. *B*, The elastic deformation of the alveolar sheet is sketched for three conditions: $\Delta p < 0$, $\Delta p = 0$, and $\Delta p > 0$. The relaxed thickness h_0 of the sheet is equal to the relaxed length of the posts. Under a positive internal (transmural) pressure, the thickness of the sheet increases; the posts are lengthened; the membranes deflect from the planes connecting the ends of the posts; and the mean thickness becomes $\bar{h}$.

the pressure gradient in an alveolar sheet at small Reynolds number can be presented in the form

$$\text{grad } p = -\frac{\mu U}{h^2} k(\frac{w}{h}) f(S, \frac{h}{\epsilon}, \frac{\epsilon}{a}, \theta, N_R, \ldots) \tag{7}$$

where p is pressure, μ is the apparent coefficient of viscosity, U is the mean velocity of flow, h is the sheet thickness, k is a dimensionless function of the ratio of the width of the sheet, w, to the sheet thickness, and f is the so-called geometric friction factor, which is a dimensionless number defined by the VSTR (here written as S), the thickness-to-postal-diameter ratio h/ϵ, the cell orientation, θ, the Reynolds number $N_R = \rho U h/\mu$, and whatever other dimensionless parameters define the configuration of the flow. The function k is well known (see, for example, Purday, 1949). When $h/w < 0.2$, it is given by the equation

$$k = 12/(1 - 0.63\frac{h}{w})$$ (8)

Hence for all practical purposes k can be replaced by 12. The function f has been analyzed by Lee (1969) and confirmed by Yen and Fung (1973).

But blood is not a Newtonian fluid. It is entirely possible that because of the particulate nature of the suspension and the narrowness of the vessel, the pressure–flow relationship becomes nonlinear and the Newtonian fluid results have no application whatsoever. The quickest way to decide this is to make a model experiment in which both kinematic and dynamic similarities are maintained. Yen and Fung (1973) made such a model and it is fortunate that the pressure–flow relationship was found to be linear in the ranges of parameters of interest to normal physiology. (Figure 7).

Therefore it is possible to reduce the experimental data according to Eq. 7. In other words, we measure grad p, U, h, k, f and compute a value of μ according to Eq. 7. This value is defined as the *apparent viscosity* of blood in a pulmonary alveolar sheet.

The ratio of the apparent viscosity of blood to that of the plasma is defined as the *relative viscosity*. Both the apparent viscosity and the relative viscosity must be defined for a specific system, and cannot be used for other systems. For example, the apparent viscosity of blood in a pulmonary alveolar sheet is different from that in a circular cylindrical tube. In the latter case, we use the Hagen–Poiseuille formula

$$\frac{\Delta p}{\Delta L} = \frac{8\mu}{\pi a^4}\dot{Q}$$ (9)

to compute the apparent viscosity μ, where Δp is the pressure drop in a length ΔL, a is the radius of the tube, and $\dot{Q}$ is the volume rate of flow.

Yen and Fung's (1973) results are shown in Figure 8, in which the mean values of the relative viscosity are plotted against the hematocrit, H.

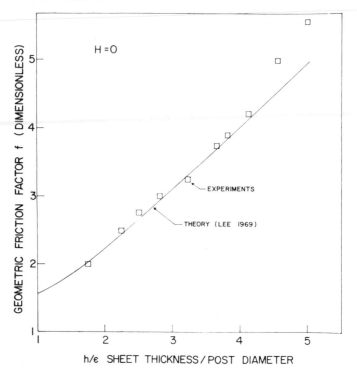

Figure 7. Comparison of theoretical and experimental "geometric friction factor." From Yen and Fung (1973). Reprinted by permission.

The regression line may be represented by the equation

$$\mu_{\text{relative}} = 1 + a\,H + b\,H^2 \tag{10}$$

Applying this result to blood, we have

$$\mu_{\text{blood in alv}} = \mu_{\text{plasma}}(1 + a\,H + b\,H^2) \tag{11}$$

Since we have accounted for the geometric factors k and f for pulmonary alveoli, the apparent viscosity of plasma (when it alone is used as a perfusing fluid) is the same as the coefficient of viscosity of the plasma as a homogeneous fluid measured in a conventional viscometer. The values of the constants a and b in Eq. 10 are listed in Figure 8.

In principle, the parameters a and b are functions of those dimensionless parameters that define the effect of red cells on the flow characteristics of the blood. The task of determining these functions relative to

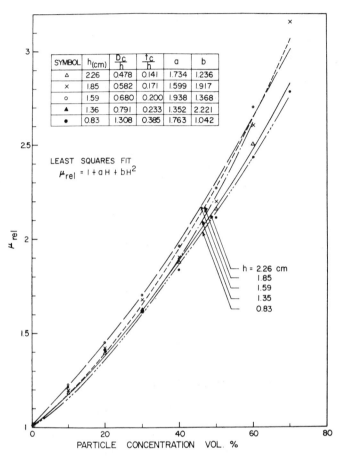

Figure 8. Plot of relative viscosity versus particle concentration. From Yen and Fung (1973). Reprinted by permission.

all the variables will be an exceedingly difficult and extensive one. What is offered above is merely a simplified view with most of the variables fixed. The most severe failing in our simulation is that our pellets are too rigid compared with the red blood cells. Future improvements are desired in this respect.

1.4 "Sluicing" or "Waterfall" Phenomenon

"Sluicing" or "waterfall" phenomenon refers to a condition of flow in a collapsible tube in such a manner that the volume flow rate is independent of the downstream condition, just as the flow over a waterfall does not depend on how high the waterfall is. This condition occurs when the pressure outside the tube is lower than the pressure of the fluid at the entry into the tube, but higher than the pressure at the exit. A tube like this was first used by Starling in his heart–lung machine in 1915, and is known as a Starling resistor, or a Starling mechanism. We experimented on the Starling mechanism because it was considered by Permutt and his associates to be a principal feature of the pulmonary alveolar blood flow, particularly in West's zone II, in which the blood pressure in the pulmonary artery is higher than the alveolar air pressure, whereas that in the pulmonary vein is lower than the air pressure. We show theoretically that the character of the flow depends on the Reynolds number. When the Reynolds number is large, the flow in an elastic vessel is governed by a wave equation. When the Reynolds number is small, it is governed by a diffusion equation. In the pulmonary alveolar septa the Reynolds number is very small, in the range of 10^{-2} to 10^{-4}. Theoretically, the flow at such a small Reynolds number is stable. This is verified by a model experiment. We show that whereas the model flutters at a large Reynolds number, it does not flutter when the Reynolds number is small. The Starling mechanism operates statically, which provides a great simplification to further analysis. Details are given in Fung and Sobin (1972b).

2 FORMULATION OF THE ANALYTICAL PROBLEMS

2.1 "Local Mean Flow" and "Local Mean Disturbances"

To analyze the blood flow in an alveolar sheet, we introduce first the concept of local mean velocity of flow. The detailed flow field is, of course, very complicated when the disturbances of individual posts, red cells, membrane deflections, and other phenomena are considered. Therefore mathematically it is expedient to separate the flow field into two parts: a local mean flow and local disturbances. It is expected that the local mean flow field will be relatively smooth and can be determined from the boundary conditions. The present chapter is concerned with the local mean flow. When the mean flow field is known, the local disturbances can be computed separately in a much simplified manner.

To be precise, we now define the local mean flow and the perturbations. Let us first define a Cartesian frame of reference x, y, z. We take the origin at a point on the midplane of the sheet, x, y axes in the sheet, and z

axis perpendicular to the sheet. At a point x,y,z the velocity vector has three components $u(x,y,z)$, $v(x,y,z)$, $w(x,y,z)$ in the directions of the coordinate axes. We break u,v,w into two parts, and write

$$u(x,y,z) = U(x,y) + u'(x,y,z)$$

$$v(x,y,z) = V(x,y) + v'(x,y,z) \qquad (12)$$

$$w(x,y,z) = W(x,y) + w'(x,y,z)$$

where $U(x,y)$, $V(x,y)$, $W(x,y)$ are functions of x,y alone. We call $U(x,y)$, $V(x,y)$ the local mean velocity if they represent the average value of $u(x,y,z)$, $v(x,y,z)$ over a small volume around $(x,y,0)$; i.e., if

$$U(x,y) = \frac{1}{Ah} \iint_{A(x,y)} dx'dy' \int_{-h/2}^{h/2} u(x',y',z)\, dz \qquad (13)$$

$$V(x,y) = \frac{1}{Ah} \iint_{A(x,y)} dx'dy' \int_{h/2}^{h/2} v(x',y',z)\, dz \qquad (14)$$

The mean velocity $W(x,y)$, defined by a similar equation, vanishes when the area A is chosen large enough. In these equations, h is the thickness of the sheet, $A(x,y)$ is a domain of integration containing the point (x,y), and A is the area of $A(xy,y)$ as illustrated in Figure 5. The points (x',y') lie in the area A. The domain A is chosen to be large enough that it contains a number of posts and red cells so that the velocities U and V represent the smoothed-out velocity field, and yet small enough that the variation of U, V over the entire alveolar sheet still reflects the significant features of the flow field. In practical calculations an area containing, say, 10 posts would be satisfactory for such a local averaging.

The velocity components $u'(x,y,z)$, $v'(x,y,z)$, $w'(x,y,z)$ in Eq. 13 are called the local perturbations. According to Eq. 14 the mean values of the local perturbations $u'(x,y,z)$, $v'(x,y,z)$ are zero.

The local mean pressure and the mean sheet thickness can be defined in a similar manner.

In the development of our theory, the first basic relation we seek is that relating the local mean pressure $\bar{p}(x,y)$ to the velocities $U(x,y)$, $V(x,y)$. This can be derived from the basic equations of hydrodynamics, or alternatively by model testing with the help of dimensional analysis. As it is shown in Section 1.3, the arguments of dimension analysis lead to the general form Eq. 7 or

$$\frac{\partial \bar{p}}{\partial x} = -\frac{\mu U}{h^2} k\, f_x\left(\frac{h}{a}, S, \ldots\right)$$

$$\frac{\partial \bar{p}}{\partial y} = -\frac{\mu V}{h^2} k\, f_y\left(\frac{h}{a}, S, \ldots\right)$$

(15)

In this equation, μ is the apparent viscosity of blood, h is the sheet thickness, and the numerical factors k, f_x, f_y are functions of L/h, h/z, S, etc., which depend on the detailed geometry of the alveolar sheet, the number, size and shape of the posts, the red cells, the hematocrit, etc. k is equal to 12 in practical cases, and f lies in the range 2–3.

The second basic relation we need is one that describes the conservation of mass. Consider a small rectangular element of the alveolar sheet (see Figure 9). Blood enters the left-hand side and leaves the right-hand side. In a time interval dt the mass entering the left-hand side is equal to the product of the density, velocity, area, and dt. The velocity is U and the area is $h \cdot dy$, h being the thickness of the sheet and dy the length of the edge. The density is ρ. Hence

$$\text{mass inflow at left} = \rho h U\, dy\, dt$$

On the right-hand side, the density, thickness, and velocity differ from those on the left-hand side by the amount

$$\Delta(\rho h U) = \frac{\partial(\rho h U)}{\partial x} dx$$

(16)

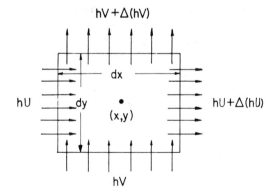

Figure 9. A rectangular element of the sheet showing the balance of the flow. From Fung and Sobin (1969). Reprinted by permission.

Hence the mass outflow on the right in the same interval is

$$\left[\rho h U + \frac{\partial(\rho h U)}{\partial x}\, dx\right] dy\, dt$$

Similarly, the mass inflow at the bottom edge is $\rho h V\, dx\, dt$, and the outflow at the top is

$$\left[\rho h V + \frac{\partial(\rho h V)}{\partial y}\, dy\right] dx\, dt$$

Summing up all the inflow and outflow, we have

net mass outflow = $\left[\rho h U + \dfrac{\partial(\rho h U)}{\partial x}\, dx\right] dy\, dt - \rho h U\, dy\, dt$

Hence

$\quad + \left[\rho h V + \dfrac{\partial(\rho h V)}{\partial y}\, dy\right] dx\, dt - \rho h V\, dx\, dt$

net mass outflow = $\left[\dfrac{\partial(\rho h U)}{\partial x} + \dfrac{\partial(\rho h V)}{\partial y}\right] dx\, dy\, dt$ $\qquad$ (17)

By the law of conservation of mass, this net mass outflow must be equal to the net decrease of the mass of the element. For a *steady flow* there can be no change in the mass of the element; hence we must have

$$\frac{\partial(\rho h U)}{\partial x} + \frac{\partial(\rho h V)}{\partial y} = 0 \qquad (18)$$

If the sheet thickness h is variable, then the equation of continuity (Eq. 18) combined with the constitutive equation (Eq. 15) yields the following equation:

$$\frac{\partial}{\partial x}\left(\frac{h^3}{k f_x}\frac{\partial \bar{p}}{\partial x}\right) + \frac{\partial}{\partial y}\left(\frac{h^3}{k f_y}\frac{\partial \bar{p}}{\partial y}\right) = 0 \qquad (19)$$

Now $\bar{p}$ is related to h by Eqs. 5a–5d. Using Eq. 5b or 5d, we obtain

$$\frac{\partial}{\partial x}\left(\frac{h^3}{k f_x}\frac{\partial h}{\partial x}\right) + \frac{\partial}{\partial y}\left(\frac{h^3}{k f_y}\frac{\partial h}{\partial y}\right) = 0 \qquad (20)$$

If we ignore the spatial variation of k and f, and assume $f_x = f_y$ for practical purposes, we obtain

$$\frac{\partial}{\partial x}\left(h^3\frac{\partial h}{\partial x}\right) + \frac{\partial}{\partial y}\left(h^3\frac{\partial h}{\partial y}\right) = 0 \qquad (21)$$

or

$$\left(\frac{\partial^2}{\partial x^2} + \frac{\partial^2}{\partial y^2}\right) h^4 = 0 \qquad (22)$$

Thus the fourth power of h is governed by a harmonic equation. Expressed in terms of pressure, we have, on defining

$$\Phi = h^4 = [h_0 + \alpha(\bar{p} - p_A)]^4, \qquad (23)$$

the result

$$\left(\frac{\partial^2}{\partial x^2} + \frac{\partial^2}{\partial y^2}\right) \Phi = 0 \qquad (24)$$

This completes the mathematical formulation for the steady-state case of sheets with impermeable wall.

2.2 Generalization to Nonstationary Case and Permeable Vessel

For a nonstationary flow and in the case where fluid movement in or out of the endothelium of the capillary blood vessel takes place, the equation of continuity (Eq. 18) must be modified. This modification can be obtained by considering the balance of inflow and outflow in a control volume that consists of the sides x = const., x = const. + dx, y = const., y = const. + dy, and the membranes $z = \pm h/2$. The mass transfer from the sides is expressed by the equation

$$\text{net mass outflow} = \left[\frac{\partial(\rho \bar{h} \bar{U})}{\partial x} + \frac{\partial(\rho \bar{h} \bar{V})}{\partial y}\right] dx \, dy \, dt \qquad (25)$$

This must be balanced by changes that take place in the membranes at the top and bottom—changes due to (a) the transient change in thickness $\bar{h}$, and (b) the filtration across the blood–tissue barrier. The rate of increase of thickness is $\partial \bar{h}/\partial t$, which induces, in a time interval dt, an increase of control volume equal to $(\partial \bar{h}/\partial t)dt \, dx \, dy$. The mass transfer across the blood–tissue barrier may be assumed to obey Starling's hypothesis[1] $\dot{m} = K_p(\Delta p - \sigma \Delta \pi)$, where $\dot{m}$ is the rate of mass transfer per unit time per unit

---

[1] This is a linear phenomenologic law for mass transport across a membrane. A general discussion of equations of this type from the point of view of irreversible thermodynamics is given by Katchalsky and Curran (1965). The general idea of fluid transport across blood vessels embodied in this formula (though not in this form) was first presented by Starling (1896).

area, K_p is the filtration coefficient, Δp is the difference in hydrostatic pressure on the sides of the barrier, $\Delta \pi$ is the corresponding difference in osmotic pressure, and σ is the reflection coefficient. Since our attention is focused on the flow of blood, we may write

$$\dot{m} = K_p(\bar{p} - p^*),\tag{26}$$

where $\bar{p}$ refers to the local mean pressure in the blood, and

$$p^* = \sigma \Delta \pi + \text{pressure in tissue space}\tag{27}$$

Summing up both contributions and noting that by the law of conservation of mass what leaves the sides of control volume must enter the top and bottom faces, we obtain

$$\left[\frac{\partial(\rho \bar{h} \bar{U})}{\partial x}\right] + \left[\frac{\partial(\rho \bar{h} \bar{V})}{\partial y}\right] = -\rho\left(\frac{\partial h}{\partial t}\right) - 2K_p(\bar{p} - p^*)\tag{28}$$

The factor 2 in the last term is added because the capillary wall area is about twice the area of the sheet. Eliminating $\bar{U}$, $\bar{V}$ from Eqs. 28 and 15, we obtain

$$\frac{\rho}{\mu}\left[\frac{\partial}{\partial x}\left(\frac{\bar{h}^3}{kf_x}\frac{\partial \bar{p}}{\partial x}\right) + \frac{\partial}{\partial y}\left(\frac{\bar{h}^3}{kf_y}\frac{\partial \bar{p}}{\partial y}\right)\right] = \rho\left(\frac{\partial \bar{h}}{\partial t}\right) + 2K_p(\bar{p} - p^*)\tag{29}$$

To complete the analysis we again use the equation that describes the elasticity of the alveolar sheet in the physiologic range when $\bar{p} - p_{\text{alv}}$ is positive:

$$\bar{h} = h_0 + \alpha(\bar{p} - p_{\text{alv}})\tag{5b}$$

Accordingly, we obtain the following basic equation when blood flow exists:

$$\frac{\partial}{\partial x}\left(\frac{\bar{h}^3}{kf_x}\frac{\partial \bar{h}}{\partial x}\right) + \frac{\partial}{\partial y}\left(\frac{\bar{h}^3}{kf_y}\frac{\partial \bar{h}}{\partial y}\right) = \mu\alpha\left[\frac{\partial \bar{h}}{\partial t} + \frac{2}{\rho}K_p\left(\frac{\bar{h} - h_0}{\alpha} - p^* + p_{\text{alv}}\right)\right]\tag{30}$$

This is a nonlinear "diffusion" equation, basically different from the usual "wave" equation that describes pulsatile flow in large arteries. The impedance characteristics of the capillaries are therefore different from those of the arteries.

In general, we may use the approximation $f_x = f_y = f$. If the variation of $\bar{h}$ is not too large, we may regard k and f as constant and simplify Eq. 30 to

$$\left(\frac{\partial^2}{\partial x^2} + \frac{\partial^2}{\partial y^2}\right)\bar{h}^4 = 4\,\mu k f \alpha\left[\frac{\partial \bar{h}}{\partial t} + \frac{2K_p}{\rho \alpha}(\bar{h} - h^*)\right], \qquad (31)$$

where

$$h^* = h_0 + \alpha(p^* - p_{\text{alv}}) \qquad (32)$$

Solutions of these equations are considered in the next section.

3 THEORETIC PREDICTIONS AND COMPARISON WITH RESULTS OF PHYSIOLOGIC EXPERIMENTS

The sheet-flow equation contains a great deal of information that can be revealed through solutions with various boundary conditions. This equation is nonlinear. But the nonlinearity is a special kind, through the fourth power of h which is operated on by the Laplace operator. We illustrate the features of the solution for the simplest problem in Section 3.1, which deals with the steady-state flow in a "one-dimensional" sheet. In Section 3.2 we demonstrate the same for a somewhat more general situation: the "two-dimensional" case. In subsequent sections we discuss more realistic problems that can be tested in the laboratory.

3.1 An Elementary Analog of the Theory

The nature of the solution can be brought out easily if we use a one-dimensional analog. Consider two uniform, parallel, horizontal, elastic strings as shown in Figure 10. At finite intervals these strings are tied by vertical cross members. If we pull on the horizontal strings with a tension T, the strings are stretched uniformly, and the ratio of the lengths of segments bc and ac remains a constant. This ratio is an analog of VSTR: the segments ab and cd are analogs of the posts, and bc and de are the analog of the alveolar–capillary membrane.

On the other hand, if the post segments were replaced by springs of different compliance than the strings, then the VSTR (bc/ac) would change with the tension T (Figure 10B). The constancy of VSTR observed in the pulmonary alveolar sheets of the cat suggests that the elasticity of the postal region (segments ab, cd, etc.) is represented by the analog shown in Figure 10A.

Let the strings be loaded by an internal vertical loading of Δp per unit

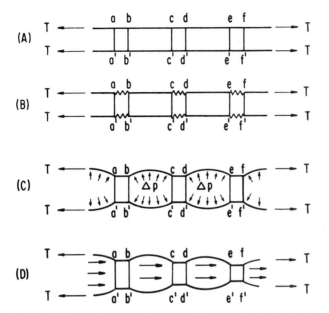

Figure 10. Simplified one-dimensional analog of the alveolar sheet. *A*, Stretching of the membrane. *B*, Stretching of the post. *C*, Deflection under internal pressure. *D*, Deflection due to variable internal pressure when blood flows in the channel. From Fung and Sobin (1972). Reprinted by permission.

length, as shown in Figure 10C. The equilibrium of the string requires that

$$T \times \text{curvature of string} = \Delta p$$

If the tension remains constant and the deflection is small, then the vertical deflection of the string is proportional to Δp.

The change of the average distance between the strings (analog of the sheet thickness) is given by the sum of the distention of the posts aa', bb', etc. and the average deflection of the strings.

Now consider flow in a channel of unit width represented by Figure 10D (replace the strings by channel walls). Let the average speed of flow be U, the volume flow rate per unit width be Q, the local thickness be h, and the pressure be p. Then

$$U = -\frac{h^2}{8\mu} \frac{dp}{dx} \tag{33}$$

$$Q = hU \tag{34}$$

In the range of p in which $h = h_0 + \alpha p$, we have

$$\frac{dh}{dx} = \alpha \frac{dp}{dx} \tag{35}$$

Hence

$$Q = -\frac{h^3}{8\mu\alpha}\frac{dh}{dx} = -\frac{1}{32\mu\alpha}\frac{dh^4}{dx} \tag{36}$$

For a steady flow Q is a constant. Differentiating Eq. 36 with respect to x, we obtain, because $dQ/dx = 0$, the differential equation

$$\frac{d^2 h^4}{dx^2} = 0 , \tag{37}$$

which is a special case of the sheet-flow equation (Eq. 22). This differential equation is easily integrated. The general solution is

$$h^4 = c_1 x + c_2 \tag{38}$$

where c_1, c_2 are arbitrary constants. To determine c_1, c_2, we notice the boundary conditions

(a) at the "arteriole," $x = 0$, the thickness of the "sheet" is h_a.

(b) at the "venule," $x = L$, the thickness of the "sheet" is h_v.

Hence

$$h_a^4 = c_2, \qquad h_v^4 = c_1 L + h_a^4 \tag{39}$$

Solving for c_1, c_2 and substituting into Eq. 38, we obtain

$$h^4 = h_a^4 - (h_a^4 - h_v^4) \, x/L \tag{40a}$$

or

$$h = [h_a^4 - (h_a^4 - h_v^4) \, x/L]^{1/4} \tag{40b}$$

This is the full solution. For various combinations of h_a and h_v the distribution of the thickness h is shown in Figure 11. It is seen that the exponent $\frac{1}{4}$ makes h rather flat near the arteriole, and constricts rather rapidly toward the venule if h_v is small.

We can obtain the flow Q from Eq. 36. If the channel length is L, then

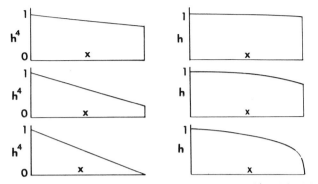

Figure 11. Plot of Eqs. 40a and 40b showing the variation of h^4 and h with x. With an appropriate choice of units, we assume that the thickness h_a is 1. $h_v{}^4$ at $x = L$ is assumed to be 0.75, 0.25, and 0 for the three cases shown in the figure. The corresponding values of h_v are 0.931, 0.707, and 0, respectively.

the mean flow in the whole channel is

$$\frac{1}{L}\int_0^L Q\, dx = \frac{1}{32\mu\alpha L}\,[h^4(0) - h^4(L)] \tag{41}$$

For a one-dimensional channel flow the conservation of mass requires that Q be constant. Hence the left-hand side of Eq. 41 is exactly Q. In this case, we can also integrate Eq. 36 to obtain

$$h^4 = -32\mu\alpha Qx + \text{constant}$$

But $h = h_a$ when $x = 0$. Hence the constant equations h_a^4, and we have the channel thickness distribution:

$$h(x) = (h_a^4 - 32\mu\alpha Qx)^{1/4}$$

which is, of course, equivalent to Eq. 40b. When $x = L$, the thickness h becomes h_v, and we obtain the exact result

$$Q = \frac{h_a^4 - h_v^4}{32\mu\alpha L} \tag{42}$$

The last equation is a remarkable result. It shows that the flow depends on the difference of the fourth power of the sheet thickness at the arteriole from the fourth power of the sheet thickness at the venule. Thus if h_v is considerably smaller than h_a, its influence on the volume flow rate would be small. This is exhibited in Figure 12, in which we have plotted the dimensionless volume flow rate

$$q = \frac{32\mu\alpha L}{h_a^4} \dot{Q} \tag{43a}$$

against the ratio h_v/h_a. From Eqs. 42 and 43a we have, obviously,

$$q = 1 - \left(\frac{h_v}{h_a}\right)^4 \tag{43b}$$

It is seen clearly that q is significantly reduced by h_v only if h_v approaches h_a. If h_v is less than one-half of h_a, q differs from 1 by less than 6%; hence the flow is controlled essentially by h_a, the sheet thickness at the arteriole.

The Exit Conditions   The formulas above are derived in the range of applicability of Eq. 5b, in which $h = h_0 + \alpha p$. Therefore, the smallest permissible value of h_v is h_0. If, however, p is allowed to become negative, then h can become smaller. In the range $-\epsilon < p < 0$, we may use Eq. 5d, so that

$$h = h_0 + (h_0/\epsilon)p \tag{44a}$$

Then Eq. 36 becomes

$$Q = -\frac{\epsilon}{32\mu h_0} \frac{d}{dx} h^4, \tag{44b}$$

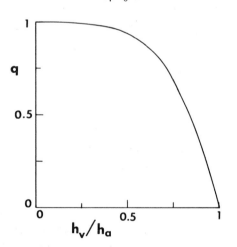

Figure 12. The variation of the volume flow rate with the thickness ratio h_v/h_a. q is dimensionless, defined by Eq. 43a. h_v and h_a are sheet thickness at the venule and arteriole, respectively.

whereas Eq. 37 remains valid. The solution in the range $-\epsilon < p < 0$ is the same Eq. 38. Now consider the following case with boundary conditions:

$$\text{at } x = 0: \qquad h = h_a,$$

$$\text{at } x = L_1: \qquad h = h_0,$$

$$\text{at } x = L_1 + \Delta L: \quad h = 0 \tag{45a}$$

Then the solution is

$$\text{for } 0 \leqslant x \leqslant L_1: \qquad h = [h_a^4 - (h_a^4 - h_0^4)x/L]^{1/4} ,$$

$$\text{for } L_1 \leqslant x \leqslant L_1 + \Delta L: \ h = h_0(1 - \frac{\xi}{\Delta L})^{1/4}, \quad \text{where } \xi = x - L_1 \tag{45b}$$

The volume flow per unit width Q is

$$Q = \frac{1}{32\mu\alpha L_1}(h_a^4 - h_0^4) = \frac{\epsilon}{32\mu h_0 \Delta L} h_0^4$$

If we define a new path length L so that

$$Q = \frac{1}{32\mu\alpha L}h_a^4 , \tag{46}$$

we see that

$$L = L_1 \left(1 + \frac{h_0^4}{h_a^4 - h_0^4}\right) \tag{47}$$

Thus, if the thickness at the arteriole, h_a, is sufficiently larger than h_0 (for example, when $h_a = 2h_0$), then L is approximately equal to L_1.

Equation 46 represents the largest flow possible from a given arteriolar pressure p_a (remember that $h_a = h_0 + \alpha p_a$). It is obtained by continuously lowering the exit pressure p_v until it becomes $-\epsilon$, at which valve $h \to 0$. The thickness h tends to zero like a cusp as shown in Eq. 45b. Further discussion on this matter is given in Section 3.3.

3.2 General Features of Sheet Flow. Examples of Rapid Variation of Sheet Thickness at the Venule, and Nearly Uniform Hydrostatic Pressure near the Arteriole

In the more general case, the nature of the solution may be illustrated by an idealized example as shown in Figure 13. In Fig. 13A we have a sheet of alveolar wall opened to an arteriole and a venule at regularly spaced intervals. The pattern is periodic and three segments are shown in the

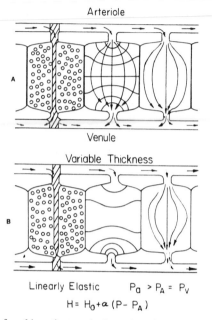

Arteriole

Venule

Variable Thickness

Linearly Elastic $P_a > P_A = P_V$

$H = H_0 + \alpha (P - P_A)$

Figure 13. A type of problem that can be investigated theoretically. With given sheet dimensions and boundary conditions, the variation of the average sheet thickness, velocity distribution, and pressure distribution can be computed. Figure shows streamlines and pressure contours. From Fung and Sobin (1969). Reprinted by permission.

figure. At the left are shown a plan view and a vertical cross section. The thickness of the sheet is assumed to be constant. At the right are shown the streamlines, i.e., the lines tangential to the velocity vectors. In the center are shown the lines of constant blood pressure. These contours of equipressure lines are drawn at intervals of constant pressure drop. The pressure at the horizontal line in the middle is halfway between the arteriole pressure and venule pressure. Other equipressure lines are orthogonal to the streamlines. The pressure gradient is inversely proportional to the distance between the equipressure lines. The velocity of flow is inversely proportional to the spacing between streamlines. These contours thus show the velocity and pressure distribution in the alveolar walls.

In Figure 13B we consider a different situation. We relax the assumption that the alveolar wall is rigid and assume instead that the sheet thickness varies linearly with the difference between the blood pressure and the air pressure in the alveolar space. In this case the pressure and velocity distributions are significantly modified. Figure 13B is drawn for the case in which the arteriole pressure is greater than the airway pressure, but the venule pressure is equal to the airway pressure. In the left panel the sheet thickness is seen to contract rapidly in the neighborhood of the venule. In the middle panel the equipressure contours are seen to crowd toward the venule. The pressure in the sheet is much more uniform than that in Figure 13A except in the neighborhood of the venule, where rapid pressure drop occurs. The streamlines shown in the figure on the right show a similar increase in the velocity near the drain into the venule.

The detailed information on velocity and pressure distribution has important bearings on pulmonary physiology. The velocity distribution is relevant to the blood transit time in alveoli and oxygenation of the red cells. The pressure distribution is important to the question of fluid transport across the alveolar wall and hence is relevant to the question of edema and homeostasis. The thickness distribution is directly related to the flow resistance, and to the regional stratification of blood flow in the lung.

The mathematical details of the solution are given in Fung and Sobin (1969).

3.3 Pressure–Flow Relationship

We have derived a nonlinear pressure–flow relationship in the very simple case of one-dimensional flow in Section 3.1. We have shown by the examples given in Section 3.2 that the features of two-dimensional sheets are quite similar to the one-dimensional case. By integrating the equation of motion along the streamlines over the entire field, we now derive an expression for the average flow over a sheet in the general, two-dimensional case.

We have shown (Eq. 7) that the mean flow velocity in a pulmonary alveolar sheet is

$$U = -\frac{1}{\mu k f} \, \bar{h}^2 \, \text{grad} \, \Delta p \qquad (48)$$

Here Δp stands for the transmural pressure, $\bar{p} - p_{\text{alv}}$, μ is the coefficient of viscosity of the blood, k and f are numerical factors that depend on the details of the sheet structure and red cell characteristics, $\bar{h}$ is the local mean thickness, and the symbol "grad" stands for the gradient operator. The flow per unit width is therefore

$$\dot{Q} = \bar{h}U = -\frac{1}{\mu kf} \bar{h}^3 \, \text{grad} \, \Delta p \tag{49}$$

Applying this to a streamline, using Eq. 5b, which holds in the linear range of elasticity, and integrating from the arteriole to the venule, we obtain, with ds representing length along the streamline,

$$\int \dot{Q} \, ds = -\int \frac{1}{\mu kf} \, [h_0 + \alpha \Delta p]^3 \, \frac{d\Delta p}{ds} \, ds \tag{50}$$

Let $L = \int ds$ be the length of the streamline; then assuming μkf to be constant, we obtain the average flow per unit width along a streamline,

$$\dot{Q}_{\text{avg}} = \frac{1}{4\mu kfL\alpha} \left[(h_0 + \alpha \Delta p_{\text{art}})^4 - (h_0 + \alpha \Delta p_{\text{ven}})^4 \right] \tag{51}$$

Here the subscripts "art" and "ven" refer to arteriole and venule, respectively.

Equation 51 shows that the average velocity of blood flow along a streamline connecting an arteriole and a venule is inversely proportional to the length of the streamline and the viscosity of the blood. This feature is common to all blood vessels. But the dependence of the blood flow on pressure is quite unique in the pulmonary alveoli as compared with that in a rigid tube. Thus, instead of following Poiseuille's law, according to which Q_{avg} is directly proportional to the pressure drop ($p_{\text{art}} - p_{\text{ven}}$), we see that in the pulmonary capillaries

$$\dot{Q}_{\text{avg}} = \frac{.1}{4\mu kfL} (p_{\text{art}} - p_{\text{ven}}) \left[(h_0 + \alpha \Delta p_{\text{art}})^3 + (h_0 + \alpha \Delta p_{\text{art}})^2 (h_0 + \alpha \Delta p_{\text{ven}}) \right.$$
$$\left. + (h_0 + \alpha \Delta p_{\text{art}}) (h_0 + \alpha p_{\text{ven}})^2 + (h_0 + \alpha \Delta p_{\text{ven}})^3 \right] \tag{52}$$

The factor in the brackets is the *conductance* of the flow and depends on the blood pressure.

Because a field of flow can be wholly covered by streamlines, we can sum up all the streamlines between an arteriole and a venule to obtain the flow between these two vessels. Let A be the area of alveolar sheet in question and S be the vascular-space–tissue ratio; then the total vascular space is SA, and the total flow is

$$\frac{SA\dot{Q}_{ave}}{\bar{L}} = \frac{SA}{4\mu k f \bar{L}^2 \alpha} \left[(h_0 + \alpha\Delta p_{art})^4 - (h_0 + \alpha\Delta p_{ven})^4 \right] \quad (53)$$

Expressed in terms of sheet thickness, this is

$$\text{Flow} = \frac{1}{C} \left[h_a^4 - h_v^4 \right], \quad (54)$$

where $\bar{L}$ is the average length of the streamlines in this field, and

$$C = \frac{4\mu k f \bar{L}^2 \alpha}{SA} \quad (55)$$

$$h_a = h_0 + \alpha\Delta p_{art}, \quad h_v = h_0 + \alpha\Delta p_{ven}, \quad (56a)$$

$$\Delta p_{art} = p_{art} - p_{alv}, \quad \Delta p_{ven} = p_{ven} - p_{alv}. \quad (56b)$$

We may compute $\bar{L}$ by associating each streamline with a specific value of the stream function, ψ, and compute

$$\frac{1}{\bar{L}} = \frac{1}{\psi_2 - \psi_1} \int_{\psi_2}^{\psi_1} \frac{1}{L(\psi)} d\psi, \quad (57)$$

where ψ_1 and ψ_2 are the dividing streamlines that enclose the whole field of flow between the arteriole and venule in question.

Equation 53 provides an explicit formula of blood flow in the pulmonary alveoli as related to the blood rheology (through μ), alveolar area (A), alveolar structural geometry (through k, f, which depend on a, c, etc.), the vascular-space—tissue ratio (S), the arteriole and venule transmural pressures (p_{art}, p_{ven}), the average length of streamlines between an arteriole and a venule ($\bar{L}$), the compliance of the alveolar sheet with respect to blood pressure (α), and indirectly, through α, to the tension of the alveolar septa (T, which is the sum of tissue stress and surface tension).

If we write Eq. 53 in the form

$$p_{art} - p_{ven} = R \cdot (\text{Flow}), \quad (58)$$

then R can be called the *resistance* of the capillary blood vessels. If both Δp_{art} and Δp_{ven} are positive, the resistance is given by

$$R = \frac{C}{h_a^3 + h_a^2 h_v + h_a h_v^2 + h_v^3} \quad (59)$$

So far we have not explicitly dealt with the discontinuity of the thickness–pressure relationship at zero pressure at which the governing equation changes from Eq. 5b to Eq. 5d, and then at $p = -\epsilon$ changes further to Eq. 5a.

If the transmural pressure at the venule is negative and less than $-\epsilon$, the sheet thickness is zero and there is no flow. If the pressure is greater than $-\epsilon$ but less than zero, the differential equation remains the same ($\nabla^2 h^4 = 0$). The solution for h requires no change. A change is needed only when we compute Δp from h: we have to use Eq. 5b if $h > h_0$, and we use Eq. 5d if $h < h_0$. The pressure–flow relationship, Eq. 49, remains valid. But $\bar{h}$ as a function of Δp depends on the value of Δp (either Eq. 5b or 5d); and if the pressure at venule is negative, the integral in Eq. 50 must be replaced by

$$\int \dot{Q}\, ds = \frac{1}{\mu k f}\left[\int_{\Delta p_{\text{ven}}}^{0}\left(h_0 + \frac{h_0}{\epsilon}\Delta p\right)^3 d\Delta p + \int_{0}^{\Delta p_{\text{art}}}(h_0 + \alpha\Delta p)d\Delta p\right] \quad (60)$$

Equations 51–53 will become more complex.

The case of real interest is $p_{\text{ven}} \to -\epsilon$ or $h_v \to 0$. In this case, we have shown in the one-dimensional case (in Section 3.1, Eq. 46) that the flow can be written as

$$\dot{Q} = \dot{Q}_{\text{max}} = \frac{1}{C}h_a^4 = \frac{1}{C}(h_0 + \alpha\Delta p_{\text{art}})^4 \quad (61)$$

This is the maximum flow that can be obtained from a given arteriolar pressure. To achieve this maximal flow the downstream (left atrium) pressure must be so low as to make the pressure at the venule equal to $-\epsilon$.

Actually, the maximum given by Eq. 61 is not quite achievable, because as $h \to 0$ the velocity of flow becomes very large, and the Stokes flow approximation Eq. 33 ceases to be valid. The effect of convective inertia must be added. Dawson and Elliott (1974) point out that in a convergent–divergent channel flow there is a limiting velocity of flow: the maximum velocity of flow at the throat cannot exceed the velocity of the pulse wave in the vessel. (This is analogous to the sonic throat of a supersonic wind tunnel, or the Laval nozzle in stream turbine.) By imposition of such a velocity limitation and the addition of inertia effects, the maximum flow is somewhat smaller than that given in Eq. 61. We use Eq. 61, because of its simplicity, as an upper bound of the pulmonary blood flow.

To display these relationships graphically, we may consider the variation of flow and resistance with independent changes of arteriolar pressure, p_{art}, the venular pressure, p_{ven}, and the alveolar pressure, p_{alv}. In anticipation of a possible comparison with experimental data on the pulmonary vascular resistance of the dog, we take $h_0 = 2.5$ μ and $\alpha = 0.122$ μ/cm H_2O. Figure 14 shows the results for the case in which the left atrium pressure is fixed at 3 cm H_2O (in all the figures the pressure is in units of cm H_2O), the alveolar air pressure is 0, 7, 17, or 23 cm H_2O, and the pressure difference between the arteriole and left atrium is varied. The pleural pressure is assumed to be zero in the cases of positive inflation and negative in the cases of negative inflation represented by the curve for $p_{alv} = 0$. In the case of positive inflation, the left atrium pressure is smaller than the alveolar air pressure. The pulmonary veins are subjected to negative transmural pressures. The transmural pressure at the venule is likely to be negative. Therefore we calculate the flow first with Eq. 53

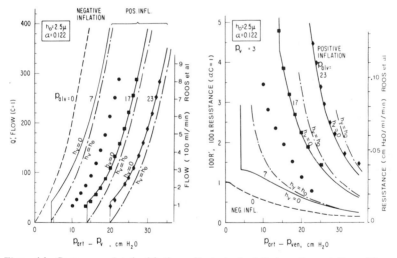

Figure 14. Curves associated with the ordinate to the left show the variation of flow and resistance with pressure head, $p_{art} - p_{ven}$, at a constant venule pressure of 3 cm H_2O. The alveolar pressures are 23, 17, and 7 cm H_2O for positive inflation, with pleural pressure equal to 0. For negative inflation, p_{alv} is 0, while pleural pressure is negative. Q' is the flow when $C = 1$ and $R' = \alpha R$ in units of $(\mu)^4$ and $(\mu)^{-3}$, respectively. Points associated with the ordinate to the right correspond to experimental data by Roos et al. (1961) on dogs with left atrium pressure equal to 3 cm H_2O, pleural pressure equal to 0, and alveolar pressure equal to 23 (♦), 17 (■), and 7 (●) cm H_2O. From Fung and Sobin (1972a). Reprinted by permission.

under the assumption $h_v = h_0$, i.e., $\Delta p_{ven} = 0$, and then with Eq. 56 under the assumption that $h_v = 0$, i.e., $\Delta p_{ven} = -\epsilon$. The actual flow will be between these bounds. The values of Q' and R' plotted in Figure 14 are, respectively, the flow and the product αR in units of $(\mu)^4$ and $(\mu)^{-3}$. To obtain flow in ml/min and R in cm H_2O ml^{-1} min, one should divide Q' by 10^{16} C and multiply R' by 10^{16} C/α with C in units of centimeter minutes and α in $\mu m/cm$ H_2O.

The features of the positive inflation curves in Figure 14 may be explained as follows. Consider the case $p_{alv} = 23$ cm H_2O. Because $p_{LA} = 3$ cm H_2O, p_{art} is smaller than 23 cm H_2O when the pressure head, $p_{art} - p_{LA}$, is smaller than 20 cm H_2O. Hence when $p_{art} - p_{LA} < 20$ cm H_2O, there is no flow and the resistance is infinite. When $p_{art} > p_{alv}$ there is flow. If $p_{LA} = 3$ cm H_2O and $p_{alv} = 23$ cm H_2O as assumed, Q is bounded either by the solid curves ($h_v = 0$, the maximal flow) or by the dash–dot curves ($h_v = h_0$) in Figure 14.

We would like to compare these results with experiments. Roos et al. (1961) experimented on dog's lung in 1961 and obtained the pressure–flow relationship. Strictly speaking, we have no right to compare their results directly with ours, because p_{art} is not the pulmonary artery pressure, and p_{ven} is not the left atrium pressure; the whole lung is a summation of all sheets with varying p_{art} and p_{ven}. But if we assume that the pulmonary arteries and veins are linearly elastic, and then sum up all the sheets of the lung to account for the effect of gravity, we find that the equation named above should hold approximately if p_{art} and p_{ven} are replaced by pressures in the pulmonary artery and vein, respectively. We do not know the constant C, which depends on the sheet compliance and area. But if we accept the formula, then the value of C can be computed by identifying one experimental point with the theoretic value. This we did by plotting the results of Roos et al. on the same graph, except with a scale (ordinate on the right-hand side) so adjusted that one of the experimental point falls exactly on the theoretic curve. Figure 14 shows that when this is done, the entire set of experimental data on positive inflation agrees with the theory. The trend seems correct also for negatively inflated lung, but obviously it requires a different constant C.

Permutt et al. (1969) performed an interesting experiment on dog's lung. They perfused the lung with a constant-flow pump, and measured the pulmonary arterial pressure (P_{PA}) for various values of controlled left atrium pressure (p_{LA}). We can predict the outcome with our formula if we make the same allowances named above. Figure 15 shows how the predic-

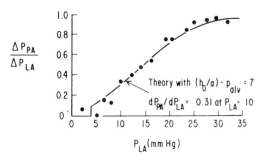

Figure 15. The fitting of experimental data on dog's lung perfused at constant flow and constant transpulmonary pressure from the work of Permutt et al. (1969) by a theoretic curve computed according to Eq. 54. From Fung and Sobin (1972b). Reprinted by permission.

tion compares with the experimental result. It shows again that if one of the experimental points is made to agree with the theory (thus determining the constant C), then the entire set of experimental results falls on the theoretic curve.

3.4   The Arteriolar and Venular Pressure. The Exit Condition of the Sheet

The lungs of human or other larger animals are so large that the hydrostatic pressure due to gravitation plays a dominant role. In considering the effect of gravity, the alveolar gas pressure is used as the gauge standard, and we set $p_{alv} = 0$. All pressures are referred to levels above the alveolar gas pressure.

We recall that p_{art} and p_{ven} denote, respectively, the pressure in the flowing blood at the points of arteriolar entry into an alveolar sheet and venular exit from the sheet. Undoubtedly, p_{art} and p_{ven} are related to the pressures at the pulmonary artery, p_{PA}, and at the left atrium, p_{LA}. They differ because of the hydrostatic pressure head and the hemodynamic resistance. Let the pulmonary artery be located at the level z_0. Let z (or z_{LA}) be the height of an alveolar sheet (or the left atrium) above $z = z_0$, measured along the direction of gravitational acceleration. Then we have

$$p_{art} = p_{PA} - \rho g z - \Sigma(\Delta p_a)_i \quad \text{(summation over arteries)} \quad (62)$$

$$p_{ven} = p_{LA} - \rho g(z - z_{LA}) + \Sigma(\Delta p_v)_i \quad \text{(summation over veins)} \quad (63)$$

where ρ is the density of the blood, g is the gravitational acceleration, $(\Delta p_a)_i$ is the pressure drop in the ith generation of the arteries, $(\Delta p_v)_i$ is that in the ith vein. $(\Delta p_a)_i$ is equal to the product of the flow in the ith vessel and the resistance in that vessel, which, for an elastic vessel, is itself pressure dependent. Therefore, to calculate p_{ven} from p_{LA} one must account for the flow.

Because of the last term in Eq. 63, one must not conclude that $p_{ven} \leqslant 0$ whenever $p_{LA} - \rho g(z - z_{LA}) \leqslant 0$. This is an important point if one wishes to understand the connection between the sheet flow and the "waterfall" of Permutt, Bromberger-Barnea, and Bane (1962) or the "sluicing" of Bannister and Torrance (1960).

We have shown in Section 2.4 that in pulmonary capillaries the Reynolds number is much less than 1 and flutter cannot arise in the pulmonary interalveolar septa. Therefore, when the boundary conditions are steady state, the solution is also steady state. Accordingly, as long as there is flow the alveolar sheet thickness cannot be zero (except possibly for a singular point). Thus following Eqs. 5a–5d, p_{ven} must be greater than $-\epsilon$. Hence we conclude that in the so-called "zone 2" condition, when $p_{LA} - \rho g(z - z_{LA}) < 0 < p_{art}$, the sum of the pressure drops in the veins, $\Sigma (\Delta p_v)_i$, must be so large that the pressure at the venule is sufficient to open the alveolar sheet ($p_{ven} > -\epsilon$). The "waterfall" or "sluicing," if it takes place, is to take place in the pulmonary veins. Most likely, however, under negative pressure the pulmonary vein will deform and buckle, thus increasing the resistance to flow.

From the discussions above it is clear that in the zone 2 condition it is not immediately possible to say what the pressure at the venular exit is. Let us consider the sequence of events when the left atrium pressure is continuously lowered. (Assume that arteriolar pressure exceeds 0 and alveolar pressure equals 0.) Let us begin with $p_{LA} = p_{art}$. At first, as p_{LA} decreases the flow increases. This continues until the pressure in the pulmonary vein becomes smaller than the alveolar pressure. At sufficiently large negative pressure the vein buckles. Further decrease of p_{LA} causes more severe and more widely spread buckling and consequently reduces the cross-sectional area of the veins and increases their resistance to flow. Whether the flow will continue to increase or not when p_{LA} decreases further depends on which of the two contending factors wins: the increase in pressure gradient, or the increase in resistance. Eventually, when buckling becomes very severe the flow will become very small. Thus when the left atrium pressure is decreased continuously from p_{art}, the flow increases, reaches a peak, and then decreases. The maximum value of the flow at the peak is bounded by the Q given in Eq. 61.

3.5 Other Comparisons with Experiments

3.5.1 Effect of Gravity
·Regional blood flow.
·Smooth merging of zone 2 and zone 3.

The effect of gravity on the blood, which creates a hydrostatic pressure gradient throughout the lung, can be examined by calculating p_{art} and p_{ven} as function of height and sum over the alveolar sheets of the lung. The regional differences expounded by West (1970) can be studied in theoretic detail. One of the particular results obtained is that there should be no hemodynamic line of demarcation between zone 2 and zone 3. In other words, zone 2 and zone 3 merge smoothly. The rate of increase of blood flow down a vertical lung has no sudden change at the junction of zone 2 and zone 3. This agrees with the observations of Hughes et al. (1968) in a vertical lung.

3.5.2 Transit Time Distribution of Flow in Sheet
·Convolution with flow in arteries and veins.

Because the solution of the differential equation provides a detailed picture of the blood velocity in the interalveolar sheets, we can calculate the transit time distribution in these sheets. This is found to be a sum of a delta function and a decaying exponential function (χ^2 distributions of degrees of freedom 0 and 2 respectively), as shown in the middle of the left-hand panel of Figure 16. The transit time distribution of blood through pulmonary arteries has been given by Cumming et al. (1969). As it is sketched at the top of the left-hand panel in Figure 16, it can be approximated by a χ^2 distribution of degree 6. The transit time distribution in the pulmonary vein has not been reported, but we assume that it is approximately the same as that in the arteries. The resultant transit time distribution of blood from the pulmonary artery to the left atrium is obtained by convolution of these three distribution functions. If we use the approximations named above, the resultant transit time distribution function is a sum of two χ^2 distributions of degrees of freedom 12 and 14 (6 + 0 + 6 and 6 + 2 + 6 respectively). The theoretic result is shown in the middle panel of Figure 16, which may be compared with the experimental curves of Maseri et al. (1970) shown on the right-hand side for two different heart rates.

3.5.3 Pulmonary Blood Volume
·Correlates with arteriolar pressure.
·Does not correlate with venular pressure.

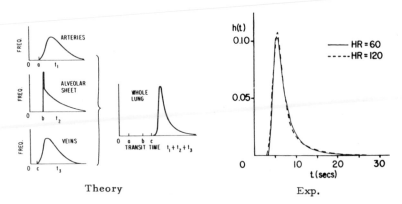

Theory   Exp.

Figure 16. *Left middle,* theoretic transit time distribution for blood flow in an alveolar sheet that is illustrated in Figure 13. Computation gives the histogram that is fitted by a curve $f(\tau)$. τ is the ratio of transit time to the minimum transit time through the sheet. From Fung and Sobin (1972*b*). *Left upper,* transit time distribution in pulmonary arteries, from Cumming et al. (1969). *Left lower,* transit time distribution in pulmonary vein, assumed to be the same as that in the arteries. *Middle panel,* convolution of transit times, t_1, t_2, and t_3, of blood in the pulmonary arteries, capillaries, and veins, respectively. From Fung and Sobin (1972*b*). *Right-hand panel,* the frequency function, $h(t)$, of transit times in pulmonary circulation in open-chest dogs at constant cardiac output and left atrial pressure, showing the lack of effect of heart rate. From Maseri et al. (1970, p. 537). Reprinted by permission.

By integrating the sheet thickness over the sheet area, we obtain the vascular volume. The features shown in Figure 13 and section 3.2 above suggest that the alveolar blood volume would be directly related to the pulmonary arterial pressure, whereas the pulmonary venous pressure would have only a minor effect, because any decrease in sheet thickness due to a lowering of p_{ven} is localized to the immediate neighborhood of the venule.

A theoretically predicted pulmonary capillary blood volume as a function of p_{art}, p_{ven}, and p_{alv} is shown in the left-hand panel of Figure 17, with the constants and geometry pertinent to dog's lung. It is seen that the blood volume varies almost linearly with $p_{\text{art}} - p_{\text{alv}}$, whereas very little effect is shown by $p_{\text{ven}} - p_{\text{alv}}$. This result may be compared with the experimental results of Permutt et al. (1969), which are shown on the right-hand side of Figure 17. The pulmonary blood volume shown here, however, is the total pulmonary blood volume obtained by the indicator-dilution method, not merely the capillary blood volume. But the related work of Permutt et al. (1969) on the steady-state carbon-monoxide

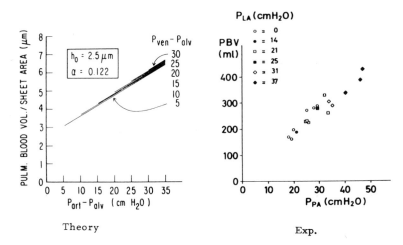

Figure 17. *Left*, Theoretic relationship between the pulmonary alveolar blood volume and the arterial and venous pressures. Ordinate is the pulmonary blood volume per unit area of the sheet. Abscissa is the transmembrane pressure at the arteriole end of the sheet. The transmembrane pressure at the venule end is seen to have only a minor effect on the blood volume. Data correspond to Figure 4 of Fung and Sobin (1972*b*). *Right*, Experimental results showing the relationship between pulmonary blood volume and pulmonary artery pressure in one dog at a variety of left atrial pressures. From Permutt et al. (1968). Reprinted by permission.

diffusing capacity, which is proportional to the capillary blood volume, shows the same trend.

4 FLUID IN THE INTERSTITIAL SPACE OF THE PULMONARY ALVEOLAR SHEET

If edema or the movement of water across the endothelium is considered, the vascular space is no longer bounded by impermeable walls, and the more general differential equation for sheet flow, Eqs. 30 or 31, must be used. Consideration of this problem reveals another feature of the sheet flow.

The very extensive literature on pulmonary edema is somewhat controversial. Some of the most recent thoughts are contained in Fishman (1972), Fishman and Hecht (1969), and Giuntini (1971). Staub et al. (1967) have examined the sequence of fluid accumulation in dog's lung when edema was induced. They showed that in the initial stage of fluid leak, fluid flows to the extra-alveolar interstitial space around the conducting vessels and airways. Next, the alveolar wall thickens, and fluid collects at the lines of juncture of alveolar sheets. Finally, some alveoli begin to be filled completely, while others remain dry, in a random manner which the authors called "quantal." The first and the third phases are not considered in the present paper, but the second is relevant. Staub, Nagano, and Pearce (1967) showed that in edema induced by high pressure or by alloxan, the dog's interalveolar septa thicken somewhat, say, in the upper zone, from $4.0 \pm 0.8 \mu$ at no edema to $4.3 \pm 1.3 \mu$ when there was light edema, to $6.1 \pm 1.2 \mu$ at moderate edema, and 5.0 ± 1.0 or $5.6 \pm 1.7 \mu$ (in different experiments) at severe edema. This thickening is due to an increase of vascular space, the swelling of the cells, and an increase of the interstitial space. Staub et al. estimated the maximum thickening of the alveolar-capillary membrane to be about 1μ on each side of the wall. Schultz (1959) has shown by electron microscopy such a thickening of interstitial space. However, the total volume of the intra-alveolar interstitial space must be quite small, because it is only a fraction of the alveolar sheet wall. This is consistent with the findings of Guyton and Lindsey (1959), who measured the weight increase of the extravascular lung tissue as a function of the left atrium pressure and found that below a critical pressure at which edema sets in, the change in total extravascular water was small.

No experimental value is known for the intra-alveolar interstitial water volume. The multiple indicator-dilution method measures an extravascular water volume that includes the cellular water. The method of comparing wet and dry weights measures, in addition, extra-alveolar water, and water in various degrees of association with proteins and mucopolysaccharides. For this reason it would be interesting to see what the theory would predict.

We assume that water moves across the blood—tissue barrier according to the equation

$$\dot{m} = K_{bt}[p_{blood} - p_{tissue} - \sigma(\pi_{blood} - \pi_{tissue})], \qquad (64)$$

where p and π are, respectively, the hydrostatic and osmotic pressures, $\dot{m}$ is the rate of water movement per unit area per unit time, K_{bt} is the filtration constant of the blood—tissue barrier, and σ is the reflection coefficient of Staverman (1951). When $\dot{m}$ is in units of g/sec cm^2, p and π in units of dynes/cm^2, K_{bt} is in units of sec/cm.

The tissue pressure in the equation above refers to the hydrostatic pressure of "free" water in the interstitial space. If a tissue is exposed to bulk water, we define the tissue pressure at the interface as equal to the pressure in the bulk water. Inside the tissue we define the gradient of tissue pressure as the driving force for water movement according to a constitutive equation such as Darcy's law, Eq. 68, below. Thus the tissue pressure is defined operationally by a constitutive equation and a boundary condition. Such a method of defining tissue pressure may seem artificial, but it is actually common to the concept of pressure in all incompressible fluids.

The equation governing the sheet thickness is Eq. 30, or the simpler version, Eq. 31:

$$\left(\frac{\partial^2}{\partial x^2} + \frac{\partial^2}{\partial y^2}\right) h^4 = 4\mu k f\alpha \left[\frac{\partial \bar{h}}{\partial t} + \frac{2K_{bt}}{\rho\alpha}(\bar{h} - h^*)\right], \qquad (65)$$

where

$$h^* = h_0 + \alpha(p^* - p_{alv}) \qquad (66)$$

$$p^* = \sigma(\pi_{blood} - \pi_{tissue}) + p_{tissue} \qquad (67)$$

The parameters p^* and h^* are of paramount importance in our problem. p^* is the pressure that counteracts the hydrostatic pressure of the blood in forcing water to permeate through the capillary membrane. h^* is a hypothetic thickness of the sheet if the counteracting pressure p^* were applied as a distending transmural pressure inside the blood vessel. We call p^* the *counteracting pressure* and h^* the *counteracting thickness.*

The equation governing the movement of water in the tissue space is not definitely known. The interstitium being a structural gel, it is natural to assume that the same equations governing porous media apply (Darcy, 1856; Scheidegger, 1957; Lew and Fung, 1970). A commonly accepted equation is Darcy's law (1856), which states that the velocity of fluid motion is proportional to the negative pressure gradient:

$$u_i = \sum_{j=1}^{3} K_{ij} \left(-\frac{\partial p}{\partial x_j}\right) \qquad (i = 1,2,3,), \qquad (68)$$

where u_1, u_2, u_3 are the macroscopic velocity components in the direction of rectangular Cartesian coordinates x_1, x_2, x_3, and $k_{11}, k_{12}, \ldots, k_{33}$ are a set of permeability constants. If we assume that the porosity does not change with time and location, then the conservation of mass is expressed by the equation of continuity,

$$\sum_{i=1}^{3} \frac{\partial u_i}{\partial x_i} = 0 \qquad (69)$$

On substituting Eq. 68 into Eq. 69, we obtain

$$\sum_{i=1}^{3} \sum_{j=1}^{3} \frac{\partial}{\partial x_i} \left(K_{ij} \frac{\partial p}{\partial x_j} \right) = 0 \qquad (70)$$

To solve the problem we must determine how the tissue pressure and osmotic pressure vary with interstitial water. In the tissue space, van't Hoff's law does not apply, and the nonlinear relationship between the osmotic pressure and the concentration of proteins and hyaluronates must be determined experimentally. Wiederhielm (1971) presented such an interaction curve. Let W be the volume of the interstitial water, and let W_0 be that at a standard state that corresponds with Wiederhielm's concentration c_0 (= 2.7% albumin and 1.0% hyaluronate). Then, in the range $0.7 < W/W_0 < 1.3$ and for $\alpha = 0.122 \ \mu/\text{cm H}_2\text{O}$ and $h_0 = 2.5 \ \mu$, we may represent Wiederhielm's data by an equation

$$F = (\alpha/h_0)\pi_{\text{tissue}} = 1.364 - 2.11[(W/W_0) - 1] + 2.222[(W/W_0) - 1]^2 \quad (71)$$

The factor (α/h_0) is used to normalize the expression into a dimensionless form.

Next, consider p_{tissue}. Three approaches can be taken. (1) Solve the problem exactly as is done by Tang and Fung (1975); however, the solution is very complicated. (2) Leave p_{tissue} as an open parameter and examine its effect. (3) Follow Guyton, Granger, and Taylor (1971) and Wiederhielm (1968) to write

$$p_{\text{tissue}} = (W - W_0)/C_{\text{tissue}}, \qquad (72)$$

where C_{tissue} is called the "compliance constant" for the tissue pressure. This is based on the idea that the interstitial water is embedded in an elastic matrix and a container. If we consider the balance of stresses at the boundary of the interstitial water and the container, and assume that the tension in the container vanishes when $W = W_0$, then Eq. 72 follows.

The mathematical solution is given in Fung (1974). A brief outline is presented below. We limit ourselves to the two-dimensional case (Figure 18) in which an alveolar sheet stretches between parallel arterioles and venules. Let the x axis be perpendicular to the arteriole. We assume that everything is a function of x alone and not of y. If the flow is *steady* and the walls are *impermeable,* the solution is given in Section 3.1. Let us indicate that solution with a subscript SI to signify steady and imper-

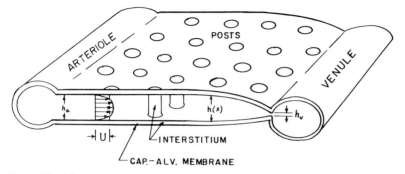

Figure 18. Schematic of an alveolar sheet. Vascular space bounded by capillary-alveolar membranes which are connected by posts. From Fung (1974). Reprinted by permission.

meable:

$$h_{SI}(x) = [h_a^4 - (h_a^4 - h_v^4)x/L]^{1/4} \tag{73}$$

where h_a, h_v are, respectively, the thickness of the alveolar sheet at the arteriole $(x = 0)$ and venule $(x = L)$.

With permeable walls the solution of Eq. 65 can be posed in the form

$$h(x,y) = h_{SI}(x,y) + \Phi(x) \tag{74}$$

The last term, $\Phi(x)$, accounts for the effect of permeability at the wall. Because fluid filtration across the capillary wall is very small compared with the blood flow, it is justified to assume $\Phi < h_{SI}$, so that Eq. 65 can be linearized to obtain, for the two-dimensional case,

$$\frac{d^2}{dx^2} (h_{SI}^3 \Phi) = (2\mu k f K_{bt}/\rho)(h_{SI} - h^*) \tag{75}$$

At this point it is convenient to introduce dimensionless variables. We take the sheet thickness at zero pressure, h_0, as a characteristic thickness, and the distance between arteriole and venule, L, as a characteristic length, and define the dimensionless parameters:

$$\begin{aligned}
\tilde{x} = x/L, \quad &\tilde{z} = z/h_0, \\
\tilde{h} = \bar{h}/h_0, \quad \tilde{h}^* = h^*/h_0, \quad \tilde{h}_{SI} = h_{SI}/h_0, \quad &\tilde{\Phi} = \Phi h_0, \\
\tilde{p} = \bar{p}/(h_0/\alpha), \quad \tilde{q}_x = (\mu k f \alpha L/h_0^4)\bar{h}\bar{U}, \\
\epsilon = 2\mu k f L^2 K_{bt}/(\rho h_0^3) &
\end{aligned} \tag{76}$$

Note that $\tilde{z}$, the coordinate normal to the sheet, is defined with respect to h_0. Then Eq. 75 becomes

$$\frac{d^2(\tilde{h}_{SI}^3\Phi)}{d\tilde{x}^2} = (\tilde{h}_{SI} - \tilde{h}^*), \tag{77}$$

whereas the pressure and flow are given by

$$\begin{aligned} \tilde{p} &= \tilde{p}_{SI} + \tilde{\Phi}, \\ \tilde{q}_x &= \tilde{q}_{xSI} - \partial\tilde{\Phi}/\partial\tilde{x} \end{aligned} \tag{78}$$

Here $\tilde{p}_{SI}, \tilde{q}_{xSI}$ are values corresponding to $\tilde{h}_{SI}$.

The rate at which water permeates through the blood–tissue barrier per unit area of the barrier is given by Eq. 64, which may be written

$$\dot{m} = \frac{K_{bt}h_0}{\alpha} \, [\tilde{h}_{SI} + \tilde{\Phi} - \tilde{h}^*] \tag{79}$$

The boundary conditions associated with Eq. 77 must be specified. It seems reasonable that the small amount of fluid permeation does not affect the arterial pressure and flow. Hence we specify

$$\tilde{\Phi} = \frac{d}{d\tilde{x}} \, [\tilde{h}_{SI}^3\tilde{\Phi}] = 0 \qquad \text{at } \tilde{x} = 0 \tag{80}$$

Equation 77 can then be solved to yield

$$\tilde{\Phi}(\tilde{x}) = \frac{\epsilon}{\tilde{h}_{SI}^3(\tilde{x})} \int_0^{\tilde{x}} (\tilde{x} - \xi)[\tilde{h}_{SI}(\xi) - \tilde{h}^*(\xi)] \, d\xi \tag{81}$$

An insertion of Eq. 81 into Eq. 79 yields the total fluid transfer per unit time per sheet with area A:

$$2\iint \dot{m} \, dx \, dy = \frac{2K_{bt}Ah_0}{\alpha} \, (E_1 + \epsilon E_2), \tag{82}$$

where

$$E_1 = \int_0^1 [\tilde{h}_{SI}(\xi) - \tilde{h}^*(\xi)] \, d\xi, \tag{83}$$

$$E_2 = \frac{1}{\epsilon}\int_0^1 \tilde{\Phi}(\tilde{x}) \, d\tilde{x} = \int_0^1 \frac{d\tilde{x}}{\tilde{h}_{SI}^3(\tilde{x})} \int_0^{\tilde{x}} (\tilde{x} - \xi)[\tilde{h}_{SI}(\xi) - \tilde{h}^*(\xi)] \, d\xi \tag{84}$$

4.1   The Condition of Steady State

At a steady state, the influx of water from the vascular space into the interstitial space must be equal to the sum of the efflux into the alveolar space through the tissue–alveolar barrier and the drainage into the lymph system. For a normal lung these effluxes are very small. As a first case to investigate we assume that they are negligible so that the condition at steady state is that the total efflux across the blood–tissue barrier is zero. Thus from Eq. 84 we have the condition for steady state,

$$E_1 + \epsilon E_2 = 0 \tag{85}$$

E_1, E_2 are functions of the static sheet thickness distribution $\bar{h}_{SI}$ and the counteracting thickness $\bar{h}^*$, which in turn depend on the arterial pressure, the alveolar pressure, the osmotic pressures (the concentration of solutes and the volume of extravascular water in the tissue space), and the tissue pressure.

One thing we learned from the lengthy solution of the hydrodynamics problem of flow in a channel bounded by porous layers (see Tang and Fung, 1975) is that if the ratio of the thickness of the porous layer to the channel width lies in the range of 0.05–1 (a physiologic range), then the "tissue" pressure in the porous layer is essentially a constant, i.e., it is essentially uniform. Now, we must recall the morphology of the interstitial space on pulmonary alveolar sheets. Remember that much of the interstitial space is concentrated at the "posts," which are continuous with the narrow interstitium between the basement membranes between the endothelial and epithelial layers. Thus, the posts are where the interstitial water would normally be stored, while these storage centers communicate with each other through the space between the basement membranes. Thus we consider two limiting cases:

1. The communication channels between posts are wide open, in which case we assume the tissue pressure to be constant.
2. The communication channels between posts are closed, in which case the tissue pressure in each post is determined by local equilibrium with the vascular fluid.

The real condition lies between these extremes. It is interesting that the major results to be presented below apply to both extremes, and, hence, are likely to be true for the intermediate case.

4.2 Equilibrium when Communication Between Posts is Open

When the communication is open, p^* and h^* are constants, and E_1, E_2 are functions of $\bar{h}_a$, $\bar{h}_v$, $\bar{h}^*$. Equation 85 can then be solved for $\bar{h}^*$. This solution shall be designated as $\bar{h}_{ss}^*$, to signify its importance as a *counteracting thickness at steady state*. A numerical analysis brings out the remarkable fact that the steady-state values of the counteracting thickness are almost directly proportional to the arteriolar thickness $\bar{h}_a$ and are rather insensitive to variations in the venular thickness $\bar{h}_v$ and the "permeability parameter" ϵ. In other words, at a steady state, the counteracting pressure p^* is proportional to the arteriolar pressure, p_{art}, and is insensitive to variations in the venular pressure p_{ven}, and the permeability of the blood–tissue barrier, K_{bt}. It is this result that leads to the almost linear correlation between the pulmonary alveolar blood volume and the volume of interstitial water, as is shown below.

4.3 The Volume of Interstitial Water
in Case of Open Communication Between Posts

Knowing $\bar{h}_{ss}^*$, we can go back to Eqs. 66, 67, 71, and 72 to evaluate the volume of interstitial water, W. The results can be presented in two forms. If we use tissue pressure as a free parameter, we may write

$$\bar{h}^* = G - F(W/W_0), \tag{86}$$

where

$$G = 1 + (\alpha/h_0)(\pi_{blood} - p_{alv} + p_{tissue}) \tag{87}$$

If we express tissue pressure in terms of tissue compliance, as in Eq. 72, then we write

$$\bar{h}^* = G' - F(W/W_0) + \theta[(W/W_0) - 1] \tag{88}$$

where

$$G' = 1 + (\alpha/h_0)(\sigma\pi_{blood} - p_{alv}) \tag{89}$$

$$\theta = \alpha W_0/(h_0 C_{tissue}) \tag{90}$$

In either case, we can plot $\bar{h}^*$ versus W/W_0. Then we can compute the volume of interstitial water at a steady state by equating $\bar{h}^*$ to $\bar{h}_{ss}^*$. The results are shown in Figures 19 and 20. It is seen that the interstitial water increases with increasing arteriolar pressure, but is not greatly affected by the membrane permeability (ϵ) and the venular pressure ($\sim\bar{h}_v$). The

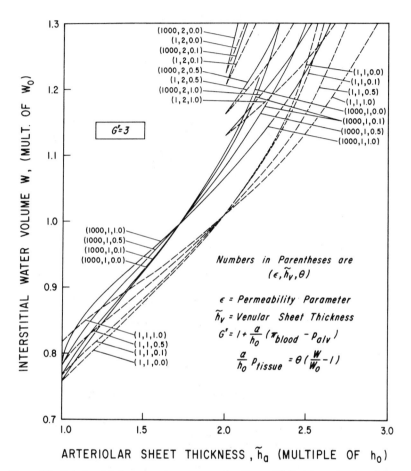

Figure 19. Relationship between the extravascular (interstitial) water volume and the arteriolar thickness (pressure) when communication between posts is open. The values of the permeability constant ϵ, the venular thickness (pressure) $\tilde{h}_v$, and the tissue pressure compliance parameter θ (see Eq. 90) are enclosed in parentheses. These curves refer to a fixed value of $G' = 3$, which is related to the osmotic pressure in blood and tissue pressure as defined in Eq. 89. From Fung (1974). Reprinted by permission.

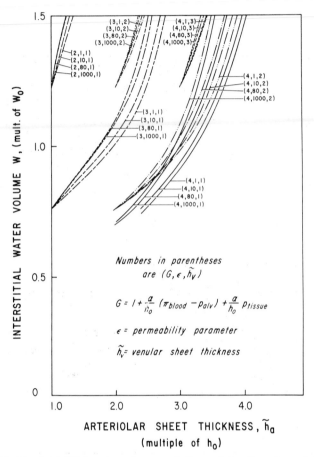

Figure 20. The interstitial water volume as influenced by the values of $G = 1 - (\alpha/h_0)(\pi_{blood} - p_{alv}) + (\alpha/h_0)p_{tissue}$, permeability parameter ϵ, and venular thickness $\tilde{h}_v$. Communication channels between posts open. Tissue pressure is treated as an independent variable. From Fung (1974). Reprinted by permission.

osmotic pressure of the blood and the tissue pressure have considerable effect as shown through the parameter G'.

4.4 Correlation of Interstitial Water Volume with Capillary Blood Volume

The pulmonary capillary blood volume per sheet (PCBV/sheet) is given by integrating the product of local thickness with area:

$$\text{PCBV/sheet} = (\text{sheet area}) \cdot h_0 \int_0^1 [\tilde{h}_{SI}(\tilde{x}) + \tilde{\Phi}(\tilde{x})] \; d\tilde{x}$$

$$= (\text{sheet area}) \cdot h_0 \left[\int_0^1 \tilde{h}_{SI}(\tilde{x}) \, d\tilde{x} + \epsilon E_2 \right] \tag{91}$$

The integral in the bracket is the value of E_1 when $\tilde{h}^*$ is zero. The second term in the bracket is, according to Eq. 85, equal to $E_1(\tilde{h}^*)$. Because at a steady state $\tilde{h}^* = \tilde{h}_{ss}^*$, we have

$$\text{PCBV/sheet} = (\text{sheet area}) h_0 [E_1(0) - E_1(\tilde{h}_{ss}^*)], \tag{92}$$

where $E_1(0)$ and $E_1(\tilde{h}_{ss}^*)$ are the values of E_1 when $\tilde{h}^* = 0$ and $h^* = h_{ss}^*$, respectively.

Combining these solutions, we can demonstrate the correlation between the interstitial water volume and the capillary blood volume. Figure 21 shows the correlation for specified values of the venular sheet thickness (venular pressure) and permeability parameter. It is seen that they are simply correlated over wide ranges of variations in the arteriolar and venular pressures and capillary permeability. The effect of varying the parameter G is shown in Figure 22 where the tissue pressure is considered as an independent variable. It is seen that the tissue pressure has considerable effect on the interstitial water volume.

4.5 Equilibrium When Communication Between Posts is Closed

At another extreme let us assume that the space between the basement membranes under the endothelial cells and epithelial cells is so narrow that the tissue fluid flow is entirely negligible and no communication between posts exists. In this case each post must be in equilibrium with the blood in its immediate neighborhood. Because at any point in an alveolar sheet the pressure does not vary across the thickness and because the diameter of each post is small compared with the length of the sheet, we see that each post may be regarded as situated in a uniform surrounding. Therefore all points on the surface of the post are equivalent. If there is an inflow into the post at one point, there must be uniform inflow at every point; similarly for an outflow. Since at a steady state there can be no net flow over the entire post, there can be no flow at all.

Therefore when there is no communication between the posts, the condition of equilibrium is $\dot{m} = 0$ (Eq. 64). It follows from Eqs. 79 and 77 that $\Phi = 0$ and

$$\tilde{h}^*(\tilde{x}) = \tilde{h}_{SI}(\tilde{x}) \tag{93}$$

Thus $\tilde{h}^*$ is a function of $\tilde{x}$. Returning to Eq. 86 or 88, we see that when communication between posts is closed the interstitial water is distributed

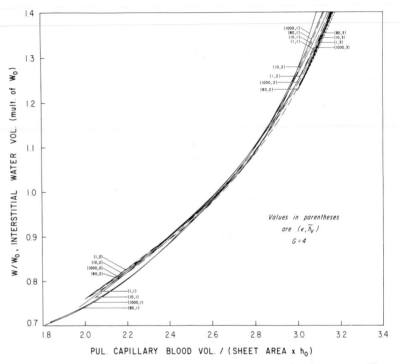

Figure 21. Correlation between interstitial water volume and pulmonary capillary blood volume, when communication channels are open. For a fixed value of G (which includes the tissue pressure), the correlation seems indifferent to the membrane permeability and venular pressures. Values of ϵ, $\bar{h}_v$ are enclosed in parentheses. From Fung (1974). Reprinted by permission.

according to the equation

$$\bar{h}_{SI}(\tilde{x}) = 1 + (\alpha/h_0)(\pi_{\text{blood}} - \pi_{\text{alv}}) - F(W/W_0) + (\alpha/h_0)(W - W_0)/C_{\text{tissue}} \tag{94}$$

The solution of this equation yields the ratio W/W_0 as a function of the location of the post $\tilde{x}$. A summation over all the posts gives the total volume of free water in the tissue space.

An approximate solution can be obtained if we ignore the last term. Then on solving Eq. 94 for W/W_0 and integrating, we obtain

$$\text{Interstital water per sheet} \doteq W_0 \left\{ 1 + ((1/b) \int_0^1 [\bar{h}_{SI}(\tilde{x}) - (J - a)] \, d\tilde{x} \right\}, \tag{95}$$

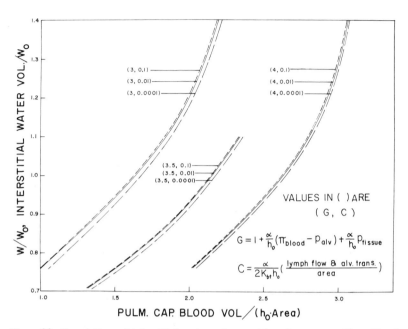

Figure 22. Correlation of interstitial water volume with pulmonary capillary blood volume as the parameter G varies. $G = 1 + (\alpha/h_0)(\pi_{blood} - p_{alv}) + (\alpha/h_0 p_{tissue})$. Because the correlation is indifferent to ϵ and h_v, only curves referring to a single set of these parameters ($\epsilon = 1$, $\bar{h}_v = 1$) are shown to make the graph more readable. Case of open communication channels. The parameter C refers to lymph flow and alveolar transudation which is discussed later in connection with Eq. 97. From Fung (1974). Reprinted by permission.

where $a = 1.364$, $b = 2.11 + (\alpha/h_0)(W_0/C_{tissue})$, and $J = 1 + (\alpha/h_0)(\pi_{blood} - \pi_{alv})$. The first integral in Eq. 95 is the value of E_1 at $\bar{h}^* = 0$. Comparing Eq. 92 and noticing that $E_2 = 0$ because of Eq. 93, we obtain

$$\text{Interstitial water} \doteq (W_0/b)\left[\left(\frac{\text{pul. cap. blood vol.}}{h_0 \cdot \text{area}}\right) - J + a\right] + W_0 \quad (96)$$

This equation beautifully exhibits a linear correlation between the interstitial water volume and pulmonary capillary blood volume.

A heuristic derivation of these results is given in Fung (1974).

4.6 Effect of Lymph Flow and Alveolar Transudation

If lymph drainage and transudation across the tissue–alveolar barrier are not negligible, let them be expressed in terms of an average total flow per unit sheet area. Equation 85 is now upset and must be replaced by

$$E_1 + \epsilon E_2 = [\alpha/(2K_{bt}h_0)] \cdot (\text{lymph \& alv. trans./area}) \equiv C \qquad (97)$$

To estimate the size of the dimensionless constant C, let us assume that the lymph and alveolar transudation is as massive as 1 ml/sec. If the alveolar area is 80 m^2, then the drainage flow is 1.25×10^{-6} g/sec cm^2. The compliance coefficient α is of the order of 0.1 μm per cm H_2O pressure or 10^{-8} $cm^2 sec^2$/g mass. h_0 is of the order 2.5 μm. K_{bt} lies in the range of 10^{-10} to 10^{-7} sec/cm. Then C lies in the range of 10^{-3} to 0.5.

The effect of this new parameter on the steady state counteracting thickness $\bar{h}_{ss}^*$ turns out to be quite small. Its effect on the alveolar blood volume is also quite negligible. In Figure 22, the effect of C on the correlation between the interstitial water volume and the capillary blood volume is shown. It is seen that it is not an important parameter.

4.7   Discussion

Guyton and Lindsey (1959) showed the existence of a critical left atrial pressure for edema formation. For a subcritical left atrial pressure the accumulation of lung water is negligible. This is consistent with our concept that the interstitial space in the alveolar sheet is small compared with that of the lung tissue. Our calculation shows that the sheet's interstitium remains small even in the supercritical pressure range, but its volume varies with the blood pressure. In the supercritical range it is reasonable to suppose that the permeability of the epithelial–alveolar barrier is increased so that fluid accumulates in the alveoli. The great effect of alloxan on edema formation, as shown by Staub et al. (1967) and Goetzman and Visscher (1969), is undoubtedly associated with the change of the permeability of the same barrier. In our analysis, the rate of edema formation is expressed in terms of the constant C in Eq. 97. Figure 22 shows that the water that remains in the interstitium of the alveolar sheet is almost independent of C. Therefore, the water in the interstitium remains about the same whether edema forms rapidly or not.

Our conclusions are as follows:

1. For a given set of tissue pressure, alveolar pressure, and plasma colloidal osmotic pressure, the interstitial water volume in the alveolar sheets increases with increasing pulmonary blood volume. This correlation is practically independent of the pressures in the pulmonary artery and left atrium, the membrane permeability of the blood–tissue barrier, and fluid transudation into the lymph and the alveoli.

2. Over a wide range of left atrium pressure, the interstitial water volume in the alveolar sheets is almost linearly correlated with the pulmonary arteriolar blood pressure. The membrane permeability, lymph flow, and fluid transudation into the alveoli have only minor effects on this correlation. At a given arteriolar pressure the interstitial water volume increases if the parameter $G = 1 + (\alpha/h_0)[\sigma\pi_{blood} + p_{tissue} - p_{alv}]$ decreases.

3. These conclusions are derived for pulmonary alveolar sheet that (a) obeys a linear thickness–pressure relationship, (b) has open vascular space whenever the arteriolar pressure exceeds the alveolar pressure, (c) obeys Starling's hypothesis at the blood–tissue barrier, and Darcy's law in the tissue space.

5 PULMONARY MICROVASCULAR IMPEDANCE

Bergel and Milnor (1965), Milnor, Bergel, and Bargainer (1966), Wiener et al. (1966), Skalak (1969), Pollack, Reddy, and Noordergraaf (1968), and many others have analyzed the pulmonary vascular impedance in dog and man. Theoretic analyses by these authors show a general agreement with experimental results, although not in all details. In these articles the capillary blood vessels are represented by parallel circular cylindrical tubes; the unrealistic geometric representation of the capillaries and the uncertainty about their compliance constitute perhaps the weakest link in their model of the pulmonary vascular bed. A more realistic model can be based on the sheet-flow theory.

The basic equation for a transient flow, Eq. 31, becomes, on neglecting permeability of water across the endothelium,

$$\left(\frac{\partial^2}{\partial x^2} + \frac{\partial^2}{\partial y^2}\right) \bar{h}^4 = 4\mu k f\alpha \frac{\partial \bar{h}}{\partial t} \tag{98}$$

This is a nonlinear differential equation and does not have a harmonic solution with respect to time. Hence, strictly speaking, the usual concept of impedance does not apply. Only in small perturbations can the basic equations be linearized and the concept of impedance be useful. Linearization can be justified if and only if the amplitude of the thickness fluctuations is small compared with the mean pulmonary alveolar sheet thickness. This condition is met if the amplitude of the pressure oscillation is small compared with the mean pulmonary arterial pressure. We proceed under this restriction.

The solution of Eq. 98 is set in the following form:

$$h(x, y, t) = h_{SI}(x, y) + e^{i\omega t}H(x, y) \tag{99}$$

We assume $H(x, y)$ to be much smaller than $h_{SI}(x, y)$, which is the solution of the equation for a steady flow between impervious walls:

$$\left(\frac{\partial^2}{\partial x^2} + \frac{\partial^2}{\partial y^2}\right) h_{SI}^4 = 0 \tag{100}$$

Equation 100 has been treated in Sections 3.1–3.2. The subscripts SI stand for steady and impervious. Substituting Eq. 99 into Eq. 98, and retaining only the first powers of H, we obtain the basic equation,

$$\left(\frac{\partial^2}{\partial x^2} + \frac{\partial^2}{\partial y^2}\right) h_{SI}^3 H = \mu k f \alpha \omega i H \tag{101}$$

Similar to Eq. 99, the pressure and flow per unit width (with components q_x, q_y) can also be represented as the sum of the steady-impervious terms and the oscillatory terms

$$\bar{p}(x,y,t) = p_{SI}(x,y) + e^{i\omega t}P(x,y),$$

$$q_x(x,y,t) = \bar{U}\bar{h} = q_{x_{SI}}(x,y) + e^{i\omega t}Q_x(x,y), \tag{102}$$

$$q_y(x,y,t) = \bar{V}\bar{h} = q_{y_{SI}}(x,y) + e^{i\omega t}Q_y(x,y)$$

For further work we use dimensionless variables defined as follows:

$$\tilde{x} = x/L, \quad \tilde{y} = y/L,$$

$$\tilde{h}_{SI} = h_{SI}/h_0, \quad \tilde{H} = H/h_0, \tag{103}$$

$$\tilde{p} = p/(h_0/\alpha),$$

$$\tilde{q} = (\mu k f \alpha L/h_0^4)q, \quad \tilde{Q} = (\mu k f \alpha L/h_0^4)Q,$$

where L is a typical length of the sheet, and h_0 is the constant in Eq. 5b that represents the sheet thickness as the transmural pressure tends to zero from positive values. We introduce further the dimensionless frequency parameter:

$$\Omega = \mu k f \alpha \omega L^2/h_0^3 \tag{104}$$

Equation 101 becomes

$$\left(\frac{\partial^2}{\partial \tilde{x}^2} + \frac{\partial^2}{\partial \tilde{y}^2}\right) \tilde{h}_{SI}^3 \tilde{H} = i\Omega\tilde{H}, \tag{105}$$

and the pressure, flow, and thickness relations become

$$\tilde{p} = \tilde{p}_{SI} + \tilde{H} e^{i\omega t}$$

$$\tilde{Q}_x = -\frac{\partial}{\partial \tilde{x}}(\tilde{h}_{SI}^3 \tilde{H}), \quad \tilde{Q}_y = -\frac{\partial}{\partial \tilde{y}}(\tilde{h}_{SI}^3 \tilde{H}) \tag{106}$$

5.1 Impedance

Blood enters each sheet at the arteriole and exits at the venule. Let there be oscillatory components of pressure and flow superimposed on the steady component. Let the circular frequency be ω, and let the oscillatory pressure and flow at the arteriole and venule edges of the sheet be denoted by P_a, Q_a, P_v, Q_v, respectively. The relationship between these quantities (all nondimensionalized according to Eq. 103) can be expressed in the following matrix form:

$$\begin{Bmatrix} P_a \\ P_v \end{Bmatrix} = \begin{Bmatrix} Z_{11} & Z_{12} \\ Z_{21} & Z_{22} \end{Bmatrix} \begin{Bmatrix} Q_a \\ Q_v \end{Bmatrix}, \tag{107}$$

$$\begin{Bmatrix} \tilde{Q}_a \\ \tilde{Q}_v \end{Bmatrix} = \begin{Bmatrix} Y_{11} & Y_{12} \\ Y_{21} & Y_{22} \end{Bmatrix} \begin{Bmatrix} \tilde{P}_a \\ \tilde{P}_v \end{Bmatrix}, \tag{108}$$

$$\begin{Bmatrix} \tilde{P}_a \\ \tilde{Q}_a \end{Bmatrix} = \begin{Bmatrix} A_{11} & A_{12} \\ A_{21} & A_{22} \end{Bmatrix} \begin{Bmatrix} \tilde{P}_v \\ \tilde{Q}_v \end{Bmatrix} \tag{109}$$

With P as the analog of voltage and Q the analog of current, we can use the terminology of the "four-terminal" network theory and call the Z_{ij} *impedances*, the Y_{ij} *conductances*, and the A_{ij} the elements of a *transfer matrix* (i,j = 1 and 2). For example, $Z_{11} = P_a/Q_a$ when $Q_v = 0$; hence it is the impedance between the arterial pressure and arterial flow when oscillation in venous flow is eliminated. $Z_{12} = \tilde{P}_a/\tilde{Q}_v$ when $\tilde{Q}_a = 0$; hence it is the transfer impedance between arterial pressure and venous flow when there is no fluctuation in arterial flow. Other coefficients can be similarly interpreted. The A matrix is the most useful, because with it the capillary network can be inserted between arteries and veins and thus completing the circuit.

It is also instructive to consider the following impedances:

$Z_{oa} = \tilde{P}_a/\tilde{Q}_a$ = input impedance at arteriole with $\tilde{Q}_v = 0$ (open-circuit at venule),

$Z_{ov} = \tilde{P}_v/\tilde{Q}_v$ = input impedance at venule with $\tilde{Q}_a = 0$ (open-circuit at arteriole),

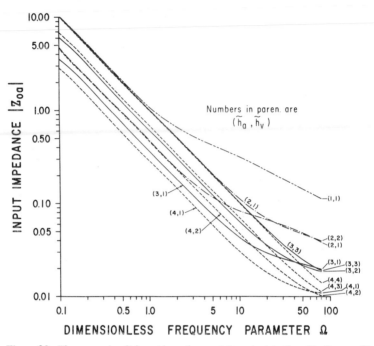

Figure 23. The open-circuit input impedance at the arteriole Z_{oa}. No flow oscillation at the venule end. Absolute value of Z_{oa} versus the frequency parameter. From Fung (1972). Reprinted by permission.

$Z_{sa} = \tilde{P}_a/\tilde{Q}_a$ = input impedance at arteriole when $\tilde{P}_v = 0$ (short-circuit at venule),

$Z_{sv} = \tilde{P}_v/\tilde{Q}_v$ = input impedance at venule when $\tilde{P}_a = 0$ (short-circuit at arteriole)

$$(110)$$

Clearly, we have

$$Z_{oa} = A_{11}/A_{21}, \qquad Z_{ov} = A_{22}/A_{21},$$
$$Z_{sa} = A_{12}/A_{22}, \qquad Z_{sv} = A_{12}/A_{11}$$

$$(111)$$

5.2 Impedance of Two-Dimensional Alveolar Sheets

Let us consider the case in which the arteriole and venule feeding a sheet are essentially parallel; see Figure 18. In this case we choose the x axis

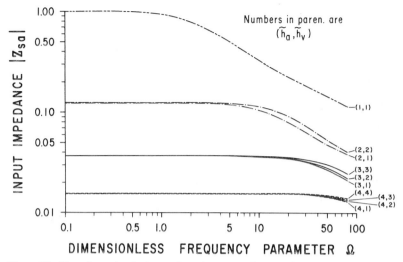

Figure 24. The short-circuit input impedance at the arteriole Z_{sa}. No pressure oscillation at venule end. Absolute value of Z_{sa} versus the frequency parameter. From Fung (1972). Reprinted by permission.

perpendicular to the arteriole and y axis parallel to it. Then all the derivatives with respect to y vanish, and we have (see Section 3.1)

$$\tilde{h}_{SI} = [\tilde{h}_a^4 - (\tilde{h}_a^4 - \tilde{h}_v^4)\tilde{x}]^{1/4} \tag{112}$$

where $\tilde{h}_a$ is the steady-state sheet thickness at the arteriole inlet, $\tilde{h}_v$ is that at the venule outlet (both in units of h_0), and $\tilde{x}$ is the distance measured from the inlet (in units of the length L between the arteriole and venule).

The solution of Eq. 105 is complex-valued and depends on the frequency parameter Ω. Let us write $\tilde{H} = \tilde{H}_R + i\tilde{H}_I$; then

$$(d^2/d\tilde{x}^2)(\tilde{h}_{SI}^3\tilde{H}_R) = -\Omega\tilde{H}_I,$$
$$(d^2/d\tilde{x}^2)(\tilde{h}_{SI}^3\tilde{H}_I) = \Omega\tilde{H}_R \tag{113}$$

Let the fundamental set of solutions $\tilde{H}^{(1)}$ and $\tilde{H}^{(2)}$ be defined by the boundary conditions

$$\tilde{H}_R^{(1)} = \tilde{H}_I^{(1)} = 0, \quad (d/d\tilde{x})(\tilde{h}_{SI}^3\tilde{H}_R^{(1)}) = -1, \quad (d/d\tilde{x})(\tilde{h}_{SI}^3\tilde{H}_I^{(1)}) = 0, \quad \text{at } \tilde{x} = 1$$
$$H_R^{(2)} = \tilde{H}_I^{(2)} = 0, \quad (d/d\tilde{x})(\tilde{h}_{SI}^3\tilde{H}_R^{(2)}) = -1, \quad (d/d\tilde{x})(\tilde{h}_{SI}^3\tilde{H}_I^{(2)}) = 0, \quad \text{at } \tilde{x} = 0 \tag{114}$$

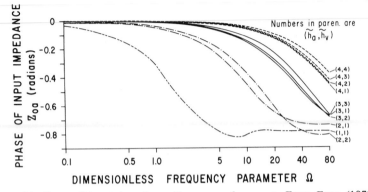

Figure 25. Phase of input impedance Z_{oa} versus frequency. From Fung (1972). Reprinted by permission.

Routine programs for integrating Eq. 105 from initial values specified in Eq. 114 exist in most computing centers. The general solution is a linear combination of these two solutions. The integration constants are determined by the boundary values of pressure at the arteriole inlet and venule outlet of the sheet. The results can be illustrated in Figures 23–26. In

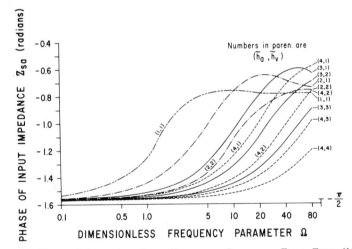

Figure 26. Phase of input impedance Z_{sa} versus frequency. From Fung (1972). Reprinted by permission.

Figures 23 and 24 the absolute values of the input impedances at the arteriole Z_{oa} and Z_{sa} are plotted against the frequency parameter Ω, both in logarithmic scales. Figure 23 refers to open-circuit impedances (no flow oscillation at venous end, $\tilde{Q}_v = 0$). Figure 24 refers to short-circuit impedances (no pressure oscillation at the venous end, $\tilde{P}_v = 0$). The corresponding phase angles of the impedances are plotted against Ω in Figures 25 and 26. The symbol $(\bar{h}_a, \bar{h}_v)$ means the combination of the parameters $\bar{h}_a$ and $\bar{h}_v$. For example, $(2, 1)$ means $\bar{h}_a = 2$, $\bar{h}_v = 1$; $(4, 3)$ means $\bar{h}_a = 4$, $\bar{h}_v = 3$.

We have reduced a very complex problem involving many variables to a dimensionless form involving directly only one parameter, Ω, and indirectly, through $\bar{h}_{SI}$, two parameters, $\bar{h}_a$ and $\bar{h}_v$, which in turn are simply related to the tissue elasticity, sheet structure, and transmural pressures at the arteriole and venule.

The nondimensional parameter Ω is equal to $\mu k f \alpha \omega L^2 / h_0^3$. If $\mu = 0.04$ poise $= 0.04$ dyne·sec/cm^2, $K = 12$, $f = 2.5$, $\alpha = 0.12$ μm/cm H$_2$O $= 0.12 \times 10^{-4}$ cm/(g/cm^2) $= 0.12 \times 10^{-7}$ cm^3/dyne, $L = 250$ μm, $h_0 = 2.5$ μm then

$$\Omega = 0.04 \times 12 \times 2.5 \times 0.12 \times 10^{-7} \left(\frac{250}{2.5}\right)^2 \frac{1}{2.5 \times 10^{-4}} \, 2\pi \times (\text{freq in Hz})$$

$$= 3.62 \times \text{freq in Hz} \tag{115}$$

Hence at 10 Hz the value of Ω is 36.

Further details and extension to three-dimensional cases are presented in Fung (1972).

CONCLUDING REMARKS

The things that we have looked into so far seem to unify quite well around the basic point of view of a red cell moving in an underground garage-like sheet flow. We have tried to introduce a minimum number of hypotheses. The geometry is realistic. The elasticity was measured. The blood viscosity and Reynolds number are pertinent to the mammalian lung. To these we have added only the principles of conservation of mass and momentum. We have observed the rule of economy of hypotheses, but further extension is needed to bring in the realistic particulars of each animal, especially man. Then there remains a very large area of pathologic conditions. Only when these extensions are understood can the theory claim to be useful.

GENERAL REFERENCES

Comroe, Julius H. 1965. Physiology of Respiration. Year Book Medical Publishers, Chicago.

Cumming, G., and S. J. Semple. 1973. Disorders of the Respiratory System. Blackwell Scientific Publishers, London.

Daly, I. de Burgh, and Catherine Hebb. 1966. Pulmonary and Bronchial vascular systems. Williams and Wilkins, Baltimore.

Fenn, W. O., and H. Rahn. 1965. Handbook of Physiology, Section 3. Respiration. 2 Vol. American Physiological Society, Washington, D.C.

Fishman, A. P. 1963. Dynamics of the pulmonary circulation. In W. H. Hamilton and P. Dow (eds.), Handbook of Physiology, Section 2, Vol. II, pp. 1667–1743. American Physiological Society, Washington, D.C.

Fishman, A. P., and H. H. Hecht (eds.), 1968. The Pulmonary Circulation and Interstitial Space. University of Chicago Press, Chicago.

Folkow, B., and E. Neil. 1971. Circulation. Oxford University Press, New York.

Giuntini, O. C. (ed.). 1971. Central Hemodynamics and Gas Exchange: With Emphasis on the Measurement of Pulmonary Extravascular Water. Proc. of a Sym. held in Pisa, May 1970. Minerva Medica, Torino.

Guyton, A. (ed.). 1974. Cardiovascular Physiology. MTP International Review of Science. Physiology. Ser. 1, Vol. 1. University Park Press, Baltimore.

Harris, P., and D. Heath. 1962. The Human Pulmonary Circulation. Williams and Wilkins, Baltimore.

Lighthill, M. J. 1975. Mathematical Biofluiddynamics. Society for Industrial and Applied Mathematics, Philadelphia.

Miller, W. S. 1947. The Lung. Charles C Thomas, Springfield, Ill.

Mountcastle, V. B. (ed.), 1968. Medical Physiology. C. V. Mosby, St. Louis.

Nagaishi, Chuzo. 1972. Functional Anatomy and Histology of the Lung. University Park Press, Baltimore.

von Hayek, H. 1966. The Human Lung. Hefner Publishing, New York.

Weibel, E. R. 1963. Morphometry of the Human Lung. Academic Press, New York.

West, J. B. 1970. Ventilation/Blood Flow and Gas Exchange. 2d Ed. F.A. Davis, Philadelphia.

West, J. B. 1974. Respiratory Physiology–the Essentials. Williams and Wilkins, Baltimore.

Wolstenholme, G. E. W., and Knight, J. (eds.), 1969. Circulatory and Respiratory Mass Transport. Little and Brown, Boston.

Yu, Paul N. 1969. Pulmonary Blood Volume in Health and Disease. Lea & Febiger, Philadelphia.

LITERATURE CITED

Agarwal, J. B., R. Paltoo, and W. A. Palmer. 1970. Relative viscosity of blood at varying hematocrits in pulmonary circulation. J. Appl. Physiol. 29: 866–871.

Bannister, J., and R. W. Torrance. 1960. Effects of the tracheal pressure upon flow: pressure relations in the vascular bed of isolated lungs. Quart. J. Exp. Physiol. 45: 352–367.

Bergel, D. H., and W. R. Milnor. 1965. Pulmonary vascular impedance in the dog. Circ. Res. 16: 401–415.

Chen, P. C. Y., and Y. C. Fung. 1973. Extreme-value statistics of human red blood cells. Microvasc. Res. 6: 32–43.

Cramer, H. 1946. Mathematical methods of statistics. Princeton University Press, Princeton.

Cumming, G., R. Henderson, K. Horsfield, and S. S. Singhal. 1969. The functional morphology of the pulmonary circulation. In A. Fishman and H. Hecht (eds.), The pulmonary circulation and interstitial space. pp. 327–338. University of Chicago Press, Chicago.

Darcy, H. 1856. Les fontaines publiques de la villa de dijon. Dalmont, Paris.

Dawson, S. V., and E. A. Elliott. 1974. Expiratory flow limitation at wave speed. (Abstract). Fed. Proc. 33: 324.

Einstein, A. 1906. Eine neue bestimmung der molekuldimensionen. Ann. Physik. 19: 289–306.

Elias, Hans. 1957. De structura glomeruli renalis. Anat. Anz. 104: 26–36.

Fishman, A. P. 1972. Pulmonary edema: the water-exchanging function of the lung. Circulation 46: 390–408.

Fung, Y. C., and S. S. Sobin. 1967. A sheet-flow concept of the pulmonary alveolar microcirculation: morphometry and theoretical results. 20th Annual Conf. Eng. Med. Biol., Boston, Mass. (Abstr.).

Fung, Y. C. 1969. Studies on the blood flow in the lung. In Proceedings of the Second Canadian Congress of Applied Mechanics, Waterloo, Canada. pp. 433–454.

Fung, Y. C., and S. S. Sobin. 1969. Theory of sheet flow in lung alveoli. J. Appl. Physiol. 26: 472–488.

Fung, Y. C. 1972. Theoretical pulmonary microvascular impedance. Ann. Biomed. Eng. 1: 221–245.

Fung, Y. C. B., and S. S. Sobin. 1972a. Elasticity of the pulmonary alveolar sheet. Circ. Res. 30: 451–469.

Fung, Y. C. B., and S. S. Sobin. 1972b. Pulmonary alveolar blood flow. Circ. Res. 30: 470–490.

Fung, Y. C. 1973. Stochastic flow in capillary blood vessels. Microvasc. Res. 5: 34–48.

Fung, Y. C. 1974. Fluid in the interstitial space of the pulmonary alveolar sheet. Microvasc. Res. 7: 89–113.

Gaar, K. A., A. E. Taylor, L. J. Owens, and A. C. Guyton. 1967.

Pulmonary capillary pressure and filtration coefficient in the isolated perfused lung. Am. J. Physiol. 213: 910–914.

Glazier, J. B., J. M. B. Hughes, J. E. Maloney, and J. B. West. 1967. Vertical gradient of alveolar size in lungs of dogs frozen intact. J. Appl. Physiol. 23: 694–705.

Glazier, J. B., J. M. B. Hughes, J. E. Maloney, and J. B. West. 1969. Measurements of capillary dimensions and blood volume in rapidly frozen lungs. J. Appl. Physiol. 26: 65–76.

Goetzman, B. W., and M. D. Visscher. 1969. The effects of alloxan and histamine on the permeability of the pulmonary alveolocapillary barrier to albumin. J. Physiol. 204: 51–61.

Goldsmith, H. L., and S. G. Mason. 1967. The microrheology of dispersions. In F. R. Eirich (ed.), Rheology, Theory and Applications. Vol. 4, pp. 85–250. Academic Press, New York.

Gregersen, M. I., C. A. Bryant, W. E. Hammerle, S. Usami, and S. Chien. 1967. Flow characteristics of human erythrocytes through polycarbonate sieves. Science 157: 825–827.

Guyton, A. C., and A. W. Lindsey. 1959. Effect of elevated left atrial pressure and decreased plasma protein concentration on the development of pulmonary edema. Circ. Res. 7: 649–657.

Guyton, A. C., H. J. Granger, and A. E. Taylor. 1971. Interstitial fluid pressure. Physiol. Rev. 51: 527–563.

Happel, J., and H. Brenner. 1965. Low Reynolds number hydrodynamics with special application to particulate media. Prentice-Hall, Englewood Cliffs, N.J.

von Hayek, H. 1960. The Human Lung. Translated by V. E. Krahl. Hafner, New York.

Horsfield, K., and G. Cumming. 1968. Morphology of the bronchial tree in man. J. Appl. Physiol. 24: 373–383.

Hughes, J. M. B., J. B. Glazier, J. E. Maloney, and J. B. West. 1968. Effect of extra-alveolar vessels on distribution of blood flow in the dog lung. J. Appl. Physiol. 25: 701–712.

Katchalsky, A., and P. F. Curran. 1965. Nonequilibrium Thermodynamics in Biophysics. Harvard University Press, Cambridge, Mass.

Kenner, T. 1972. Flow and pressure in the arteries. In Y. C. Fung, N. Perrone, and M. Anliker (eds.), Biomechanics: Its Foundations and Objectives. pp. 381–434. Prentice-Hall, Englewood Cliffs, N.J.

Krahl, V. E. 1964. In vivo microscopy of the rabbit's lung. Biblio. Anat., Fasc. 4: 400–410.

Krahl, Vernon E. 1964. Anatomy of the mammalian lung. In W. O. Fenn and H. Rahn (eds.) Handbook of physiology. Section 3, Respiration, Vol. 1, pp. 213–284. American Physiology Society, Washington, D.C.

Lee, J. S., and Y. C. Fung. 1968. Experiments on blood flow in lung alveoli modes. pp. 1–8. Paper No. 68-WA/BHF-2, American Society of Mechanical Engineers.

Lee, J. S. 1969. Slow viscous flow in a lung alveoli model. J. Biomech. 2: 187–198.

Lew, H. S., and Y. C. Fung. 1970. Formulation of a statistical equation of motion of a viscous fluid in an anisotropic non-rigid porous solid. Int. J. Solid Structure 6: 1323–1340.

Lloyd, Thomas C., Jr. 1967. Analysis of the relation of pulmonary arterial or airway conductance to lung volume. J. Appl. Physiol. 23: 887–894.

Lloyd, Thomas C., Jr., and A. J. L. Schneider. 1969. Relation of pulmonary arterial pressure to pressure in the pulmonary venous system. J. Appl. Physiol. 27: 489–497.

Lunde, P. K. M., and B. A. Waaler. 1969. Transvascular fluid balance in the lung. J. Physiol. 205: 1–18.

Maloney, J. E., and B. L. Castle. 1969. Pressure–diameter relations of capillaries and small blood vessels in frog lung. Respir. Physiol. 7: 150–162.

Maseri, A., P. Caldini, S. Permutt, and K. L. Zierler. 1970. Frequency function of transit times through dog pulmonary circulation. Circ. Res. 26: 527–543.

Maseri, A., C. Giuntini, F. Fazio, and A. L'Abbate. 1971. Intravascular pressures and interstitial water space in the lung. In C. Giuntini (ed.), Central Hemodynamics and Gas Exchange. pp. 163–173. Minerva Medica, Turin, Italy.

Maseri, A., P. Caldini, P. Harward, R. C. Joshi, S. Permutt, and K. L. Zierler. 1972. Determinants of pulmonary vascular volume: recruitment versus distensibility. Circ. Res. 31: 218–228.

Milnor, W. R. 1972. Pulmonary hemodynamics. In D. H. Bergel (ed.), Cardiovascular Fluid Dynamics, Vol. 2, pp. 299–340. Academic Press, New York.

Milnor, W. R., D. H. Bergel, and J. D. Bargainer. 1966. Hydraulic power associated with pulmonary blood flow and its relation to heart rate. Circ. Res. 19: 467–480.

Milnor, W. R., C. R. Conti, K. B. Lewis, and M. F. O'Rourke. 1969. Pulmonary arterial pulse wave velocity and impedance in man. Circ. Res. 25: 637–649.

Naimark, A., B. W. Kark, and W. Chernecki. 1971. Regional water volume, blood volume, perfusion of the lung. In C. Giuntini (ed.), Central Hemodynamics and Gas Exchange. pp. 143–160. Minerva Medica, Turin, Italy.

Ogston, A. G., and C. F. Phelps. 1961. The partition of solutes between buffer solutions and solutions containing hyaluronic acid. Biochem. J. 78: 827–833.

Oliver, D. R., and S. G. Ward. 1953. Relationship between relative viscosity and volume concentration of stable suspensions of spherical particles. Nature (London) 171: 396–397.

Patel, D. J., F. M. de Freitas, and D. L. Fry. 1963. Hydraulic input impedance to aorta and pulmonary artery in dogs. J. Appl. Physiol. 18: 134–140.

Permutt, S., B. Bromberger-Barnea, and H. N. Bane. 1962. Alveolar pressure, pulmonary venous pressure, and the vascular waterfall. Med. Thorac. 19: 239—260.

Permutt, S., and R. L. Riley. 1963. Hemodynamics of collapsible vessels with tone: the vascular waterfall. J. Appl. Physiol. 18: 924—932.

Permutt, S., P. Caldini, A. Maseri, W. H. Palmer, T. Sasamori, and K. L. Zierler. 1969. Recruitment versus distensibility in the pulmonary vascular bed. In A. Fishman and H. Hecht (eds.), The Pulmonary Circulation and Interstitial Space. pp. 375—387. University of Chicago Press, Chicago.

Pollack, G. H., R. V. Reddy, and A. Noordegraaf. 1968. Input impedance, wave travel, and reflections in the human pulmonary arterial tree: studies using an electrical analog. IEEE Trans. Biomed. Eng. BME-15, 151—164.

Purday, H. F. P. 1949. An Introduction to the Mechanics of Viscous Flow. Dover, New York. pp. 16—18.

Reid, L. 1967. The embryology of the lung. In A. V. S. de Reuck and R. Porter (eds.), Ciba Foundation Symposium. Little, Brown & Co., Boston. pp. 109—130.

Rhodin, Johannes A. G. 1968. Ultrastructure of mammalian venous capillaries, venules and small collecting veins. J. Ultrastructural Res. 25: 452—500.

Roos, A., L. J. Thomas, Jr., E. L. Nagel, and D. G. Prommas. 1961. Pulmonary vascular resistance as determined by lung inflation and vascular pressures. J. Appl. Physiol. 16: 77—84.

Scheidegger, A. E. 1957. The Physics of Flow Through Porous Media. University of Toronto Press, Toronto.

Schmid-Schoenbein, G. W., Y. C. Fung, and B. W. Zweifach. 1975. Vascular endothelium-leucocyte interaction: sticking shear force in venules. Circ. Res. 36: 173—184.

Schultz, H. 1959. The Submicroscopic Anatomy and Pathology of the Lung. Springer, Berlin.

Skalak, R. 1969. Wave propagation in the pulmonary circulation. In A. P. Fishman and H. H. Hecht (eds.), The Pulmonary Circulation and Interstitial Space. pp. 361—373. University of Chicago Press, Chicago.

Sobin, S. S. 1965. The vascular injection method and the functional geometry of the microcirculation. In Symposium on Vascular Diseases of the Eye. Investigative Ophthalmology 4: 1105—1110.

Sobin, S. S. 1966. Vascular injection methods, p. 233—238. In R. F. Rushmer (ed.), Methods in Medical Research. Vol. 11, pp. 233—238. Year Book, Chicago.

Sobin, S. S., M. Intaglietta, W. G. Frasher, and H. M. Tremer. 1966. The geometry of the pulmonary microcirculation. Angiology 17: 24—30.

Sobin, S. S., and Herta M. Tremer. 1966. Functional geometry of the microcirculation. Fed. Proc. 25: 1744—1752.

Sobin, S. S., H. M. Tremer, and Y. C. Fung. 1970. The morphometric basis of the sheet-flor concept of the pulmonary alveolar microcirculation in the cat. Circ. Res. 26: 397—414.

Sobin, S. S., Y. C. Fung, H. M. Tremer, and T. H. Rosenquist. 1972. Elasticity of the pulmonary alveolar microvascular sheet in the cat. Circ. Res. 30: 440–450.

Starling, E. H. 1896. On the absorption of fluid from the connective tissue spaces. J. Physiol. 19: 312–326.

Starling, E. H. 1918. The Linacre Lecture on the Law of the Heart, given at Cambridge, 1915. Longmans, Green & Co., London. 27 pp. *In* C. B. Chapman and J. H. Mitchell (eds.), Starling on the Heart (facs. reprints). Dawsons, London, 1965.

Staub, N. C., H. Nagano, and M. L. Pearce. 1967. Pulmonary edema in dogs, especially the sequence of fluid accumulation in lungs. J. Appl. Physiol. 22: 227–240.

Staub, N. C., and E. L. Schultz. 1968. Pulmonary capillary length in dog, cat and rabbit. Resp. Physiol. 5: 371–378.

Staverman, A. J. 1951. The theory of measurement of osmotic pressure. Rec. Trav. Chim. 70: 344–352.

Tancredi, R., and K. L. Zierler. 1971. Indicator-dilution, flow-pressure and volume-pressure curves in excised dog lung. Fed. Proc. 30: 380 (Abstr.).

Tang, H. T., and Y. C. Fung. 1975. Fluid movement in a channel with permeable walls covered by porous media (a model of lung alveolar sheet). J. Appl. Mech. 42: 45–50.

Wagenvoort, C. A., D. Heath, and J. E. Edwards. 1964. The pathology of the pulmonary vasculature. Charles C Thomas, Springfield, Ill.

Wagner, W. W., Jr., and L. P. Latham. 1975. Pulmonary capillary recruitment with hypoxia in the dog. J. Appl. Physiol. 39: 900–905.

Wearn, J. T., A. C. Ernstene, A. W. Bromer, J. S. Barr, W. J. German, and L. J. Zschiesche. 1934. Normal behavior of the pulmonary blood vessels with observations on the intermittence of the flow of blood in the arterioles and capillaries. Am. J. Physiol. 109: 236–256.

Weibel, E. R., and R. A. Vidone. 1961. Fixation of the lung by formalin stream in a controlled state of air inflation. Am. Rev. Respir. Dis. 84: 856–861.

Weibel, E. R. 1963. Morphometry of the Human Lung. Academic Press, New York. p. 124.

West, J. B. 1970. Ventilation/Blood Flow and Gas Exchange. 2d Ed. F.A. Davis, Philadelphia.

West, J. B., C. T. Dollery, and A. Naimark. 1964. Distribution of blood flow in isolated lung; relation to vascular and alveolar pressure. J. Appl. Physiol. 19: 713–724.

West, J. B., and C. T. Dollery. 1965. Distribution of blood flow and the pressure–flow relations of the whole lung. J. Appl. Physiol. 20: 175–183.

West, J. B., C. T. Dollery, C. M. E. Matthews, and P. Zardini. 1965. Distribution of blood flow and ventilation in saline-filled lung. J. Appl. Physiol. 20: 1107–1117.

West, John B., Alan M. Schneider, and Mark M. Mitchell. 1975. Recruitment in networks of pulmonary capillaries. J. Appl. Physiol. 39: 976–984.

Wiederhielm, C. A. 1968. Dynamics of transcapillary fluid exchange. J. Gen. Physiol. 52: 29–63.

Wiederhielm, C. A. 1971. The interstitial space. *In* Y. C. Fung, N. Perrone, and M. Anliker (eds.), Biomechanics. pp. 273–286. Prentice-Hall, Englewood Cliffs, N.J.

Wiener, F., E. Morkin, R. Skalak, and A. P. Fishman. 1966. Wave propagation in the pulmonary circulation. Circ. Res. 19: 834–850.

Womersley, J. R. 1955. Oscillatory motion of a viscous liquid in a thin-walled elastic tube: I. The linear approximation for long waves. Phil. Mag. 46: 199–221.

Yen, M. R. T., and Y. C. Fung. 1972. Apparent viscosity of blood in pulmonary alveolar sheet. Presented at the 2nd Annual Meeting of the Society of Biomedical Engineering, April 7, 1972. Baltimore, Md.

Yen, Rong-Tsu, and Yuan-Cheng Fung. 1973. Model experiments on apparent blood viscosity and hematocrit in pulmonary alveoli. J. Appl. Physiol. 35: 510–517.

Zweifach, B. W., and M. Intaglietta. 1968. Mechanics of fluid movement across single capillaries in the rabbit. Microvasc. Res. 1: 83–101.

Cardiovascular Flow Dynamics and Measurements
Edited by N. H. C. Hwang and N. A. Normann
Copyright 1977   University Park Press   Baltimore

chapter 18

DRUG ACTIONS ON CARDIOVASCULAR DYNAMICS

Joseph P. Buckley, Regis R. Vollmer,
Mustafa Lokhandwala, and Bhagavan S. Jandhyala

ABSTRACT

Chemicals can affect cardiovascular dynamics by modifying the activity of various sites within the central nervous system, as well as by affecting various peripheral components of the cardiovascular system. For example, interference with ganglionic transmission can markedly lower blood pressure and modify flow to various organ systems. Compounds acting directly on α- and/or β-adrenergic receptors can affect both myocardial activity and the tone of various vascular beds. Hormones such as angiotensin II can affect vascular tone and cardiac activity through direct actions and via the central nervous system. Recently, there have been several reports supporting the existence of central α-adrenergic mechanisms that produce a sympathoinhibitory function, and both α-methyldopa and clonidine appeared to produce a decrease in blood pressure through stimulation of these receptors. In addition, α-methyldopa appears to inhibit sympathetic activity peripherally, thereby altering cardiovascular dynamics. Prolonged administration of compounds interfering with adrenergic neuronal transmission such as reserpine and guanethidine produce effects in cardiovascular function that are markedly different from those obtained on acute administration.

INTRODUCTION

Chemicals can affect cardiovascular dynamics by modifying the activity of various sites within the central nervous system, as well as by directly affecting various components of the cardiovascular system.

Arterial blood pressure can be considered to be a summation of cardiac

731

output, that is, the amount of blood ejected by the left ventricle in a given period of time, and peripheral resistance, that is, intravascular volume or arterial tone. Arterial smooth muscle lacks the intrinsic tone found in other smooth muscle structures and depends upon continuous bombardment by the sympathetic division of the autonomic nervous system to maintain the arterial tone necessary for the regulation of arterial blood pressure. The myocardium, on the other hand, possesses both intrinsic tone and contractility; however, both the tone and the rate and contractile force are modified by the autonomic nervous system. In addition, both the vasculature and the myocardium are greatly influenced by reflexogenic mechanisms. Drugs can interfere with autonomic activity and thereby greatly modify cardiovascular dynamics. For example, compounds that interfere with ganglionic transmission, such as the bisquaternary ammonium compounds (pentolinium, chlorisondamine, trimethidinium) and mecamylamine, lower arterial blood pressure through a specific paralysis of transmission at ganglionic synapses. Since the tone of the vasculature is maintained by sympathetic activity, the result is an inhibition of this activity and dilation of arterial vasculature. The mechanism of action is that of competitive inhibition in that these compounds block impulses at autonomic ganglia by raising the threshold of the ganglion cells to acetylcholine release at preganglionic nerve endings.

Because the compounds inhibit all autonomic ganglia, the parasympathetic division is also blocked. As the arterial blood pressure drops, the baroreceptors in the carotid sinus area and the aortic arch are activated; impulses forwarded to the medulla oblongata result in an increase in sympathetic outflow from the central nervous system. However, because the efferent outflow involves two neurons, that is, the preganglionic and postganglionic sympathetic fibers, reflexogenic activity is blocked.

Compounds can alter vascular tone by affecting postganglionic adrenergic neuronal activity. Reserpine and other rauwolfia alkaloids deplete peripheral stores of catecholamines and thereby interfere with sympathetic neuronal transmission. Although reserpine releases large quantities of norepinephrine, the sympathetic activity is not enhanced, because the norepinephrine passively diffuses from its storage sites within the neuronal endings and is deaminated by monoamine oxidase. Available data suggest that reserpine acts through at least three specific mechanisms: (1) the depletion of norepinephrine from peripheral binding sites, thus producing sympathetic blockade; (2) depression of central sympathetic outflow and stimulation of parasympathetic central outflow due to central depletion of catecholamines; and (3) central nervous system depression producing a decrease in tension and aggressiveness as well as a decreased response of the sympathetic centers to external stimuli.

Guanethidine also interferes with sympathetic transmission through the vasculature by releasing norepinephrine from peripheral sympathetic neurons. Because the compound does not pass the blood–brain barrier, it has little or no effect on norepinephrine stores in the brain. The compound accumulates in peripheral sympathetic neuronal endings, thereby blocking the release of the neuronal transmitter, norepinephrine, and to some extent inhibits the re-uptake of norepinephrine. The effects of prolonged administration of these compounds are most complex and are discussed in detail later in this chapter. The peripheral α-adrenergic receptors can be selectively blocked by α-adrenergic receptor blocking agents such as phentolamine or phenoxybenzamine, thereby blocking the action of the sympathetic neuronal transmitter, norepinephrine, and thereby producing a relaxation of vascular smooth muscle, resulting in a decrease in peripheral resistance and a marked drop in blood pressure.

Compounds such as phenylephrine and levo-norepinephrine directly stimulate α-adrenergic receptors, inducing vasoconstriction and a marked increase in arterial blood pressure.

β-Adrenergic stimulants such as isoxyprine and nylidrin stimulate both β_1 and β_2 receptors, thereby producing vasodilation, an increase in heart rate, and an increase in cardiac output, resulting in a marked increase in blood flow to practically every organ. On the other hand β-adrenergic blockers such as propranolol produce a marked decrease in cardiac rate as well as a decrease in cardiac output. It would be expected that a blockade of β-adrenergic receptors in the vasculature would produce vasoconstriction; however, propranolol produces a decrease in peripheral resistance, probably due to a mechanism unrelated to β-adrenergic blockade.

Many anticholinergic compounds such as atropine and probanthine, which are commonly used to decrease gastrointestinal activity, especially in the treatment of gastric or duodenal ulcers, produce a marked increase in cardiac rate by inhibiting vagal activity.

Because the control of the cardiovascular system is extremely complex, many of the actions of chemicals, whether endogenous or exogenous, are also complex and in many instances unpredictable. The compensatory mechanisms, such as reflexogenic control of the cardiovascular system, autoregulatory mechanisms, blood volume, and salt and water metabolism, must also be taken into consideration; alterations in intrarenal dynamics are of utmost importance when considering the effects of drugs on the cardiovascular system. For example, such compounds as guanethidine and hydrochlorothiazide produce a drop in blood pressure but increase the production of renin by the kidney. It is not the purpose of this chapter to discuss the complete pharmacologic actions and mechanisms of actions of the various drugs that affect cardiovascular dynamics. Because of the complexities of these effects and the particular interests of the authors, this discussion is limited to the effects of certain endogenous peptides and catecholamines on central and peripheral receptors and to the effects of some of the more recent compounds on the renin-angiotensin system and adrenergic receptors.

RENIN–ANGIOTENSIN SYSTEM

Renin, a proteolytic enzyme having no inherent pressor activity, is synthesized, stored, and secreted by the juxtaglomerular apparatus of the kidney. The enzyme then acts upon angiotensinogen, a glycoprotein synthesized in the liver to form the decapeptide, angiotensin I. Angiotensin I is then hydrolyzed by the converting enzyme to produce the octapeptide, angiotensin II, which is rapidly destroyed, mainly in peripheral capillary beds by angiotensinases (Oparil and Haber, 1974). Angiotensin II produces a marked increase in peripheral vascular resistance due to a direct constriction of the vascular smooth muscle. The octapeptide also produces an increase in the synthesis and release of aldosterone and therefore plays a major role in electrolyte and water metabolism.

Angiotensin II has generally been accepted as the major active hormone of the renin–antiotensin system; however, evidence has been obtained suggesting that angiotensin I also possesses physiologic activity. Peach (1971) reported that angiotensin I released adrenal catecholamines, and Solomon and Buckley (1974) suggested that angiotensin I may stimulate receptors within the central nervous system, inducing pressor effects. Goodfriend et al. (1971) suggested that the des-1-heptapeptide metabolite of angiotensin II was biologically active, and this compound has been shown to increase aldosterone synthesis and secretion (Blair-West et al., 1971).

Although the renin-angiotensin system has been implicated in the pathogenesis of essential hypertension, there has been little correlation between the concentration of angiotensin II in plasma and the blood pressure of essential hypertensive patients (Sealey et al., 1973). The complex actions of angiotensin were critically reviewed by Page and

Bumpus (1961); it is interesting to note, however, that in this excellent comprehensive review, there is little indication that there was an interaction between this polypeptide and the autonomic nervous system. Based on the data available at that time, these reviewers stated, "most investigators agree that angiotensin has a strong peripheral vasoconstrictor action and no action on the central nervous system."

Bickerton and Buckley (1961) first suggested that angiotensin II could possibly influence cardiovascular dynamics via a central mechanism. Angiotensin II in doses ranging between 0.2 and 4.0 μg/kg administered via the carotid inflow to the vascularly isolated, neurally intact recipient's head in dog cross-circulation preparations, produced pressor effects in the recipient's trunk that were approximately 40% of those obtained in the donor dog. The pressor responses to the polypeptide, 1 μg/kg, administered centrally, were blocked by the administration of piperoxan, an α-adrenergic blocker, 0.2–1.0 mg/kg, administered via the recipient's femoral vein (Buckley et al., 1963). These preliminary experiments suggested that angiotensin II stimulated central structures, resulting in an increase in sympathetic outflow from the central nervous system that was apparently responsible for the observed increase in systemic blood pressure. Halliday and Buckley (1962) reported that angiotensin II in doses of 1 μg/kg administered via the carotid inflow to the recipient's head, or femoral vein of the donor dog following bilateral denervation of the carotid sinus-body complex, produced consistent pressor responses in the recipient animal. Because vasopressin, 0.1 μg/kg, failed to induce hypertensive effects in the recipient animal when administered via the carotid inflow to the recipient's head (Buckley et al., 1963), it seems that the centrally induced pressor effects of angiotensin II were the result neither of cerebral vasoconstriction, nor of effects on the baro- or chemoreceptors. The cat lateral ventricle preparation, described by Bhattacharya and Feldberg (1958), was utilized to further study the central effects of angiotensin II and to identify possible sites of action of the peptide. The administration of angiotensin II, in doses ranging from 0.1 to 4.0 μg via the cerebral ventricular system (I.V.T.) in α-chlorolose anesthetized cats, produced dose-related hypertensive effects (Smookler et al., 1966). The minimal effective dose was 0.01 μg, which produced a mean increase in systolic blood pressure of 19 ± 5 mm Hg. Angiotensin II, 0.05 μg, produced a mean increase in systolic blood pressure of 21 mm Hg and 0.1 μg produced an increase of 35 mm Hg. Two micrograms of the peptide produced pressor effects of 45 mm Hg and, although there was no

significant difference between the pressor effects produced by doses ranging from 0.5 to 4.0 μg of angiotensin II, the 4-μg dose was used to
investigate the possible site of action of the peptide. Angiotensin II, in
doses of 2–4 μg administered I.V.T. to α-chlorolose anesthetized cats,
increased systolic and diastolic blood pressure and heart rate and induced a
contraction of the nictitating membrane (Smookler et al., 1966). C-1
section of the spinal cord essentially abolished response to I.V.T. administered angiotensin, further suggesting that the hypertensive effects were due
to a central action of angiotensin II. The administration of 4 μg of
angiotensin II I.V.T. to 32 α-chlorolose anesthetized cats produced an increase in systolic and diastolic blood pressure of 60 ± 4 and 45 ± 3 mm Hg,
respectively (Severs et al., 1966). Phenoxybenzamine, an α-adrenergic
blocker, administered via the femoral vein in a dosage of 5 mg/kg, significantly attenuated the pressor effect induced by I.V.T. administration of
angiotensin II, further confirming the hypothesis that the centrally
induced hypertensive effects of angiotensin II were due to stimulation of
central sympathetic structures. The intravenous administration of P-286
(N,N-diisopropyl-N'-isoamyl-N'-diethylaminoethylurea)   or   pronetholol
significantly reduced the hypertensive effects of I.V.T. administered angiotensin II. The inhibition of the pressor effects by pronetholol, a β-adrenergic blocking compound, could possibly be due to an inhibition of
neurogenically induced release of renin by the kidney. Cerveau Isolé
transsection abolished the centrally induced pressor response to angiotensin II. Cannulation of the cerebral aqueduct markedly attenuated the
pressor response to the peptide, suggesting that the central action of
angiotensin II, administered I.V.T., originates when the peptide leaves the
third ventricle and enters the aqueduct and the fourth ventricle. Angiotensin II failed to produce an increase in arterial blood pressure when
administered into the posterior hypothalamus in doses up to 0.5 μg (Severs
et al., 1966). These results suggested a midbrain site of the central pressor
responses to angiotensin II when the peptide was administered via the
lateral ventricles. Severs, Daniels, and Buckley (1967) investigated the
effects of I.V.T. administration of angiotensin prior to and following gross
midbrain lesions and confirmed this hypothesis because the pressor activity was essentially abolished by this procedure.

Deuben and Buckley (1970) administered, in α-chlorolose anesthetized
cats, 4 μg of angiotensin II into the aqueduct of Sylvius, 6 and 5 mm
anterior to Horsley–Clarke Zero and reported that the peptide produced
mean pressor effects of 46 and 42 mm Hg, respectively. In a separate

group of animals, the administration of the peptide 4 or 3 mm anterior to Horsley–Clarke Zero produced significantly lower pressor effects, 18 and 11 mm Hg, respectively. These results indicated that a central site of action of angiotensin II was located in the peri-aqueductal gray region of the mesencephalon between 4 and 5 mm anterior to Horsley–Clarke Zero.

Additional experiments were undertaken in which bilateral lesions were made within the peri-aqueductal gray, 4 mm anterior to Horsley–Clarke Zero. The lesions significantly reduced pressor responses produced from the I.V.T. administration of angiotensin II, whereas similar lesions placed 1 mm caudal (3 mm anterior to Horsley–Clarke Zero) did not significantly affect the pressor response (Deuben and Buckley, 1970). The subnucleus medialis of the peri-aqueductal gray was thus identified as one of the sites of action of angiotensin II within the central nervous system. This synaptic area is in close proximity to the aqueduct, and the pathway has been shown by Enoch and Kerr (1967*a,b*) to be functionally involved with the control of systemic peripheral resistance. This pathway turns abruptly in the lateral direction after synapsing in the subnucleus medialis; therefore, lesions placed below this area would not be expected to disrupt these tracts. The intrinsic pressor pathway arises in the medial, posterior region of the hypothalamus. It projects via the peri-ventricular system to the peri-aqueductal gray, pretectal and superior collicular areas, where it synapses and relays laterally to the deep tegmental nucleus of the mid-brain (Enoch and Kerr, 1967*b*).

Studies were undertaken to investigate the effects of SQ 20,881 (pyrrolididone carboxylic acid-L-tryptophyl-L-arginyl-L-prolyl-L-glutaminyl-L-isoleucyl-L-prolyl-L-proline), an inhibitor of the converting enzyme, on certain actions of angiotensin I and angiotensin II (Solomon, Cavero, and Buckley, 1974). The intravenous infusion of SQ 20,881 (100 μg or 500 μg/kg/min) produced significant inhibitory effects on the pressor responses to intravenously administered angiotensin I (0.5, 1.0, and 2.0 μg/kg) but had little effect on the hypertensive responses to angiotensin Ii (0.5, 1.0, and 2.0 μg/kg). The lower dose produced a 60.4% and the higher dose a 96.7% inhibition of the angiotensin I pressor effect. The I.V.T. administration of SQ 20,881 produced qualitatively similar effects on the hypertensive activity of angiotensin I as seen in studies of peripheral actions; however, the compound also inhibited the centrally induced pressor responses of angiotensin II. The intraventricular infusion of 100 μg/kg/min of SQ 20,881 inhibited the pressor response to angiotensin I an average of 77.6%, and the 500 mg/kg/min dose produced a 92%

inhibition. However, the inhibitor in these doses also decreased angiotensin II activity by 77.5% and 88.2% respectively. The pressor activity produced by the intraventricular infusion of angiotensin II was antagonized approximately to the same degree as that produced by angiotensin I in α-chlorolose anesthetized cats. Because the compound did not attenuate the peripheral effects of angiotensin II, it seems that the inhibition of the centrally elicited pressor effects of angiotensin II by SQ 20,881 is selective to the central nervous system receptor sites. Therefore, although the converting enzyme inhibitors have not been reported to have any effects other than blocking conversion of angiotensin I to angiotensin II, the data obtained in these studies suggest that the activity of these compounds may be more complex. If angiotensin I is in itself an active peptide and possibly important in the development of essential hypertension, then the inhibitor of the converting enzyme could be acting by inhibition of the "receptors" of angiotensin I and angiotensin II. SQ 20,881 had, by itself, no effect on mean blood pressure, nor any responses to vagal stimulation, stimulation of the innervation to the nictitating membrane, acetylcholine, bilateral carotid occlusion, or epinephrine (Solomon et al., 1974).

Saralasin acetate (1-sar-8-ala-angiotensin II) was studied for a possible inhibitory effect on the central hypertensive activity of angiotensin I and II (Solomon and Buckley, 1974). Saralasin acetate, 1.0 and 5.0 μg/kg/min, i.v., significantly attenuated the pressor effects of intravenously administered angiotensin I and angiotensin II (0.1–1.0 μg/kg) in α-chlorolose anesthetized cats. The percent inhibition of the pressor responses to angiotensin I and angiotensin II was almost identical. The I.V.T. infusion of saralasin acetate markedly attenuated the centrally induced pressor effects of both angiotensin I and angiotensin II (0.25–2.0 μg/kg). Saralasin acetate, 1.0 μg/kg/min, produced a mean inhibition of the pressor effect of I.V.T. administered angiotensin I of 48.5% and 5.0 μg/kg/min produced a mean inhibition of 83.5%. The pressor effects of angiotensin II were reduced 84.9% and 98.1% respectively. Analyzed statistically, the data demonstrated that the antagonistic action of saralasin acetate (in the lower dose) was significantly greater ($p < 0.01$) against angiotensin II than against angiotensin I. The fact that angiotensin I retained some of its activity, whereas the activity of angiotensin II is almost abolished, supports the hypothesis that angiotensin I possesses activity independent of that of angiotensin II within the central nervous system.

Extremely minute doses of angiotensin II perfused via the vertebral artery of cats (Keim and Sigg, 1971; Buckley, 1972; Gyang, Deuben, and

Buckley, 1973), dogs (Gildenberg, 1969, 1971), and rabbits (Yu and Dickinson, 1965) have been reported to produce marked pressor effects. Gildenberg (1969) demonstrated that sectioning of the dog's brain stem at the level of the mesencephalon did not alter the response to angiotensin administered via the vertebral arteries. The blood flow distribution by the vertebral arteries was altered by successively lower ligations of the basilar artery, exposed through the roof of the dog's mouth. The application of a silver clip at the lower-most portion of the basilar artery eliminated the pressor response. Gildenberg concluded that the area responsible for the central effects of angiotensin II administered via the vertebral artery was in the lower medulla. Gildenberg, Ferrario, and McCubbin (1973) infused angiotensin II into both vertebral arteries of anesthetized dogs and into the ventricular perfusion system. The pressor response to perfusion of angiotensin II into the vertebral arteries was immediately and permanently abolished by cauterization of the area postrema. Infusion of angiotensin II via the vertebral arteries following transsection of the midbrain at the level of the tentorium, instead of destroying the area postrema, failed to alter the pressor response produced by centrally administered angiotensin II. Heat coagulation of the area postrema did not alter the pressor response induced by administration of the peptide via the cerebral lateral ventricles, whereas transsection of the midbrain eliminated the pressor effect induced by intraventricular administration of the peptide. These studies indicated that there are at least two separate areas in the dog brain that respond to angiotensin, causing a rise in arterial pressure, and that the route of administration of angiotensin determines which is stimulated. The area of the midbrain responds when angiotensin is infused into the lateral ventricle, because the response is abolished when the midbrain sensors are lesioned, but not when the area postrema is destroyed. Conversely, the pressor response to perfusion of angiotensin into the vertebral arteries is eliminated by destruction of the area postrema, but not by transsection of the midbrain.

COMPOUNDS ACTING ON CENTRAL α-ADRENERGIC RECEPTORS

There have been several reports supporting the existence of central α-adrenergic mechanisms that produce sympathoinhibition (Heise and Kroneberg, 1972; van Zweiten, 1973). Phentolamine, a competitive α-receptor antagonist, perfused at rates of 50, 100, or 200 $\mu g/min$ via the lateral ventricles of α-chlorolose anesthetized cats for a period of 30 min, produced a dose-related reduction in blood pressure (Vollmer et al., 1975). The decrease in blood pressure occurred within 5 min, was maximal at the termination of the 30-min infusion period, and was not associated with significant changes in heart rate. The pressure slowly returned to control levels following cessation of the perfusion, and the duration of the depressor effect was greatest with the highest dose used. There was no evidence of measurable peripheral α-adrenergic blockade with the two lower doses; norepinephrine pressor response and contractions of the nictitating membrane to neuronal stimulation were not altered. Therefore, it is likely that the observed depressor response produced by the two lower doses was of central origin and not due to passage of the compound from the central nervous system into the peripheral circulation. Angiotensin II administration, following phentolamine perfusion, resulted in a potentiated pressor response. The three dose levels of phentolamine were equally effective in potentiating the pressor response to centrally administered angiotensin II.

Further studies involving perfusion of specific areas of the ventricular system revealed that confinement of the α-adrenergic blocker to cerebrospinal spaces rostral to the midbrain (by aqueductal cannulation) diminished the hypotensive effects observed when the entire system was perfused. When the perfusion was limited to areas caudal to the midbrain, the depressor response was not attenuated. Perfusion from a cannula placed in the cerebellar system, superior to the cisterna magna, also resulted in a depressor response equal to that obtained when the entire lateral ventricular system was perfused. Therefore, it can be concluded that the depressor response induced by the administration of phentolamine centrally is not entirely a result of an action on structures reached from the ventricular system, but appears to be mainly due to effects on sites in the ventral medulla or pons.

Centrally administered phentolamine markedly attenuated the reflex bradycardia elicited by intravenous administration of norepinephrine and angiotensin II. Because the centrally induced hypertensive effects of angiotensin II were enhanced by phentolamine also in vagotomized cats, it is unlikely that the blockade of reflexogenic bradycardia by centrally administered phentolamine could account for the enhanced response to angiotensin. On the other hand, the antagonistic effects of phentolamine on other cardiovascular reflexes may be an important factor in the enhancement of the centrally induced pressor activity of angiotensin II, because the intraventricular perfusion of phentolamine significantly diminished the reflex hypotensive and bradycardic responses to carotid sinus nerve stimulation in vagotomized cats (Buckley and Vollmer, 1975). The results of these studies suggest that central α-adrenergic mechanisms may functionally inhibit the centrally induced hypertensive effects of angiotensin II administered via the lateral ventricles. When these receptors are blocked by phentolamine there is a potentiation of the centrally induced pressor effects of angiotensin II. Similarly, the antagonistic effects produced by centrally administered norepinephrine to angiotensin II administered via the lateral ventricles, described by Smookler et al. (1966), may be explained by the activation of a sympathoinhibitory system by norepinephrine.

Two compounds, namely, clonidine and α-methyldopa, have been shown to produce hypotensive effects mainly through stimulation of central α-adrenergic receptors (van Zweiten, 1973).

α-Methyldopa

α-Methyldopa is a competitive inhibitor of amino acid decarboxylase (Sourkes, 1954) and was originally designed as a potential hypotensive agent that would deplete neuronal endings of norepinephrine by inhibiting the synthesis of this neural transmitter. Hess et al. (1961) demonstrated that α-methyldopa produced prolonged depletion of norepinephrine from the brain and myocardium of guinea pigs which could not be attributed simply to inhibition of norepinephrine synthesis. Subsequently, Levine and Sjoerdsma (1964) demonstrated that decarboxylase inhibition does not decrease tissue norepinephrine levels and that α-methyldopa is dependent on its decarboxylation to the amine for its pharmacologic and norepinephrine-depleting effects. Both methyldopamine and methylnorepinephrine were identified in the brains of α-methyldopa treated animals (Carlson and Lindquist, 1962; Porter, Totaro, and Borcin, 1965; Torchiana et al., 1965), and methylnorepinephrine has been identified in the hearts of mice and rats (Porter et al., 1965; Torchiana et al., 1965). These data suggested that methylnorepinephrine could be the principal amine involved in peripheral structures, while both amines could be involved in action on central structures. It is difficult to explain the hypotensive action of α-methyldopa by inhibition of dopa decarboxylase or the production of α-methylnorepinephrine and its activity as a false transmitter. α-Methylnorepinephrine is also an α-adrenergic receptor stimulant and therefore can act on central α-receptors. Henning and van Zweiten (1968) reported that α-methyldopa has a central depressor effect because the hypotension produced by administration via the vertebral artery was much greater than when the compound was administered intravenously. Heise and Kroneberg (1972, 1973), using perfused cerebral ventricular preparation of the cat, demonstrated that perfusion with methyldopa, methyldopamine, methylnorepinephrine, or norepinephrine produced a significant decrease in systemic blood pressure. They also reported that the blood pressure lowering effects of these amines were inhibited or abolished by perfusion with phentolamine or yohimbine, α-adrenergic blockers. These data led the authors to postulate that there are α-adrenergic receptors in the brain capable of mediating hypotensive effects upon stimulation. van Zweiten (1973) stated that the central adrenergic receptors are connected to an inhibitory neuron (possibly the bulbospinal sympathetic neuron), the activation of which brings about the depression of the peripheral sympathetic nervous system and thus a fall in blood pressure.

Finch and Haeusler (1973) found that the hypotensive effects of α-methyldopa (300 mg/kg, i.p.) could be prevented or reversed by I.V.T. administration of phentolamine (200 μg) in conscious, genetically hypertensive rats. Destruction of central sympathetic neurons by the administration of 6-hydroxydopamine intraventricularly prevented the hypotensive action of α-methyldopa whereas intravenous administration of 6-hydroxydopamine reduced, but did not prevent, the depressor effects. Finch and Haeusler concluded that the central actions of α-methyldopa were important to the hypotensive effect, although a possible peripheral effect could not be excluded.

Day, Roach, and Whiting (1973) observed that methyldopa administered to hypertensive rats produced a marked depressor effect that was not affected by peripheral dopa decarboxylase inhibition, but that was abolished by simultaneous central and peripheral inhibition of dopa decarboxylase. Administration of α-methyldopa into the cerebral ventricles of hypertensive rats produced marked depressor effects at a dose level that was 1% of that used systemically. The authors concluded that methyldopa reduced blood pressure by a central mechanism involving the production of methylnorepinephrine. Day and Roach (1974a) reported that although methylnorepinephrine infused into the lateral cerebral ventricles of conscious cats was equipotent to norepinephrine in inducing both hypotensive effects and bradycardia, the response to methylnorepinephrine was of much longer duration. This observation led the authors to postulate that this longer duration of action of the false transmitter on central α-receptors might make it more, rather than less, effective as a neurotransmitter, which would then bring about the observed hypotension following the administration of α-methyldopa (Day and Roach, 1974b). The experimental data available suggest that central α-adrenergic inhibitory receptors play an extremely important role in the mechanism by which α-methyldopa reduces systemic blood pressure.

Stone and Porter (1966) reviewed the effects of α-methyldopa on adrenergic nerve function and indicated that even large doses of methyldopa do not markedly interfere with responses to adrenergic nerve stimulation in laboratory animals. Malik and Muscholl (1969) found that pretreatment of rats with 100 mg/kg of α-methyldopa i.p., 44 hr and 18–20 hr before the experiment, decreased responses of the isolated perfused mesenteric artery preparation to electrical stimulation of the periarterial adrenergic nerves. The sensitivity of the vessels to infused norepinephrine was unaltered. Although peripheral impairment of adrenergic transmission by α-methyldopa on resistance vessels was demonstrated, these investigators indicated that it was still questionable whether this site of action is primarily responsible for the antihypertensive action of the compound. Salmon and Ireson (1970) also demonstrated that α-methyldopa caused a significant depression of peripheral sympathetic function in anesthetized rats, and that this impairment of sympathetic function had the same temporal pattern as the hypotension induced in conscious animals. These authors also concluded that, although methyldopa depresses peripheral sympathetic function, this action probably plays only a minor role in the overall hypotensive effect of the compound. Other investigators (Doxey and Scutt, 1974) reported that pressor responses induced by stimulation of the entire sympathetic outflow in the pithed rat were unaffected by acute dosage with α-methyldopa, 200 mg/kg, i.p., but significantly reduced on subchronic dosage. They also concluded that it was most unlikely that impairment of peripheral sympathetic nervous transmission plays a significant part in the observed hypotensive effects of α-methyldopa. Equipressor effects with α-methylnorepinephrine could only be achieved when the dose used in the pithed rat was twice that of norepinephrine. Kelly and Burks (1974) reported that α-methylnorepinephrine was 0.3 as potent as norepinephrine in raising blood pressure in anesthetized adult mongrel dogs.

Lokhandwala and co-workers (1975a,b) investigated the effects of α-methyldopa on regional hemodynamics and peripheral sympathetic nerve function in the dog. Administration of α-methyldopa, 100 mg/kg, p.o., twice daily for 3 days produced a significant decrease in mean blood pressure, heart rate, and renal vascular resistance and significantly impaired sympathetic neuronal function to the myocardium, hind leg vasculature, and the kidney. Chronotropic responses to cardioaccelerator nerve stimulation as well as vasoconstrictor responses to lumbar sympathetic nerve and renal nerve stimulation were significantly attenuated in the treated dogs. Pressor and chronotropic responses to bilateral carotid occlusion and to tyramine were also attenuated in the α-methyldopa treated animals. The decrease in the resting blood pressure, heart rate, and renal vascular resistance observed in the treated dogs was attributed to a reduction in the sympathetic neuronal function. These investigators found that methylnorepinephrine was significantly less potent than norepinephrine in producing an increase in mean blood pressure and in hind leg and renal vascular resistance, while the chronotropic and inotropic potency of methylnorepinephrine was approximately equal to norepinephrine. These data further suggest that in addition to a central site of action of α-methyldopa, the inhibitory effects of the compound on the peripheral sympathetic nervous system cannot be excluded in explaining the antihypertensive action of α-methyldopa. The decrease in plasma renin activity observed following treatment with methyldopa to hypertensive patients and laboratory animals is also attributed to the impairment of peripheral sympathetic neuronal function (Privitera and Mohammed, 1972).

Cohen et al. (1967) investigated the effects of α-methyldopa, 500 or 1000 mg, i.v. in hypertensive patients. In 19 patients who received 1 g of α-methyldopa, the compound significantly increased myocardial blood flow and significantly decreased coronary vascular resistance, systemic blood pressure, systemic vascular resistance, and tension time index, while cardiac output and heart rate remained essentially unchanged. Lund-Johansen (1972) investigated the hemodynamic changes following long-term α-methyldopa therapy in hypertensive patients. α-Methyldopa was administered daily in doses ranging from 500 to 1500 mg/day for a period of 11−12 mo. In contrast to the data obtained in acute studies, chronic administration of α-methyldopa resulted in a drop in blood pressure associated with a decrease in cardiac output and practically no change in total peripheral resistance. Heart rate was reduced at both rest and during exercise and there was an insignificant change in stroke index.

Clonidine

Clonidine (2-(2,6-dichlorophenylamino)-2-imidazoline hydrochloride) is one of the most interesting hypotensive compounds to be investigated in the past decade. The evidence for central α-adrenergic inhibitory receptors is mainly based on experiments with clonidine and related imidazoline compounds (Kobinger, 1974). Early studies suggested that the hypotensive effects of clonidine were primarily due to actions on the central nervous system (Kobinger and Walland, 1967; Schmitt et al., 1968; Sherman et al., 1968). Clonidine, administered intravenously, initially causes a transient rise in arterial blood pressure and is followed by a prolonged hypotensive action (van Zweiten, 1973). The initial hypertensive effect is apparently due to stimulation of peripheral α-adrenergic receptors and the subsequent decrease, due to a central action, caused by a reduction in peripheral sympathetic activity (van Zweiten, 1973). Schmitt et al. (1968) investigated the effects of clonidine on central sympathetic structures in anesthetized dogs, cats, and rats. In dogs, the compound produced bradycardia and hypertension, usually followed by hypotension. There was a decrease in sympathetic discharge from the splanchnic and inferior cardiac nerves lasting approximately 3 hr. Sherman et al. (1968) administered clonidine into the arterial inflow of the neurally intact, vascularly isolated recipient head in dog cross-circulation preparations. Minute doses of the compound produced depressor responses in the recipient animal and a transient pressor response followed by a prolonged hypotensive response in the donor animal. Clonidine produced a marked decrease in mean arterial blood pressure in the recipient in experiments in which the recipient's carotid sinus-body areas were bilaterally denervated, whereas an initial transient pressor response preceded the hypotensive effect in the donor animal. The data obtained in dog cross-circulation experiments indicated that the hypotensive effects of clonidine were due to central mechanisms. Schmitt, Schmitt, and Fenard (1971) and Kobinger and Walland (1971) presented data indicating that the mechanism of action of clonidine was stimulation of central α-adrenergic receptors that were inhibitory in nature. The central actions of clonidine could be blocked by certain α-adrenergic blocking agents such as piperoxan (Schmitt et al., 1971). Kobinger and Pichler (1975) undertook studies to localize the central site of action of clonidine in dogs. Intracisternal injection of clonidine in decerebrate or i.v. injection of the compound in bulbar animals significantly facilitated reflex bradycardia. The effect was antagonized by piperoxan. The results of the studies suggested that the facilitatory action of clonidine was mediated by α-adrenoreceptors within the medulla oblongata. Schmitt and Schmitt (1969) utilized transsection studies to identify the main site of action of clonidine in the medulla oblongata. Schmitt, Schmitt, and Fenard (1973) further investigated the sympathoinhibitory action of clonidine in anesthetized cats and reported that the main site for the hypotensive effect of clonidine is localized in the depressor medullary area at the level of the obex. Because a large destruction was necessary to decrease the sympathoinhibitory effect of clonidine and because the reduction in the sympathetic discharge induced by clonidine was never completely abolished in experiments conducted in dogs, they suggested that other sites of action, possibly the spinal cord, may also be involved.

Brod et al. (1972) investigated the acute effects of clonidine in normotensive and hypertensive patients. They reported in all patients an initial transient rise in blood pressure that was almost certainly due to generalized vasoconstriction, similar to that observed in experimental animals. Both systolic and mean blood pressure fell markedly following the initial pressor response and the cardiac index fell during the first 3 min with a further decrease within the next 30 min. Because heart rate was unaffected, the reduction in the cardiac index was due to the reduction of the stroke volume index. Total peripheral resistance did not change in most of the patients. Central venous pressure fell in all but one patient and renal vascular resistance decreased in 66% of the patients. Peripheral renin activity decreased slightly; however, the decrease was not of statistical significance. This could possibly be due to the acute nature of the studies. These authors concluded that the failure of the total peripheral resistance and heart rate to rise in response to a falling cardiac index and arterial pressure, together with the inferred diminution of cardiac contractile force, should be considered as evidence of inhibition of the sympato-adrenal system, probably at some central site. They also suggested that the inhibition was probably only partial because vasomotor response to changes in the body's position seems to be sufficiently well maintained to prevent more serious hypotension on tilting.

Investigators have reported that clonidine, like methyldopa, also suppresses renin secretion (Hokfelt, Hedeland, and Dymling, 1970; Onesti et al., 1971). This action has been reported to occur in humans and experimental animals, and it has been suggested that unlike methyldopa the suppression of renin secretion by clonidine is due to a centrally mediated decrease in sympathetic activity. Reid et al. (1975) further investigated the effects of clonidine on renin secretion and found that clonidine, 1 μg/kg, administered directly into the third ventricle of dogs, in which renal perfusion pressure was controlled by adjusting an aortic clamp, produced hypotension and bradycardia and suppressed plasma renin activity to 39% of the control value. Intraventricular clonidine produced similar alterations in blood pressure and heart rate in another group of dogs in which renal perfusion pressure was not controlled, but failed to suppress plasma renin activity. When clonidine was administered intravenously in a dose of 30 μg/kg, the compound produced a transient hypertension followed by hypotension, decreased heart rate, and suppressed plasma renin activity to 49% of the control value. Renal denervation reduced renin secretion and prevented the suppression of renin secretion produced by i.v. clonidine. The authors concluded that the suppression of renin secretion by clonidine resulted from a centrally mediated decrease in renal sympathetic neural tone.

The centrally induced hypotensive effects of phentolamine, an α-adrenergic blocker, and α-methyldopa and clonidine, central α-adrenergic stimulants, seem contradictory in nature. Furthermore, the fact that central administration of phentolamine potentiates the central hypertensive activity of angiotensin II and blocks the hypotensive activity of α-methyldopa and clonidine, indicates that there are α-adrenergic receptors located in the central nervous system capable of inducing both inhibitory and stimulatory effects. The data suggest that the inhibitory receptors are located in the lower brain stem and that the stimulatory receptors may be located in an area above the pons, possibly the hypothalamus.

Prolonged Administration of Compounds
Interfering with Adrenergic Activity

Jandhyala, Clarke, and Buckley (1974) reviewed in depth the pharmacology of reserpine and guanethidine, and therefore, the present comments are limited to the prolonged pharmacologic effects of these two compounds. Adams et al. (1971) administered reserpine, 0.137–0.274 mg/day, to mongrel dogs, orally for a period of 12 mo (18–39 μg/kg). Reserpine induced a moderate decrease in both systolic and diastolic blood pressure following 2 wk of treatment; however, blood pressure returned to pretreatment levels 4–5 wk after initiation of the experiment. There was a gradual decrease in heart rate; at the end of the experimental period, heart rates remained significantly below control levels. Prolonged reserpine treatment did not alter blood pressure responses to hypoxia, cold pressor tests, exercise using a treadmill, and intravenous administration of sodium nitrite and phenylephrine. Postural hypotension was evident when the animals were subjected to a 60° head-up position tilt. Hexamethonium produced a marked transient increase in heart rate and blood pressure in untreated dogs, followed by a prolonged depressor response. However, in the reserpine-treated dogs, the hypotensive response was absent, whereas the pressor and tachycardia responses seen in the control dogs were present in the treated animals. Since the tachycardia induced by hexamethonium in conscious animals appears to be predominantly due to vagal blockade (Lokhandwala et al., 1973), the bradycardia induced by reserpine may not be due to increased vagal activity. The phenylephrine-induced pressor responses were essentially identical in both treated and untreated groups, whereas the accompanying reflex bradycardia was markedly inhibited by prolonged reserpine treatment. Based on the pressor responses to phenylephrine, it seems that intrinsic α-adrenergic receptor activity was not altered by the prolonged administration of reserpine (Jandhyala et al., 1974). The fact that hexamethonium did not induce a depressor response in the reserpine-treated conscious dogs, nor inhibition of reflex bradycardia to phenylephrine and inhibition of tyramine pressor responses, suggested marked inhibition in sympathetic tone in the cardiovascular system. Studies conducted in the same animals under pentobarbital anesthesia (Jandhyala et al., 1971) demonstrated that under these experimental conditions the blood pressure responses to bilateral carotid occlusion and hexamethonium were markedly inhibited by prolonged administration of reserpine, together with a reduction in cardiac output and left ventricular work. In addition, there was a marked increase in contractile force and rate of tension development in the ventricular myocardium of the reserpine treated dogs, but no corresponding increases in stroke volume. Systemic function curves indicated that reserpine treatment did not alter the ability of the peripheral vasculature to return blood to the heart (Jandhyala et al., 1971). Adams et al. (1971) reported that gross pathologic examination revealed marked dilation of the right ventricle in reserpine-treated dogs. Jandhyala et al. (1971) suggested that prolonged reserpine treatment produced a diminished efficiency of the right ventricle of mongrel dogs.

Clarke, Adams, and Buckley (1970) investigated the effects of prolonged reserpine treatment on sympathetic neuronal function in the isolated perfused mesenteric vessels of dogs. They found that there was an attenuation of sympathetic nerve activity and that this decrease could be restored by infusion of norepinephrine, indicating that chronic reserpine administration failed to alter neuronal uptake mechanisms. In addition, there was no alteration in α-adrenergic receptor activity in the perfused mesenteric vessels, whereas studies conducted by Cavero, Jandhyala, and Buckley (1971) reported a twofold increase in α-adrenergic receptor activity in the femoral artery but no significant alterations were observed in the superior mesenteric artery.

Guanethidine, 2.5 mg/kg, was administered daily to beagle dogs for periods of 2 days, 7 days, and 6–8 mo. Chronic administration of guanethidine did not produce any significant alteration in body weight, blood volume, or blood pressure (Jandhyala et al., 1974). There was a slight reduction in heart rate, which was more significant in males than in females. The cardiovascular responses to tilt, mild exercise on a treadmill (12° inclination at 5 miles/hr for 4–5 min), ganglionic blockade, sodium nitrite, tyramine, angiotensin, phenylephrine, and norepinephrine were not significantly different in the treated animals as compared to controls (Jandhyala et al., 1974). The oral administration of the compound for 2 days failed to inhibit the chronotropic responses to cardiac sympathetic stimulation, whereas administration of the same dose for 7 days significantly depressed cardiac sympathetic nerve activity (Clarke et al., 1974). However, following chronic administration of the same dose for a period of 6–8 mo, cardiac sympathetic nerve function returned to normal levels. Similarly, in hind limb vasculature neurogenic tone and vasoconstrictor responses to lumbar sympathetic stimulation, which were depressed after 7 days of guanethidine treatment, were restored to normal levels after 6–8 mo of treatment with guanethidine (Jandhyala et al., 1974). In addition, there was a progressive potentiation of the sympathetic cholinergic vasodilator activity as the duration of treatment increased. Increased tolerance to guanethidine was not accompanied by alterations in adrenergic receptor activity either in the heart (Clarke et al., 1974) or in the hind limb vasculature (Jandhyala et al., 1974).

Chronic administration of guanethidine, 2.5 mg/kg/day for 7–8 mo, did not produce significant changes in blood pressure and heart rate of beagle dogs anesthetized with sodium pentobarbital (Jandhyala et al., 1975). There were a significant elevation of stroke volume and stroke work, a reduction in total peripheral resistance, and an increase in cardiac output in the treated animals. Ventricular function curves obtained in both the treated and placebo group were virtually identical and the data obtained in these studies suggested that chronic guanethidine administration did not induce any adverse effects on myocardial functions.

In contrast to the tolerance observed in cardiac sympathetic nerve activity to guanethidine after 6–8 mo, the vasoconstrictor response to periarterial nerve stimulation to the isolated perfused mesenteric arteries was abolished after 7 days and 2, 6, and 8 mo of guanethidine treatment

(Clarke et al., 1974). Although treatment for 24 hr failed to significantly alter the frequency-response curve to periarterial nerve stimulation, there was a twofold shift to the left in the dose-response curve to injected norepinephrine and this twofold shift was evident throughout the study.

SUMMARY AND CONCLUSIONS

Data have been presented indicating that angiotensin II, an octapeptide, produces marked pressor effects when administered via the cerebral ventricular system or via the vertebral arteries. Because the centrally induced pressor effects were obtained in dogs in which the buffer nerves arising from the carotid sinus-body areas of the recipient's head had been destroyed, this effect was not due to an action of angiotensin II on reflexogenic receptors. Selective perfusion studies and studies in which small, bilateral electrolytic lesions were placed within the periaqueductal gray suggest that the subnucleus medialis of the periaqueductal gray is one of the sites of action of angiotensin II within the central nervous system. This synaptic area lies in close proximity to the aqueduct, and the intrinsic pressor pathway has been shown to be functionally involved in the control of systemic peripheral resistance. Peripheral administration of α-adrenergic blocking agents in dog cross-circulation experiments and in α-chlorolose anesthetized cats blocks or markedly attenuates this centrally induced pressor effects of angiotensin II; therefore, it seems that the increase in arterial pressure was induced by increased sympathetic outflow. Investigators have reported the presence of renin and angiotensin, mainly angiotensin I, in the central nervous system of rats and dogs (Ganten et al., 1971a, b). Therefore, angiotensin II produced within the central nervous system most probably affects structures in the midbrain area. On the other hand, it does seem that angiotensin II administered via the vertebral arteries initially stimulates receptors in the area postrema. Data have also been presented suggesting that angiotensin II may not only stimulate central receptors, inducing pressor responses via increased adrenergic outflow, but may also stimulate receptors in the central nervous system capable of increasing renin production by the kidney via neuronal activation.

The administration of phentolamine, an α-adrenergic blocker, via the cerebral lateral ventricular system markedly potentiates the centrally induced pressor effects of angiotensin II. These data indicate that functional central α-adrenergic mechanisms may inhibit the centrally induced hypertensive effects of angiotensin II and offers further evidence for central sympatoinhibitory receptors. Both α-methyldopa and clonidine produce hypotensive effects through stimulation of these central α-adrenergic inhibitory receptors. In addition, it seems that α-methyldopa may also impair peripheral sympathetic neuronal function.

The pharmacology of reserpine and guanethidine differs depending on whether the data are obtained in acute or chronic studies. Although both compounds markedly deplete norepinephrine from neuronal endings, there is a marked difference between the effects of chronic administration on myocardial activity. When guanethidine was administered to beagle dogs for 6–8 mo, cardiac sympathetic nerve function and cardiac efficiency were normal. Prolonged administration of reserpine, however, produced a marked inhibition in sympathetic tone to the myocardium. In addition, reserpine decreased cardiac output and left ventricular work and induced ventricular dilation and diminished efficiency of the right ventricle.

LITERATURE CITED

Adams, H. R., H. H. Smookler, D. E. Clarke, B. S. Jandhyala, B. N. Dixit, R. J. Ertel, and J. P. Buckley. 1971. Clinicopathologic effects of chronic reserpine administration in mongrel dogs. J. Pharm. Sci. 60: 1134–1138.

Bhattacharya, B. K., and W. Feldberg. 1958. Perfusion of cerebral ventricles: effect of drugs on outflow from the cisterna and the aqueduct. Brit. J. Pharmacol. 13: 156–162.

Bickerton, R. Y., and J. P. Buckley. 1961. Evidence for a central mechanism in angiotensin induced hypertension. Proc. Soc. Exp. Biol. Med. 106: 834–836.

Blair-West, J. R., J. P. Coghlan, D. A. Denton, J. W. Funder, P. A. Scoggins, and R. D. Wright. 1971. The effects of the heptapeptide (2-8) and hexapaptide (3-8) fragments of angiotensin II on aldosterone secretion. J. Clin. Endocrinol. Metab. 32: 575–578.

Brod, J., L. Horback, H. Just, J. Rosenthal, and R. Nicolescu. 1972. Acute effects of clonidine on central and peripheral hemodynamics and plasma renin activity. Eur. J. Clin. Pharmacol. 4: 107–114.

Buckley, J. P. 1972. Actions of angiotensin on the central nervous system. Fed. Prod. 31: 1332–1337.

Buckley, J. P., R. K. Bickerton, R. P. Halliday, and H. Kato. 1963. Central effects of peptides on the cardiovascular system. Ann. N. Y. Acad. Sci. 104: 299–310.

Buckley, J. P., and R. Vollmer. 1975. Influence of angiotensin on central cardiovascular control. Proceedings of the Sixth International Congress of Pharmacology, Vol. 4, Drug Therapy, p. 59.

Carlson, A., and M. Lindquist. 1962. In vivo decarboxylation of alpha-

752   Buckley et al.

methyldopa and alpha-methyl-meta-tyrosine. Acta Physiol. Scand. 54: 87−94.

Cavero, I., B. S. Jandhyala, and J. P. Buckley. 1971. Prolonged effects of reserpine administration on adrenergic receptor activity in dogs. J. Pharm. Pharmacol. 23: 988−989.

Clarke, D. E., H. R. Adams, and J. P. Buckley. 1970. Chronic reserpine treatment on adrenergic neuronal and receptor function in the isolated perfused mesenteric blood vessels of the dog. Eur. J. Pharmacol. 12: 378−381.

Clarke, D. E., B. S. Jandhyala, I. Cavero, D. N. Dixit, and J. P. Buckley. 1974. A differential effect of chronically administered guanethidine on sympathetic neural-transmission to the dog heart and mesenteric arterial blood vessels. Can. J. Physiol. Pharmacol. 52: 641−648.

Cohen, A., J. P. Maxmen, M. Ragheb, H. Baleiron, E. J. Zaleski, and R. J. Bing. 1967. Effects of alpha-methyldopa on the myocardial blood flow, utilizing the coincidence counting method. J. Clin. Pharmacol. 7: 77−83.

Day, M. D., and A. G. Roach. 1974a. Central alpha and beta-adrenal receptors modifying arterial blood pressure and heart rate in conscious cats. Brit. J. Pharmacol. 51: 325−333.

Day, M. D., and A. G. Roach 1974b. Central adrenal receptors and the control of arterial blood pressure. Clin. Exp. Pharmacol. Physiol. 1: 347−360.

Day, M. D., A. G. Roach, and R. L. Whiting. 1973. The mechanism of antihypertensive action of alpha-methyldopa in hypertensive rats. Eur. J. Pharmacol. 21: 271−280.

Deuben, R. R., and J. P. Buckley. 1970. Identification of a central site of action of angiotensin II. J. Pharmacol. Exp. Ther. 175: 139−146.

Doxey, J. C., and A. Scutt. 1974. Effect of alpha-methyldopa on sympathetic nerve function in the pithed rat. Eur. J. Pharmacol. 29: 320−323.

Enoch, D. M., and F. W. L. Kerr. 1967a. Hypothalamic vasopressor and vessicopressor pathways. I. Arch. Neurol. 16: 290−306.

Enoch, D. M., and F. W. L. Kerr. 1967b. Hypothalamic vasopressor and vessicopressor pathways. II. Arch. Neurol. 16: 307−320.

Finch, L., and G. Haeusler. 1973. Further evidence for a central hypotensive action of alpha-methyldopa in both the rat and the cat. Brit. J. Pharmacol. 47: 217−228.

Ganten, D., A. Marquez-Julio, P. Granger, K. Hayduk, K. P. Karsunky, R. Boucher, and J. Genest. 1971a. Renin in dog brain. Amer. J. Physiol. 221: 1733−1737.

Ganten, D., J. Minnich, P. Granger, K. Hayduk, H. N. Brecht, A. Barbeau, R. Boucher, and J. Genest. 1971b. Angiotensin-forming enzyme in brain tissue. Science 173: 64−65.

Gildenberg, P. L. 1969. Localization of a site of angiotensin vasopressor activity in the brain. Physiologist 12: 235.

Gildenberg, P. L. 1971. Site of angiotensin vasopressor activity in the brainstem. Fed. Proc. 30: 432.

Gildenberg, P. L., C. M. Ferrario, and J. W. McCubbin. 1973. Two sites of cardiovascular action of angiotensin II in the brain of the dog. Clin. Sci. (London) 44: 417–420.

Goodfriend, T., D. Allmann, and K. Kent. 1971. Angiotensin's ionotropic and mitochondrial effects. Clin. Res. 19: 316.

Gyang, E. A., R. R. Deuben, and J. P. Buckley. 1973. Interaction of prostaglandin E_1 and angiotensin II on centrally mediated pressor activities in the cat. Proc. Soc. Exp. Biol. Med. 142: 532–537.

Halliday, R. P., and J. P. Buckley. 1962. Central hypertensive effects of angiotensin II. Int. J. Neuropharmacol. 1: 43–47.

Heise, A., and G. Kroneberg. 1972. Alpha sympathetic receptors stimulation in the brain and hypotensive activity of alpha-methyldopa. Eur. J. Pharmacol. 17: 315–317.

Heise, A., and G. Kroneberg. 1973. Central nervous alpha-adrenergic receptors and the mode of action of alpha-methyldopa. Naunyn-Schmiedeberg's Arch. Pharmacol. 279: 285–300.

Henning, M., and P. A. van Zweiten. 1968. Central hypotensive effects of alpha-methyldopa. J. Pharm. Pharmacol. 20: 409–417.

Hess, S. M., R. H. Connamacher, M. Ozaki, and S. Udenfriend. 1961. Effects of alpha-methyldopa and alpha-methyl-meta-tyrosine on the metabolism of norepinephrine and serotonin in vivo. J. Pharmacol. Exp. Ther. 134: 129–138.

Hokfelt, B., H. Hedeland, and J. F. Dymling. 1970. Studies on catecholamines, renin and aldosterone following Catapresan (2-(2,6-dichlorophenylamine)-2-imidazoline hydrochloride) in hypertensive patients. Eur. J. Pharmacol. 10: 389–397.

Jandhyala, B. S., I. Cavero, H. R. Adams, H. H. Smookler, B. N. Dixit, and J. P. Buckley. 1971. Cardiovascular effects of chronic reserpine administration in mongrel dogs. Eur. J. Pharmacol. 16: 261–270.

Jandhyala, B. S., I. Cavero, and J. P. Buckley. 1975. Effects of chronic guanethidine administration on cardiovascular function of dogs. Res. Commun. Chem. Path. Pharmacol. 11: 523–532.

Jandhyala, B. S., D. E. Clarke, and J. P. Buckley. 1974. Effects of prolonged administration of certain antihypertensive agents. J. Pharm. Sci. 63: 1497–1513.

Keim, K. L., and E. G. Sigg. 1971. Activation of central sympathetic neurons by angiotensin II. Life Sci. 10: 565–574.

Kelly, R. J., and T. F. Burks. 1974. Relative vasoconstrictor potencies of norepineprhine, alpha-methylnorepinephrine and octopamine. Arch. Int. Pharmacodyn. 208: 306–316.

Kobinger, W. 1974. Medicinal chemistry related to the central regulation of blood pressure II. Pharmacological Part. In N.J. Maas (ed.), Medicinal Chemistry IV. Proceedings of the Fourth International Symposium on Medical Chemistry, pp. 107–119. Elsevier, New York.

Kobinger, W., and L. Pichler. 1975. Localization in the CNS of adrenore-
ceptors which facilitate a cardioinhibitory reflex. Naunyn-Schmiedeberg's Arch. Pharmacol. 280: 371–377.

Kobinger, W., and A. Walland. 1967. Investigations into the mechanism of
the hypotensive effect of 2-(2,6-dichlorophenylamino)-2-imidazoline
HCl. Eur. J. Pharmacol. 2: 155–162.

Kobinger, W., and A. Walland. 1971. Involvement of adrenergic receptors
in central vagus activity. Eur. J. Pharmacol. 16: 120–122.

Levine, R. J., and A. Sjoerdsma. 1964. Dissociation of the decarboxylase
inhibiting and norepinephrine depleting effects of α-methyldopa, α-
ethyl-dopa, 4-bromo-3-hydroxy-benzyloxyamine and related substances. J. Pharmacol. Exp. Ther. 146: 42–47.

Lokhandwala, M. F. 1975a. Effect of methyldopa on regional hemodynamics and sympathetic nerve function in the dog. Fed. Proc. 34:
817.

Lokhandwala, M. F., J. P. Buckley, and B. S. Jandhyala. 1975b. Effect of
methyldopa treatment on peripheral sympathetic nerve function in the
dog. Eur. J. Pharmacol. 32: 170–178.

Lokhandwala, M. F., I. Cavero, J. P. Buckley, and B. S. Jandhyala. 1973.
Influence of pentobarbital anesthesia on the effects of certain autonomic blocking agents on heart rate. Eur. J. Pharmacol. 24: 274–277.

Lund-Johansen, P. 1972. Hemodynamic changes in long term alpha-
methyldopa therapy of essential hypertension. Acta Med. Scand. 192:
221–226.

Malik, K. V., and E. Muscholl. 1969. The effect of alpha-methyldopa on
the vasoconstrictor responses of the rat mesenteric artery preparation
to nerve stimulation. Arzneimittel-Forschung 19: 1111–1113.

Onesti, G., A. Schwartz, K. E. Kim, D. Paz Martinez, and C. Schwartz.
1971. Antihypertensive effect of clonidine. Circ. Res. 28–39: Suppl.
II. 53–69.

Oparil, S., and E. Haber. 1974. The renin-angiotensin system. N. Engl.
J. Med. 291: 389–401.

Page, I. H., and F. M. Bumpus. 1961. Angiotensin. Physiol. Rev. 41:
331–390.

Peach, M. J. 1971. Adrenal medullary stimulation induced by angiotensin
II and analogs. Circ. Res. 28: Suppl. II, 107–117.

Porter, C. C., J. A. Totaro, and A. Borcin. 1965. The relationship between
radioactivity and norepinephrine concentration in the brain and the
heart of mice following administration of labelled methyldopa or
6-hydroxydopamine. J. Pharmacol. Exp. Ther. 150: 17–22.

Privitera, P. J., and S. Mohammed. 1972. Studies on the mechanism of
renin suppression by alpha-methyldopa. In T. A. Assaykeen (ed.),
Advances in Experimental Medicine and Biology: Control of Renin
Secretion, Vol. 13, p. 93. Plenum Press, New York.

Reid, I. A., M. D. MacDonald, P. Pachnis, and W. F. Ganong. 1975. Studies
concerning the mechanism of suppression of renin secretion by clonidine. J. Pharm. Exp. Ther. 192: 713–721.

Salmon, G. K., and J. D. Ireson. 1970. A correlation between the hypotensive action of methyldopa and its depression of peripheral sympathetic function. Arch. Int. Pharmacodyn. 183: 60–64.

Schmitt, H., and H. Schmitt. 1969. Localization of the hypotensive effect of 2-(2,6-dichlorophenylamine)-2-imidazole hydrochloride (ST 155, Catapresan). Eur. J. Pharmacol. 6: 8–12.

Schmitt, H., H. Schmitt, J. R. Boissier, J. F. Giudicelli, and J. Fichelle. 1968. Cardiovascular effects of 2(2,6-dichlorophenylamino)-2-imidazoline hydrochloride (ST-155). II. Central sympathetic structures. Eur. J. Pharmacol. 2: 340–346.

Schmitt, H., H. Schmitt, and S. Fenard. 1971. Evidence for an alpha-sympathomimetic component in the effects of Catapresan on vasomotor centers: Antagonism by piperoxane. Eur. J. Pharmacol. 14: 98–100.

Schmitt, H., H. Schmitt, and S. Fenard. 1973. Increase in the sympathico-inhibitory action of clonidine after destruction of the sympatho-inhibitory area. Experientia 29: 1247–1249.

Sealey, J. E., F. R. Byhler, J. A. Laraoh, and E. D. Vauulan. 1973. The physiology of renin secretion in essential hypertension: Estimation of renin secretion rate and renal plasma flow from peripheral and renal vein renin levels. Amer. J. Med. 55: 391–401.

Severs, W. B., A. E. Daniels, and J. P. Buckley. 1967. On the central hypertensive effect of angiotensin II. Int. J. Neuropharmacol. 6: 199–205.

Severs, W. B., A. E. Daniels, H. H. Smookler, W. J. Kinnard, and J. P. Buckley. 1966. Interrelationship between angiotensin II and the sympathetic nervous system. J. Pharmacol. Exp. Ther. 153: 530–537.

Sherman, G. P., G. J. Grega, R. J. Woods, and J. P. Buckley. 1968. Evidence for a central hypotensive mechanism of 2-(2,6-dichloro-phenylamino)-2-imidazoline (Catapresan ST-155). Eur. J. Pharmacol. 2: 326–328.

Smookler, H. H., W. B. Severs, W. J. Kinnard, and J. P. Buckley. 1966. Centrally mediated cardiovascular effects of angiotensin II. J. Pharmacol. Exp. Ther. 153: 485–494.

Solomon, T. A., and J. P. Buckley. 1974. Inhibitory effects of the central hypertensive activity of angiotensin I and II by 1-sar-8-ala-angiotensin II (saralasin acetate). J. Pharm. Sci. 63: 1109–1113.

Solomon, T. A., I. Cavero, and J. P. Buckley. 1974. Inhibition of central pressor effects of angiotensin I and II. J. Pharm. Sci. 63: 511–515.

Sourkes, T. L. 1954. Inhibition of dihydroxyphenylalanine decarboxylase by derivatives of phenylalanine. Arch. Biochem. 51: 444–456.

Stone, C. A., and C. C. Porter. 1966. Methyldopa and adrenergic nerve function. Pharmacol. Rev. 569–575.

Torchiana, M. L., C. C. Porter, L. S. Watson, and C. A. Stone. 1965. Relationship of cardiovascular and antihypertensive effects of methyldopa with alpha-methylnorepinephrine concentrations in the hearts of rats. Pharmacologist 7: 145.

van Zweiten, P. A. 1973. Central action of antihypertensive drugs mediated via central alpha receptors. J. Pharm Pharmacol. 25: 89–95.

Vollmer, R., J. P. Buckley, T. A. Solomon, and B. S. Jandhyala, 1975. Central hypertensive actions of angiotensin. Acta Physiol. Latinoam. 24: 582.

Yu, R., and C. J. Dickinson. 1965. Neurogenic effects of angiotensin. Lancet 2: 1276–1277.

Cardiovascular Flow Dynamics and Measurements
Edited by N. H. C. Hwang and N. A. Normann
Copyright 1977   University Park Press   Baltimore

chapter 19

RED CELL MEMBRANE AND HEMOLYSIS

Shu Chien

ABSTRACT

Hemolysis is the result of damage to the red cell membrane. Biochemical, biophysical, and ultrastructural studies have shown that the red cell membrane is composed of a lipid bilayer in association with specialized protein molecules. The membrane can tolerate considerable uniaxial deformation, but an expansion of membrane area by only a few percent leads to hemolysis. These findings can be explained by a structural model in which the spectrin molecules lining the membrane endoface are postulated to form a network connected with the glycophorin molecules penetrating the thickness of the membrane. These proteins form a scaffold for the lipids and confer mechanical strength to the membrane, whereas the fluidity of the lipid bilayer permits the dynamic movements and interactions of membrane components. Hemolysis can be experimentally produced by subjecting the red blood cell to various physicochemical disturbances (e.g., osmotic, mechanical, thermal, or chemical) that produce energy changes in some regions of the red cell membrane to exceed the interaction energy that keeps together the component molecules. Hemolysis in various diseases can generally be attributed to intrinsic defects in the red cell and/or abnormal physicochemical disturbances causing membrane damage. These defective or damaged red cells are constantly subjected to mechanical stresses in the circulation and they are vulnerable to the hemolytic environment in the spleen and other regions.

INTRODUCTION

Hemolysis is the liberation of hemoglobin from the red cells (Dorlands, 1974). The membrane of the intact red blood cell (RBC, or erythrocyte)

The unpublished studies in this paper were supported by U. S. Public Health Service Research Grants HL 16851 and HL 15161 from the National Heart and Lung Institute.

757

separates the intracellular, hemoglobin-rich fluid from the extracellular
fluid medium, which is normally the blood plasma. Therefore, by definition, hemolysis is a result of failure of the RBC membrane. The intraeryth-
rocyte fluid differs from the plasma not only in its protein contents, but
also in the concentration of small molecules, particularly the electrolytes
(Table 1). This transmembrane difference in ionic composition is maintained by the selective passive permeability as well as specific active
transport processes in the membrane. The proper functioning of the RBC
membrane (including active and passive transport processes and viscoelastic deformation) depends on its normal structure in terms of biochemical constituents and molecular organization. Various physical disturbances
(e.g., mechanical, osmotic, and thermal) and chemical agents (e.g., drugs,
antibodies, and snake venom) cause alterations in membrane structure and
derangements in membrane functions. Whereas the passive permeability of
the normal RBC membrane is equivalent to "pores" with approximately 4
Å diameter (Goldstein and Solomon, 1960), the RBC membrane subjected
to sufficiently strong physicochemical disturbances develops "holes" large
enough for the diffusion of hemoglobin, and hemolysis ensues. It should
be recognized that hemolysis actually represents some type of an end-
point in RBC membrane damage and that alterations in membrane structure and function in response to physicochemical disturbances proceed in
the prelytic stage. Furthermore, small pieces of membrane may be pinched
off (fragmentation) as a result of cell damage without significant losses of
hemoglobin.

It is obvious from the foregoing discussion that an understanding of
the phenomenon of hemolysis necessitates a knowledge of the structure
and function of RBC membrane. In the following sections the morpho-

Table 1. Concentrations of some constituents in
red blood cells and plasma

	Red blood cell	Plasma
Electrolytes (meq/L)		
Na^+	9	140
K^+	88	4
Cl^-	68	103
HCO_3^-	11	27
Proteins (g/100 ml)	34	7

logic, biochemical, and biophysical properties of the RBC membrane are considered. The basic knowledge reviewed serves as a background for the discussion of various types of hemolysis produced in the laboratory and encountered in clinical conditions.

1 MORPHOLOGY AND
ULTRASTRUCTURE OF RED CELL MEMBRANE

The human RBC, in the absence of significant shearing stress, has a biconcave diskoid shape (Figure 1). The mean corpuscular volume (V) is approximately 90 μ^3 and the mean corpuscular area (A) is approximately 140 μ^2 (Evans and Fung, 1972), but considerable variations occur among the population in a given blood sample (Chen and Fung, 1973). The major diameter of the diskoid is approximately 8 μ, the rim is approximately 2.5 μ thick, and the center is thinner than 1 μ. The sphericity index (4.84 $V^{2/3}/A$) is approximately 0.7. A sphere with the same volume of 90 μ^3 has a surface area of only 97 μ^2. Therefore, the normal diskoid RBC has an excess membrane area, which allows its deformation into a wide variety of shapes (Fung, 1966; Chien, 1975). The remarkable deformability of the normal RBC is demonstrated by its ability to pass through narrow capillary channels smaller than 3 μ in diameter without changes in area or volume (Gregersen et al., 1967; LaCelle, 1970) (Figure 2).

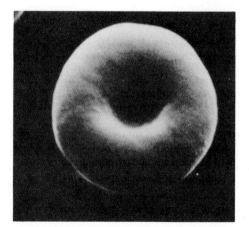

Figure 1. Scanning electron micrograph showing the biconcave diskoid shape of the normal human red cell.

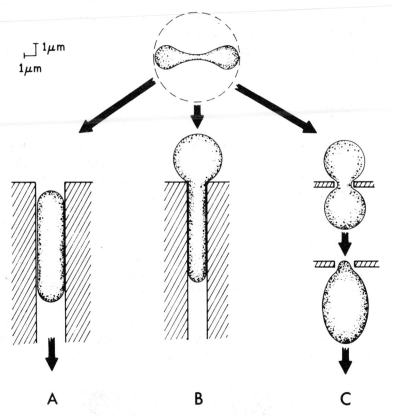

Figure 2. Passage of normal red cells (top and side views of biconcave diskoids shown at the top of the diagram) through cylindrical channels with diameters 3 μ(A) and 2 μ(B and C). The channel length was longer than 15 μ in (A) and (B), and only 0.5 μ in (C) Note that the deformation of the normal red cell allows its passage through (A) and (C), but not through (B). From Chien, 1975. Reprinted by permission.

On thin sections under high-magnification transmission electron-microscopy, the RBC membrane fixed in osmium tetroxide shows a typical trilaminar pattern (Figure 3). The triple-layered structure, which has been named the unit membrane by Robertson (1960), consists of a central electron-lucent zone separating two electron-dense lines, each approximately 25 Å in thickness, giving a total thickness of about 75 Å. These findings have been interpreted as evidence for the lipid bilayer model (Danielli and Davson, 1935) in which a central zone of the

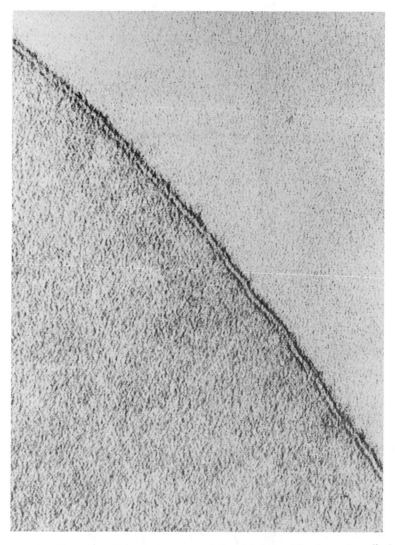

Figure 3. Thin-section electron microscopy of the triple-layered "unit membrane" of an intact human red blood cell. Cell cytoplasm is at the lower left. The cell membrane consists of a central electron-lucent zone sandwiched between two electron-dense lines. Glutaraldehyde-osmium tetroxide fixation. ×280,000. Courtesy of Dr. J. D. Robertson; from Weinstein, 1974.

hydrophobic chains of lipid molecules separates two layers of hydrophilic groups. Recent evidence, however, suggests that the trilaminar image probably is not specific for membrane lipids and may result from fixation artifacts (Weinstein and McNutt, 1970).

Considerable insight into membrane ultrastructure has been gained by the introduction of the freeze-cleavage technique (Branton, 1966; Tillack and Marchesi, 1970; Weinstein, 1974). In this method, packed red cells or

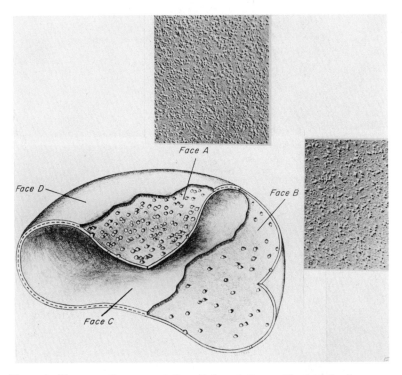

Figure 4. Diagrammatic representation of the relative positions of the four membrane "faces" that can be examined with the freeze-fracture and freeze-etch techniques. A population of small particles named "membrane-associated particles" or MAP are illustrated on face *A* and face *B*, the fracture faces that are produced by membrane splitting. The substructure of the juxtacytoplasmic surface (face *C*) and true exterior surface (face *D*) of the membrane is not represented in this highly schematic figure. Insets show replicas of freeze-fractured human red cell membranes. *A*, Freeze-fracture face *A* originating from within the interior of the membrane shows more or less randomly distributed MAP that may represent sites of integral membrane proteins. X 90,000. *B*, Face *B* has fewer MAP than face *A*. X 97,000. Modified from Weinstein, 1974; reprinted by permission.

RBC ghosts are rapidly frozen and then mechanically fractured in liquid nitrogen or in vacuo with a precooled razor blade. The cleavage follows the natural paths of low mechanical resistance, usually along the membrane interior between the two layers of lipid (Figure 4). The faces are replicated with the use of vaporized carbon and platinum in vacuo. The replicas are then examined in a transmission electronmicroscope. This method has the advantage that large areas of membranes can be examined in three-dimensional relief without removing membrane water. The freeze-cleavage procedure exposes two opposing inner surfaces, both of which exhibit particles approximately 80 Å in diameter (Figure 4). The surface remaining with the inner half of the membrane (face A in Figure 4) has 4–5 times as many of these membrane-associated particles as the surface remaining with the outer half of the membrane (face B in Figure 4). These membrane-associated particles are found in many other cell membranes but not in myelin membrane, where protein content is very low. As is mentioned again in the next section, there is evidence that these membrane-associated particles represent the protein molecules penetrating the lipid layers in the membrane.

2 BIOCHEMICAL PROPERTIES OF RED CELL MEMBRANE

The human RBC membrane is primarily composed of lipid and protein, and the two moieties are present in approximately equal amounts by weight.

2.1 Membrane Lipids

Phospholipids and cholesterol account for nearly 95% of the total lipid, and they exist in approximately equal molar ratio (Dodge and Phillips, 1967). The cholesterol in RBC membrane undergoes rapid exchange with plasma, with half of the membrane cholesterol replaced in a few hours (Hagermann and Gould, 1951; van Deenen and DeGier, 1974). This rapid exchange rate depends upon the presence of beta-lipoprotein in the plasma that binds cholesterol. Phospholipids are generally composed of a glycerol backbone in which the third carbon atom is in phosphodiester linkage to a base (e.g., choline, ethanolamine, serine, or inositol). The great majority of the phospholipids of the red cell membrane are diacyl phosphatides, in which the other two carbon atoms of the glycerol backbone are both linked to fatty acids (Figure 5), e.g., phosphatidylcholine (PC, also called lecithin), phosphatidylethanolamine (PE), or phosphatidylserine

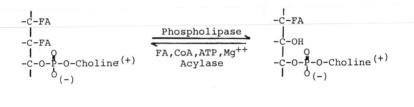

Phosphatidyl choline   Lyso-phospatidyl choline

Figure 5. Basic structures of phosphatidylcholine and lyso-phosphatidylcholine and their interconversion. FA, fatty acid.

(PS). These phosphatides are highly lipophilic and their exchange rates between RBC membrane and plasma are much slower than that of cholesterol (Reed, 1968). If only one of the carbon atoms is linked to a fatty acid (Figure 5), then the phospholipids are called lyso-phosphatides, e.g., lyso-phosphatidylcholine (L-PC, also called lysolecithin) and lyso-phosphatidylethanolamine (L-PE). Lyso-phosphatides are double-ended molecules with both hydrophilic and lipophilic properties, and such detergent qualities give rise to their ability to cause RBC membrane lysis at low concentrations. The normal RBC membrane, however, contains only very small amounts of lysophosphatides. Owing to its water solubility, lysophosphatides are exchanged rather rapidly between RBC membrane and plasma (Tarlov, 1966). There exist several mechanisms to maintain the membrane concentration of these potentially dangerous lysophosphatides at low levels (Shohet, 1972), the most important of which is the enzymatic acylation with free fatty acid to form diacyl phosphatides (Oliveira and Vaughan, 1964).

The nature of the fatty acids in the phosphatides may affect the functional manifestations of model membranes (Shohet, 1972). Thus saturated fatty acids permit stronger hydrophobic interactions, increasing the rigidity in the lipid phase of the membrane and decreasing permeability. On the other hand, unsaturated fatty acids tend to cause membrane expansion, increasing flexibility and permeability. The fluidity of cell membranes may increase with a rise in phospholipid/cholesterol ratio (Shinitzky and Inbar, 1974).

The lipids in the membrane are believed to be arranged as a bilayer (Danielli and Davson, 1935). Thus, the membrane contains two mono-molecular sheets of phospholipids with the hydrocarbon tail forming a central core and the ionized head groups (choline, ethanolamine, etc.)

facing the surfaces. The RBC membrane shows compositional asymmetry with respect to these phosphatides (Bretscher, 1973). Thus, there are more choline phospholipids (PC) on the outer half and more amino phospholipids (PE and PS) on the inner half of the lipid bilayer.

2.2 Membrane Proteins

Membrane proteins can be classified into two categories: The peripheral proteins are found on membrane surfaces with a loose attachment, whereas the integral proteins penetrate into the membrane core and are tightly bound to lipid. Hence it is difficult to extract and purify these integral proteins. Recently, an integral glycoprotein has been isolated from RBC membranes and is named glycophorin (Marchesi et al., 1973). This purified protein, which has a molecular weight of 50,000–55,000 and spans the entire thickness of the RBC membrane, can be divided into three parts. The first part consists of 90–100 amino acids to which a large number of oligosaccharide chains are attached. This part, with its negatively charged sialic acid residues and antigenic sites on the oligosaccharide chains, is found in the outer hydrophilic region of the lipid bilayer and extends beyond the membrane exoface into the external environment. The middle part is composed of about 25 amino acids without charge groups, and has been shown to be situated in the hydrophobic region of the lipid bilayer. The remainder (the carboxyl end of the chain) is rich in charged amino acids but contains no sugar residues. It resides in the inner hydrophilic regions of the lipid bilayer and protrudes beyond the membrane endoface to the cell interior. Thus the glycophorin molecule runs perpendicularly through the membrane. Each molecule may be composed of subunits forming a channel for the passage of small hydrophilic molecules through an otherwise hydrophobic core (Singer, 1975). Other integral proteins occupy only a portion of the thickness, but their biochemical properties have not been as clearly established as in the case of glycophorin. Most of these other integral proteins are located near the endoface (Bretscher, 1973). Hence the RBC membrane also exhibits compositional asymmetry with respect to proteins. The larger volume occupied by the proteins on the inner half of the membrane is probably balanced by a smaller volume of lipids, and the reverse situation exists on the outer half (Bretscher, 1973).

An important peripheral protein in the RBC membrane is spectrin (Marchesi and Steets, 1968; Kirkpatrick, 1976), which is found on the endoface and accounts for approximately one-fourth of total RBC membrane proteins. This protein can bind antibodies to the muscle protein myosin, and it has been suggested that it may have a contractile function (Singer, 1975). Spectrin molecules tend to aggregate in solution, especially in the presence of Ca^{++}, to form rodlike units. Phosphorylation of spectrin and other membrane proteins may affect their molecular conformation and interactions, contributing to the normal membrane deformability. As is discussed in the next section, spectrin may play an important role in determining the biomechanical properties of the RBC membrane.

2.3 Membrane Model

Many models have been proposed to account for the structure and function of cell membranes. The most commonly accepted model for the RBC membrane is a modified version of the bilayer model, in which the topographic and functional specializations of the protein molecules have been taken into account (Figure 6). As pointed out above, the integral protein molecules penetrate into the lipid core to various depths. Membrane proteins are amphiphatic: Their hydrophobic regions are embedded in the interior of the lipid bilayer, and their hydrophilic ends remain near the membrane surfaces. Thus these portions of the protein molecule are in contact with the corresponding components in the lipid, and protein–lipid interactions between neighboring molecules probably have an important

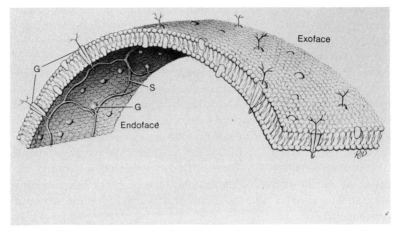

Figure 6. Schematic drawing showing the hypothetical structure of red cell membrane. S, spectrin; G, glycophorin.

influence on membrane properties. The glycophorin molecules penetrate the entire thickness of the membrane, with their hydrophobic midregion embedded in the membrane interior and their two hydrophilic ends protruding from the two surfaces. There is evidence that the midregion of the glycophorin molecule, and possibly also other embedded protein molecules, constitute the membrane associated particles obtained after freeze cleavage (Marchesi et al., 1973).

With the use of several techniques for probing molecular structure, e.g., electron spin resonance, nuclear magnetic resonance, fluorescence labeling, etc. (Chapman and Dodd, 1971), it has been shown that the lipid molecules in the membrane undergo lateral migration with great ease (Kornberg and McConnell, 1971a) and they may even flip over in the membrane, although at very low frequencies (Kornberg and McConnell, 1971a; Blank and Britten, 1973). The constant lateral diffusional motion of the lipid molecules apparently is accompanied by dynamic activities of the protein molecules embedded in the bilayer (Frye and Edidin, 1970; Singer and Nicholson, 1972). In contrast to the fluidity of the lipid bilayer, the proteins, especially the spectrin on the endoface, probably confer the mechanical strength to the RBC membrane. Spectrin molecules have a tendency to form rodlike aggregates in solution; these may join each other, as well as the integral proteins (e.g., glycophorin) protruding from the membrane, to form a reinforcing undercoating beneath the lipid bilayer (Figure 6).

2.4 Membrane Transport of Ions

Anions such as Cl^- and HCO_3^- penetrate the RBC membrane about 10^6 times faster than cations of comparable size, e.g., Na^+ and K^+. This selectiveness in passive permeability of RBC membrane to charged small molecules has been explained by the fixed-charge hypothesis (Solomon, 1960). There is evidence that fixed positive charges, probably amino groups (Passow, 1969), are present inside the membrane; these charges prevent the passage of cations without blocking the movements of anions. For the cations Na^+ and K^+, in addition to the channels for passive permeability ("leak") through the RBC membrane, there also exist parallel and independent pathways for active transport ("pump") against electrochemical gradients. The Na–K active transport system is dependent upon metabolic energy derived from the activity of Na–K-sensitive membrane ATPase (Skou, 1957). In the normal RBC, the rates of "leak" and "pump" are balanced, leading to steady-state concentrations of intracellular K^+ and Na^+ (Table 1). A disturbance of this balance causes alterations in the transmembrane distribution of these cations.

The Ca^{++} concentration is less than 10^{-6} M inside the normal RBC, as compared to the plasma concentration of 10^{-3} M. This concentration gradient is maintained because of a low membrane permeability for calcium and the operation of the calcium pump. The Ca^{++}-activated ATPase in the membrane transduces energy from ATP for the active transport of Ca^{++} against the electrochemical gradient (Schatzmann and Vincenzi, 1969). The membrane proteins on the endoface, possibly spectrin, have a high affinity for calcium (Forstner and Manery, 1971; LaCelle et al., 1973) and serve to keep the free calcium concentration very low in the intracellular fluid. The ATP in the cell membrane also chelates calcium. A reduction in ATP level would decrease the Ca pump, elevate the intracellular calcium concentration, and increase the amount of calcium bound to the proteins on membrane endoface. As a result, there may be changes in protein conformation and an increase in membrane rigidity (Weed, LaCelle, and Merrill, 1969).

3 BIOPHYSICAL PROPERTIES OF RED CELL MEMBRANE

Because hemolysis usually reflects a mechanical failure of the RBC membrane, it is reasonable to examine the material properties of this membrane in a discussion on hemolysis. In fact, the earliest quantitative studies on the rheologic properties of cell membranes were performed on red cells subjected to osmotic hemolysis (Katchalsky et al., 1960) and to mechanical hemolysis (Rand, 1964).

When a solid material responds to a mechanical disturbance, its elastic modulus describes the relation between stress (force per unit area) and strain (fractional change in geometry, i.e., deformation). For a fluid, the viscosity describes the relation between shear stress (tangential force per unit area) and strain rate (rate of deformation). The RBC membrane has viscoelastic properties and exhibits a combination of these properties and a time-dependent response to mechanical disturbance. Because the RBC membrane is not a homogeneous material, especially in the direction normal to the surface, and its relatively constant thickness is not known precisely, it is more convenient to consider membrane tension (force per unit length on a cross section of the membrane), instead of membrane stress.

3.1 Membrane Elasticity

The results of the studies by Katchalsky et al. (1960) and Rand (1964) on RBC membrane subjected to hemolysis indicate that the elastic modulus[1] is of the order of 10^2 dynes/cm. More recently, experimental studies have been carried out in which the RBC membrane is subjected to mechanical disturbances much milder than those required to produce hemolysis (Hochmuth and Mohandas, 1972), and the elastic modulus is only of the order of 10^{-2} dynes/cm. These divergent results on elastic modulus (approximately 4 orders of magnitude) have been unified by a new material model in which the rheologic behavior of the RBC membrane varies depending on the mode of stress applied (Skalak et al., 1973; Evans, 1973). Because of the presence of excess membrane area in relation to its volume, the RBC can undergo considerable deformation without a change in membrane area (see Section 1). Thus stretching of the membrane along one axis can be compensated by shortening in another direction (Hochmuth and Mohandas, 1972), and the elastic modulus for such uniaxial loading (E_L, in dynes/cm) is relatively low:

$$E_L = T_L/e_L, \tag{1}$$

where T_L is the uniaxial tension (in dynes/cm) and e_L is the uniaxial strain (dimensionless). The normal RBC membrane can tolerate large uniaxial strains (more than the original dimension in one axis) without hemolysis. In contrast, the RBC membrane is rather stiff in response to areal strain (e_A, dimensionless), and the areal modulus (E_A, in dynes/cm) is

$$E_A = T_A/e_A, \tag{2}$$

where T_A (in dynes/cm) is the isotropic tension during area change. Normal RBC membrane area can tolerate an expansion of only about 7.5% before onset of hemolysis (Evans and Fung. 1972).

Considerations of the elasticity of the RBC membrane should also include the bending energy, which may be important in determining the curvature and shape of the red cell surface (Canham, 1970). The bending stiffness of the RBC membrane has not been measured, but theoretic estimations show that it is relatively low (Skalak, 1976).

Mechanical models have been proposed to simulate the deformation of

---

[1] The membrane tension at hemolysis with a short time scale is approximately 10–25 dyn/cm (Rand, 1964) and the critical strain is probably about 0.075 (Evans and Fung, 1972). Therefore, the elastic modulus is approximately 200 dyn/cm.

RBC membrane on the basis of a network structure formed by joining pivot points or posts with belts or wires (Sirs, 1970; Bull, 1973). The spectrin matrix on the endoface, presumably formed in combination with the glycophorin posts running through the membrane (Figure 6), may provide such an arrangement in the RBC membrane. Measurements on areal modulus of protein monolayers give values of the order of 10 dynes/cm (Blank, Lucassen, and van der Tempel, 1970), whereas results on lipids are several orders of magnitude lower (White, 1974).

3.2 Membrane Viscosity

Rheologic studies on hemolysis have demonstrated a time-dependent behavior of the RBC membrane (Katchalsky et al., 1960; Rand, 1964). In such cases, the large membrane tensions near hemolysis are accompanied by rather slow rates of change of strain (on the order of minutes), and the areal viscosity (μ_A) calculated with the use of some simple viscoelastic models is of the order of $10-10^2$ dynes-sec/cm. Studies on shape change of RBC ejected from a narrow pipette have shown that the recovery time without significant area change is of the order of 0.3 sec. This relatively fast rate of recovery and the small stress involved indicate that the uniaxial viscosity (μ_L) of the membrane is considerably lower than μ_A. A general theoretic approach to the analysis of μ_L has been given by Skalak (1973). Evans and Hochmuth (1976a) have used the Kelvin model (a spring and a dashpot in parallel) to derive an estimate of μ_L from the time course of shape recovery. The result is of the order of 10^{-3} dynes-sec/cm. Thus, similar to the case in membrane elastic properties, membrane viscosity varies greatly (4–5 orders of magnitude) depending on whether the stresses applied cause area dilatation or only uniaxial loading at constant area.

As mentioned in Section 2, studies with the use of membrane molecular probes have shown that the lipid bilayer has a high fluidity, and the viscosity value is of the order of 10^{-6} to 10^{-5} dynes-sec/cm. Because this value is several orders of magnitude lower than the viscosity values of the membrane, it seems that the μ_L and μ_A of the membrane are mainly contributed by the protein components, e.g., the spectrin matrix on the endoface (Evans and Hochmuth, 1976b), or by protein–lipid interactions.

3.3 Membrane Plasticity

The viscoelastic behavior of a material is associated with reversible recovery following the removal of the stress. When the applied stress exceeds a critical level (the yield point), however, the viscoplastic behavior of a material is associated with permanent deformations. Because of the limited extent to which the RBC can increase its surface area, it is difficult to ascertain the critical tension or reversibility of deformation in experiments involving area dilatation (Rand, 1964). On the other hand, plastic deformation of RBC membrane has been observed in response to shear stresses in a variety of conditions, e.g., the formation and growth of long tethers when shear stresses are applied to RBC adhering to a boundary (Kochen, 1968; Blackshear et al., 1971; Hochmuth and Mohandas, 1972). Evans and Hochmuth (1976b) have analyzed such viscoplastic behavior of membrane tether, assuming a constant membrane area. Their analysis involves initially a viscoelastic behavior and a later transition of a region of the tether neck to a viscoplastic zone. During the growth of the tether, membrane material flows from the main part of the cell through the plastic zone to form additional tether. The estimated value for the yield tension (T_y) is 10^{-2} to 10^{-1} dynes/cm and the viscosity associated with plastic deformation (μ_p) is of the order of 10^{-2} dynes-sec/cm. Since in this analysis the area is assumed to be constant, it is possible that the μ_p value would become higher when local areas begin to increase as the hemolytic condition is approached.

The various properties of the RBC membrane, i.e., elasticity, viscosity, plasticity, and bending rigidity (Table 2), must have their structural basis in the molecular organization of the membrane. It is likely that a major contributing factor to these properties is the spectrin–glycophorin network, which serves as the supporting matrix for the lipid bilayer with a high fluidity. Thus the fluid nature of the lipids provides the substrate for dynamic interactions of membrane components, whereas the mechanical

Table 2. Material properties of human red cell membrane (approximate orders of magnitudes)

Elasticity		
Uniaxial modulus	$\sim 10^{-2}$	dynes/cm
Areal modulus	$\sim 10^{2}$	dynes/cm
Viscosity		
Uniaxial viscosity	$\sim 10^{-3}$	dynes-sec/cm
Areal viscosity	~ 10	dynes-sec/cm
Viscoplasticity		
Plastic viscosity	$\sim 10^{-2}$	dynes-sec/cm
Bending property		
Bending modulus	$\sim 10^{-11}$	dynes-cm

properties of the protein matrix afford the support for the structural stability of the membrane. It must be pointed out that the lipid and protein components should not be treated as completely separate entities and that their interactions probably are of considerable importance in determining the mechanical properties of the cell membrane.

4 HEMOLYSIS INDUCED BY EXPERIMENTAL PROCEDURES

Hemolysis can be induced by subjecting the RBC to a number of physical and chemical disturbances (Ponder, 1948). Most of these disturbances can be controlled under laboratory conditions, and such in vitro hemolytic procedures are useful as clinical diagnostic tests and in research investigations on mechanisms of hemolysis. Hemolysis results when these physico-chemical disturbances produce energy changes in some regions of the RBC membrane to exceed the interaction forces that keep the molecular constituents together. The resulting transient lesions in the membrane, which may be seen on electronmicroscopic examination, allow the escape of hemoglobin.

4.1 Osmotic Hemolysis

The release of hemoglobin from RBCs placed in hypotonic media is probably the most widely used experimental technique in studying hemolysis. This procedure has been employed to prepare RBC membrane ghosts following the hemolytic release of hemoglobin (Dodge, Mitchell, and Hanahan, 1963). In clinical tests on osmotic fragility, red cells are exposed to decreasing strengths of hypotonic NaCl solutions and the percent hemolysis is calculated from measurements on hemoglobin release. The osmotic fragility curve relating hemolysis to salt concentration generally shows a sigmoidal shape, and 50% hemolysis occurs normally at a NaCl concentration of approximately 0.4 g/dl.

Because of the relatively low permeability of K^+ and Na^+ through the RBC membrane, net water fluxes are governed by the difference in osmotic concentrations across the membrane. Thus the hypotonic saline medium causes an influx of water and osmotic swelling. The RBC membrane behaves as a good (but not perfect) osmometer in separating these cations, and a factor R can be used to indicate the degree of imperfectness (Ponder, 1948). R is the ratio of the change in cell volume actually measured to that predicted on the basis of a perfect osmometer. One of the possible reasons for the deviation of R from unity during osmotic swelling is the leakage of K^+. Seeman et al. (1969) have found that the leakage of cellular K^+ prior to hemolysis depends on the rate of swelling (i.e., the initial osmotic gradient). The prelytic leakage of K^+ is 10% for rapid hemolysis (3 sec) and 20% for slow hemolysis (15 min). The prelytic leakage of K^+ presumably results from the opening of transmembrane channels for ions, as a consequence of the mechanical strain on the RBC membrane during cell swelling. This leakage of K^+, together with a possible increase in hydrostatic pressure inside the cell, may serve to retard the osmotic influx of water and maintain a quasisteady state. Canham and Parkinson (1970) observed a period of approximately 7 min during which the RBC remains spherical before hemolyis occurs.

Because the diffusion radius of the hydrated K^+ is smaller than that of the hydrated Na^+ (Shanes, 1958), it is reasonable to expect that an outward leakage of K^+ occurs before an inward leakage of Na^+. As hypotonic swelling gradually proceeds, however, an inward leakage of Na^+ does occur later, and the RBC membrane then becomes somewhat similar to blood capillary membranes in that it has a high permeability to all the major electrolytes in the system and that the major osmotically active solutes are the proteins. Because the hemoglobin concentration inside the cell (approximately 5 mM) is considerably higher than the protein concentration in the extracellular fluid (less than 1 mM for plasma and zero for saline solution), a colloidal osmotic gradient serves to draw the extracellular fluid inward. Although the colloidal osmotic gradient is much smaller than the osmotic gradient imposed on the system by the hypotonic saline (over 150 mOsm for a 0.4% NaCl solution), inward water flux may increase rapidly as the equivalent radius of the membrane channel increases during area stretching, because Poiseuille flow varies with the fourth power of the radius.

With the progress of colloidal osmotic flow and the rise in intracellular pressure, the membrane "holes" eventually become large enough for hemoglobin molecules (diffusion radius approximately 60 Å) to escape from the RBC. This transmembrane loss occurs mostly by diffusion (Kochen, 1962; Seeman, 1967) and the rate is retarded by the presence of macromolecules in the extracellular fluid (Seeman, 1974). Other intracellular constituents, e.g., adenylate kinase, are also lost, and the relative rates of loss suggest molecular sieving (Hjelm, Ostling, and Persson, 1966; MacGregor and Tobias, 1972), probably through effective "pores" with diameters of the order of 100 Å. The permeability to hemoglobin reduces its contribution to the colloidal osmotic pressure, and the hydrostatic pressure inside the cell then causes an outward fluid filtration, together with the hemoglobin leakage. Microscopic observations indicate that the hemoglobin leaves the cell gradually in all directions in slow hemolysis experiments (Danon, 1961). In contrast, in rapid hemolysis experiments, the hemoglobin appears to be ejected from the cell in streams about 1 μ wide, and holes and slits in RBC membrane ranging from 200 Å to 1 μ can be seen by electronmicroscopy (Seeman, 1967). The membrane holes that allow the leakage of hemoglobin also permit the inward passage of various macromolecules present in the extracellular fluid, but this is a transient phenomenon (25–250 sec) because the membrane seals itself spontaneously (Seeman, 1967, 1974). The RBC subjected to slow hemolysis can also recover its normal permeability to electrolytes over a longer period (Hoffman, Tosteson, and Whittam, 1960). Such abilities of the RBC membrane to reseal itself indicate the dynamic mobility of its molecular constituents.

With the use of an improved microscopic holography technique, Evans and Fung (1972) have measured the geometry of normal human RBCs subjected to hypotonic swelling (Table 3). These results indicate that at an osmolality corresponding to approximately 50% hemolysis (131 mOsm), the RBC is a nearly perfect sphere with a volume expansion of about 75% and an area stretching of about 7.5%. Further increases in membrane area probably would cause sufficient enlargement in membrane "holes" and leakage of hemoglobin. From these data one can calculate the value of R from the equation (Ponder, 1948)

$$\frac{C_h}{C_0} = \frac{RW_0}{100[(V_h/V_0) - 1] + RW_0} \tag{3}$$

where C_h and C_0 are the hypotonic and isotonic salt concentrations (or osmolalities), respectively, V_h and V_0 are the cell volumes in these

Table 3. Geometry of normal human red cells subjected to hypotonic swelling

Osmolality	Surface area (μ^2)	Cell volume (μ^3)
300 mOsm	135 ± 16	94 ± 14
217 mOsm	135 ± 13	116 ± 16
131 mOsm	145 ± 14	164 ± 23

Means ± S.D. From Evans and Fung (1972).

corresponding media, and W_0 is the percent cell water content in the isotonic medium. Using a value of 70% for W_0, the R value for RBC in 131 mOsm medium can be calculated as 0.82.

If the RBC lyses at a critical salt concentration, C_c, when it is a sphere with a surface area of $\lambda_m A_0$, where A_0 is the surface area in the isotonic medium and λ_m is the maximal areal expansion ratio which the membrane can sustain, then Eq. 3 can be written as

$$\frac{C_c}{C_0} = \frac{R W_0}{100[(\lambda_m/SI_0)^{3/2} - 1] + R W_0} \tag{4}$$

where SI_0 is the sphericity index of the RBC in isotonic medium and is equal to $4.84\, V_0^{2/3}/A_0$. It is apparent from this equation that the osmotic fragility of the RBC is not a simple property. The osmotic fragility test can be used to detect abnormal cell shapes, i.e., variations in SI_0. Thus spherocytes (e.g., in hereditary spherocytosis, with a high SI_0 near unity) have a high osmotic fragility (high C_c). On the other hand, the flattened shape leptocytes (e.g., in thalassemia, with a low SI_0) have a high resistance to osmotic lysis (low C_c). Equation 4 indicates that the leakiness to ions (R), the initial water content in the cell (W_0, reciprocally related to corpuscular hemoglobin concentration), and the rheologic properties of the membrane (λ_m) all can influence the result of osmotic fragility tests. The value of λ_m is dependent on the molecular organization of the red cell membrane constituents and is probably reduced in many diseases that involve defects in RBC membrane, e.g., hereditary spherocytosis, and thus contribute to an increased fragility. It should be noted that Eq. 4 is based on osmotic gradients of electrolytes. As mentioned earlier, the final phase of slow osmotic hemolysis is governed by the colloidal osmotic gradient, which is not included in Eq. 4.

With the use of a servomicropipette technique (Intaglietta, 1973), the increase in intracellular pressure during osmotic swelling has been measured in RBCs of amphiuma (Usami and Chien, unpublished observations). The transmembrane pressure rises sharply after the RBC attains a spherical shape and the critical pressure for lysis is of the order of 50 mmHg. The sequence of events in osmotic hemolysis is schematically summarized in Figure 7.

4.2 Mechanical Hemolysis

Since mechanical hemolysis is treated in detail in another chapter of this book (Hellums, 1976), only a brief account is given here. The discussions

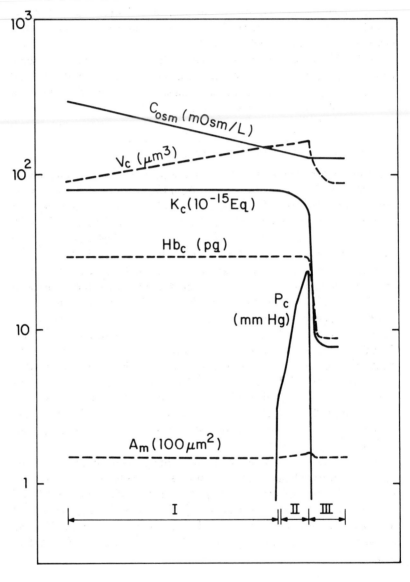

Time ⟶

in Section 3 indicate that the mechanical factors required to hemolyze RBC should vary according to the mode in which the forces are applied, i.e., whether isotropic or uniaxial deformation is involved. The terminal phase of osmotic hemolysis (Section 4.1) is actually mechanical in nature, consisting of an isotropic tension due to volume expansion. Hemolysis resulting from drawing RBC into narrow pipettes (inner radius less than 2 μ) also involves local areal strain. The critical membrane tension is approximately 10–25 dynes/cm, depending upon the speed of hemolysis (Rand, 1964).

Hemolysis in shear flow probably does not involve a significant change in total surface area, although areal strain may occur in localized regions. The mechanism of hemolysis in shear flow probably involves a local membrane stretching when the cell is subjected to tensile forces in a certain orientation in the shear field, similar to that described for liquid drops (Goldsmith, 1971). Indeed, scanning electronmicroscope pictures of RBCs fixed while subjected to high shear stresses (Sutera et al., 1975) show behavior very similar to liquid drops. Because of the low elastic modulus for uniaxial loading (approximately 10^{-2} dynes/cm), the uniaxial extension can be rather large without hemolysis. Studies on hemolysis induced by mechanical disturbance applied for very short periods of time have shown that the critical bulk shear stress is of the order of 10^4 dynes/cm^2 (Blackshear, Dorman, and Steinbach, 1965; Nevaril et al., 1968; Williams, Hughes, and Nyborg, 1970). Because of the time-dependent properties of the membrane, however, the critical shear stress required for hemolysis is lowered to 1.5×10^3 dynes/cm^2 when the duration of mechanical shearing is prolonged (Leverett et al., 1972).

Figure 7. Sequence of events during osmotic hemolysis by lowering the extracellular fluid osmolality (Cosm) from 300 to 130 mOsm, following an exponential course. The ordinate shows various parameters in logarithmic scale, and the abscissa is time in linear scale (absolute time not given, but the total period covers approximately 3 min). Phase I is crystolloid osmotic swelling, during which the cell volume (V_c) increases without any increase in membrane area (A_m), and the cell becomes increasingly spherical. The intracellular pressure (P_c) rises only very slightly toward the end of phase I. The increase in K permeability occurs at the end of phase I, and this is quickly followed by an increase in Na permeability, thus beginning the colloidal osmotic swelling (phase II). In phase II, the increase of V_c of the spherical cell is accompanied by a small expansion of A_m and a large increase in P_c. The total intracellular potassium content (K_c) decreases because of K leakage, but the total corpuscular hemoglobin (Hb$_c$) remains constant. As the increases in P_c and A_m reach critical levels, the membrane becomes permeable to hemoglobin and hemolysis (phase III) begins. The release of hemoglobin is accompanied by fluid loss (decreases in V_c and K_c), and recoveries of P_c and A_m.

Because the critical factor for hemolysis is the shearing condition at the membrane surface rather than that existing in the fluid, hemolysis in shear flow may be influenced by the geometry of the system. Shear hemolysis is enhanced by a marked narrowing in the diameter of the capillary channels through which the RBC is driven (Chien, Luse, and Bryant, 1971). This may occur in the in vivo hemolysis found in severe exercise during which skeletal muscular contraction may cause severe constriction of the narrow vessels in the exercising limb (Yoshimura, 1966). For RBCs attached to a glass surface (Hochmuth, Mohandas, and Blackshear, 1973), stress is constantly experienced by a given region of the membrane during shear, unlike the shear flow in a wide field where tensile and compressive stresses vary periodically with cell rotation. Therefore, probably less shear stress is required to induce viscoplastic flow and eventual hemolysis of such attached RBCs. The clinical test of mechanical fragility of RBCs usually involves shaking the cells in a flask with glass beads. This probably represents a shear hemolysis of RBC attached to the glass surface.

The molecular sieving behavior seen in osmotic hemolysis is also seen in mechanical hemolysis, suggesting the occurrence of similar membrane holes with an effective radius of the order of 100 Å during lysis (Chien et al., 1971).

4.3 Hemolysis due to Other Physical Factors

Hemolysis may result from the exposure of RBC to in vitro temperatures greater than 47°C (Ham et al., 1948; Kimber and Lander, 1964). The heat-treated red cells show membrane fragmentation and develop into spherocytes, which have increased osmotic and mechanical fragilities. These alterations probably result from the denaturation of membrane proteins (Rakow and Hochmuth, 1975) and the breakdown of membrane structure. Severe thermal burns of extensive body parts have been shown to cause acute hemolytic anemia (Shen, Ham, and Fleming, 1943).

Other physical factors that may cause hemolysis include laser and ultrasonic waves.

4.4 Hemolysis due to Chemical Factors

Many chemical substances with hydrophobic properties can be incorporated into the RBC membrane from the extracellular fluid. These include many local anesthetic agents and steroids (Seeman, 1966). A moderate amount of these substances serves to increase the membrane area and thus protects the RBC from osmotic hemolysis. The presence of a large concentration of these substances, however, may cause disruption of membrane structure and lead to hemolysis (Seeman, 1966). The detergent substance saponin and the polyene antibiotic filipin have a high affinity for cholesterol to form complexes (Thron, 1964; Kinsky, Luse, and van Deenen, 1966). Electron-microscopic studies on RBC membranes treated by these agents have demonstrated ringlike lesions approximately 80 Å in diameter by saponin and 150 Å by filipin (Seeman, 1974). As mentioned earlier, lyso-phosphatidylcholine has detergent qualities, and the presence of a large amount of L-PC in the extracellular fluid can raise its membrane concentration and cause hemolysis.

Membrane constituents may be affected by enzymes added to the extracellular fluid. Thus the presence of phospholipase in snake venom contributes to the hemolytic action of this poison (Condrea et al., 1964).

Prolonged storage of blood in vitro, e.g., under blood bank storage conditions beyond 4 wk, leads to a decrease in cellular ATP (Simon, Chapman, and, Finch, 1962). As a result, membrane calcium is released from ATP chelation to induce changes in membrane protein conformation (LaCelle, 1970) and losses of membrane lipid and membrane area (Haradin, Weed, and Reed, 1969). These membrane alterations enhance the hemolysis of stored RBC in vitro and following their transfusion in vivo.

The RBC membrane can be coated by many specific or nonspecific substances, which may be simultaneously bound to another surface (e.g., glass or another cell). If the binding force is very strong, the progressive increase in surface of contact may impose sufficient mechanical strain on the free membrane surface to cause hemolysis. An example of this is found in the hemolysis of RBC at glass surface when the extracellular medium contains polylysine, protamine, or other polycations (Nevo, DeVries, and Katchalsky, 1955). Strong electrostatic bonding forces exist between the positive charge groups of the polycation molecule and the negative charges on the glass and on the RBC surface (sialic acid). The removal of sialic acid from the RBC surface reduces such bonding (Jan and Chein, 1973), and prevents the hemolysis induced by polycations. Hemolysis can also result from covalent bonding of red cell surfaces by macromolecules.

The attachments of appropriate antibodies and complement to the RBC surface cause rearrangement of the normal components of the membrane, and hemolysis occurs when complement components beyond C5 are present (Polley, Müller-Eberhard, and Feldman, 1971). Electronmicroscopic examinations of RBC membrane after immune hemolysis have demonstrated the presence of surface ring structures approximately 100 Å in diameter (Borsos, Dourmashkin, and Humphrey, 1964). With the use of the freeze-cleavage technique, Iles et al. (1973) have shown that the membrane associated particles fuse together in units of three or four and that the number of these aggregate units generally equals the number of surface rings (Figure 8). The surface rings do not extend through the entire thickness of the membrane, but they may represent the transient holes that have been resealed on the inner half. Ferritin added to extracellular fluid before lysis can be demonstrated inside the RBC after hemolysis, but no ferritin is found inside the RBC ghost if added after immune lysis has already taken place (Iles et al., 1973). The final sequence of events in immune hemolysis has been postulated to be due to colloidal osmotic hemolysis (Iles et al., 1973).

5 HEMOLYSIS IN DISEASE

Normal human RBCs have an average life span of 120 days, and the removal of senescent cells from the circulation may be considered as the result of hemolysis under physiologic conditions. In many diseases the rate of hemolysis is accelerated, leading to premature destruction of RBCs. Anemia may result if the rate of destruction is considerably faster than the rate of RBC production. Red cell destruction in vivo differs in several aspects from hemolysis in vitro. Thus red cells flowing in the circulation are continuously subjected to mechanical stresses and undergo considerable deformations, especially in regions where the channel for passage is narrow. The capillaries in the spleen contain myriads of small fenestrations, through which RBC must squeeze to return to the circulation (Weiss and Tavassoli, 1970). The spleen has not only a unique microcirculatory architecture, but also the metabolic environment and phagocytic activities to cause entrapment and lysis of abnormal RBCs. Because of the sluggishness of the splenic circulation, the concentrations of glucose and other energy-yielding substrates in the RBC are reduced, with a consequent decrease in ATP level. This reduction in cellular ATP, together with low P_{O_2} and pH in the splenic blood, causes an increase in cell rigidity, further retarding the transit of RBC through the spleen (LaCelle, 1970). The reduction in ATP may also affect the energy-dependent lipid renewal pathways and cause an accumulation of lyso-phosphatidylcholine in the membrane (Jandl and Aster, 1967). All of these changes, together with the

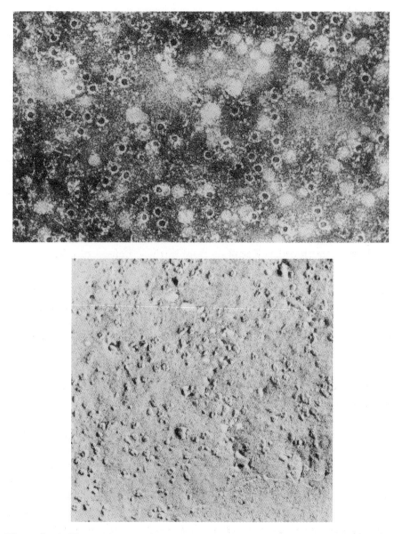

Figure 8. *A,* Negatively stained membranes of a sheep erythrocyte membrane that had been lysed by the complete system of rabbit complement and antisheep erythrocyte antibody. Note the surface rings, having outer and inner diameters of about 195 and 105Å, respectively. ×257,000. *B,* Freeze-cleave-etch appearance of sheep erythrocytes that had been lysed by the complete system of antibody and complement. The lower right-hand portion shows the intracellular surface of the cell membrane. The majority of the micrograph reveals the cleavage face of the extra-cellular leaflet, containing globule aggregates. Each aggregate appears to consist of 3 or 4 globules fused together. × 176,000. From Iles et al., 1973; reprinted by permission.

phagocytic activities of the mononuclear cells, tend to enhance hemolysis of even mildly abnormal RBC following erythrostasis in the spleen. Therefore, the spleen is usually the major site of hemolysis in vivo, although this process can also occur in the liver or other regions, especially when the RBC abnormality is severe (Jacob and Jandl, 1962). Because of the existence of various hemolytic factors in vivo, RBCs from patients with hemolytic anemias, e.g., autoimmune hemolytic anemia, sometimes do not exhibit the same hemolytic tendency in vitro.

Hemolytic disorder may result from intrinsic defects in the RBC or factors acting on the membrane from extracellular origin, or a combination of these mechanisms. Some examples are given for each type of hemolysis. The reader is referred to hematology texts (Wintrobe et al., 1974) for a more complete classification of hemolytic anemias.

5.1 Hemolytic Disorders Resulting from Intrinsic Defects of RBC

5.1.1 Membrane Defects   The pathology of erythrocyte membrane in various types of hemolytic anemias has been the subject of several reviews (Weed, 1968; LaCelle, 1970; Jacob, 1975). In these disorders, the deformability of the RBC is generally reduced because of an increase in sphericity and/or a change in the rheologic property of the membrane. As a result, the rigid, but fragile, RBCs are trapped and lysed in the reticuloendothelial system, especially the spleen.

A typical example of hemolytic anemia due to RBC membrane defect is hereditary spherocytosis. This is a congenital disorder in which the erythrocytes are more spherical in shape with a reduced membrane area (Figure 9). These spherocytes have an increased osmotic fragility, a reduced deformability, and a tendency to lose membrane by a budding process when incubated in vitro. The spherocytes are easily trapped in the spleen and undergo hemolysis, and splenectomy is usually the treatment of choice in this type of hemolytic anemia. The total and relative amounts of the various lipids are normal, and the membrane defect appears to lie in the protein moiety (Jacob, 1974). Extracts of membrane proteins from spherocytes differ from those of normal RBC in that the spherocytic proteins do not polymerize in response to an increase in ionic strength by adding K^+ or Ca^{++}. Furthermore, the phosphorylation of proteins from spherocytic membrane is abnormally sluggish. There is also an increased sodium permeability.

Abetalipoproteinemia (acanthocytosis) is a hereditary disorder in which the lack of plasma betalipoprotein is accompanied by the spicule,

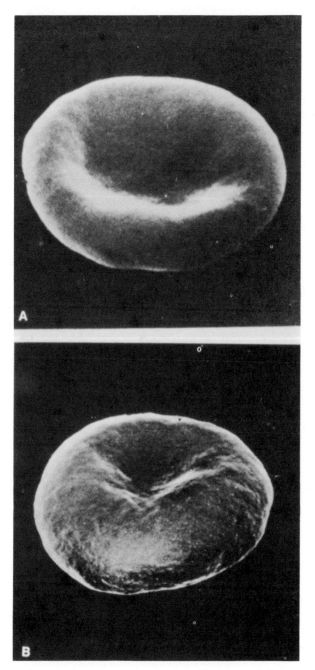

Figure 9. Scanning electron micrograph showing (A) a normal biconcave diskoid human RBC and (B) an RBC from a patient with hereditary spherocytosis. Note the loss of central depression. From Bessis et al., 1973; reprinted by permission.

thorny shape of RBC (acanthocyte) (Figure 10). The decrease in plasma beta-lipoprotein leads to a decrease in the turnover rate of the cholesterol in the RBC membrane, but the membrane cholesterol content shows only a slight increase (McBride and Jacob, 1970). Membrane phosphatidyl choline content and the PL/cholesterol ratio are significantly reduced (Ways, Reed, and Hanahan, 1963).

In fulminating liver diseases, the red cells may assume an appearance similar to the acanthocytes, and the condition is referred to as spur-cell anemia (Silber et al., 1966). The spur cell membrane also shows a decrease in PL/cholesterol ratio, but this results from a massive accumulation of cholesterol, rather than a decrease in PL as in the case of acanthocytosis (Cooper, 1969). The degree of hemolysis is greater in spur-cell anemia than in acanthocytosis. Cation permeability is not increased in either condition (Hoffman, 1962).

5.1.2 Enzyme Deficiencies There are several types of "inborn errors" of metabolism involving the glycolytic, energy-yielding pathways of RBC (Valentine, 1971). One of the possible mechanisms underlying the congenital hemolytic anemia is an impaired ability of RBC to generate ATP, with consequent alterations in the molecular organization and permeability of the membrane. In general, the blood contains irregularly crenated RBC, some with spicule forms. During in vitro incubation, the RBC tends

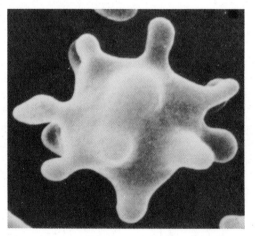

Figure 10. Scanning electron micrograph of an acanthocyte from a patient with abetalipoproteinemia. From Bessis et al., 1973; reprinted by permission.

to lose K^+ rather than, as in the case of hereditary spherocytosis, gain Na^+. Splenectomy is beneficial, but not as much as in hereditary spherocytosis. Examples of this group of hemolytic anemias are pyruvate kinase deficiency and hexokinase deficiency.

5.1.3 Hemoglobinopathies Abnormalities in globin peptide synthesis may cause secondary membrane alterations and hemolysis because of membrane–hemoglobin interactions. A classical example is sickle cell anemia (HbSS disease). The paracrystalline formation of hemoglobin S following deoxygenation (Bertles and Dobler, 1969) imparts a stress on the RBC membrane and distorts the cell into the characteristic sickle shape (Figure 11). Such deoxygenated sickle cells have a reduced deformability, especially in traversing narrow channels (Jandl, Simmons, and Castle, 1961; Messer and Harris, 1970; Usami, Chien, and Bertles, 1975). As a result these cells may cause microvascular obstruction in several parts of the body. The deoxygenated sickle cells also have increases in membrane permeability to Na^+ and K^+ (Tosteson, 1955) and to Ca^{++} (Eaton et al., 1973).

The HbSS cells may recover the normal biconcave shape following reoxygenation, but repeated sickling–unsickling due to cyclic oxygenation–deoxygenation may cause sufficient membrane damage to result in irreversibly deformed sickle cells (ISC) (Shen, Fleming, and Castle, 1949). These cells maintain the sickle shape even when the internal HbS becomes fluid following full oxygenation, indicating that the membrane has suffered irreversible damage (Bertles and Milner, 1968). There is an increase in intracellular Ca^{++} in these cells (Eaton et al., 1973), and the membrane area is probably reduced because of fragmentation during repeated sickling. Rheologic tests indicate that these ICSs have a reduced deformability (Chien, Usami, and Bertles, 1970). Freeze-cleavage examinations have demonstrated the distortion of internal membrane surfaces in ISC (Lessin, 1973). Instead of the normally occuring 100 Å membrane-associated particles, many discoid particles with diameter of approximately 500 Å are observed (Figure 12), which have been interpreted as denatured hemoglobin molecules bound to altered membrane proteins (Lessin, 1973). The membrane changes in deoxygenated sickle cells and in ISCs render them vulnerable to hemolysis in vivo.

5.2 Hemolytic Disorders Resulting from Factors Extrinsic to RBC

The various physicochemical stresses used to induce hemolysis in vitro, probably with the exception of osmotic hemolysis, can also operate in vivo

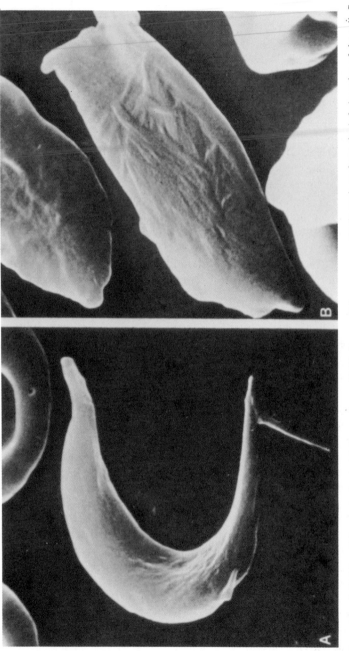

Figure 11. *A*, Sickle cell from a patient with homozygous HbSS disease. *B*, The surface patterning of this Hb-S cell may be indicative of the distribution of fascicles of intracytoplasmic Hb-S rods (see text). SEM preparation. From Bessis et al., 1973; reprinted by permission.

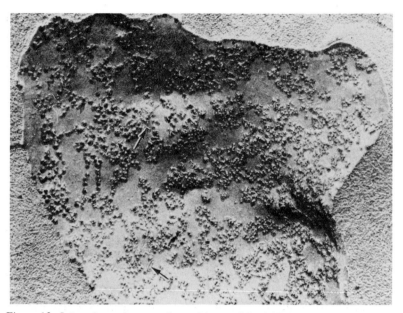

Figure 12. Internal membrane surface of irreversibly sickled cell. Membrane from ISC ghost preparation showing internal surface markedly distorted by large number of adherent microbodies. Occasional filaments (arrows) are also seen (× 105,000). From Lessin, 1973; reprinted by permission.

to cause premature RBC destruction. These disturbances can either cause hemolysis directly or they may induce sublethal damage in the RBC, which is then trapped and lysed in the spleen.

5.2.1 Extrinsic Physical Factors Cardiac patients with prosthetic heart valves, particularly aortic valve prosthesis, often develop hemolytic anemia (Stohlman et al., 1956; Brodeur et al., 1965). The onset of hemolytic anemia often corresponds to the occurrence of valvular leaks (Rogers and Sabiston, 1969), suggesting that regurgitated blood flow through a small opening at a high pressure gradient imparts the high stress for cell damage. The material properties of the valve surface may also have an important influence, because RBCs attached to the foreign surface would be subjected to high stresses for long periods of time.

The term microangiopathic anemia has been used to describe mechanical hemolysis in association with microvascular disorders, such as those found in malignant hypertension, cancer, disseminated intravascular coagulation, and polyarteritis (Brain, Dacie, ahd Hourihane, 1962). In these conditions, fibrin deposition on the inner wall of the arterioles forms a loose network in the lumen. RBCs tend to be attached to the fibrin mesh and are then damaged by the shear stress.

5.2.2 Hemolysis Induced by Chemical Agents Some drugs and poisons, e.g., snake venom (Condrea et al., 1964), can induce changes in the molecular composition of the membrane and cause hemolysis of normal RBCs. Other drugs, e.g., the oxidant primaquine, act on RBCs from patients with glucose-6-phosphate dehydrogenase (G-6-PD) deficiency to induce intracellular precipitation of hemoglobin as Heinz bodies (Jacob, 1970). This results from oxidation of the sulfhydryl groups of hemoglobin and the formation of mixed disulfide with glutathione or membrane proteins, causing the denaturation of hemoglobin and its precipitation in association with membrane proteins (Allen and Jandl, 1961), possibly spectrin. The red cells containing Heinz bodies have a reduced deformability and encounter difficulties in negotiating the narrow channels in the spleen (Rifkind, 1965). Because the oxidant acts specifically on RBCs with G-6-PD deficiency, this type of hemolysis represents the result of a combination of intrinsic and extrinsic factors. Heinz body formation also occurs in RBCs of patients with inherited unstable hemoglobins and thalassemia, even in the absence of oxidant drugs (Heller, 1966).

Freeze cleavage of Heinz-body containing RBC has shown a distortion of inner membrane surfaces (Lessin, 1973). The *A* face associated with the inner half of the membrane is markedly deformed by multiple domelike elevations of the Heinz bodies (Figure 13). The membrane-associated particles often become aggregated over the dome and rarified in other regions. Filamentous extensions from the underlying Heinz bodies to the inner membrane surface are often seen, suggesting that these bodies may bind to spectrin or other components of the membrane endoface (Lessin, 1973).

5.2.3 Immunohemolytic Anemia Because of immunologic reactions, antibody (immunoglobulin) or complement can be attached to red cell membrane and induce hemolysis. Depending on the nature of the immunologic process, hemolysis may result from intravascular lysis, agglutination, or selective destruction by the reticuloendothelial system (Cooper and Jandl, 1972). Intravascular hemolysis results when the antibody is able to induce the fixation of complement component beyond C5 to the RBC membrane. Under these circumstances, membrane holes probably open transiently to allow hemoglobin escape (see Section 4.4). In this regard, it

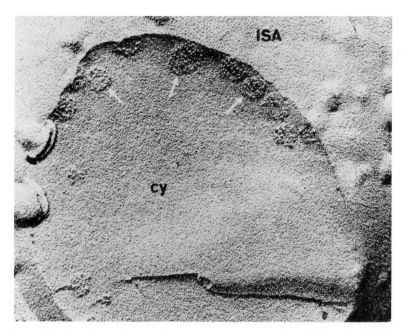

Figure 13. Relation of Heinz bodies to intramembrane surfaces. Heinz body containing erythrocytes showing face *A* (ISA) with subsurface Heinz bodies (arrows) within the cell interior (Cy). Membrane distortion by the Heinz bodies is evident and the close association of Heinz bodies with the internal aspect of the membrane is seen (× 38,000). From Lessin, 1973; reprinted by permission.

should be pointed out that lysis by complement-fixing antibodies is uncommon in human hemolytic disorders, except in ABO incompatible transfusion (Cooper and Jandl, 1972).

The antibodies of the IgM class can bridge RBCs and cause agglutination. The relatively strong bridging force exerted by IgM probably induces membrane tension on the agglutinated RBCs (see Section 4.4). Furthermore, the agglutinates, because of their large size, cannot pass through the narrow channels in the spleen, where cell trapping and lysis occur (Jandl, Jones, and Castle, 1957). Antibodies of the IgM type are not recognized by phagocytic cells (LoBuglio, Cotran, and Jandl, 1967).

Because of the existence of electrostatic repulsive force over the negatively charged surfaces of adjacent red cells (Chien and Jan, 1973), incomplete antibodies of the IgG class do not induce RBC agglutination in peripheral blood. Agglutination of IgG-coated RBCs, however, is found in the spleen (Jandl et al., 1957), probably because of the existence of a high cell concentration, a low shear rate, and an unusual metabolic environment. It has been found that IgG-coated RBCs can adhere to monocytes and to splenic macrophages (LoBuglio et al., 1967). Therefore, the unique environment in the spleen may cause the entrapment of IgG-coated RBCs and their hemolysis.

6 CONCLUSIONS

Hemolysis results from a disturbance of force balance in the red cell membrane. That is, the intermolecular attractive force in the membrane is exceeded by extrinsic physicochemical forces that tend to cause separation of the component molecules. An understanding of the molecular organization and biophysical behavior of the red cell membrane serves to elucidate the pathogenic mechanisms of hemolysis in many diseases. Investigations on hemolytic disorders, in turn, provide valuable insights into the normal properties of the red cell membrane. Further advances in our knowledge on the structure and function of cell membranes depend on interdisciplinary investigations including areas such as biochemistry, bioengineering, biophysics, hematology, physiology, and ultrastructure.

ACKNOWLEDGMENT

The author wishes to thank Professors Richard Skalak and Kung-ming Jan for helpful discussions.

LITERATURE CITED

Allen, D. W., and J. H. Jandl. 1961. Oxidative hemolysis and precipitation of hemoglobin. II. Role of thiols in oxidant drug action. J. Clin. Invest. 40: 454–475.
Bertles, J. F., and J. Dobler. 1969. Reversible and irreversible sickling: a distinction by electron microscopy. Blood 33: 884–898.
Bertles, J. F., and P. F. A. Milner. 1968. Irreversibly sickled erythrocytes: a consequence of the heterogeneous distribution of hemoglobin types in sickle-cell anemia. J. Clin. Invest. 47: 1731–1741.
Blackshear, P. L., F. D. Dorman, and J. H. Steinbach. 1965. Some mechanical effects that influence hemolysis. Trans. Am. Soc. Art. Int. Organs 11: 112–117.
Blackshear, P. L., R. J. Forstrom, F. D. Dorman, and G. O. Voss. 1971. Effect of flow on cells near walls. Fed. Proc. 30: 1600–1609.

Blank, M., and J. S. Britten. 1973. Comments on the molecular basis of fluidity in membranes. Chem. Phys. Lipids 10: 286–288.

Blank, M., J. Lucassen, and M. van den Tempel. 1970. The elasticities of spread monolayers of bovine serum albumin and of ovalbumin. J. Colloid Interface Sci. 33: 94–100.

Borsos, T., R. R. Dourmashkin, and J. H. Humphrey. 1964. Lesions in erythrocyte membranes caused by immune haemolysis. Nature 202: 251–252.

Brain, M. C. 1970. Microangiopathic hemolytic anemia. Ann. Rev. Med. 21: 133–144.

Brain, M. C., J. V. Dacie, and D. O'B. Hourihane. 1962. Microangiopathic hemolytic anemia: the possible roles of vascular lesions in pathogenesis. Brit. J. Haematol. 8: 358–374.

Branton, D. 1966. Fracture faces of frozen membranes. Proc. Natl. Acad. Sci. U.S. 55: 1048–1056.

Bretscher, M. S. 1973. Membrane structure: some general principles. Science 181: 622–629.

Brodeur, M. T. H., D. W. Sutherland, R. D. Kiler, A. Starr, J. A. Kinsey, and H. E. Griswold. 1965. Red blood cells survival in patients with aortic valvular disease and ball-valve prosthesis. Circulation 32: 570–581.

Bull, B. 1973. Red cell biconcavity and deformability. A macromodel based on flow chamber observations. In M. Bessis, R. I. Weed, and P. F. Leblond (eds.), Red Cell Shape, pp. 115–124. Springer-Verlag, New York.

Burt, D. H., and J. W. Green. 1971. The sodium permeability of butanol-treated erythrocytes: the role of calcium. Biochim. Biophys. Acta 225: 46–55.

Canham, P. B. 1970. The minimum energy of bending as a possible explanation of the biconcave shape of the human red blood cell. J. Theor. Biol. 26: 61–81.

Canham, P. B., and D. R. Parkinson. 1970. The area and volume of single human erythrocytes during gradual osmotic swelling to hemolysis. Can. J. Physiol. Pharmacol. 48: 369–376.

Chapman, D., and G. H. Dodd. 1971. Physicochemical probes of membrane structure. In L. I. Rothfield (ed.), Structure and Function of Biological Membranes, pp. 13–83. Academic Press, New York.

Chau-Wong, M., and P. Seeman. 1971. The control of membrane-bound Ca^{2+} by ATP. Biochim. Biophys. Acta 241: 473–482.

Chen, P. C. Y., and Y. C. Fung. 1973. Extreme-value statistics of human red blood cells. Microvasc. Res. 6: 32–43.

Chien, S. 1975. Biophysical behavior of red cells in suspension. In D. M. Surgenor (ed.), The Red Blood Cell, 2nd Ed. Vol. II, pp. 1031–1133. Academic Press, New York.

Chien, S., and K. M. Jan. 1973. Red cell aggregation by macromolecules: roles of surface adsorption and electrostatic repulsion. J. Supramol. Struct. 1: 385–409.

Chien, S., S. A. Luse, and C. A. Bryant. 1971. Hemolysis during filtration through micropores: a scanning electron microscopic and hemorheologic correlation. Microvasc. Res. 3: 183–189.

Chien, S., S. Usami, and J. F. Bertles. 1970. Abnormal rheology of oxygenated blood in sickle cell anemia. J. Clin. Invest. 49: 623–634.

Condrea, E., F. Mammon, S. Aloof, and A. DeVries. 1964. Susceptibility of erythrocytes of various animal species to the hemolytic and phospholipid splitting action of snake venom. Biochim. Biophys. Acta 84: 365–375.

Cooper, R. A. 1969. Anemia with spur cells: a red cell defect acquired in serum and modified in the circulation. J. Clin. Invest. 48: 1820–1831.

Cooper, R. A. 1970. Lipids of human red cell membrane: normal composition and variability in disease. Semin. Hematol. 7: 296–322.

Cooper, R. A., and J. H. Jandl. 1972. Destruction of erythrocytes. In W. J. Williams, E. Beutler, A. J. Erslev, and R. W. Rundles (eds.), Hematology, p. 181. McGraw-Hill, New York.

Danielli, J. F., and H. Davson. 1935. A contribution to the theory of permeability of thin films. J. Cell. Comp. Physiol. 5: 495–508.

Danon, D. 1961. Osmotic hemolysis by a gradual decrease in the ionic strength of the surrounding medium. J. Cell. Comp. Physiol. 57: 111–117.

Dodge, J. T., C. Mitchell, and D. J. Hanahan. 1963. The preparation and chemical characterization of hemoglobin-free ghosts of human erythrocytes. Arch. Biochem. 110: 119–130.

Dodge, J. T., and G. B. Phillips. 1967. Composition of phospholipids and of phospholipid fatty acids and aldehydes in human red cells. J. Lipid Res. 8: 667–675.

Dorlands Illustrated Medical Dictionary. 1974. 25th Ed. Saunders, Philadelphia.

Eaton, J. W., T. D. Skelton, H. S. Swofford, C. E. Kolpin, and H. S. Jacob. 1973. Elevated erythrocyte calcium in sickle cell disease. Nature 246: 105–106.

Evans, E., and Y. C. Fung. 1972. Improved measurements of the erythrocyte geometry. Microvasc. Res. 4: 335–347.

Evans, E. A. 1973. A new material concept for the red cell membrane. Biophys. J. 13: 926–940.

Evans, E. A., and R. M. Hochmuth. 1976a. Membrane visco-elasticity. Biophys. J. 16:1–11.

Evans, E. A., and R. M. Hochmuth. 1976b. Membrane visco-plastic flow. Biophys. J. 16: 13–26.

Forstner, J., and J. F. Manery. 1971. Calcium binding by human erythrocyte membranes. Biochem. J. 124: 563–571.

Frye, C. D., and M. Edidin. 1970. The rapid intermixing of cell surface antigens after formation of mouse-human heterokaryons. J. Cell. Sci. 7: 319–333.

Fung, Y. C. 1966. Theoretical considerations of the elasticity of red cells and small blood vessels. Fed. Proc. 25: 1761–1772.

Goldsmith, H. L. 1971. Deformation of human red cells in tube flow. Biorheology 7: 235–242.

Goldstein, D. A., and A. K. Solomon. 1960. Determination of equivalent pore radius for human red cells by osmotic pressure measurement. J. Gen. Physiol. 44: 1–17.

Gregersen, M. I., C. A. Bryant, W. Hammerle, S. Usami, and S. Chien. 1967. Flow characteristics of human erythrocytes through polycarbonate sieves. Science 157: 825–827.

Hagermann, J. S., and R. G. Gould. 1951. The in vitro interchange of cholesterol between plasma and red cells. Proc. Soc. Exp. Biol. Med. 78: 329–332.

Ham, T. M., S. C. Shen, E. M. Fleming, and W. B. Castle. 1948. Studies on the destruction of red blood cells. IV. Thermal injury. Blood 3: 373–403.

Haradin, A. R., R. I. Weed, and C. F. Reed. 1969. Changes in physical properties of stored erythrocytes. Transfusion 9: 229–237.

Heller, P. 1966. Hemoglobinopathic dysfunction of the red cell. Am. J. Med. 41: 799–814.

Hellums, J. D. 1976. Damage of blood by mechanical forces. In N. H. C. Hwang (ed.), Cardiovascular Flow Dynamics. (this volume). University Park Press, Baltimore.

Hjelm, M., S. G. Ostling, and A. E. G. Persson. 1966. The loss of certain cellular components from human erythrocytes during hypotonic hemolysis in the presence of dextran. Acta Physiol. Scand. 67: 43–49.

Hochmuth, R. M., and N. Mohandas. 1972. Uniaxial loading of the red cell membrane. J. Biomech. 5: 501–511.

Hochmuth, R. M., N. Mohandas, and P. L. Blackshear, Jr. 1973. Measurement of the elastic modulus for red cell membrane using a fluid mechanical technique. Biophys. J. 13: 747–762.

Hoffman, J. F. 1962. Cation transport and structure of the red cell plasma membrane. Circulation 26: 1201–1213.

Hoffman, J. F., D. C. Tosteson, and R. Whittam. 1960. Retention of potassium by human erythrocyte ghosts. Nature 185: 186–187.

Iles, G. H., P. Seeman, D. Naylor, and B. Cinader. 1973. Membrane lesions in immune hemolysis. Surface rings, globule aggregates and transient openings. J. Cell Biol. 56: 528–539.

Intaglietta, M. 1973. Pressure measurements in the microcirculation with active and passive transducers. Microvasc. Res. 5: 317–323.

Jacob, H. S. 1970. Mechanisms of Heinz body formation and attachment to red cell membrane. Semin. Hematol. 7: 93–106.

Jacob, H. S. 1974. Dysfunctions of the red cell membrane. In D. M. Surgenor (ed.), The Red Blood Cell, 2nd Ed. Vol. I, pp. 269–292. Academic Press, New York.

Jacob, H. S. 1975. Pathologic states of the erythrocyte membrane. In G. Weissman and R. Claiborne (eds.), Cell Membranes: Biochemistry, Cell Biology and Pathology, pp. 249–255. HP Publishing, New York.

Jacob, H. S., and J. H. Jandl. 1962. Effects of sulfhydryl inhibition on red blood cells. II. Studies in vivo. J. Clin. Invest. 41: 1514–1523.

Jan, K. M., and S. Chien. 1973. Role of surface electric charge in red blood cell interaction. J. Gen. Physiol. 61: 638–654.

Jandl, J. H., and R. H. Aster. 1967. Increased splenic pooling and the pathogenesis of hypertension. Am. J. Med. Sci. 253: 383–398.

Jandl, J. H., A. R. Jones, and W. B. Castle. 1957. The destruction of red cells by antibiotics in man. I. Observations on the sequestration and lysis of red cells altered by immune mechanisms. J. Clin. Invest. 36: 1428–1459.

Jandl, J. H., R. L. Simmons, and W. B. Castle. 1961. Red cell filtration and the pathogenesis of certain hemolytic anemias. Blood 18: 133–148.

Katchalsky, A., O. Keden, C. Klibansky, and A. DeVries. 1960. Rheological considerations of the haemolysing red blood cell. In A. L. Copley and G. Stainsby (eds.), Flow Properties of Blood and Other Biological Systems, pp. 155–164. Pergamon Press, New York.

Kimber, R. J., and H. Lander. 1964. The effect of heat on human red cell morphology, fragility and subsequent survival in vivo. J. Lab. Clin. Med. 64: 922–933.

Kinsky, S. C., S. A. Luse, and L. M. van Deenen. 1966. Interaction of polyene antibiotics with natural and artificial membrane systems. Fed. Proc. 25: 1503–1510.

Kirkpatrick, F. H. 1976. Spectrin: current understanding of its physical, biochemical, and functional properties. Life Sci. 19: 1–18.

Kochen, J. A. 1962. Structural disturbances during red cell lysis. Am. J. Dis. Child. 104: 537–538.

Kochen, J. A. 1968. Viscoelastic properties of the red cell membrane. In A. L. Copley (ed.), Hemorheology, pp. 455–463. Pergamon Press, London.

Kornberg, R. D., and H. M. McConnell. 1971a. Lateral diffusion of phospholipids in a vesicle membrane. Proc. Nat. Acad. Sci. U.S. 68: 2564–2568.

Kornberg, R. D., and H. M. McConnell. 1971b. Inside–outside transitions of phospholipids in vesicle membranes. Biochemistry 10: 1111–1120.

LaCelle, P. L. 1970. Alteration of membrane deformability in hemolytic anemias. Semin. Hematol. 7: 355–371.

LaCelle, P. L., F. H. Kirkpatrick, M. P. Udkow, and B. Arkin. 1973. Membrane fragmentation and Ca^{++}-membrane interaction: potential mechanisms of shape change in the senescent red cell. In M. Bessis, R. I. Weed, and P. F. Leblond (eds.), Red Cell Shape, pp. 69–78. Springer-Verlag, New York.

Lessin, L. S. 1973. Membrane ultrastructure of normal, sickled and Heinz-body erythrocytes by freeze-etching. In M. Bessis, R. I. Weed, P. F. Leblond (eds.), Red Cell Shape, pp. 151–168. Springer-Verlag, New York.

Leverett, L. B., J. D. Hellums, C. P. Alfrey, and E. C. Lynch. 1972. Red blood cell damage by shear stress. Biophys. J. 12: 257–273.

Lichtman, M. A., and R. I. Weed. 1973. Divalent cation content of normal and ATP-depleted erythrocytes and erythrocyte membranes. *In* M. Bessis, R. I. Weed, and P. F. Leblond (eds.), Red Cell Shape, pp. 77–93. Springer-Verlag, New York.

LoBuglio, A. F., R. S. Cotran, and J. H. Jandl. 1967. Red cells coated with immunoglobulin G: binding and sphering by mononuclear cells in man. Science 158: 1582–1585.

MacGregor, R. D., II, and C. A. Tobias. 1972. Molecular sieving of red cell membrane during gradual osmotic hemolysis. J. Membrane Biol. 10: 345–356.

McBride, J. A., and H. S. Jacob. 1970. Abnormal kinetics of red cell membrane cholesterol in acanthocytosis: studies in genetic and experimental abetalipoproteinemia and in spur cell anemia. Brit. J. Haematol. 18: 383–397.

Marchesi, V. T., and E. Steers, Jr. 1968. Selective solubilization of a protein component of the red cell membrane. Science 159: 203–204.

Marchesi, V. T., R. L. Jackson, J. P. Segrest, and I. Kahane. 1973. Molecular features of the major glycoproteins of the human erythrocyte membrane. Fed. Proc. 32: 1833–1837.

Messer, M. J., and J. W. Harris. 1970. Filtration characteristics of sickle cells: rates of alteration of filterability after deoxygenation and reoxygenation, and correlation with sickling and unsickling. J. Lab. Clin. Med. 76: 537–547.

Mulder, E., J. W. O. vanden Berg, and L. L. M. van Deenen. 1965. Metabolism of red-cell lipids. II. Conversions of lysophosphoglycerides. Biochim. Biophys. Acta 106: 118–127.

Nathan, D. G., F. A. Oski, V. W. Sidel, F. H. Gardner, and L. K. Diamond. 1966. Studies of erythrocyte spicule formation in haemolytic anemia. Brit. J. Haematol. 12: 385–395.

Nevaril, C. G., E. C. Lynch, C. P. Alfrey, Jr., and J. D. Hellums. 1968. Erythrocyte damage and destruction induced by shearing stress. J. Lab. Clin. Med. 71: 784–790.

Nevo, A., A. DeVries, and A. Katchalsky. 1955. Interaction of basic amino acids with the red blood cell. I. Combination of polylysine with single cells. Biochim. Biophys. Acta 17: 536–547.

Oliveira, M. M., and M. Vaughan. 1964. Incorporation of fatty acids into phospholipids of erythrocyte membranes. J. Lipid. Res. 5: 156–162.

Passow, H. 1969. Passive ion permeability of the erythrocyte membrane. Prog. Biophys. Mol. Biol. 19 (2): 423–467.

Polley, M. J., H. J. Müller-Eberhard, and J. D. Feldman. 1971. Production of ultrastructural membrane lesions by the fifth component of complement. J. Exp. Med. 133: 53–62.

Ponder, E. 1948. Hemolysis nad Related Phenomena. Grune and Stratton, New York.

Rakow, A. L., and R. M. Hochmuth. 1975. Thermal transition in the human erythrocyte membrane: effect on elasticity. Biorheology 12: 1–3.

Rand, R. P. 1964. Mechanical properties of the red cell membrane. II. Viscoelastic breakdown of the membrane. Biophys. J. 4: 303–316.

Reed, C. F. 1968. Phospholipid exchange between plasma and erythrocytes in man and the dog. J. Clin. Invest. 47: 749–760.

Rifkind, R. A. 1965. Heinz body anemia: an ultrastructural study. II. Red cell sequestration and destruction. Blood 26: 433–448.

Robertson, J. D. 1960. The molecular structure and contact relationships of cell membranes. Prog. Biophys. Biophys. Chem. 10: 343–418.

Rogers, B. M., and D. C. Sabiston, Jr. 1969. Hemolytic anemia following prosthetic valve replacement. Circulation 39 (Suppl. I): I155–I161.

Rosenthal, A. S., F. M. Kregenow, and H. L. Mosle. 1970. Some characteristics of Ca^{++} dependent ATPase activity associated with a group of erythrocyte membrane proteins which form fibrils. Biochim. Biophys. Acta 196: 254–262.

Schatzmann, H. J., and F. F. Vincenzi. 1969. Calcium movements across the membrane of human red cells. J. Physiol. 201: 369–395.

Seeman, P. 1966. Erythrocyte membrane stabilization by local anesthetics and tranquilizers. Biochem. Pharmacol. 15: 1753–1766.

Seeman, P. 1967. Transient holes in the erythrocyte membrane during hypotonic hemolysis and stable holes in the membrane after lysis by saponin and lysolecithin. J. Cell. Biol. 32: 55–70.

Seeman, P. 1974. Ultrastructure of membrane lesions in immune lysis, osmotic lysis and drug-induced lysis. Fed. Proc. 33: 2116–2124.

Seeman, P., D. Cheng, and G. H. Iles. 1973. Structure of membrane holes in osmotic and saponin hemolysis. J. Cell Biol. 56: 519–527.

Seeman, P., T. Sauks, W. Argent, and W. O. Kwant. 1969. The effect of membrane-strain rate and of temperature on erythrocyte fragility and critical hemolytic volume. Biochim. Biophys. Acta 183: 476–489.

Shanes, A. M. 1958. Electrochemical aspects of physiological and pharmacological action in excitable cells. Pharmacol. Rev. 10: 59–164.

Shen, S. C., T. H. Ham, and E. M. Fleming. 1943. Mechanism and complication of hemoglobinuria in patients with thermal burns: spherocytosis and increased osmotic fragility of red blood cells. N. Engl. J. Med. 229: 701–713.

Shen, S. C., E. M. Fleming, and W. B. Castle. 1949. Irreversibly sickle erythrocytes: their production in vitro. Blood 4: 498–504.

Shinitzky, M., and M. Inbar. 1974. Difference in microviscosity induced by different cholesterol levels in the surface membrane lipid layer of lymphocytes and malignant lymphoma cells. J. Molec. Biol. 85: 603–615.

Shohet, S. B. 1972. Hemolysis and changes in erythrocyte membrane lipids. N. Engl. J. Med. 286: 577–583, 638–644.

Silber, R., E. Amorosi, J. Lhowe, and J. J. Kayden. 1966. Spur-shaped erythrocytes in Laennec's cirrhosis. N. Engl. J. Med. 275: 639–643.

Simon, E. R., R. G. Chapman, and C. A. Finch. 1962. Adenine in red cell preservation. J. Clin. Invest. 41: 351–359.

Singer, S. J. 1975. Architecture and topography of biological membranes.

In G. Wasserman and R. Claiborne (eds.), Cell Membranes: Biochemistry, Cell Biology and Pathology, pp. 35–44. HP Publishing, New York.

Singer, S. J., and G. L. Nicholson. 1972. The fluid mosaic model of the structure of cell membranes. Science 175: 720–732.

Sirs, J. A. 1970. Structure of the erythrocyte. J. Theor. Biol. 27: 107–115.

Skalak, R. 1973. Modelling the mechanical behavior of red blood cells. Biorheology 10: 229–238.

Skalak, R. 1976. Rheology of red blood cell membrane. *In* Proceedings of First World Congress on Microcirculation. Toronto, June 1975. Plenum Press, New York. In press.

Skalak, R., A. Tozeren, R. P. Zarda, and S. Chien. 1973. Strain energy function of red cell membranes. Biophys. J. 13: 245–264.

Skou, J. C. 1957. The influence of some cations on an adenosine triphosphatase from peripheral nerves. Biochim. Biophys. Acta 23: 394–401.

Solomon, A. K. 1969. Red cell membrane structure and ion transport. J. Gen. Physiol. 43 (Suppl. 1): 1–15.

Stohlman, F., Jr., S. J. Sarnoff, R. B. Case, and A. T. Ness. 1956. Hemolytic syndrome following the insertion of a lucite ball valve prosthesis into the cardiovascular system. Circulation 13: 586–591.

Sutera, S., M. Mehrjardi, and N. Mohandas. 1975. Deformation of erythrocytes under shear. Blood Cells 1: 369–376.

Tarlov, A. R. 1966. Lecithin and lysolecithin metabolism in rat erythrocyte membranes. Blood 28: 990–991.

Thron, D. C. 1964. Hemolysis by holothurin A, digitonin and wuillaia saponin: estimates of the required cellular lysin uptakes and free lysin concentrations. J. Pharmacol. Exp. Ther. 145: 194–202.

Tillack, T. W., and V. T. Marchesi. 1970. Determination of the outer surface of freeze-etched red blood cell membranes. J. Cell. Biol. 45: 649–653.

Tosteson, D. C. 1955. The effect of sickling on ion transport. II. Effect on sodium and cesium transport. J. Gen. Physiol. 39: 55–67.

Tosteson, D. C., and J. F. Hoffman. 1960. Regulation of cell volume by active cation transport in high and low potassium sheep red cells. J. Gen. Physiol. 44: 169–194.

Usami, S., S. Chien, and J. F. Bertles. 1975. Deformability of sickle cells as studied by microsieving. J. Lab. Clin. Med. 86: 274–282.

Valentine, W. N. 1971. Deficiencies associated with Embden–Meyerhof pathway and other metabolic pathways. Semin. Hematol. 8: 348.

van Deenen, L. L. M., and J. DeGier. 1974. Lipids of the red cell membrane. *In* D. M. Surgenor (ed.), The Red Blood Cell, 2nd Ed. Vol. I, pp. 147–211. Academic Press, New York.

Ways, P., C. F. Reed, and D. J. Hanahan. 1963. Red-cell and plasma lipids in acanthocytosis. J. Clin. Invest. 42: 1248–1260.

Weed, R. I. 1968. The cell membrane in hemolytic disorders. Plenary

Session Papers, XII. Congr. Internat. Soc. Hemat., New York, pp. 81–92.

Weed, R. I., P. L. LaCelle, and E. W. Merrill. 1969. Metabolic dependence of red cell deformability. J. Clin. Invest. 48: 795–809.

Weinstein, R. S. 1974. The morphology of adult red cells. *In* D. M. Surgenor (ed.), The Red Blood Cell, 2nd Ed. Vol. I, pp. 213–268. Academic Press, New York.

Weinstein, R. S., and N. S. McNutt. 1970. Ultrastructure of red cell membranes. Semin. Hematol. 7: 259–274.

Weiss, L., and M. Tavassoli. 1970. Anatomical hazards to the passage of erythrocytes through the spleen. Semin. Hematol. 7: 124–133.

White, S. H. 1974. Comments on "Electrical breakdown of bimolecular lipid membranes as an electrochemical instability." Biophys. J. 14: 155–158.

Williams, A. R., D. E. Hughes, and W. L. Nyborg. 1970. Hemolysis near a transversely oscillating wire. Science 169: 871–873.

Wintrobe, M. M., C. R. Lee, D. R. Boggs, T. C. Bithell, J. W. Athens, and J. Foerster (eds.). 1974. Clinical Hematology, 7th ed., Lea & Febiger, Philadelphia.

Yoshimura, H. 1966. Sports anemia. *In* K. Evang and K. L. Anderson (eds.), Physical Activity in Health and Disease, pp. 74–78. Universitets Forlaget, Oslo.

Cardiovascular Flow Dynamics and Measurements
Edited by N. H. C. Hwang and N. A. Normann
Copyright 1977   University Park Press   Baltimore

chapter 20

BLOOD CELL DAMAGE BY MECHANICAL FORCES

J. David Hellums and Clarence H. Brown, III

ABSTRACT

Blood damage problems sometimes limit the usefulness of various devices involving blood flow such as artificial cardiac valves, artificial hearts, and extracorporeal circulation systems. Therefore, there is considerable interest in establishing the mechanism of damage. A series of studies has been made using rotational viscometers of special design in an effort to establish the effects of shear stress in the absence of other complications. Above a threshold stress level, red cell damage is revealed in hemolysis, morphologic changes, and in shorter life span in vivo. The exposure time—shear stress plane is divided into two distinct regimes. In the regime of relatively low stresses and exposure times there is relatively little damage, and the damage is dominated by solid surface interaction effects. In the other regime, at high stresses and exposure time, stress effects alone dominate and very high rates of hemolysis occur. The experimental findings of several workers are shown to be consistent when interpreted in this way. Much lower stresses stimulate the platelet reaction and subsequent aggregation. The sensitivity of platelets to stress raises the possibility that thrombus formation in patients with artificial heart valves or other cardiac prostheses could result from the effects of shearing stress on circulating platelets.

INTRODUCTION

Comments on the Problem

The research on which this chapter is based is directed toward the problem of prosthesis—blood interaction with resulting blood trauma. To understand the need for the work one can suppose for a moment that complete information is available on blood damage. That is to say, suppose that for

799

a given prosthesis we have established the levels of all the various blood changes incurred, and we have established all the physiologic effects of these blood changes. Even in this extreme case, where all this information is supposed to be known, it can be seen that we lack the answer to the most important question: What changes in the design or operation of the prosthesis will yield improvement in the effects on the subject? Without a relatively fundamental approach, progress can only be made through trial-and-error experiments guided by intuitive arguments. Hence, the need for studies on the mechanics of blood damage.

Consider a small element of blood as it moves with the flow through a prosthesis. The element is subjected to normal stresses (pressure[1]) and to tangential or shear stresses (due to viscosity and the velocity gradients). If the observer is supposed to move with the element of blood, these stresses will change with time as the element passes through the various regions—even for flows at steady state. If the flow is turbulent, additional changes in the stresses occur that fluctuate in both space and time. In addition, the element will be subjected to various physical and biochemical effects as it changes in proximity to (and perhaps comes in contact with) various interfaces and other blood components. The effect of solid interfaces is of most interest in the applications considered here, although of course gas interfaces are known to have important effects. The solid-interface effects are strongly influenced by shear stress or shear rate in general, because the shear rate is of primary importance in determining transport rates near solid interfaces.

In summary, when we speak of the mechanics of blood damage, we are referring to the effects of the stress distribution in the fluid with the understanding that the effects may depend on at least two primary parameters in addition to magnitude of stresses: proximity to solid surfaces, and time of application of the stress (more accurately one should speak of the time history, rather than simply time of application).

Rotational Viscometers

Studies involving complicated flows such as those in a prosthesis cannot be expected to lead to an understanding of the mechanics of blood damage.

---

[1]On the flows under consideration the shear rate and dimensions are such that for most practical purposes blood may be considered to be Newtonian, and the normal stress may be assumed to equal the pressure.

The stress effects can be determined only from much simpler flows in which the stress distributions are known simple functions of time and of position. From previous work (Nevaril et al., 1968, 1969) it seems that the normal stress is of secondary importance; we therefore concentrate on the effects of shear stress.

Rotational viscometers have several important properties useful for studies on shear degradation of biological fluids. The most important property is that the shear stress is known and approximately constant in a certain fluid region. However, conventional concentric cylinder viscometers have some other characteristics that make them imperfectly suited for such studies. A schematic drawing of a conventional design of platens (the parts that contact the specimen) for such devices is given in Figure 1. The specimen of blood occupies both the narrow gap between the two concentric cylinders and about half the volume of the reservoir (the wide gap between the outer cylinder and the shaft at the top is here designated as the reservoir). With reference to this figure it is possible to explain certain difficulties in using such instruments.

First, in Figure 1 it should be noted that there is a substantial area of blood—air interface at the top of the reservoir. Furthermore, this interface is in rapid motion when high shear rates are employed. Some workers have neglected blood damage at such interfaces. Our results of a study on this damage and the related mixing problem (Leverett et al., 1972) suggest that the hemolysis due to blood—air interaction at the interface is of the same order as that due to all other causes. Hence the suggestion is that this hemolysis, which often has been neglected, seriously clouds the interpretation of results. It seems that some workers who have reported effects of shear stress unknowingly have included a large contribution from the blood—air interface.

Second, in Figure 1 it should be noted that the blood subjected to the known uniform shear stress is that in the narrow gap, whereas that in the reservoir is subjected to relatively low shear stress. This difference causes no difficulty in ordinary rheologic work. One simply may neglect the stress in the reservoir and base the calculations on the torque transmitted through the narrow gap. However, in shear degradation studies no such simplifying assumptions can be invoked. Even if one could neglect the blood damage in the reservoir, there is always mixing of an unknown degree between the specimen in the narrow gap and that in the reservoir. This mixing problem has been studied and found to be important in some

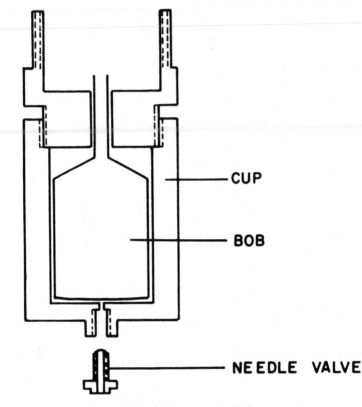

Figure 1. Head of a conventional viscometer.

viscometers (Leverett et al., 1972). Hence the neglect of the effects associated with the reservoir should be viewed with caution in interpreting results.

Third, it should be noted that in such instruments narrow gaps are usually employed between the two platens. Thus the blood—solid interfacial area is significant in relation to the small volume of blood. There is no question that shear stress and solid interfaces interact in their various effects on the blood—at least over some ranges of the parameters. Hence in any studies of very general applicability, we would like to be able to vary the stress and the surface area independently. Apparently there have been only two studies (Croce, 1972; Leverett et al., 1972; Sutera et al., 1972) wherein the surface-to-volume ratio was varied independently of the shear stress. Otherwise, previous workers using rotational viscometers seem to have used a fixed configuration. In these cases it is difficult or impossible to establish the importance of blood–solid interaction.

The three factors listed above served as the stimuli for the development in our laboratories of an instrument that we have called The Rice Viscometer. In 10 years of working in blood damage-related problems we have developed several similar instruments; the most recent model incorporates several features that make it uniquely suited to shear degradation studies. The head of this instrument is shown in Figure 2. The instrument has the following important properties:

1. Drive Belt
2. Cup
3. Thermocouple Well
4. Sample Port
5. Cooling Fins
6. Torque Shaft
7. Height Adjustment
8. Bob

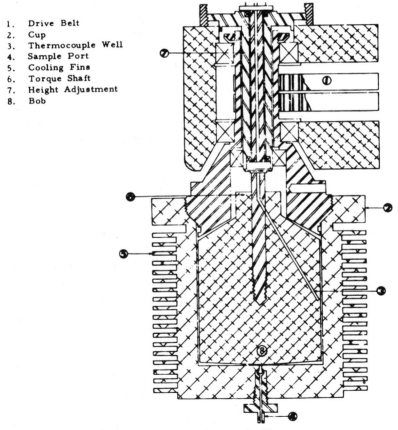

Figure 2. Head of the Rice University Viscometer.

1. The unsheared reservoir at the top of the instrument has been eliminated. In its place, as shown in Figure 2, we have a cone-and-cone section. The (upper) cone-and-cone section, the (middle) concentric cylinder section, and the (bottom) cone-and-plate section are all carefully designed so that the specimen in all three sections is subjected to the same shear rate. This design has the added advantage of greatly reducing the blood—air interfacial area.

2. The instrument is extremely flexible. It is capable of imposing shear rates much higher than ordinary viscometric equipment (up to 200,000 sec^{-1}). The driving and control system have accurate, rapid response. Start up time of only about 3 sec is required with only 10% overshoot of the desired stress level. This rapid response is essential in studies on time dependence. The instrument has a sheared sample volume large enough for evaluation of a number of parameters of blood response.

3. The instrument has three different configurations so that solid interfacial area can be varied independently of shear rate.

In summary this special-purpose instrument (Figure 3) has the properties needed for establishing the shear stress—blood—solid interface effects while minimizing other complications. More detailed discussion of the design of the instrument is given by MacCallum et al. (1973).

Applications

Experimental determination of blood damage in complex flows cannot be used to determine the mechanics of blood damage. In general, it is not possible to take overall measurements, and from them to determine the amount of damage attributable to the diverse phenomena taking place at various positions in the flow. However, the converse case is possible, and indeed that is the main point of the work: Given sufficient understanding of the mechanics of blood damage, it is possible to predict the overall damage that would take place in any complicated flow. One can estimate the velocity and stress distribution in a complicated flow, relying in part on empirical correlations and on measurements as needed. Then from the known mechanics, the rates of change per unit volume can be estimated throughout the fluid. Integration of these rates over the total volume yields the desired overall result. This approach is basically the same as that often applied in the analysis of chemical reactions and transport processes in cases where variations in space and time are important.

It should be pointed out that the case described in the preceding

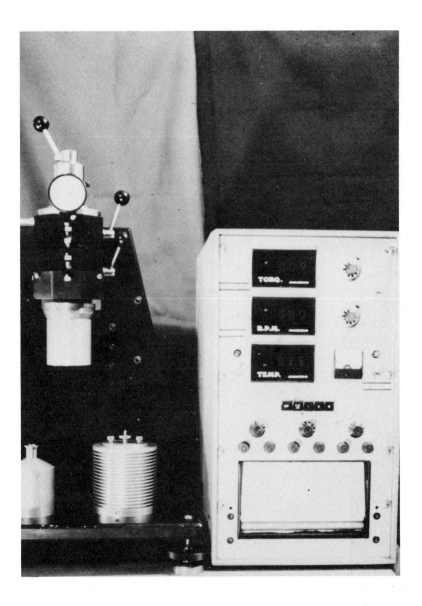

Figure 3. Overall view of the Rice University Viscometer.

paragraph is highly idealized for purposes of illustration. Sufficiently detailed studies to make complete analysis possible are probably not necessary, because adequate approximations usually suffice. However, studies on a sound engineering basis appear to be essential to long-term progress in circulation assistance. At the present time the effects of some variables are not known with certainty even to the nearest order of magnitude.

ERYTHROCYTE TRAUMA STUDIES

Previous Research in These Laboratories

In the research program now under discussion, studies have been carried out on three physical forces that might result in injury to red blood cells, i.e., (1) pressure changes, (2) impact due to crushing of erythrocytes between solid surfaces, and (3) shearing stress.

The response of erythrocytes has been evaluated by the measurement of the release of hemoglobin into the plasma, by morphologic examination of traumatized red blood cells, and by the determination of the survival of traumatized erythrocytes in vivo. The studies to date have led to the following conclusions and findings:

1. When erythrocytes are subjected to a shear stress above a critical value (approximately 1500 dynes/cm^2 for human blood for 2-min exposures) hemolysis occurs, observable morphologic changes occur, and in vivo survival of cells is decreased. Below this critical shear stress relatively little hemolysis occurs.

2. Quantitative measurements were made of morphologic changes due to shear stress. Significant morphologic changes may occur at stresses that produce relatively little plasma hemoglobin.

3. Evidence was obtained of rapid removal of damaged cells from the circulation, principally by the spleen. The erythrocyte removal from the circulation is consistent on a quantitative basis with the morphologic changes.

4. The morphologic changes induced by exposure of erythrocytes to shear stress are similar to those observed in patients with hemolytic anemia associated with artificial valves.

5. From fluid mechanical considerations, it has been shown that the shear stresses associated with a jet (as might be found with a regurgitant

flow about an aortic valvular prosthesis) may exceed the critical shear stress necessary to injure erythrocytes in vitro. This finding, together with the previous ones, shows consistency between clinical observations and the in vitro work.

6. Pressure fluctuations of the magnitude of those associated with the normal cardiovascular system produce little or no red cell trauma. This conclusion is based on measurements and calculations corresponding to the major pressure differences known to occur. However, more study is needed on high-frequency fluctuations as would be associated with the "ringing" of prosthetic valves and with turbulent flow. More study is also needed at low pressures where cavitation bubbles may occur.

7. An evaluation of the effect of crushing (as would result from valve seating upon erythrocytes) was performed in vitro with a simulated Starr—Edward valve. Repeated apposition of the ball against the valve seat resulted in some release of hemoglobin but did not cause morphologic changes of significance or effect survival of erythrocytes in vivo. The magnitude of the hemolysis was below that thought to be important clinically.

8. A series of careful studies was made on various secondary effects in a rotational viscometer. Specific attention was focused on the effects of solid surface interaction, centrifugal force, air—interface interactions, cell—cell interaction (effect of hematocrit), viscous heating, and mixing of sheared and unsheared sample. The results show that for stress above the threshold level, 1,500 dynes/cm^2 for 2-min exposure, there is extensive cell damage that is directly due to shear stress. In this regime the various secondary effects listed above were negligible in the particular instrument used.

9. Erythrocytes containing Hb SS are very fragile in venous preparation (the critical shear stress is less than 400 dynes/cm^2). When oxygenated, Hb SS cells are more shear-stress resistant but still much more fragile than normal cells (the critical shear stress is 500 dynes/cm^2).

10. Pathologic erythrocytes differ in shear resistance from normal cells and may be ordered in increasing resistance: sickle cell anemia, iron deficient, thalassemia minor, pyruvate kinase deficient, normal, and hereditary spherocytosis.

11. A study has been completed in which the shear resistance of cohort-labeled cells was determined at various times throughout the lifetime of the cells. It appears that cell shear fragility, at least up to ages very near the cell normal life span, decreases with increasing age of the cell.

12. The effect of exposure time to shear stress was studied in the rotational viscometer over the time range 15–600 sec. It seems that the rate of hemolysis (expressed as a fraction of the cells exposed) is almost independent of exposure time. That is to say, the plasma hemoglobin increases approximately linearly with time until substantial amounts of hemolysis occur (in which case the rate of increase of plasma hemoglobin is proportional to the hematocrit).

These findings are discussed in more detail by Nevaril et al. (1968, 1969), Leverett et al. (1972), MacCallum et al. (1973, 1975). In addition, the correlation with work of others and the effect of exposure time are reviewed in the following section.

Other Previous Work

The importance of studying the mechanics of cell damage has been realized for some time and several studies have been carried out using relatively simple flows. Here we briefly summarize the findings and reproduce part of Leverett et al. (1972) where we have been able to organize much of this previous work.

Red cell studies employing rotational viscometers have been carried out by several workers in recent years (Bernstein, Blackshear, and Kelley, 1967; Nevaril et al., 1968, 1969; Knapp and Yarborough, 1969; Shapiro, 1970; Steinbach, 1970; Champion et al., 1971; Croce, 1972; Leverett et al., 1972; Sutera et al., 1972; MacCallum et al., 1973, 1975; Nanjappa, Chang, and Glomski, 1973). A number of interesting and important changes have been shown to take place in erythrocytes subjected to shear stress. The interpretation of results in some cases has been subject to question to a degree since, as explained previously, there are some difficulties in determining the effect of shear stress independently of that of the blood–air interface and of the blood–solid interface interaction. There have been five (Nevaril, et al., 1968; Champion et al., 1971; Leverett et al., 1972; Sutera et al., 1972; Sutera and Mehrjardi, 1975) studies that employed shear rates above the level where stress effects alone are thought to dominate. In some work (Sutera et al., 1972) a viscometer with a rotating inner cylinder has been used. This configuration has a higher tendency to secondary flow and turbulence than the case of rotating outer cylinder. In other work (Champion et al., 1971) high stresses were obtained by suspending cells in high-viscosity dextran solutions.

Several workers have investigated the high-stress regime using equipment other than the concentric cylinder viscometer. Rooney (1970) used a pulsating gas bubble immersed in the blood, and Williams, Hughes, and Hyborg (1970) carried out a similar study using an oscillating wire. In both cases the authors analyzed the flow and were able to estimate the maximum shear stress in the flow field. They found a threshold stress for damage of 5,600 dynes/cm^2 for the bubbles.

Indelgia et al. (1968) and Blackshear (1972a) used jets of blood and jets of other liquids into blood to study the effect of shear stress. In the jet device there is no completely satisfactory way of characterizing the shear stress. The stress depends strongly on position and there is no well-defined maximum stress. Near the entrance, in the high-stress region of most interest, the stress varies approximately as $1/x^2$ where x is distance from the entrance (Schlichting, 1968a). Using a stress based on an average inlet velocity gradient, the authors reported a threshold stress of 40,000 dynes/cm^2. This figure is not directly comparable to those from other devices in which the maximum stress is known; however, the calculated stress presumably is a valid order of magnitude estimate. The high threshold stress is in the direction one might expect because the cells are subjected to stress for very short periods of time in the jet.

Keshaviah (1970) and Blackshear (1972a) studied hemolysis in canine blood flow through capillaries and reported results in terms of velocity. The maximum shear stress can be calculated for these flows. The resulting threshold values are about 4,500 dynes/cm^2 for ordinary capillaries and about 7,000 dynes/cm^2 for capillaries with a smooth, tapered entrance.

Bacher and Williams (1970) used capillary tubes in studies on bovine blood. There is some difficulty in comparing this work with others because the authors stated that the age of the blood made it more susceptible to damage than fresh blood. This work shows a threshold for damage of about 5,000 dynes/cm^2. The authors give some arguments in favor of a cell–solid surface mechanism although their data seem insufficient to give clear support to arguments on the mechanism.

Blackshear (1972a, b) has written two reviews covering various aspects of hemolysis in flowing blood.

The Effect of Exposure Time on Hemolysis

The time of exposure to shearing stress is an important variable that has sometimes received inadequate attention. We have investigated the time effect at several shear stress levels. The time range of 3–120 sec was investigated. As can be seen by the typical results in Figure 4 the

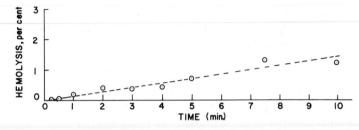

Figure 4. Effect of exposure time on erythrocytes for a shear stress of 1920 dynes/cm^2.

destruction is approximately linear in time, at least for relatively low levels of hemolysis. Morphologic abnormalities also increase with exposure time. This behavior is consistent with the concept of a threshold shear stress that depends on exposure time.

In addition to this experimental work in rotational viscometers we have collected and analyzed the previous work on hemolysis with attention focused on the exposure time (Figure 5). Exposure time is measured directly in the concentric cylinder viscometer. In other equipment estimates of the time are more difficult, but in even the most complex flows it is possible to make an order of magnitude estimate. For the oscillating wires and bubbles the exposure time was taken to be the boundary-layer

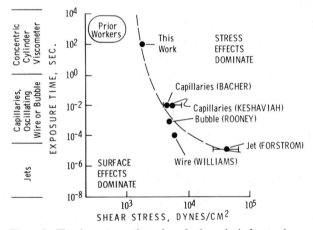

Figure 5. The shear stress–time plane for hemolysis due to shear.

length divided by the product of the maximum shear rate and the bound-ary-layer thickness. For the jet experiments the exposure time was based on the time required for the stress on a cell to decay by one order of magnitude, based on a simple analysis of the turbulent jet (Schlichting, 1968a).

A summary of the state of studies on red blood cell damage is given in Table 1. This table brings all the results together in a way that makes it easy to see why there have been numerous disagreements among various workers as to the mechanism and threshold levels for damage. Exposure time and stress level are the two primary parameters. In the high-stress region the threshold level may be seen to vary in a monotonic way with exposure time. At stresses below 1,500 dynes/cm^2 there is little direct damage due to shear stress. Solid-surface interaction and other shear rate-related phenomena (such as air-interface interaction) predominate in the low-stress regime and the levels of hemolysis per unit time are rela-tively low. Hence it seems that the primary reason for disagreements among previous workers is that different workers have studied different regimes of the exposure time–stress domain. Most individual studies are insufficiently detailed to establish mechanisms for damage.

The results are presented in Figure 5 in which the division of the shear stress–time domain into two distinct regimes is displayed. The curve represents our estimate of the threshold for extensive shear stress damage. Considering the diverse flows and different bloods and conditions used by the various workers, the results are remarkably consistent. The envelope designated "prior workers" pertains to previous workers using the concen-tric cylinder viscometer. The times and the stresses are, of course, only order of magnitude estimates for the more complicated flows. Even this accuracy, however, is more than has been previously available, and this accuracy is adequate for many applications in the design and analysis of prostheses.

It should be pointed out that until recently there was uncertainty among some workers on implications of the findings as presented here. Both Sutera et al. (1972) and Blackshear (1972a, b) felt that solid-surface interaction might play a predominant role in hemolysis in viscometric flows, even at stresses above the threshold locus presented in Figure 5. Some important light was cast on this question from an interesting study by Sutera and Mehrjardi (1975). They used glutaraldehyde for fixation of erythrocytes while the cells were suspended in a viscometric flow. Then

Table 1. Summary of effect of shear stress on hemolysis

Type of exposure	Order of magnitude of exposure time (sec)	Threshold level of damage (dynes/cm^2)	Refs. and comments
Turbulent jet	10^{-5}	40,000	Indelgia et al. (1968); Black-shear (1972a)
Oscillating wire	10^{-4}	5,600	Williams et al. (1970) (human and canine)
Oscillating bubble	10^{-3}	4,500	Rooney (1970) (human and canine)
Capillary flow	10^{-2}	5,000	Bacher and Williams (1970) (bovine blood)
Capillary flow	10^{-2}	4,500–7,000	Keshaviah (1970) and Black-shear (1972b) (canine blood)
Concentric cylinder	10^{2}	1,500	This work
Concentric cylinder	10^{3}	1,000–2,000	Sutera et al. (1972)
Cone and plate	10^{3}	1,000	Williams et al. (1970) (in dextran solution)
Concentric cylinder, maximum stress, 600 dynes/cm^2	10^{2}–10^{3}	Relatively little hemolysis per unit time	Shapiro and Williams (1970) (surface effects dominate)
Concentric cylinder, maximum stress, 250 dynes/cm^2	10^{3}	Relatively little hemolysis per unit time	Knapp and Yarborough (1969) (surface effects dominate)
Concentric cylinder, maximum stress, 600 dynes/cm^2	10^{3}	Relatively little hemolysis per unit time	Steinbach (1970) and Black-shear (1972a) (surface effects dominate)

the fixed cells were examined by scanning electron microscopy. The observations indicated that shear stress fragmentation occurred at a threshold level ($2,000-2,500$ dynes/cm^2) consistent with that reported here.

Shear Stress Levels in Valves

It was pointed out previously that the high-velocity flows associated with insufficient aortic valves can result in shear stress sufficiently high to cause hemolysis. Recently, Roschke, Harrison, and Blankenhorn (1975) have shown that such stress levels can be reached even in a normally functioning prosthetic valve. They studied measurements of flow and poppet velocity and calculated wall shear stresses based on a parabolic velocity profile (which gives a conservatively low estimate of shear stress). The principal results are given in Figure 6, reproduced from their paper. From the velocities we can establish that the time of flight of an erythrocyte through the valve aperture is of the order of 10^{-3} sec. From the threshold curve in Figure 5 corresponding to an exposure time of 10^{-3} sec we see that shear stress hemolysis would be expected at a stress level of about 5×10^3 dynes/cm^2. This stress on Figure 6 falls above the curve representing the natural valve but below those representing prosthetic valves. Thus we should expect some shear stress hemolysis in prosthetic valves but none in natural valves. The levels of hemolysis would not necessarily be high

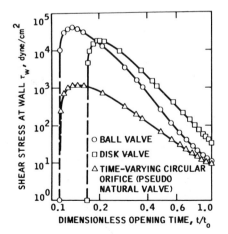

Figure 6. Estimated shear stress in aortic valves. From Roschke, Harrison, and Blankenhorn (1975); reprinted by permission.

because only the cells that pass near a solid surface are subjected to the maximum stress. These findings are consistent with clinical observations. Roschke et al. called attention to the fact that even very mild hemolysis may not be as innocuous as once thought, because gallstones may form in such cases (Merendino and Manhas, 1973).

The shear stress estimates of Roschke et al. (1975) and those of most other workers are based on flows near smooth solid surfaces. These estimates are of obvious value but care should be used in their interpretation because they can only yield a lower bound to the stress. At a given average fluid velocity the (often unknown) detailed shape of the surfaces can have a profound effect on the maximum stresses developed. Even the texture or roughness of the surfaces is extremely important. For example, Schlichting (1968b) shows that surface roughness can increase the wall shearing stress by as much as an order of magnitude in flow by a flat surface at a given average velocity. Thus it is not surprising that fabric-covered prostheses sometimes result in more blood trauma than similar, smooth devices. It is also not surprising that there may at times be difficulty in determining the mechanism of blood cell damage: solid-surface contact versus bulk shear stress. Such difficulties presumably will be more pronounced in studies on platelets, which are much more surface sensitive than erythrocytes.

PLATELET TRAUMA STUDIES

A Preliminary Viscometric Study

Since thrombosis is a serious complication associated with prosthetic circulatory devices, we have been studying the effects of physical forces, especially shearing stress, on platelets to determine if these forces are capable of promoting platelet activation resulting in the formation of platelet aggregates, perhaps the initial event in thrombus formation. The studies have employed the concentric viscometer described in the previous section. Fresh human blood was centrifuged at $1400\,g$ for 5 min to remove the red and white cells, leaving a platelet-rich plasma (PRP). This PRP was then subjected to graded levels of shearing stress for varying periods of time.

The number of platelets in the sheared samples fell remarkably (Figure 7). The maximum decrease in platelet count occurred between 100 and 200 dynes/cm^2, whereas higher shearing stresses resulted in less of a

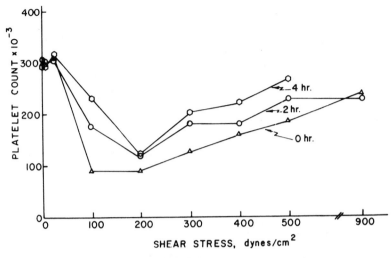

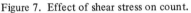

Figure 7. Effect of shear stress on count.

depression in counts. When counts were again determined 2 and 4 hr after shearing stress was applied, there was a tendency for the counts to be higher than those obtained immediately after shearing was discontinued. We determined that the fall in counts is due to the formation in specimens of platelet aggregates and that these aggregates are able to partially disaggregate over a period of 2–4 hr. The higher counts at higher shear are due to aggregates and individual platelets being broken apart by the shearing forces. We have formed these conclusions based on examination of the specimens with electron microscopy.

Figure 8 shows an electron micrograph of PRP that was subjected to shearing stress at a level below that which results in a fall in platelet count. Note that platelets are single entities in this specimen.

Figure 9 shows the appearance of a specimen sheared at 100 dynes/cm^2, the shear force that results in severe depression in platelet count. Note the larger aggregate of platelets. All of the platelets in this clump are excluded from the platelet count because counts are performed with an electronic particle counter that is designed to enumerate only particles of 3–30 μ diameter.

At a much higher shear stress (Figure 10) we found some small aggregates but, more importantly, we noted fragmented and distorted platelets that did not participate in aggregation.

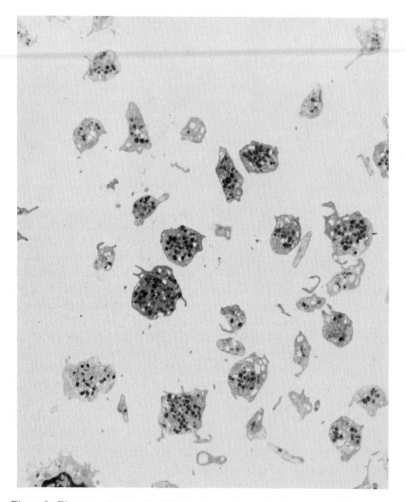

Figure 8. Electron micrograph of PRP subjected to a shearing stress of 8 dynes/cm^2.

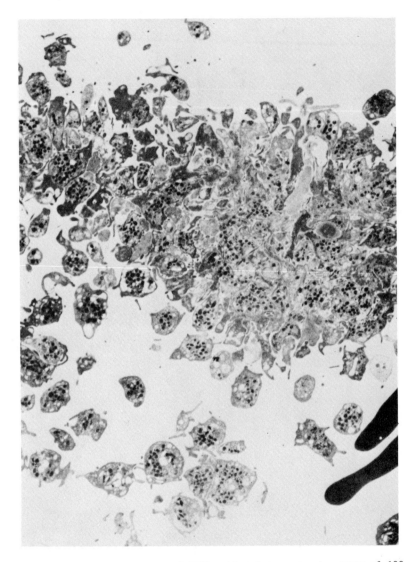

Figure 9. Electron micrograph of PRP subjected to a shearing stress of 100 dynes/cm².

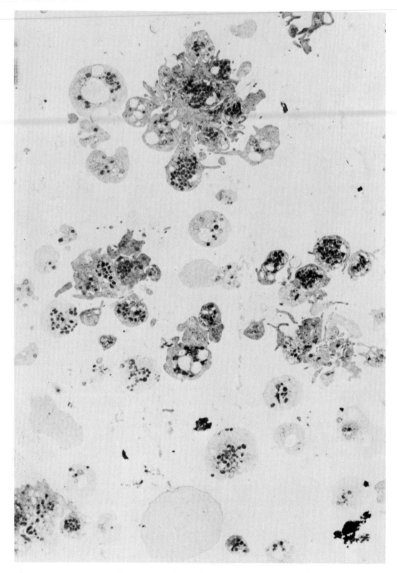

Figure 10. Electron micrograph of PRP subjected to a shearing stress of 200 dynes/cm².

The next question was, "What biochemical alterations occur in platelets that might account for aggregation?" Platelets contain within their granules and cytoplasm a number of constituents that, when extruded into the plasma, promote aggregation. Among these are serotonin and adenine nucleotides such as adenosine diphosphate (ADP).

We determined that the serotonin content of platelets fell during shearing (Figure 11) and that ADP and ATP are released into the plasma during shearing stress with a corresponding fall in the content of ADP and ATP remaining in the platelets (Figure 12). By radiolabeling studies we found that radioactive ATP and ADP are released into the plasma (Figure 13). This occurs with both EDTA and citrate.

From these studies it can be concluded that the origin of some of the ATP and ADP extruded into the plasma even at low stresses (50 dynes/cm^2) is the cytoplasmic or metabolically active pool of nucleotides which can be released to plasma only by lysing the platelet. Additional (unlabeled) nucleotide is elaborated by stimulation of the so-called release reaction or secretory function of platelets.

These studies seem to show that platelets can be altered by low levels of shearing stress and that this damage or stimulation may lead them to form aggregates that could be the initial step in thrombus formation. We are continuing the studies with varying conditions of plasma environment and in systems where whole blood will be used in order that we might, for example, determine the capability of platelets to experience the changes

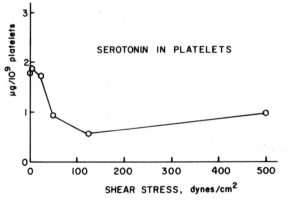

Serotonin Release from Platelets by Shear Stress to PRP

Figure 11. Serotonin release from platelets by shear stress to PRP.

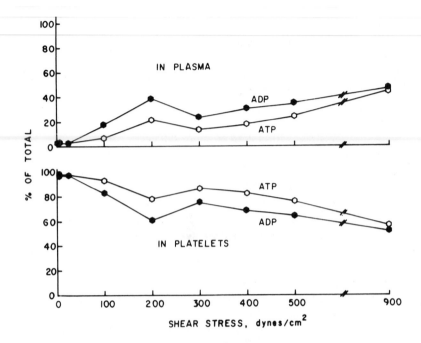

Figure 12. Nucleotide release from platelets by shear stress to PRP.

described here when red cells and white cells are present. Additional work is also underway at smaller exposure times analogous to the previously described work on red cells. Some additional results and more details on the studies have been reported elsewhere (Brown et al., 1975a and b).

Relationship to Other Work

As indicated above, our preliminary finding is that platelets are much more sensitive to shearing stress than erythrocytes. However, it must be recognized that these findings are only at relatively high exposure times. Furthermore, the effects of solid-surface interaction have been inadequately studied as yet. There is some evidence that in the practical range of exposure time (perhaps 10^{-5} to 10^{-1} sec or so) we will find that platelets are more resistant than erythrocytes, contrary to the results at long exposure times.

Some clinical evidence supports this point of view. For example, Manohitharajah and co-workers (1974) have studied 28 patients with homograft and prosthetic valves and found that the platelet survival time

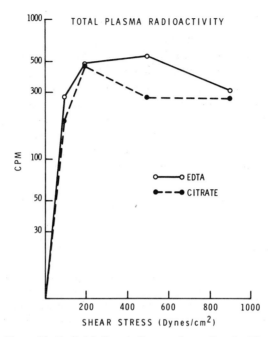

Figure 13. Radiolabeling studies on release of nucleotide.

was not influenced by the presence or severity of hemolysis. This case (the prosthetic valve) is of particular interest because, presumably, solid-surface area effects would be much less than in devices with large surface areas, a good example of which is the various devices involving extracorporeal circulation, which have a much more important effect on platelets—presumably surface related.

Bernstein and co-workers (Johnston, Marzec, and Bernstein, 1975; Bernstein et al., 1976) have studied platelets using a jet device that subjects the specimen to very high stresses (10^5 to 10^6 dynes/cm^2) for very short exposure times (on the order of 10^{-5} sec). Their results indicate that platelets are more resistant to stress than erythrocytes. They have also subjected platelets to lower shear fields in the Fleisch Hemoresistometer for relatively long exposure times (1–60 min) with results that seem to be consistent with those reported here from use of the rotational viscometer. Direct comparison is difficult, however, because the stress field in the Fleisch device is not as well characterized but is estimated to be less than 50 dynes/cm^2.

In summary, there is an apparent contradiction between the findings on platelet response to shear stress between those in the rotational devices (long exposure times), and those from very short exposure times. There are two probable explanations for the difference. First, exposure time is an important variable associated with the viscoelastic properties of the cell material, and it may be possible to organize the results at various exposure times by simply recognizing the importance of that variable—much as was the case in the study on erythrocytes. A second possibility is that the platelet response in the rotational viscometer is strongly influenced by cell—solid surface interaction. Bernstein (Johnston et al., 1975; Bernstein et al., 1976) feels that this is the case in his work with the Fleisch Hemoresistometer.

It is clear that additional work is needed on the effects of both exposure time and solid-surface interaction.

LITERATURE CITED

Bacher, P. P., and M. C. Williams. 1970. Hemolysis in capillary flow. J. Lab. Clin. Med. 76: 485.

Bernstein, E. F., P. L. Blackshear, and K. H. Kelley. 1967. Factors in flowing erythrocyte destruction in artificial organs. Am. J. Surg. 114: 126.

Bernstein, E. F., U. Marzec, M. D. Clayman, S. Swanson, and G. G. Johnston. 1976. Platelet function following surface injury and shear stress: Adhesion, aggregation, release and factor 3 activity. J. Clin. Invest. (to be published).

Blackshear, P. L. 1972a. Mechanical hemolysis in flowing blood, In Y.C. Fung (ed.), Biomechanics, pp. 501—528. Prentice-Hall, Englewood Cliffs, N.J.

Blackshear, P. L. 1972b. Hemolysis at prosthetic surfaces. In Marcel Hair (ed.), Chemistry of Biosurfaces, Vol. 2, chapter 11. New York.

Brown, C. H., L. B. Leverett, C. W. Lewis, C. P. Alfrey, and J. D. Hellums. 1975a. Morphological, biochemical and functional changes in human platelets subjected to shear stress. J. Lab. Clin. Med. 86: 462—471.

Brown, C. H., R. F. Lemuth, J. D. Hellums, L. B. Leverett, and C. P. Alfrey. 1975b. Response of human platelets to shear stress. Trans. Am. Soc. Artif. Int. Org. 21: 35—38.

Champion, J. V., P. F. North, W. T. Coakley, and A. P. Williams. 1971. Shear fragility of human erythrocytes. Biorheology 8: 23.

Croce, Paul A. 1972. Hemolysis of erythrocyte in linear and turbulent shear flows. Ph.D. Thesis, Washington University.

Indelgia, R. A., M. A. Shea, R. Forstrom, and E. F. Bernstein. 1968. Influence of mechanical factors on erythrocyte sublethal damage. Trans. Amer. Soc. Artif. Int. Org. 14: 264.

Johnston, G. G., U. Marzec, and E. F. Bernstein. 1975. Effects of surface injury and shear stress on platelet aggregation and serotonin release. Trans. Am. Soc. Artif. Int. Org. 21: 413–421.

Keshaviah, P. 1970. M. S. Thesis, University of Minnesota, Minneapolis.

Knapp, Charles F., and K. A. Yarborough. 1969. Experimental investigation of the mechanism of hemolysis in Couette flow. ICMB, Chicago 18–20.

Leverett, L. B., J. D. Hellums, C. P. Alfrey, and E. C. Lynch. 1972. Red blood cell damage by shear stress. Biophys. J. 12, No. 3: 257–273.

MacCallum, R. N., W. O'Bannon, J. D. Hellums, C. P. Alfrey, and E. C. Lynch, 1973. Viscometric instruments for studies on red blood cell damage. *In* H. L. Gabelnick and Michell Litt (Eds.), Rheology of Biological Systems, pp. 70–84. Charles C Thomas, Springfield, Ill.

MacCallum, R. N., E. C. Lynch, J. D. Hellums, and C. P. Alfrey. 1975. Erythrocyte fragility evaluated by response to shear stress. J. Lab. Clin. Med. 85: 67–74.

Manohitharajah, S. M., A. N. Rahman, R. J. Donnelly, P. B. Deverall, and D. A. Watson. 1974. Platelet survival in patients with homograft and prosthetic valves. Thorax 29: 639–642.

Merendino, K. A., and D. R. Manhas. 1973. Man-made gallstones—a new entity following cardiac valve replacement. Ann. Surg. 177: 694–703.

Nanjappa, B. N., H. K. Chang, and C. A. Glomski. 1973. Trauma of the erythrocyte membrane associated with low shear stress. Biophys. J. 13.

Nevaril, C. G., E. C. Lynch, C. P. Alfrey, and J. D. Hellums. 1968. Erythrocyte damage and destruction induced by shearing stress. J. Lab. Clin. Med. 71: 784–790.

Nevaril, C. G., J. D. Hellums, E. C. Lynch, and C. P. Alfrey. 1969. Physical factors in blood trauma. A.I.Ch.E.J. 15: 707–711.

Rooney, J. A. 1970. Science 196: 869.

Roschke, E. J., E. C. Harrison, and D. H. Blankenhorn. 1975. Fluid shear stresses during the opening sequence of prosthetic heart valves. Proc. 28th Annual Conf. Engr. Med. Bio., p. D5.4.

Schlichting, Herman. 1968a. Boundary Layer Theory. McGraw-Hill, New York. p. 699.

Schlichting, Herman. 1968b. Boundary Layer Theory. McGraw-Hill, New York. p. 611.

Shapiro, S. I., and M. L. Williams. 1970. Hemolysis in simpler shear flows. A.I.Ch.E.J. 16: 575.

Steinbach, J. 1970. M. S. Thesis, University of Minnesota, Minneapolis.

Sutera, S. P., P. A. Croce, and M. Mehrjardi. 1972. Hemolysis and subhemolytic alterations of human RPC induced by turbulent shear flows. Trans. Am. Soc. Artif. Int. Org. 18: 335.

Sutera, S. P., and M. N. Mehrjardi. 1975. Deformation and fragmentation of human RBC in turbulent shear flow. Biophys. J. 15: 1–10.

Williams, A. R., D. E. Hughes, and W. L. Hyborg. 1970. Science 196: 873.

Cardiovascular Flow Dynamics and Measurements
Edited by N. H. C. Hwang and N. A. Normann
Copyright 1977   University Park Press   Baltimore

chapter 21

FLOW DYNAMICS OF NATURAL VALVES IN THE LEFT HEART

Ned H. C. Hwang

ABSTRACT

Detailed measurements of velocity distributions downstream from a set of natural human mitral and aortic valves were made with a pair of cylindrical X-sensors. The measurements were carried out in a transparent Plexiglas chamber fabricated to reproduce both the geometry of a human left ventricular chamber at end diastole and a portion of the aortic root. The set of natural human mitral and aortic valves, procured from the same heart that the chamber geometry was based on, was carefully sutured into the prefabricated Plexiglas valve section in the chamber to reproduce the flow fields. Flow visualization techniques were used, both with cine film and still photographs, to observe the flow patterns in the chamber and to select sites for hot-film measurements. The statistical characteristics of transient disturbances in the flow at a selected location in the chamber are herein presented. The measured axial turbulent intensity, $\langle u'(t)\rangle$; the transverse turbulent intensity, $\langle v'(t)\rangle$; and the Reynolds shear stress, $\rho\langle u'v'\rangle$, are discussed in the interests of their qualitative representation rather than their absolute magnitudes. Similar measurements were also carried out in the region downstream from the aortic valve. Two planes, both normal and in the direction of the main aortic flow, were surveyed by the hot-film probes.

Much of the experimental work reported in this chapter was carried out at the Flow Dynamics Laboratory, the Baylor College of Medicine, Houston, Texas, under the support of a Heart and Lung Institute USPHS, Grant HL13330-P5 during the period I served as the Principal Investigator. The turbulent flow data were analyzed in the Engineering Systems Simulation Laboratory in Cullen College of Engineering, the University of Houston supported by Research Grant RG 743 from the Scientific Affairs Division, NATO.

825

INTRODUCTION

The set of two relatively simple, unidirectional check valves in the left heart has probably been studied by more investigators than any other kind of valve in history. Documented investigations can be dated back at least to Leonardo da Vinci (1513), whose ingenious description of the heart valve's anatomy and the role of vortices in the functioning of the heart valves has indeed stimulated many later studies on the subject. Interests in valvular dynamics in modern medicine are usually related to the generation of heart sounds and the development of certain pathologic conditions. Since the onset of open-heart surgery in the 1950s, new interests in analyzing the dynamics of blood flow through natural valves or artificial valve prostheses have risen among engineers and physicians, as it becomes directly of clinical significance.

Viewed hydraulically, the left heart consists of two chambers: the upper chamber (left atrium) collects the oxygenated blood from the lung and drains it into the lower chamber (left ventricle). Blood enters the left ventricle through the atrioventricular (mitral) valve during atrial systole while the ventricular chamber gradually dilates. Immediately following the end-diastolic period, ventricular contraction begins. The ventricular pressure rapidly rises to close the mitral valve and then to open the aortic valve through which the blood is expelled into the aorta for systemic distribution. The function of these valves is to effectively maintain the unidirectional flow of blood under physiologic pressure relationships.

In the past 10 yr, the ready availability of various types of sophisticated instruments has made it possible for more detailed studies to be carried out.

In this chapter we review some of the previous work on valvular dynamics. In addition, the techniques and results of our recent measurements of the turbulent characteristics and Reynolds stresses downstream from the human mitral and aortic valves are discussed. Our interest in studying the mechanics of the natural valves was primarily prompted by our close working relations with the clinical aspects of heart valve replacements. In spite of the large volume of literature on the subject, we feel that there is a gap between the available sophisticated technology and our basic understanding of the biologic phenomenon. This is particularly true in regard to the characteristics of the highly disturbed, if not exactly turbulent, flow through the natural heart valves and that through the various designs of their replacements. Although many investigators suspected that the highly disturbed flow through a heart valve prosthesis may be traumatic to the blood cells transported, no quantitative information is yet available to substantiate the facts.

FUNCTIONAL ANATOMY OF THE VALVES

Although the two valves in the left heart perform basically the same functions in maintaining the unidirection of blood flow through the heart, the anatomy of the two valves is quite dissimilar. A normal mitral valve consists of two leaflets projecting from the fibrous ring at the atrioventricular opening into the ventricular chamber, while a normal aortic valve consists of three equal-sized cusps that open into the aortic root.

The two leaflets of the mitral valve are not of the same size. The anteromedial (near the aortic valve) leaflet is much larger and fulfills most of the function of the valve, while the smaller, posterolateral (near the posterior wall) leaflet plays a supporting role in the closing of the atrioventricular opening during ventricular systole.

Two pillars of papillary muscles arise from the lower part of the ventricular wall to anchor the bundles of chordae tendineae that are attached on the downstream surface of both leaflets in such a way that the anterior muscle, through its tendons, controls the anterior leaflet, and the posterior muscle controls the corresponding posterior part. The papillary muscles apply tension to the chordae tendineae during ventricular systole. This action ensures that the free edges of the two leaflets come together and remain in the sealed position under the great pressure difference between the ventricle and the atrium during ventricular systole. An artist's sketch illustrating the left ventricular chamber with the columns of papillary muscles, chordae tendineae, and mitral valve leaflets in opening positions is shown in Figure 1.

At early diastole, ventricular pressure falls below atrial pressure, the mitral valve opens, and blood flow commences to fill the ventricular chamber. The flow continues throughout most of the diastolic phase. While the mitral valve opens, the annulus is enlarged and a moderate amount of tension exists at the base of the leaflets. This action takes up some of the leaflet area by elongating its base, which results in a shortening of the axial length measured between the base and its free margin (an analogy of the Poisson effect). Because of the difference in axial-to-base-length ratio in the two leaflets, the posterior leaflet (small axial-to-base-length ratio) experiences a greater reduction in its axial length and

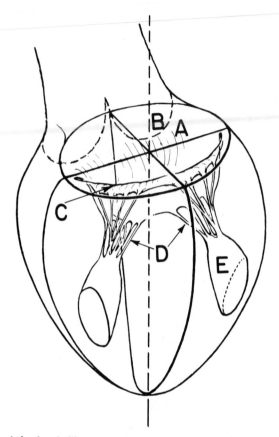

Figure 1. Artist's sketch illustrating the relative positions of anterior leaflet (*A*), posterior leaflet (*C*), chordae tendineae (*D*), papillary muscles (*E*), and the aortic valve (*B*).

consequently presents less obstruction to the flow. The axial length of the anterior leaflet, however, is not significantly affected by this base elongation and hence serves as the primary guide to direct the bloodstream (Davila, 1961; Wieting, Hwang, and Kennedy, 1971). The movements of the mitral valve were carefully studied by Brockman (1966).

The normal aortic valve consists of three equal-sized, semilunar cusps, each of which is supported at its base by a near cylindrical cuff (Figure 2). In the closed phase, the free margins of the leaflets come together and seal to each other when the left ventricular pressure falls below aortic pressure

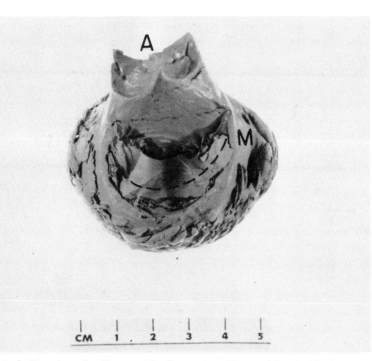

Figure 2. Top view of a silicone rubber impression of human left ventricle shows the base of the aortic leaflet support (A) and the base of mitral valve support (M). The dotted line shows approximately the position of the anterior and posterior leaflets of the mitral valve when closed.

during ventricular diastole. Davila (1961) showed, with photographs of successive frames of cine films, that the aortic leaflets do not actually open fully in systole. He explained the observation by arguing that during systole the circular orifice in which the valve lies is enlarged by aortic distention. Thus the total (sum) length of the leaflets' margin, which in closing is equal to the circumference of the diastolic orifice, is now less than the circumference of the distended circle. The opened leaflets lie as three cords within the circle, forming a triangular orifice. With a similar technique, however, Bellhouse and Talbot (1969) showed that aortic leaflets do open fully during systole and provide almost no obstacle to the blood flow. The difference apparently resulted from the fact that the latter included the geometry of the three sinuses of valsalva in their experiment, while the former probably did not. The three sinuses at the aortic root, one corresponding to each of the three aortic leaflets, have been shown to perform important hydrodynamic functions in the valve mechanisms.

The valve leaflets are thin and extremely pliable. Their surface properties are the same as those of the endocardial lining. The tissues of the leaflets have specific gravities nearly equal to that of blood. The leaflets practically "float" in the bloodstream. Very small changes in the direction of the pressure gradient in the bloodstream can set the leaflets in motion in accordance with the changes.

WHAT DO WE KNOW ABOUT THE FLUID MECHANICS OF NATURAL HEART VALVES?

We know very little about the fluid mechanics of the two valves in the right heart. As for the two valves in the left heart, however, we have learned a great deal from the fruitful research carried out by various investigators.

Bellhouse and his colleagues published a series of papers on the subject of fluid mechanics of the aortic valve (see Bellhouse, 1972 for a summary). The major discovery by the group was the hydrodynamic effect of the sinus of valsalva on the closing mechanism of the aortic leaflets. A fluid vortex trapped within each sinus was found to play an essential role in the early phase of valve closing. Using frame-by-frame cine film analysis, Bellhouse showed that at the beginning of heart systole the valve leaflets relax and the acceleration of the bloodstream from the ventricle sweeps the leaflets toward the aortic wall. As the free margins of the leaflets approach the circumference of the aorta, part of the bloodstream is intercepted by the sinus ridge, and the sinus vortices form. The entire opening procedure (leaflets move from closed to fully opened position) takes place in about 15% of the systolic time, followed by a "quasisteady phase" in which the leaflets remain fully open. This phase occupies approximately 55% of the systolic time and is regarded as mechanically identical to that of the steady flow, although the sinus ridge pressure was found to vary slowly with time.

The aortic flow begins to decelerate when the ventricle relaxes. An adverse axial pressure gradient is established in the aorta, which makes the pressure on the sinus side of the leaflet exceed that on the aortic side. At this time, the cusps start to move toward their closing position. The cavity space behind the leaflet increases as they begin to move away from the sinuses. The additional fluid needed to fill the space continues to come from upstream through the opening between the leaflet free margin and the sinus ridge. This mechanism pushes the vortex streamlines downstream from the leaflet free margin and exploits the axial pressure gradient in order to close the valve three-quarters of the way before forward aortic flow ceases. During ventricular diastole, the aortic pressure exceeds the ventricular pressure, and the leaflets seal tightly to each other to resist reverse flow.

According to Bellhouse's observations, the total reverse flow necessary for closing a normal aortic valve is only about 5% of the total forward flow, while a reversal of 25% of the total forward flow is needed to close a similar valve without the sinuses of Valsalva.

In a recent model study, Spaan et al. (1975) investigated the axial pressure gradient within the aorta due to the deceleration. This gradient results in a torque that causes the leaflet to rotate. The sinus contents then push the leaflets into the aorta. With a thin Lucite plate, rotatable around an axis at the center of a half-cylindrical shaped model "sinus" in a two-dimensional, rectangular model "aorta," the authors found that the torque was so strong that the vortex, formed during the "quasisteady" phase, was not essential for the closure of the aortic valve during systole.

Spaan's finding could well be complementary to Bellhouse's instead of contradictory. The vortex mechanism definitely provides a very logical explanation, while the torque due to the axial pressure gradient must also be real. The two mechanisms may likely exist simultaneously in the field. The combinational effect could only make the natural aortic valve an even more efficient device than we previously thought.

Hung and Schuessler (1976) recently presented a mathematical model to investigate the hemodynamic characteristics of the aortic valve during the incipient period of the aortic flow. Their numerical results support Bellhouse's data on the pressure–flow relationship through the valve. In addition, the model predicts the speed and shape of the aortic leaflets at every phase of the entire cycle of the aortic opening and closing processes. The model also predicts the aortic flow rate, the pressure drop, and the area of the open aortic orifice as functions of time.

Maximum stresses in an aortic valve leaflet occur during heart diastole. Several models have been proposed to study the stress distributions. A three-dimensional model based on membrane theory was developed in our laboratory (Chong et al., 1973). The computed results predict tensile stress distribution in the aortic leaflet during diastole. The result covered ranges of membrane radius of curvature ratio, R_2/R_1, between 0.6 and 0.9, and the subtending angle between $180°$ and $230°$. The basic geometry of this model is shown in Figure 3.

The mitral valve opens when ventricular pressure drops below atrial pressure during heart diastole. Because of the diastolic enlargement of the mitral orifice, the valve annulus is elongated, as is the base of the two mitral leaflets. As a result, the axial dimensions of the leaflets are effectively reduced. The posterior leaflet, having a much longer base and smaller axial length than the anterior leaflet, is more drastically reduced. Consequently, the posterior leaflet presents very little obstruction to the mitral flow, while the anterior leaflet, not significantly affected by its base elongation, serves as the primary guide to the direction of bloodstream.

By analyzing the flow pattern reproduced in a transparent plexiglas chamber built to simulate the geometry of a dilated adult human ventricle, we found that the leaflets guide the fluid to form a large counterclockwise vortex behind the anterior leaflet, while a much smaller, clockwise vortex is visible behind the posterior leaflet (Figure 4). It is postulated that these transient vortices in the filling ventricular cavity serve important roles in closing the mitral valve and thoroughly "washing" the chamber during ventricular systole (Wieting, Hwang, and Kennedy, 1971; Stripling, 1972). Based on our observation, the vortices begin to push the leaflets toward the closing position before the rise of ventricular pressure. This presystolic

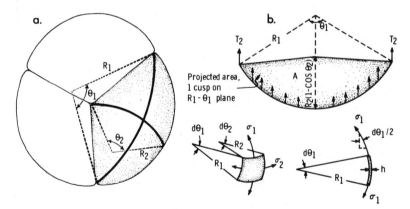

Figure 3. Geometry of an aortic leaflet stress model (Chong et al., 1973). The two principal radii, R_1 and R_2, and their subtending angles, θ_1 and θ_2. The four parameters define the geometry of an element area in the aortic leaflet during closure. σ_2 and σ_1 are the corresponding tensile stresses in the leaflet membrane.

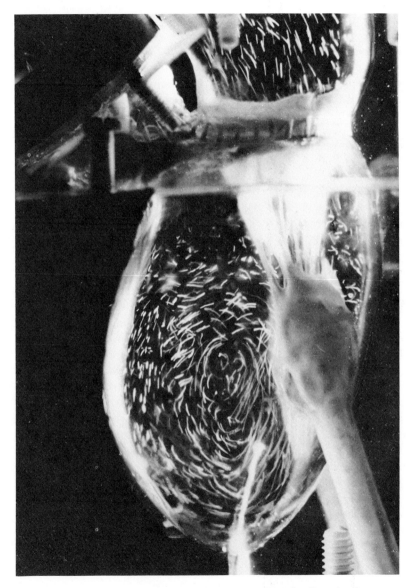

Figure 4. Ventricular vortices as seen through a Plexiglas flow chamber.

closure of the mitral valve helps to prevent blood regurgitation caused by the fast rising, high ventricular pressure.

The presystolic closure of the mitral valve was also observed by Brockman (1966). By sequentially performing a complete atrioventricular heart block on each of the 28 adult mongrel dogs, he was able to show a sequence of two closing movements of the mitral leaflets in every cardiac cycle until the heart rate was increased to about 200 beats per minute by means of sinus tachycardia.

Bellhouse and Bellhouse (1969) also reported the vortex forming in a model left ventricle. Their early model was built with a bag-shaped transparent rubber diaphragm that was alternately expanded and contracted by applying external forces. The mitral valve in their model was simulated by a sleeve of thin, flexible membrane that projected about 30 mm into the model ventricular cavity in dilated position. As the model ventricle filled, they noticed that the sleeve-like mitral valve guided the incoming fluid to form a jet that struck the apex of the ventricular bag, spreading outward and upward to generate a vortex ring behind the sleeve-like ventricle valve. Although we question the reality of simulating the mitral valve leaflets with a sleeve-like structure, the formation of a major vortex behind each of the mitral leaflets is certainly in agreement. Their model was later modified, and a large, spherical Hill vortex was observed during diastole, similar to that reported in Weiting, Hwang, and Kennedy (1971).

With a catheter-tip Doppler ultrasonic flowmeter probe, Desser and Benchimol (1974) measured the phasic velocity of mitral blood flow in 30 conscious human adults. With the right or left brachial artery and a medial antecubital vein isolated, a flowmeter-tipped catheter was introduced into the artery and passed in retrograde fashion under fluoroscopic observation into the ascending aorta. The catheter was then advanced across the aortic valve into the left ventricle and positioned at the mitral valve. Their measurements showed that the mitral valve flow velocity is characterized by a large pandiastolic wave followed by a smaller systolic component. High-frequency velocity fluctuations can be clearly seen in their ventricular flow tracings.

TURBULENT FLOW IN THE LEFT VENTRICLE?

Highly disturbed, if not definitely turbulent, flows have been measured in the aorta and other arteries in both humans and in animals (e.g., Bergel et al., 1970; Clark and Schultz, 1973; Nerem et al., 1974). Disturbed flows with high-frequency velocity fluctuations have been detected distal to the mitral valves in dogs by using catheter-tip mounted ultrasound Doppler flowmeter probes (Desser and Benchimol, 1974) and by electromagnetic flowmeters sutured in the mitral annulus (Laniado et al., 1973). Through a series of in vitro measurements, we have conducted an investigation to quantify the characteristics of the disturbance in the flow through the natural mitral valve. A detailed discussion of the flow measurement technique (with orthogonally oriented hot-film probes) and the procedure in analyzing the random hot-film signals is presented in this chapter. This technique was also used in a limited extent to measure the flow characteristics through the aortic valve. The results are also discussed.

The X-Array Hot-Film Sensors

The hot-film anemometer sensor (Figure 5) used in this experiment consists of a pair of very fine platinum cylinders orthogonally oriented but electrically insulated from each other. An electric current is used to heat each film, which is, at the same time, cooled by the flowing fluid. A fast feedback system immediately compensates the loss by feeding more current into the film to keep it at a preset constant temperature, and thus there is a constant electric resistance in each film. The feedback system changes the electric current through the film as soon as a variation in flow velocity (thus heat loss from the film) occurs. The varying electric current and the constant resistance in the film produce a varying voltage signal that is calibrated against the instantaneous flow velocity in the close vicinity of the film.

Ideally, a very thin, heated cylinder of infinite length is only sensitive to fluid velocity component normal to the cylinder and loses no heat to the velocity component in the parallel direction (Champagne, Sleicher, and Wehrmann, 1967). The film cylinders used for measurements in liquid, however, have finite length-to-diameter ratios. The sensitivities to the normal and parallel velocity components varies from one cylinder to another. Through a proper calibration procedure (which is discussed later), the sensitivities can be approximately determined for each individual cylinder. The fluctuating signals produced by the two sensors exposed to a turbulent flow field are jointly analyzed to obtain turbulent quantities such as the axial turbulent intensity, $\langle u \rangle$, the radial turbulent intensity, $\langle v \rangle$, and the Reynold shear stress, $\rho \langle uv \rangle$ (Hinze, 1975).

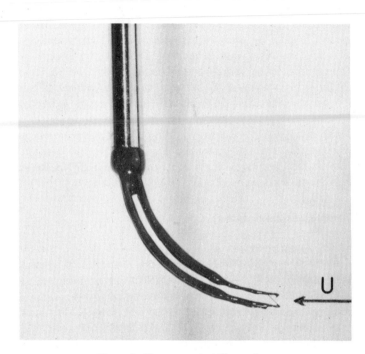

Figure 5. The x-array hot-film probe.

The Flow Model Chamber

In designing a model chamber for orthogonal hot-film measurement of mitral flow, two basic requirements are called to our attention: First, in analyzing the random signals, it is required that the sensor cylinders must always be oriented at approximately 45° and 135°, respectively, from the mean flow direction; therefore, we must be able to identify the direction of the mean flow stream throughout the entire heart cycle, or at least over that portion during which the flow measurements are considered to be meaningful. Second, to simulate the flow motions inside a small chamber enclosed by a moving boundary, such as the left ventricle, one must be able to simulate the motion of the boundary itself.

The first requirement was fulfilled by fabricating the flow chamber with transparent Plexiglas walls and a specially designed plane light system (Wieting, 1969) that illuminates one selected cross-sectional plane in the chamber. Two-dimensional flow patterns across the mitral valve were made visible by suspending small spherical plastic beads in a clear testing fluid (36.7% glycerol in water, by volume). The flow patterns, recorded by a 16 mm movie camera, were carefully analyzed before installation of the hot-film probe into the chamber.

The second requirement, however, has been the subject of considerable controversy because a meaningful reproduction of the left-ventricular wall motions is indeed a very difficult task. Generally speaking, dynamics simulation of a motion consists of the descriptions of three basic time-dependent vectors: displacement, velocity, and acceleration. Simulation of the ventricular wall motion, therefore, not only must reproduce the distances each wall element traveled during a heart cycle, but also the speed at which the element traveled and the rate of change of speed (acceleration) of the element throughout the heart cycle. Any unilateral description of one or two of the variables without proper consideration of the others would inevitably introduce erroneous information that may not be relevant to the actual situations investigated.

Several mathematical models have been proposed for studying the ventricular behavior (Beneken, 1965; Sallin, 1969; Streeter et al., 1969). However, quantitative simulation of the complex ventricular wall motions, with a physical model, for detailed flow studies is yet to be achieved.

In our experiment, a rigid model was fabricated to reproduce the geometry of a dilated left-ventricular cavity in an adult human. The model is designed to study the mitral flow during heart diastole while the ventricular wall is known to be relatively motionless. In a normal heart, this period begins approximately at the time while ventricular pressure falls below the atrial pressure and opens the mitral valve, and ends at the end of the isovolumic contraction of the ventricle when the aortic valve opens. This period covers roughly 50% of a cardiac cycle (Brockman, 1966). During this period, the ventricular flow is strong, and we expected that the transient disturbance in the flow field may also be at its maximum strength.

The construction of the left-ventricular chamber began with injection of liquid state RTV silicone rubber into the left ventricle of an isolated, adult human heart at low, near physiologic, pressure. The material solidified inside the heart after a 24-hr curing period. The heart tissue was then dissolved in a corrosive agent. What remained was the sudden impression of the left-ventricular cavity in full dilation. The rubber mold was suspended in an upright position inside a small metal box into which a liquid-state clear casting resin was filled to approximately 1 cm below the mitral annulus. After removing the mold, the solidified resin forms a chamber that reproduces the geometry of the lower ventricular cavity in dilation.

The same technique was used to produce the upper chamber section into which a set of natural human mitral and aortic valves was sutured. The two valves were dissected from a postmortem adult human heart as a unit to preserve the geometry. The mitral valve was excised along with its chordae tendineae and the papillary muscles intact (Figure 6A). Figure 6B shows the valve section of the chamber with the set of natural valves in place. Pumping action was carried out by a diaphragm attached to one side (parallel to the plane of photographs) as shown in Figure 7, which also shows the top view of the completed flow chamber.

Flow patterns were photographed from two planes orthogonal to that shown in Figure 7 and carefully compared to determine the locations and

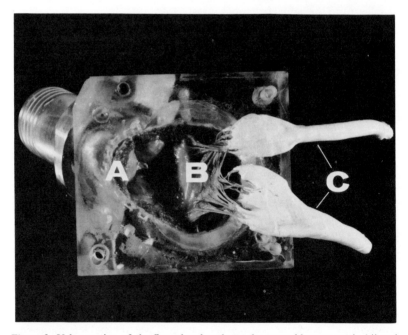

Figure 6. Valve section of the flow chamber shows the natural human aortic (A) and mitral (B) valves in position. Chordae tendineae are attached to the "papillary muscles" (C).

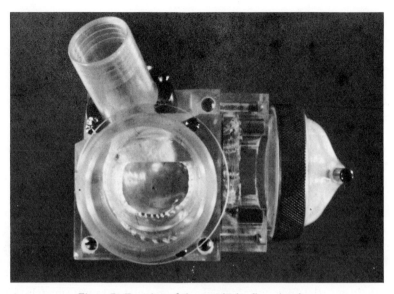

Figure 7. Top view of the ventricular flow chamber.

orientation of the hot-film probes. Because of the inherent limitations of the chamber and the sensitivity of the cylindrical hot-film probes towards the flow directions, it was expected that there would be only a limited region in the chamber where the flow measurement was meaningful. The biplane flow visualization technique revealed that, immediately downstream from the mitral valve, the flow field provided a reasonably large area where the hot-film probes could be safely applied. Only the turbulence data obtained in this area are presented here for discussion, although the entire field was surveyed by the probes.

THE FLOW LOOP AND THE MEASUREMENT SYSTEMS

The chamber was installed in a mock-up flow loop that was designed to simulate the ventricular load and return. The system consists basically of an adjustable, linear resistance unit (Westerhof, Elzinga, and Simpkama, 1971), a capacitance unit, a supply reservoir, a rotameter, a filter, and a thermal bath to control the fluid temperature. The system was manually adjusted until physiologic wave forms were obtained before any measurement was taken. Throughout the experiment, the system was adjusted to maintain a flowrate of 5 liters/min at a constant heart rate of 72 beats/min.

The "left atrial" pressure remained at about 5 mm Hg, while the "left ventricular" pressure remained at 120/0 mm Hg. Mean flow rates (equivalent to cardiac output) were measured with a Fisher Porter rotameter and the pulsatile flow rates were registered by an on-line Caroline square-wave electromagnetic flowmeter probe. A Statham P-23 H differential pressure transducer was used to measure the pressure drop across the mitral valve. All the "physiologic" signals were monitored by an Electronics for Medicine unit.

The hot-film anemometer used in the experiment was a two-channel, constant-temperature system (TSI Model 1053B). A two-channel segmental linearizer (TSI Model 1055) was used to condition the hot-film outputs. The hot-film sensors used in the mitral flow measurement are a pair of quartz-coated platinum films, formed in cylinders of approximately 1 mm long; they have a length-to-diameter ratio of 20:1. The two sensor cylinders are oriented in orthogonal directions, as described earlier. In this experiment, the films were heated to a temperature approximately $5°C$ (7% over heat) above the $28.2°C$ ambient temperature.

The sensors were calibrated in a straight, 3-m-long towing tank equipped with an electric timer and a temperature bath. During calibration, testing fluid filled into the tank was warmed to the loop temperature, and each probe was towed through the reach in directions both perpendicular and longitudinal to its axis at several speeds. The output voltages were plotted as a function of the normal velocity for each sensor.

The sensor output is proportional to the convective heat loss from the sensor to the moving medum. Ideally, a long, slender cylinder is only sensitive to cooling velocity normal to the cylinder, V_x, and not affected by the parallel velocity component V_z. In our experiment, however, the sensor cylinders used have a length-to-diameter ratio of 20, for which a significant heat loss due to V_z is expected. A correction term must be introduced to account for the additional heat loss. The term "effective cooling velocity" was suggested and defined as

$$V_{eff}(\alpha) = V(\cos^2 \alpha + k^2 \sin^2 \alpha)$$

The value of k was experimentally determined in this study. The constant value of $k = 0.18$ was used for all velocity and angular ranges measured.

A small slit cut along the posterior wall of the flow chamber allowed the installation of the hot-film probes into the ventricular cavity. Measurements were made with the probe throughout the entire Plane I (plane of photograph), upon which flow pattern visualizations were made by cine films after the completion of the hot-film survey.

EXPERIMENTAL PROCEDURE AND DATA REDUCTION

Because of the directional sensitivity of the film sensors used and the inherent limitation of the rigid chamber design, not all the measurements made at all the positions in the chamber were physically meaningful. Out of the 169 positions surveyed in Plane I, only a few points were selected for the data analyses. The selections were based on careful study of the phasic velocity patterns by means of the flow visualization technique.

The periodic nature of the flow and its oscillations defy the conventional statistical methods available for treatment of steady turbulent flow such as the time average, the root-mean-square, etc. For example, the conventional root-mean-square velocity does not provide any meaningful characterization of the flow, because the deviation of the velocity signal from its time average is not a random velocity fluctuation. For this type of flow, the concept of phase average (Hussain and Reynolds, 1970) is the appropriate approach. This average provides the deterministic part of the periodic signal. Deviation from this average is therefore the random velocity fluctuations.

For each of the selected points, the sensor outputs recorded in the FM analog tapes were digitized at 2,000 bits per channel per second, in expectation of a upper random frequency limit of 1,000 Hz. Two hundred continuous "heart" waves were analyzed to obtain the statistical averages. An IBM 360/44 digital computer was used to process the digital data and to obtain the phase average of the mean axial velocity,

$$\langle U(t)\rangle = \frac{1}{200} \sum_{n=1}^{200} U(t + nT),$$

the phase averages of axial and transverse turbulent velocities,

$$\langle u'(t)\rangle = \left(\frac{1}{200} \sum_{n=1}^{200} [u(t + nT)]^2\right)^{1/2},$$

$$\langle v'(t)\rangle = \left(\frac{1}{200} \sum_{n=1}^{200} [v(t + nT)]^2\right)^{1/2},$$

and the phase-average Reynold stress,

$$\rho\langle u'v'(t)\rangle = \frac{\rho}{200} \sum_{n=1}^{200} [u(t + nT)]\,[v(t + nT)]$$

Here, T is the average period of an average heart beat.

In processing the data, the recorded periodic pressure drop across the mitral valve was used as a signal trigger. A new period begins when the pressure drop falls below a certain preset threshold value, as shown in Figure 8. A periodic signal, say, $f(t)$, is sampled at time t from the beginning of the first cycle and at the same t from the beginning of each of the subsequent 199 cycles to obtain the average value. This average technique was repeated for all t in the range $0 \leqslant t \leqslant T$ to obtain the phase-average value $\langle f(t)\rangle$.

RESULTS AND DISCUSSION

Because the rigid wall ventricular chamber was fabricated to reproduce the dilated ventricular cavity, the flow pattern produced in the chamber may

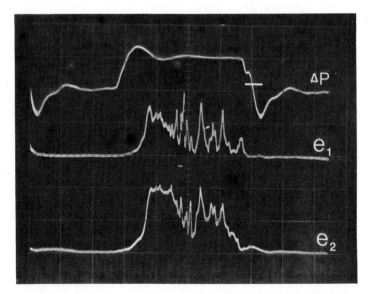

Figure 8. Traces of pressure drop across the mitral valve, and hot-film signals.

only simulate the natural flow pattern in left ventricle during diastolic phase. Discussion of the flow phenomena, therefore, is limited to those that take place in the diastolic period.

Figure 9 shows the axial velocity distribution in the left-ventricular cavity during peak diastole as registered by the hot-film probe. Because of the orientation of the probe and other inherent difficulties of the rigid chamber, the measurements are quantitatively accurate only in the regions immediately downstream from the mitral valve. For example, the maximum, peak velocity of 102 cm/sec through the mitral valve compared well with measurement obtained from other models (Stripling, 1972). The formation of a large vortex in the left-ventricular cavity during diastole is evident by both the hot-film measurement (Figure 9) and the flow visualization technique (Figure 4). We believe that this vortex plays an important role in the closing of mitral valve by helping the leaflets move back to their closing positions prior to the onset of ventricular systole (Wieting, Hwang, and Kennedy, 1970).

To discuss the transient turbulent characteristics of the mitral flow, we selected a sample point of characteristic importance 1.8 cm downstream from the mitral orifice. The data obtained at this location are discussed in the light of a representation of the mitral flow field.

From the flow signal traces shown in Figure 8, the periodic nature of the flow phenomenon during the cardiac cycle and the intermittently "turbu-

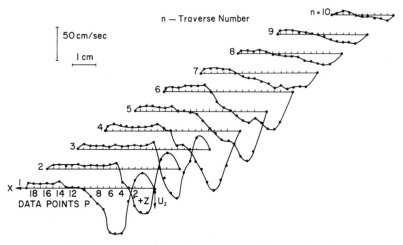

Figure 9. Mean velocity distribution of ventricular flow during diastole.

lent" flow is evident. The diastolic and systolic phases of the cardiac cycle are indicated by the pressure drop (top trace). Notice that the pressure drop is positive during diastole when the mitral valve remains open, its opening being initiated by the small hump of positive pressure. The valve starts closing at the beginning of systole because of a sudden pressure reversal; the pressure drop stays negative during systole. The hot-film traces show that the velocity at the probe location increases rapidly with the opening of the valve and becomes highly disturbed when the maximum velocity is reached. With the beginning of the systole, the velocity decreases and the transient "turbulence" disappears. Clearly, the periodic turbulent nature of the flow is indeed well correlated with the periodic diastole–systole cycle.

The phase average of the longitudinal velocity component, $\langle U(t) \rangle$, is shown in Figure 10A for the cardiac cycle. The average velocity increases nearly exponentially with time from the beginning of the diastolic phase, reaches a maximum, and then starts dropping. It drops to approximately 40% of its maximum value at the end of the diastolic phase; the velocity decrease continues in the systolic phase. Somewhere in the middle of the systolic phase, the velocity reaches the minimum value and stays relatively constant at that value until the end of that phase.

Figures 10B and 10C show that the phase-average turbulent velocities $\langle u'(t) \rangle$ and $\langle v'(t) \rangle$ while $\langle U(t) \rangle$ is still near its maximum. The intensity again increases near the end of the diastolic phase before reaching the low values near the middle of the systolic phase. The maximum turbulent intensity is about 10 times the minimum value during the cardiac cycle.

Notice that the transverse turbulent intensity varies in a qualitatively similar manner except that, even though the minimum value of $\langle v'(t) \rangle$ is about equal to the minimum value of $\langle u'(t) \rangle$, the maximum value of $\langle v'(t) \rangle$ is somewhat lower.

The phase-average Reynolds stress, as shown in Figure 10D, is nearly zero during the systolic phase but has a large value during the diastolic phase. The Reynolds stress during the diastolic phase has two peaks: during the acceleration and deceleration of the flow through the mitral valve. At the full open position of the mitral valve, the Reynolds stress is low even though the mean velocity is at its maximum.

Measurement of Aortic Flow Patterns

The x-array, hot-film sensors were also used to measure the velocity distribution and transient disturbances in the flow immediately down-

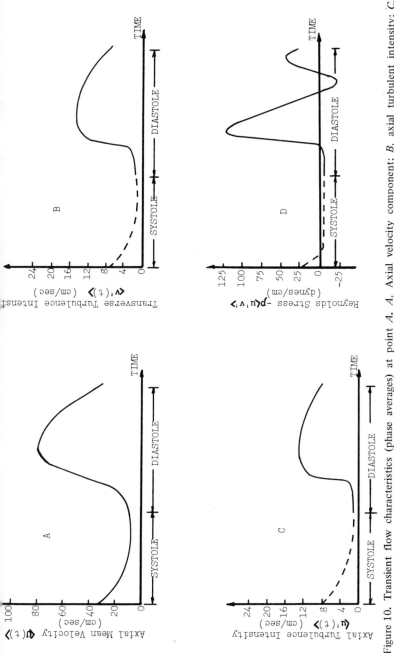
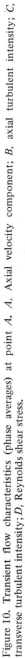

Figure 10. Transient flow characteristics (phase averages) at point *A*. *A*, Axial velocity component; *B*, axial turbulent intensity; *C*, transverse turbulent intensity; *D*, Reynolds shear stress.

stream from a natural human aortic valve. Mounted at the exit of the left-ventricular flow chamber, as previously described, the valve was sutured into the prefabricated valve section together with the mitral valve (Figure 6).

A specially designed elbow was connected to the aortic outlet, to allow installation of the hot-film sensors. With this configuration, the mean aortic flow was thus confined to the longitudinal direction in the region measured. Any secondary flow currents that may have existed under physiologic conditions were ignored in this study because our main interest was to obtain basic information concerning the characteristics of the transient disturbances in the aortic flow in the close proximity of the aortic valve. The cylindrical hot-film sensors were both oriented at 45° from the normal of the aortic valve plane.

Two parallel planes were surveyed by the hot-film sensors. On each plane, five equal spacing points across the aortic diameter were selected for the measurement. These points were located in a straight line situated directly behind the line of intersection of two of the aortic leaflets while closing, and the line bisecting the third leaflet in the same position (see the upper right corner of Figure 11).

Figure 11 shows the axial velocities as functions of time for all five locations in Plane I, which is located approximately 3 cm downstream from the aortic root. For the cardiac output of 5 liters/min and the heart

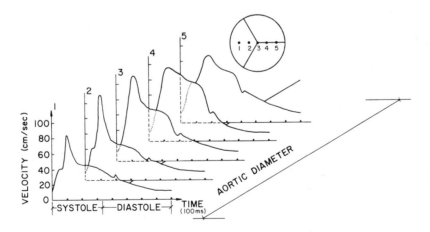

U(t)

Figure 11. Axial velocity distribution of aortic flow immediately downstream from the aortic valve.

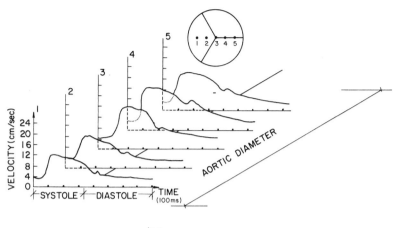

u'(t)

Figure 12. Axial turbulent intensity, $<u'(t)>$, measured downstream from a natural human aortic valve.

rate of 72 beats/min, the maximum peak velocity of approximately 110 cm/sec was recorded at both positions 1 and 3. The mass of the fluid, however, passes through the cross section with a slower speed and a much broader front. After the piercing velocity opens the leaflet seal, the main stream apparently flows through a near triangular area represented largely by 3, 4, and 5, and their corresponding points along the other two lines of

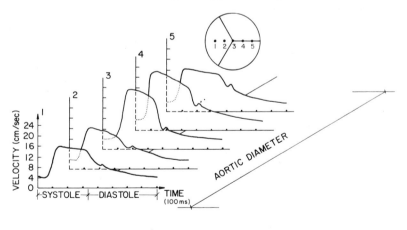

v'(t)

Figure 13. Radial turbulent intensity, $<v'(t)>$, measured downstream from a natural human aortic valve.

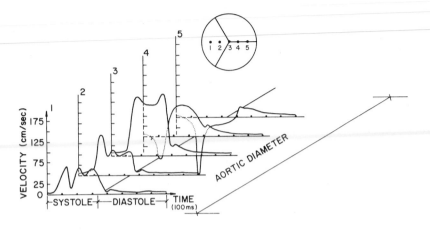

Figure 14. Reynolds shear stress, $\rho<u'v'>$, measured downstream from a natural human aortic valve.

leaflet junctions. A small, inverted notch is clearly seen on each of the five curves, indicating the event of complete closure of the aortic valve. The small-velocity wave is apparently caused by the aortic leaflets' response to the sudden loading on them at the snap closing of the valve.

Figures 12 and 13 represent the fluctuating velocity components in the axial and radial directions respectively. The higher level of fluctuation intensities coincides fairly well with the mean velocity pattern (Figure 11) in both space and in time as expected. This trend is more clearly seen in the transverse fluctuation component as shown in Figure 13.

The measured Reynolds stress levels are shown in Figure 14. As the signs of the stress are only indications of the correlation that existed between the axial and the transverse fluctuation components, we see the absolute valves rise to the level of approximately 150 dynes/cm² at both positions 3 and 5. However, these values do not peak at the same phase in a cardiac cycle. Unfortunately, it is not possible for us to elaborate on the distributions of the Reynolds stress until more detailed measurements are available.

ACKNOWLEDGMENTS

This chapter represents a collective effort and hours of diligent, hard work by my students and laboratory staff, particularly Dr. Travis E. Stripling,

Mr. P. W. Hui, Mr. Ralph E. King, and Mr. Benno L. Dunn. Two of my colleagues, Dr. D. W. Wieting, who first introduced the flow visualization technique, and Dr. A. K. M. F. Hussain, who suggested the phase-average analysis, deserve special credit for the results presented here.

LITERATURE CITED

Bellhouse, B. J., and L. Talbot. 1969. The fluid mechanics of the aortic valve. J. Fluid Mech. 35: 4, 721.
Bellhouse, B. J., and F. H. Bellhouse. 1969. Fluid mechanics of the mitral valves. Nature (Lond.) 224: 615.
Bellhouse, B. J. 1972. The fluid mechanics of heart valves. *In* D. H. Bergel (ed.), Cardiovascular Flow Dynamics, Vol. 1, p. 261. Academic Press, London.
Beneken, J. E. W. 1965. A mathematical approach to cardiovascular function. Int. Rep. 2.4 5/6. Inst. of Med. Physics, TNO, Utrecht, The Netherlands.
Bergel, D. H., C. Clark, D. L. Schultz, and P. Turnstall. 1970. The measurement of instantaneous blood velocity and calculation of total mechanical energy expenditure in ventricular pumping. Paper No. 19, AGARD Conf. Proc. No. 65, Fluid Dynamics of Blood Circulation and Respiratory Flow, NATO, Naples, Italy, 1970.
Brockman, S. K. 1966. Mechanism of the movements of the atrioventricular valves. Am. J. Cardiol. 17: 682.
Champagne, F. H., C. A. Sleicher, and O. H. Wehrmann. 1967. Turbulence measurements with inclined hot-wire. Part I. Heat transfer experiments with inclined hot-wire. J. Fluid Mech. 28: 1, 153.
Chong, K. P., D. W. Wieting, N. H. C. Hwang, and J. H. Kennedy. 1973. Analysis of normal human aortic valve leaflets during diastole. J. Biomat. Med. Dev. Art. Org. 1: 307–321.
Clark, C., and D. L. Schultz. 1973. Velocity distribution in aortic flow. Cir. Res. 7: 601.
Davila, J. C. 1961. The mechanics of cardiac valves. *In* K. A. Merendino (ed.), Prosthetic Valves for Cardiac Surgery. Charles C. Thomas, Springfield, Ill.
Desser, K. B., and A. Benchimol. 1974. Blood flow velocity measurement at the mitral valve of man. Am. J. Cardiol. 33: 541.
Haize, X. X. 1975.
Hinze, O. J. 1975. Turbulence. 2nd Ed. McGraw-Hill, New York.
Hung, T. K., and G. B. Schuessler. 1976. An analysis of the hemodynamics of the opening of aortic valves. J. Biomech. (to be published).
Hussain, A. K. M. F., and W. C. Reynolds. 1970. The mechanics of an organized wave in turbulent shear flow. J. Fluid Mech. 41(2): 241–258.
Laniado, S., E. L. Yellin, H. Miller, and R. W. M. Frater. 1973. Temporal relation of the first heart sound to closure of the mitral valve. Circulation 47: 1006.

Leonardo da Vinci. 1513. Quaderni d'Anatomica II, 9.

Nerem, R. M., J. A. Rumberger, D. R. Gross, R. L. Hamlin, and G. L. Geiger. 1974. Hot-film anemometer velocity measurements of arterial blood flow in horses. Circ. Res. 34: 193.

Sallin, E. A. 1969. Fibre orientation and ejection fraction in human left ventricle. Biophys. J. 9: 954.

Spaan, J. A. E., A. A. von Steenhoven, P. J. von der Schaar, M. E. H. von Dongen, P. T. Smulders, and W. H. Leliveld. 1975. Hydrodynamical factors causing large mechanical tension peaks in leaflets of artificial triple leaflets valves. Trans. Am. Soc. Artif. Int. Organs. 21: 396.

Streeter, D. D., H. M. Spotmitz, D. J. Patel, J. Ross, and E. H. Sonneblick. 1969. Fibre orientation in the canine left ventricle during diastole and systole. Circ. Res. 24: 339.

Stripling, T. E. 1972. Left ventricular flow characteristics of a healthy human heart. M. S. Thesis, University of Houston.

Westerhof, N., G. Elzinga, and P. Simpkama. 1971. An artificial arterial system for pumping hearts. J. Appl. Physiol. 31, 5: 776.

Wieting, D. W. 1969. Dynamic flow characteristics of heart valves. Ph.D. dissertation, University of Texas at Austin.

Wieting, D. W., N. H. C. Hwang, and J. H. Kennedy. 1971. Fluid mechanics of the human mitral valve. AIAA paper No. 71-102, New York.

Wieting, D. W., T. E. Stripling, and N. H. C. Hwang. 1972. An improved chamber for in vitro study of heart valves. Proc. ACEMB 14: 114.

Cardiovascular Flow Dynamics and Measurements
Edited by N. H. C. Hwang and N. A. Normann
Copyright 1977   University Park Press   Baltimore

chapter 22

PROSTHETIC HEART VALVES

Corrado Casci,
Roberto Fumero, and Franco Montevecchi

ABSTRACT

Valve replacement still represents one of the cardiac operations of larger application: in fact, by valve replacement it is not only possible to restrain disease development; in most instances it is possible for patients to attain an amazing functional recovery. Indications for artificial valves, application, and some typical clinical results are reported in this chapter.

The mortality causes, especially of late deaths, show that biologic compatibility problems are the most important questions to be solved. In this respect, links between the fluid dynamical situation and materials, and hemolysis and coagulation, are discussed.

As regards valve evaluation criteria, the ventricle output valves and the ventricle input valves, of which an efficiency and a filling coefficient are defined, are separately examined as a fluid-mechanical device. While examining the valves as interacting with biologic tissues, the structural differences between natural valves and artificial ones are made evident; these differences give precise indications for future development in artificial valve design. Valve testing philosophy and optimization are finally discussed and an experimental apparatus which is a replication of the cardiovascular system to test artificial valves is illustrated.

INTRODUCTION

In 1960, cardiac valve surgery received a boost with the clinical use of artificial valve prostheses. Currently, valve replacement represents one of the most important procedures in cardiac surgery; in fact, by valve replacement, it is possible not only to restrain disease development, but also in most instances to attain striking functional recovery of the patient.

The order of frequency of valve replacement is the mitral valve, the aortic valve, the tricuspid valve, and occasionally the pulmonary valve. Frequently, malfunction in valves concerns two or three valves simultaneously; the most common combination is the mitral and aortic valves. Malfunction can be described in nearly all cases as stenosis, insufficiency, or some combination of the two.

Stenosis occurs as a stricture or a stiffening of the valve leaflets, interfering with the normal blood flow during the valve opening phase, with a consequent increase of the pressure gradient across the valve. Insufficiency involves failure of the valve leaflets to close completely during the valve closing phase, with a consequent regurgitation of blood. The two conditions are often associated, especially when the mitral valve is involved.

In most cases, the primary cause of malfunction must be ascribed to rheumatic diseases. Valve lesions caused by other pathologic conditions, such as congenital defects, bacterial endocarditis, and syphilis, are considerably less common. Naturally, cardiac function is affected by the presence of these valve diseases, and the malfunctions might therefore affect other organs, with serious repercussions on the patient's health.

INDICATIONS FOR VALVE
REPLACEMENT AND CLINICAL RESULTS

The decision to perform corrective surgery or prosthetic implantation is often made on the basis of an evaluation of functional impairment according to the classification (Table 1) proposed by the New York Heart Association (N.Y.H.A.). Usually, surgery is limited to patients belonging to classes III and IV. In order to stress the risks connected with these operations and the degree of patient recovery, statistics from the period 1964–74 of "Divisione di Chirurgia Toracica e Cardiovascolare A. De Gasperis" (Ospedale Maggiore di Milano, Marcazzan et al., 1975) are quoted in Tables 2–4. These figures are similar to those of other authors (Aston and Mulder, 1971; Starr, 1971; Barclay, Reid, and Stevenson, 1972; Kirklin, 1972; Cooley, Okies, and Wulkasch, 1973; Soulie et al., 1973; Barchek, Anderson, and Starr, 1974).

Total hospital mortality was 13.2% in earlier years. This rate has now decreased to approximately 7%. Long-term survival rates of various combinations of valve replacements are listed in Figures 1–4. The data are more pessimistic than reality because the curves have not been corrected by subtracting natural death rates.

Table 1. Classes of organic heart disease

Class 1 (0–15% impairment)	Class 2 (20–40% impairment)	Class 3 (50–70% impairment)	Class 4 (80–95% impairment)
Organic heart disease exists, but without resulting symptoms	Organic heart disease exists, but without resulting symptoms at rest	Organic heart disease exists, but without resulting symptoms at rest	Organic heart disease exists with symptoms even at rest
Walking, climbing stairs freely, and the performance of the usual activities of daily living do not produce symptoms	Walking freely on the level, climbing at least one flight of stairs, and the performance of the usual activities of daily living do not produce symptoms	Walking more than one or two blocks on the level, climbing one flight of ordinary stairs, or the performance of the usual activities of daily living produce symptoms	The performance of any of the activities of daily living beyond the personal toilet or its equivalent produces increased discomfort
Prolonged exertion, emotional stress, hurrying, hill-climbing, recreation,[a] or similar activities do not produce symptoms	Prolonged exertion, emotional stress, hurrying, hill-climbing, recreation, or similar activities produce symptoms	Emotional stress, hurrying, hill-climbing, recreation, or similar activities produce symptoms	Symptoms of cardiac insufficiency or of the anginal syndrome may be present even at rest
Signs of congestive heart failure are not present	Signs of congestive heart failure are not present	Signs of congestive heart failure may be present, and if so, are usually relieved by therapy	Signs of congestive heart failure, if present, are usually resistant to therapy

[a]Prophylactic restriction of activity such as strenuous competitive sports does not exclude a patient from class 1.

Table 2. Valve replacements

Mitral	877
Mitral and tricuspid annuloplasty	122
Aortic	585
Tricuspid	10
Pulmonary	4
Mitral and aortic	276
Mitral, aortic, and tricuspid annuloplasty	32
Mitral and tricuspid	67
Aortic and tricuspid	3
Mitral, aortic, and tricuspid	31
Total	2,007

Table 3. Classification after mitral valve replacements

N.Y.H.A. Preoperative		N.Y.H.A. Postoperative	
IV	60%	IV	—
III	40%	III	5%
II	—	II	51%
I	—	I	18%
		Exitus	26%
Total	100%		100%

Table 4. Classification after aortic valve replacements

N.Y.H.A. Preoperative		N.Y.H.A. Postoperative	
IV	35%	IV	—
III	65%	III	2%
II	—	II	40%
I	—	I	45%
		Exitus	13%
Total	100%		100%

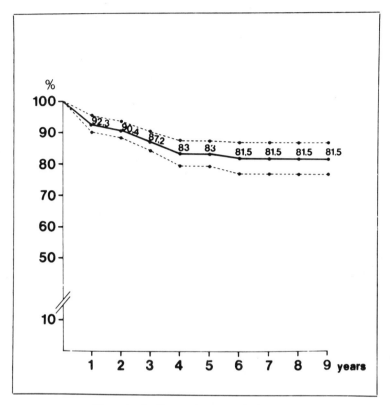

Figure 1. Aortic prostheses: survival curves.

From our point of view, it is interesting to examine the relationships between the degree of patient recovery, and the pre- and postoperative risks and prosthetic efficiency. From a clinical point of view, it is evident that, according to N.Y.H.A. classification, patients who have undergone this type of operation are greatly improved, especially in the case of aortic valve replacements; most of these patients become asymptomatic.

Another factor allowing objective evaluation of the operation is the radiologic determination of heart size. The heart is usually enlarged in patients with valvular disease but decreases in size after the first 6 months after surgery. This decrease is 15–25%, depending on the original pathology, and is particularly remarkable in aortic replacements (Meriggi, Mar-

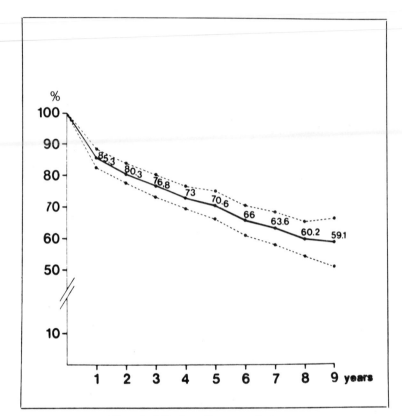

Figure 2. Mitral prostheses: survival curves.

cazzan, and Valsecchi, 1970; Bendet, Atamanyuk, and Zelenko, 1972), after which the patient's heart returns to its normal size.

From a strictly functional viewpoint, the goal of prosthetic implantation is the reinstatement of a normal hemodynamic situation. In this sense, the values of atrial, ventricular, and aortic pressures after implantation are very similar to normal values. This is achieved if prosthetic design and implantation do not cause regurgitation or pressure drops that are greater than those of natural valve leaflets. Also contributing to normal hemodynamics is the fact that the role of cardiac valves in hemodynamics is a passive one; as a matter of fact, the relative simplicity of artificial valves facilitated their development compared with other prostheses.

Although, on the whole, the results obtained by this therapy may be

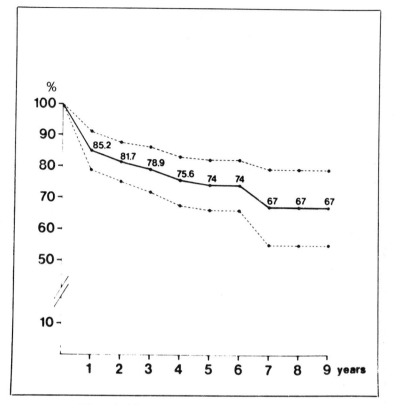

Figure 3. Mitro-aortic prostheses: survival curves.

judged satisfactory (thanks to the improvement of surgical techniques and postoperative care), and although hospital mortality may be considered acceptable (especially if considered relative to the patient's preoperative clinical conditions), it is impossible to ignore the negative aspects pertaining to the artificial nature of prosthetic valves. One must not forget that prosthetic valves are immersed in a flowing "tissue" that is chemically unstable (Davila, 1968) and must not be subjected to excessive imbalance. It possesses a clotting mechanism that must not be activated by the valve, and it transports vital cells that must not be traumatized. The valve must open and close an orifice that continuously changes in size and provides little mechanical support between the pulsatile, irregular chambers. The motion of the valves depends on cardiac action and must be coordinated

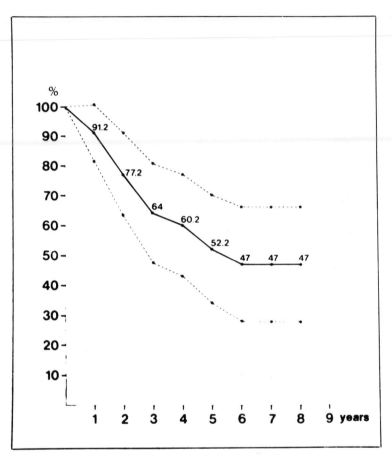

Figure 4. Mitro-tricuspid prostheses: survival curves.

with cardiac structural changes. Finally, the valvular apparatus must withstand the stress of beating more than forty million times a year during the life span of the subject, with part of its structure connected to living tissue.

BIOLOGIC COMPATIBILITY PROBLEMS

The causes of mortality, especially late deaths, confirm what was previously stated, that embolism and mechanical failure are primary causes. On the other hand, one must admit that the technologic improvement of the latest valves and the experience acquired with anticoagulants are causing a progressive decrease in the incidence of embolism. Still, the patient with a valvular prosthesis is obliged to undergo anticoagulant treatment that necessitates continuous evaluation of his general clinical status; such an evaluation is not always possible in the different national health services. This is why many physicians prefer to operate only on symptomatic patients, that is, patients belonging to class III and IV (N.Y.H.A.). In their opinion, patients belonging to other classes could also undergo surgery, but only in cases where the prostheses would not require anticoagulants. Therefore, the connection between the coagulation phenomena and structural valve design plays the leading role with respect to therapeutic goals.

Although it is impossible to say that coagulation phenomena associated with artificial prostheses are well quantified, it is possible to identify two factors strictly connected with coagulation: the chemical and physical nature of the material, and the fluid-dynamic situation. Under the same mode of ventricular contraction, flow characteristics are determined by valve geometry and, more precisely, by flow passage area and configuration of the moving part. Vorhauer and Tarnay's experiments support this assertion (Vorhauer and Tarnay, 1967). After introducing different geometric models into the descending aorta of dogs, they measured the weight of blood clots appearing in connection with these obstacles. Results are reported in Figure 5. In spite of the limitations of these experiments, the connection between the presence of wake vortices and thrombi formation is evident, emphasizing the importance of streamlined flow behavior.

As previously stated, it has not been proved what mechanisms, such as vortices, cavitation, and velocity gradients in general, may facilitate the activation of the main clotting factors. One of the most likely suppositions is that a small degree of hemolysis can release clotting factors that enhance wall adhesion (Johnson, 1970). For this reason we examine hemolysis associated with prosthetic valves, and also because this phenomenon may have clinical consequences by itself (Blackshear, 1970). Hemolysis caused by prosthetic valves was first reported by Ross et al. (1954) and was subsequently confirmed in numerous other publications. Further studies confirmed the presence of intravascular hemolysis. Most of the studies showed a significant reduction in red cell life spans and an increase in fragmentation (Bernstein et al., 1966; Hjelm, Ostling, and Persson, 1966). Both in valvular heart disease and with prostheses, aortic valves produce greater hemolysis than mitral valves.

Many authors have called attention to the similarity of the fragments

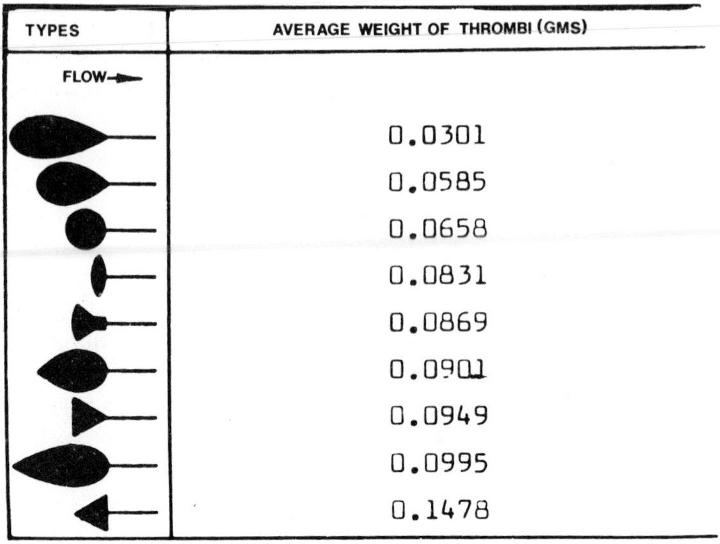

TYPES	AVERAGE WEIGHT OF THROMBI (GMS)
FLOW→	
	0.0301
	0.0585
	0.0658
	0.0831
	0.0869
	0.0901
	0.0949
	0.0995
	0.1478

Figure 5. Valve geometry effects.

found in patients with prosthetic valves and in patients with microangio-pathic hemolytic anemia (Alfrey and Lynch, 1968; Brain, 1969). The specific causes of hemolysis are not yet fully understood. Some interesting observations have been reported (Marsh, 1964; Stevenson and Baker, 1964) which reveal that blood from prosthetic-valve patients displays a normal life span when transferred into a normal, compatible recipient. This suggests that the hemolysis observed is probably intravascular and is not preceded by irreversible sublethal injury to the cell. In cases of hemolysis severe enough to cause anemia, there is usually a leak allowing backflow to occur. This observation, in view of the fact that in leaky natural valves hemolysis is slight, is relevant in interpreting the role of the prosthetic material. In reviewing the levels of hemolysis in prosthetic valves we conclude that (Blackshear, 1970)

1. All prosthetic valves produce sufficient hemolysis to exacerbate an already severe clotting problem.

2. Most prosthetic valves presently used do not tax the kidney or the ability of the bone marrow to compensate.

3. In the presence of paravalvular leaks, prosthetic valves can cause hemolysis so severe that total anemia may result.

As previously stated, these qualitative considerations are the result of the following observations: in the case of natural stenotic valves, hemolysis seems to be greater in the aortic valve, less in the mitral valve, and undetectable by ^{51}Cr half-life measurements when both valves are insufficient (Gehrman, Bleifeld, and Kaulen, 1964). Red cell fragments containing hemoglobin are found in the circulating blood in approximately 30% of the patients reported. Hemolysis is greater in patients with aortic prosthetic valves and less in patients with mitral prosthetic valves, provided they are not insufficient. In patients with mitral and aortic valvular insufficiency, hemolysis occurs so that reoperation is frequently indicated. Fragments are seen in approximately half of the patients examined.

As shown by in vitro tests, the in-bulk lysis is not present in valvular disease nor with prostheses except for trace amounts. On the other hand, it is well known that high-turbulence valves connected with high-velocity gradients give rise to wall hemolysis, either at the diseased surface of natural valves or at the prosthetic surface of artificial valves. It is possible to conclude that hemolysis in prosthetic valves is by wall hemolysis in which the excitation of the clotting factors by the local release of cell contents makes wall adhesion worse (Blackshear, 1970).

All this shows the importance of evaluating the fluid-dynamic situation by convenient methods, both in the design phase and in the evaluation phase, before implanting the prosthesis in the patient. This subject is examined below.

It has been previously observed that the other factor intimately connected with coagulation and thromboembolism is the chemical and physical nature of the valve prosthesis material. Taking into consideration all types of prostheses in contact with blood, Hufnagel et al. (1968) have identified certain factors that decrease the incidence of thrombosis. They are a hemorepellant surface, a lack of water absorption, a lack of toxic plasticizers and stabilizers, total polymerization of the plastic without residual monomers or catalysts, the lack of leeching of toxic materials, a mechanical smoothness of the surface of the material in prosthetic biologic interface, and a high degree of biologic tolerance by the host to the implanted material.

When implants are placed in the arterial tree, it is important to prevent thrombosis by preventing the production of a tissue injury potential in the region where the prosthesis is adjacent to the tissue. When materials must be employed that do not in themselves have these characteristics, it has been found that coating the material in such a way as to bring about the

desirable properties improves the performance. The use of silicone compounds to coat certain metallic surfaces is an example of this. An artificial
valve is more complex to alter than a prosthesis replacing arterial segments;
the characteristics allowing the valve to withstand special mechanical
stresses must be added to the above-mentioned characteristics. From an
engineering point of view, practically all types of artificial valves are
formed by three main parts: a moving part (ball, disk, lens, plunger,
centrally hinged flap valves, etc.), an apparatus restraining the moving part,
and a means of connection with the living tissue.

These three parts are subjected to fatigue from mechanical stresses
resulting from the functional frequency and the required geometry. On the
other hand, the different functions of these three parts require the use of
different materials for each of them. Therefore, while it is suitable to use
tissues such as Dacron felt or other polymers, which are supposed to promote
the formation of a pseudo intima (Leininger, Falb, and Grode, 1968; Lyman, 1968; Sauvage et al., 1968), for the part providing the connection with
living tissue, for the working parts we choose various materials on the basis
of impacts to which they will be subjected; such impacts could cause
breakage with the release of fragments of the pseudo intima into the blood
flow.

Mechanical solutions for the connection with living tissue, such as the
one proposed by Magovern–Cromie valve, seem to be, at least for the time
being, disregarded because of the surgical constraints. For the moving parts,
the general tendency is to use materials such as Teflon, silicone rubber or,
occasionally, something like titanium hollow balls. Recently, pyrolytic
carbon has been the material used for the moving part of disk valves
(Fernandez et al., 1974). In practically all types of existing valves the part
restraining the valve's moving part has been metal. The problem of using
metals for implantation has been studied by many authors (Laing, 1966;
Matthews, 1968; Sawyer, 1968; Weisman, 1968), but results are incon-
clusive, as shown by the lack of standards in many countries. The general
trend is to consider metals such as cast or wrought cobalt–chromium
alloys, some types of stainless steel, and unalloyed titanium, as more
suitable for this use, and to emphasize the surface finish.

VALVE EVALUATION CRITERIA

When reading the literature on the subject, apart from some naive proposi-
tions that are often nothing more than a qualitative description of the
valve operation, it is easy to find rather long lists of desirable valve

characteristics accompanied, in the best cases, with a definition of a corresponding parameter or index. Valve evaluation thus encompasses many, we would rather say too many, details without any possibility of a reasonable merging of the results into a final evaluation. Valve operation, in fact, has to be described from two basic points of view: fluid-mechanical and biologic.

Valve as Fluid-Mechanical Device

As a fluid-mechanical device, the artificial prosthetic valve has to be considered as a device with the task of allowing for the best mutual fluid-mechanical interaction of the heart and the circulation. This requires that each of the four possible positions of the valves has to be considered separately, especially as to whether the position is atrium-to-ventricle or ventricle-to-artery.

Ventricle Output Valves The fluid-mechanical efficiency of the valve can be defined as an index correlating the ratio of blood flow output to the power expenditure of the ventricle

$$\eta_m = \eta_m \left(\frac{SV}{\int_{\text{systole}} P_v dV} \right)$$

and varying with the stroke volume *(SV)* and the ventricular pressure exerted by the heart muscle fibers. The range of valve operation, and consequently the range of definition and determination of the fluid-mechanical efficiency of the prosthetic valve, is thus defined, and, in broad terms, is chiefly determined by the peripheral resistance of the arterial bed and by the heart rate and contractility. In more precise terms, the determining factors for the valve fluid-mechanical efficiency are all those parameters that define the model of ventricle contraction build-up, of vessel bed capacitance, and of control and regulatory mechanisms.

Thus we find that the complexity we shunned at the beginning by our definitions is now replaced by a complexity that is better defined and can be logically organized. Two factors are of main importance: physical scaling *(S)* and pathology *(P)*. Adding one index for the activity, for instance, metabolic index *(MI)*, we can organize a definition for the fluid-mechanical efficiency of a prosthetic artificial valve:

$$\eta_m = \eta_m \ (S, P, MI)$$

We stress that scaling and pathology are intended to define all the intrinsic parameters of cardiac contraction, vessel mechanics, flow resistance, and of the regulatory system transfer functions, while the metabolic index is related to blood flow needs of the body.

From these considerations we can make several statements. First, the fluid-mechanical quality of a prosthetic valve is, at least in theory, dependent upon physical size of the natural organs, conditions of contractility of the heart, conditions of compliance of blood vessels, and required range of operation. Second, regurgitation, delay in opening and closing, pressure drop across the valve, etc. are not to be considered in isolation, but as factors determining the blood flow output, given a mechanical energy expenditure in myocardium contraction. Thus, we define two related, but distinct, fields of analysis: valve fluid-mechanical optimization, which is concerned with obtaining better η_m values over the range of utilization of the valve, and valve operation analysis, which is concerned with the analysis of the fluid-mechanical phenomena involved in the opening, rising, staying, coming down, and closing phases of valve operation. Third, the importance of heart contraction mechanics, vessel mechanics, and cardiac control and regulation has been greatly underestimated in interactions with the operational characteristics of the artificial valves.

Ventricle Input Valves The fluid-mechanical efficiency cannot be linked to energetic consideration and has to be settled on the basis of the capability of filling the ventricle until the output valve opens. Thus we do not strictly define an efficiency but a filling coefficient $X_m = V/V_i$, where V is the corrected volume of blood in the ventricle just before the opening of the output valve, and V_i is an ideal filling volume. We would suggest for V_i, the filled volume of a ventricle at a certain pressure, 0 mm Hg. In fact, in this way we make the valve dependent on the behavior of all the venous vascular structures and the atrium ahead of the ventricle. This approach seems justified because the valve itself is not necessarily "good" or "bad"; rather, the result may depend on the matching with a particular vascular filling system.

Similarly, the input valves are characterized by a variation of the filling coefficient, X_m, over the range of operation depending upon the same parameters

$$X_m = X_m(S, P, MI)$$

The definitions stated above determine a particular corresponding approach to fluid-mechanical valve testing and to the presentation of evaluation indexes.

Before going into a more detailed discussion on this point, we should consider the extent to which these definitions contain uncertainties and difficulties. Note that according to the statements above, it is easy to test the fluid-mechanical behavior of ideal valves in isolation but that more definitions are needed when looking at a real operation involving atrial regurgitation during systole, etc. It could be useful to provide for a fluid-mechanical identification of systole and diastole (different from the physiologic identification). From a truly fluid-mechanical viewpoint, there would be no difficulty in assuming that systolic and diastolic phases are those associated with flow through output and input valves, respectively. Consistant with this definition, diastolic and systolic phases can possibly overlap due to regurgitation; furthermore, because bouncing in closure and instability can occur in some cases, the fluid-mechanical phase can be split in several bits before the final ending.

It is therefore convenient to extend the evaluation of the efficiency and filling coefficient of a prosthetic valve to each time period that corresponds, respectively, to blood output and input. To take into account the interactions of each definition, corrections have to be made to idealize the behavior of the components not under examination. For systole and output efficiency, that means that the power expenditure of the ventricle has to be corrected by subtracting the power waste caused by atrial regurgitation:

$$\int_{\text{systole}} p_v d V_{\text{atrium}}$$

The blood output also has to be corrected owing to diastolic regurgitation, and SV has to be the corrected blood output per beat:

$$\eta_m = \eta_m \ \frac{SV_{\text{corrected}}}{\int_{\text{systole}} p_v d V_{\text{atrium}}}$$

$$\eta_m = \eta_m \ \frac{SV_{\text{corrected}}}{\int_{\text{systole}} p_v d V_{\text{output}}}$$

For the filling efficiency, no correction to the proposed definition is needed for output valve regurgitation, because it at least substitutes for ventricle–atrial filling.

As for the definition of beginning systole needed in the filling coefficient evaluation, it is reasonable to associate it with the opening of the output valve, because this instant is usually clear and easy to identify. The blood volume regurgitated into the atrium during systole has to be subtracted from the ventricle fill-volume and, consequently, the corrected ventricle volume V has to be intended as the physical ventricle volume at the beginning of systole minus $\int_{\text{systole}} dV_{\text{atrium}}$.

All these definitions and the associated corrections are to be applied when studying and comparing natural and artificial valves with reasonably correct operational behavior. The proposed corrections are likely to be effective in correcting small deviations, but not large variations due, e.g., to pathologic natural valves. From a fluid-mechanical viewpoint, it has been relatively easy to define efficiency and coefficients in order to analyze and compare artificial valves; the biologic analysis is far more difficult and cannot be so easily organized.

Valve Interaction With Biologic Tissues

In considering valve interaction with biologic tissues, it is useful to distinguish at least between mechanical and chemical interactions. Mechanical interaction occurs in the regions where the valve seat is linked to the natural tissues and is in contact with the blood. At present, blood damage and the consequently high incidence of embolism are the preeminent problems in biomechanical interaction. Because it is not possible, within the limits of this chapter, to give a comprehensive summary of all the work that examines factors related to the mode of mechanical interaction of the current prosthetic valves with blood, we restrict our discussion to the most important considerations.

If for brevity we can exclude chemical problems, the simple question to be posed is why there is so great a difference between natural valves and artificial valves with respect to hemolytic effects. The answer is surprisingly simple: Because they are substantially different. Because this fact has been grossly underestimated, we stress the point by deciding what kinds of differences are present and what mechanical stresses they are likely to impose on the blood.

The most important difference is the mass of the moving parts, which can easily be one order of magnitude greater in artificial valves. The difference is even more unfavorable if we consider that a correct comparison index would be the ratio of the surface to the mass of the moving parts. In fact, the forces exchanged with the blood needed during the operation are diluted along the surface and are proportional to the mass.

If we define a pressure index, Ip, as mass/surface, we find that an aortic Starr Edwards valve has a value of 0.9 g/cm^2. When compared with a value of around 0.0075 g/cm^2 for natural valves, there is less than a

1:100 ratio; no comment is necessary. Disk valves have an *Ip* closer to that of natural valves but it is still 10 times greater.

The second difference in most artificial valves is the presence of some means or device to limit the motion of the moving body to a fixed open position and a fixed closed position. In most cases, these limits are associated with rapid decelerations of the moving body, which cause high stresses on the blood due to changes in the velocity across the surfaces limiting the flow. These features also cause great stresses on the artificial structures and are related to the mechanical failure problems.

It is not easy to evaluate local stresses on the blood and the value of frequent depressions associated with bouncing of the moving body; certainly, an important fraction of blood damage occurs in this manner. The energy dissipation associated with these operational phases is also an important index and is easier to evaluate both theoretically and experimentally. It would also be important to know the volume of blood associated with this dissipation, but again, this is a difficult parameter to evaluate. Another important difference associated with limiting devices is the rigidity of the contact areas of the valve where it closes. In natural valves, closure is not associated with rigid position of all the moving surfaces; in this case, closure is a well-dampened, low-inertia phenomenon.

In considering artificial valves it is useful to remind designers of the normal aortic valve operation. Upon opening, the cusps are moved by the blood and begin to move outward from the center of the stream, thus assuming the function of a vessel themselves. In this way, the relative motion of the blood increases gradually and the absolute motion of the moving surfaces remains low, especially at the end of opening. The sinus wall gives rise to a corrective vortex that favors dampening and stabilization of the open position of the cusps.

Near the end of systole, the cusps begin to close because of the differential pressure on the inner and outer surfaces; they are not moved by backflow. During closure, the vortices distract backflow from the center and favor closure. When closure is completed, because of its large flexible surface, the whole closed valve structure can displace a consistent travel back into the ventricle. This sustains oscillations of blood in the aorta, because of the ending of systole, without stressing the cusps zone of attachment and, of course, the blood itself.

It is no wonder that natural valves work so well; they have better materials, better attachment to other natural tissues, and better design. Artificial valves today cannot match the flexible attachment of the natural valves, but could be improved by the use of compatible structures that are flexible and reliable. Until then, the differences previously discussed will remain, and the valves will be relatively insensitive to more refined design techniques. As long as a rigid, moving body is limited in its motion by rigid cages, results can be only marginally improved.

To summarize, in this criticism of artificial valves we have underlined the difficulties in obtaining results comparable to those with natural valves. The only possible advantage of artificial devices, i.e., that metals can sustain high mechanical stresses, is of no use in this application. In fact, insofar as the existence of high stresses in the prosthetic structures implies that high stresses are imposed on living tissues, stress concentration has to be considered an undesirable design feature. For the attachment to the natural tissues and the utilization of self-restoring membranes, natural valves are clearly superior to any conceivable artificial device. The natural valve conformation is certainly the best possible one since it is the device with the best attachment features and with very sophisticated fluid-mechanical sensitivity, as determined by evolution.

In this situation it is surprising how distant in basic philosophy and how uninfluenced by the experience of nature are the designs available for artificial valves. Maybe it is too provoking a remark, but, in our opinion, not all artificial valve designers have the necessary knowledge of natural valve conformation and operational behavior. Furthermore, apart from some very fine works on natural valves, fluid-dynamic bioengineering does not sufficiently direct its attention toward the examination of natural valves. The result is that we know something about the aortic valve, less about the mitral valve, and even less about the right ventricle valves. Until new, flexible materials are available for use in artificial valves, clinical results will not dramatically improve from present standards; nevertheless, we have to emphasize what can be done under present limitations.

Improving biologic, fluid-dynamic interactions requires better understanding of the flow associated with valve operation and better knowledge of local stresses in boundary layers around cage elements. In cavitating zones, closing elements may trap particles; fast pressure variations, especially depressions, are associated with discontinuity in the motion of the moving body. Deterioration of blood is also a fatigue process that is not fully understood as biologically oriented insights need to match more closely the fluid-mechanical analysis. Research is in progress and we do not dwell on this subject; instead, we offer evidence of the links that make biomechanical damage and valve fluid-mechanical efficiencies mutually dependent, as we have defined them. Even if there is no one-to-one relationship between these factors, it is certain that high fluid-mechanical efficiencies are associated with low energy dissipations and low stresses imposed on the blood.

VALVE TESTING PHILOSOPHY AND OPTIMIZATION

Lacking a very detailed local analysis, a careful evaluation of mechanical efficiencies is an indirect measure of mechanical stresses on blood. However, this has to be done over the whole range of valve operations manifesting instabilities and particular fluid-dynamic patterns associated with all the operating points of the device.

This type of examination is best carried out largely by physical experiments, while mathematical models are needed to explain and give insight into local phenomena and flow peculiarities. A physical replica of the cardiovascular system necessitates a rather sophisticated actuation philosophy, taking into account all the regulatory parameters. Most fluid-dynamic test beds developed for artificial valves lack this capability and cannot, with fidelity, cope with all the operative ranges an artificial valve has to sustain.

For the aortic valve, this situation requires a very accurate physical model of the aorta capable of taking into account the physiologic pressure pulse reflections and the oscillations of the blood mass. At the present time, few experimental apparatuses are sufficiently developed for testing artificial valves; the one we have developed offers some interesting features and an organization specifically oriented toward control. As shown in Figure 6, systemic and pulmonary circulations are pumped by two ventricles and controls for both peripheral vascular resistance and blood flow to the organs are provided for. Because of an on-line contraction model for the ventricles and a peripheral resistance control simulation, flow is varied according to natural control patterns. An external variable causes a transitory phenomenon after which, if a stable situation has to occur, a new operating point is obtained. In this way the operation of artificial devices inserted into the vascular bed can be examined for its overall characteristics. Figure 7 shows a top view of the set-up, and Figures 8 and 9 show details of the actuator. The computer-controlled portion of the cardiovascular simulator is capable of responding, with reasonable power output, to 40–50-Hz input signals and can therefore closely follow any physiologic contraction pattern that can be imposed.

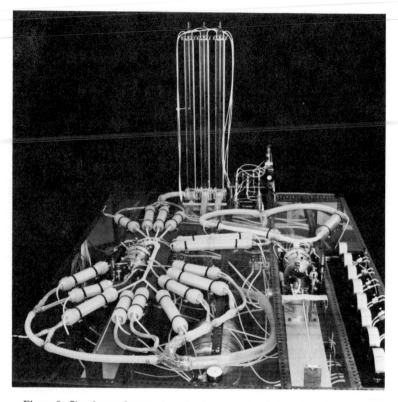

Figure 6. Simulator of systemic and pulmonary circulations for valve testing.

If we remember that, at the beginnings of experimental fluid-mechanical testing of artificial valves, the pulse generation was rather crude, and the rigid vascular and ventricular structures caused many uncontrollable reflections, we can appreciate the increasing sophistication in valve test beds as a shift from analyzing simple operational principles of the device to the physiologic research of cardiovascular system operation—with application to artificial valves. The validity of the device is therefore dependent on the validity of the matching between physiologic and artificial components, while limiting factors, especially embolism activation, constitute the most effective constraints on current devices.

Interaction between fluid-mechanical conditions and blood damage is actually a widely unresearched field in which some confusion exists about

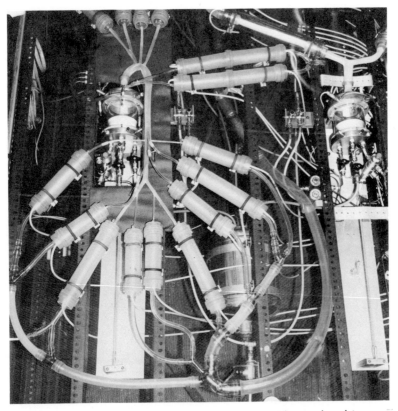

Figure 7. Simulation of left ventricle, aorta, and peripheral systemic resistances.

scientific methods and approaches. While testing of particular flow conditions, shears, stable vortices, pressure oscillations, etc., is certainly capable of giving information about blood cell life and deterioration, a reasonable and sound application of these data to a theoretic fluid-mechanical flow analysis is not at present a reliable method for forecasting biologic interactions of a prosthetic device.

Thus theoretical valve optimizations are, for some time yet, likely to be based on average values for energy losses, pressure drops, etc., without, by this approach, having the possibility of eradicating local damaging flow patterns. Having this detailed knowledge at hand, we have always maintained that without more sophisticated, flexible materials, an improvement

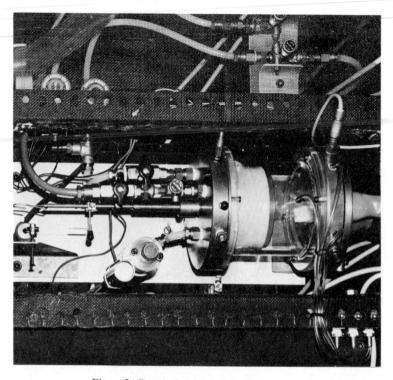

Figure 8. Detail of simulator actuating system.

in artificial valve characteristics is not foreseeable. Theoretic flow analysis capable of predicting microconditions of flow will certainly be necessary for flexible artificial valve optimization and will be the task of bioengineering design efforts. At such a time, we feel that a limited variety of possible designs will be close to the natural valve conformation and will be the subject of examination and comparison.

Fluid-mechanical and biologic optimization represent an extremely sophisticated field of research and application, since the individual conditions and conformations of the patients are very sensitive parameters for artificial valve selection and optimization. We can also imagine that the valve choice will in some cases be the result of an automated process involving ultrasound and scintigraphic examinations; medical staff and bioengineers will collaborate on individual cases and evaluate the prognosis after implantation. In this situation, valve operation, ventricular contrac-

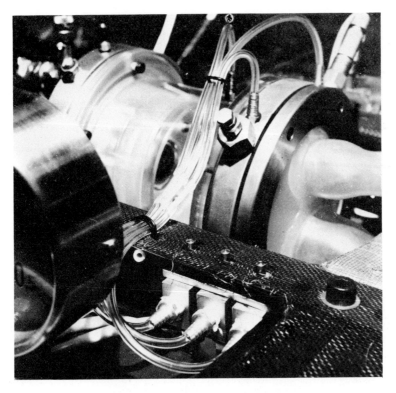

Figure 9. Detail of simulator actuating system.

tility, and all the physiologic data pertinent to cardiovascular phenomena may well be looked on as a system of models with higher levels of optimization.

LITERATURE CITED

Alfrey, C., and E. Lynch. 1968. Erythrocyte fragmentation: A diagnostic clue in hemolytic anemias. Ann. Thorac. Surg. 6: 199.

Aston, S. J., and D. G. Mulder. 1971. Cardiac valve replacement: A seven year follow-up. J. Thorac. Cardiovasc. Surg. 61: 547.

Barchek, I., R. P. Anderson, and A. Starr. 1974. Mitral valve replacement with cloth-covered composite-seat prosthesis. J. Thorac. Cardiovasc. Surg. 67,1: 93−109.

Barclay, R. S., J. M. Reid, and J. G. Stevenson. 1972. Long term follow-up

874   Casci et al.

of mitral valve replacement with Starr–Edwards prosthesis. Brit. Heart
J. 34:2: 129–133.
Bendet, Y. A., M. Y. Atamanyuk, and E. F. Zelenko. 1972. Changes of the
relative volume of the heart at a distant period after valve prosthetics
in acquired defects. Kardiologiya 12/9: 102–107.
Bernstein, E., R. Indeglia, M. Shea, and R. Varco. 1966. Sublethal damage
to the red blood cell from pumping. Circulation 35 and 36; Suppl. I:
1–226.
Blackshear, P. L., Jr. 1970. Mechanical hemolysis in flowing blood. In Y.
C. Fung, N. Perrone, and M. Anliker (eds.), Biomechanics. Prentice-
Hall, Englewood Cliffs, N.J.
Brain, M. C. 1969. Microangiopathic hemolytic anemia. N. Engl. J. Med.
281: 15.
Cooley, D. A., J. E. Okies, and D. C. Wulkasch. 1973. Ten year experience
with cardiac valve replacement: result with a new mitral prosthesis.
Ann. Surg. 177/6: 818–826.
Davila, J. C. 1968. The mechanics of the cardiac valves. In K. A. Meren-
dino (ed.), Prosthetic Valves for Cardiac Surgery. Charles C Thomas,
Springfield, Ill.
Fernandez, J., et al. 1974. Results of use of the pyrolytic carbon tilting
disc Byörk-Shiley aortic prosthesis. Chest 65: 640–645.
Gehrman, G., W. Bleifeld, and D. Kaulen. 1964. Hertzklappenfeheler und
Hämolysen. Klin. Woch. 44: 1229.
Hjelm, M., S. Ostling, and A. Persson. 1966. The loss of certain cellular
components from human erythrocytes during hypotonic hemolysis in
the presence of dextran. Acta Physiol. Scand. 67: 43.
Hufnagel, C. A., P. W. Conrad, J. F. Gillespie, R. Pifarre, A. Ilano, and T.
Yokoyama. 1968. Characteristics of materials for intravascular applica-
tion. In S. N. Levine (ed.), Materials in Biomedical Engineering. Ann.
N.Y. Acad. Sci.
Johnson, S. A. 1970. Platelets in hemostasis. In W. H. Seegers (ed.), Blood
Clotting Enzymology. Academic Press, New York.
Kirklin, J. W. 1972. Replacement of the mitral valve for mitral incompe-
tence. Surgery 72: 827.
Laing, P. G. 1966. Corrosion and failures in surgical implants. Presented at
Conference on Materials in Biomedical Engineering. The New York
Academy of Sciences, June 9.
Leininger, R. I., R. D. Falb, and G. A. Grode. 1968. Blood-compatible
plastics. In S. N. Levine (ed.), Materials in Biomedical Engineering.
Ann. N. Y. Acad. Sci.
Lyman, D. J. 1968. Biomedical polymers. In S. N. Levine (ed.), Materials
in Biomedical Engineering. Ann. N. Y. Acad. Sci.
Marcazzan, E., G. Mombelloni, A. Pellegrini, B. Peronace, E. Respighi, and
C. Santoli. 1975. Sostituzioni valvolari con protesi artificiali: risultati
immediati e a distanza. L'Osp. Magg. Milano, n. 1.
Marsh, G. W. 1964. Intravascular hemolytic anemia after aortic valve
replacement. Lancet 2: 986.

Matthews, D. B. 1968. Electrochemical aspects of the interaction of human plasma with metals. *In* S. N. Levine (ed.), Materials in Biomedical Engineering. Ann. N.Y. Acad. Sci.

Meriggi, A., E. Marcazzan, and F. Valsecchi. 1970. Le modificazioni radiologiche dopo sostituzioni valvolari protesiche. Atti XXXI Congr. Soc. It. Cardiol. Vol. II, Sorrento.

Ross, J. C., C. Hufnagel, C. Freis, W. Harvey, and E. Partenope. 1954. The hemodynamic alterations produced by a plastic valvular prosthesis for severe aortic insufficiency in man. J. Clin. Invest. 33: 891.

Sauvage, L. R., R. F. Viggers, S. B. Robel, S. J. Wood, K. Berger, and S. A. Wesolowski. 1968. Prosthetic heart valve replacement. *In* S. N. Levine (ed.), Materials in Biomedical Engineering. Ann. N.Y. Acad. Sci.

Sawyer, P. N. 1968. The effect of various metal interfaces on blood and other living cells. *In* S. N. Levine (ed.), Materials in Biomedical Engineering. Ann. N.Y. Acad. Sci.

Soulie, P., J. Valty, A. Heulin, M. Perrotin, J. Fouchard, Ch. Pauly Lambry, J. Deridda, and M. Degeorges. 1973. Résultats du remplacement de l'appareil mitral (165 prothéses). Arch. Mal. Coeur 66: 689.

Starr, A. 1971. Mitral valve replacement with ball valve prostheses. Brit. Heart. J. 33: 47.

Stevenson, T. D., and H. J. Baker. 1964. Hemolytic anemia following insertion of Starr-Edwards valve prosthesis. Lancet 2: 982.

Vorhauer, B. W., and T. J. Tarnay. 1967. Artificial heart valve design: Effect of valve profile on clotting. The 7th International Conference on Medical and Biological Engineering. Stockholm, Sweden, August.

Weisman, S. 1968. Metals for implantation in the human body. *In* S. N. Levine (ed.), Materials in Biomedical Engineering. Ann. N. Y. Acad. Sci.

Cardiovascular Flow Dynamics and Measurements
Edited by N. H. C. Hwang and N. A. Normann
Copyright 1977   University Park Press   Baltimore

chapter 23

OPERATIONAL ASPECTS OF MECHANICAL CIRCULATORY ASSIST

Nils A. Normann

ABSTRACT

Mechanical circulatory assist involves a complex interplay of physical-chemical, flow dynamic, and operational variables. Operational optimization of system performance and safety must be based on: (1) precise system information, (2) purposeful data processing, (3) effective mechanisms for control and safety, and (4) functional compatibility with respect to patient disease state.

In this chapter, current circulatory assist practices are briefly reviewed, and examples of efforts to attain operational optimization are presented. The described developments involve on-line intra-aortic balloon data processing, automatic control of roller-pumps in direct and in reservoir-coupled partial (left heart) bypass, and a monitor-control system for pulsatile pneumatic blood pumps. Effects of mechanical circulatory assist on arterial baroreceptors and neuro-humoral, cardiovascular control mechanisms are discussed.

INTRODUCTION

In this chapter, no attempt is made to review a rather voluminous literature. Furthermore, at the outset, it needs to be emphasized that progress in the field is the result of efforts by numerous individuals and research teams. Some recent, in-house developments discussed in this chapter

Work performed at Baylor College of Medicine was supported by Grants HL-13330 and HL-17269, both from the National Heart and Lung Institute.

represent extensions of work that has been going on for more than a decade within our institution (DeBakey, Liotta, and Hall, 1966*b*).

The advent of the heart–lung machine, providing the basis for present-day cardiac surgery, gave impetus to the development of cardiopulmonary support systems for use outside the operating room. The major obstacle in this development has been, and still is, the critical interface between blood and a foreign, artificial surface, involving a complex interplay between three basic parameters: (1) the physical, chemical properties of surfaces; (2) the composition of blood, including the role of pharmacologic agents; and (3) flow dynamics, as it affects blood composition, surface property, and blood–surface interactions. Topics relevant to the problems of blood composition and blood flow dynamics are discussed elsewhere in this book. With respect to the hemocompatibility of surfaces, there is general disagreement as to the importance of the various factors; the materials and surfaces used today, with some degree of success, are to a great extent based on empirical observations and happenstance. (For review, see Bruck, 1975.)

Generally, at the present time, indications for the employment of temporary, mechanical, circulatory assist are based on the premise that one deals with cardiac pathophysiologic processes that are, at least partly, reversible. The two most common clinical entities are myocardial infarction and cardiac pump failure after cardiac surgery. Operationally, from a pumping point of view, mechanical circulatory assist devices may provide circulatory support either indirectly, by improving the pumping capability of the heart, or directly, by pumping more or less of total output necessary for adequate tissue perfusion.

INTRA-AORTIC BALLOON COUNTERPULSATION (IABCP)

Introduced in 1962 (Moulopoulos, Topaz, and Kolff, 1962), this method is currently the only form for mechanical cardiac support that has attained general clinical acceptance. An elongated balloon of 30–40 cm^3 capacity is introduced through a femoral artery and placed in the proximal portion of the descending aorta, just distal to the left subclavian artery, as illustrated in Figure 1. The balloon is mounted on a catheter which, via tubing, is connected to a pneumatic power source. Triggered by the *R* wave in the ECG, the balloon is synchronized to stay inflated during a certain portion of cardiac diastole. By having the inflation occur shortly after closing of the aortic valve, the sudden increase in volume causes increased pressure in the proximal aorta, commonly termed diastolic

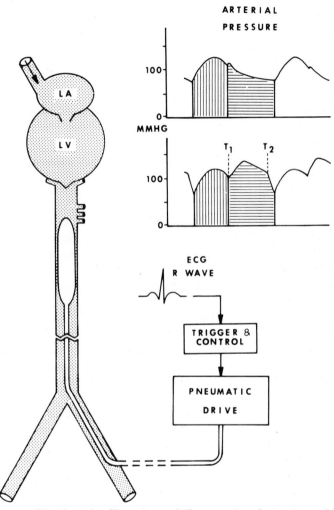

Figure 1. IABCP schematic. *Upper insert,* balloon passive. *Lower insert,* balloon active. T_1, balloon inflation; T_2, balloon deflation. Shading emphasizes systolic and diastolic pressure areas.

(pressure) augmentation. Conversely, the deflation of the balloon toward the end of diastole causes a presystolic reduction in pressure. In this manner, one seeks (1) to create a higher coronary perfusion pressure during diastole, and (2) to achieve a lowering of the pressure load on the left ventricle (LV). The intended result of this phase shifting is to alter, in a favorable direction, the ratio between oxygen supply and oxygen demand of the myocardium, thereby improving pump performance of the heart. Assuming that the optimal size balloon has been introduced, the main operational variable is the timing of the balloon. Logically, inflation is timed to occur shortly after cardiac systole, i.e., as soon as the aortic valve has closed (T_1 in Figure 1). Optimal timing of balloon deflation (T_2) is not that obvious. Relatively early deflation of the balloon provides maximal lowering of the presystolic pressure; relatively late deflation provides maximal diastolic pressure augmentation. Timing of deflation may thus represent a compromise, which, in turn, is dependent on length of the heart period, i.e., heart rate. The two basic effects of balloon assist, on LV pressure development and on diastolic pressure area, are surprisingly often evaluated simply by visual observation of an oscilloscopic pressure tracing. Since evaluation on this basis is likely to be rather inaccurate, we designed and constructed a system, depicted in the block diagram in Figure 2, for electronic integration of areas under systolic and diastolic pressure curves (Normann et al., 1972). Two points in time are needed; the first is obtained from ECG, the second from the negative slope of left ventricular pressure signal or from drive system trigger-pulse at end of systole. The experimental record reproduced in Figure 3 illustrates results obtained with the arterial pressure integrator. In the beginning of the record, the balloon was deflated relatively early in diastole, leading to a significant lowering of presystolic pressure in the proximal aorta. In the middle portion of the record, the balloon was inactive, and in the right portion of the record the balloon was deflated shortly before opening of the aortic valve. In this second control mode, the diastolic pressure area was 20% greater than in the first mode, but this was at the cost of a 10% higher left ventricular pressure development; the effect of the latter, however, was partly offset by an 8% lower heart rate. It is likely that optimum balloon timing varies with pathophysiology of the patient; whether it can be deduced from commonly used indices (cardiac output, arterial pressure, left atrial pressure, pulmonary artery wedge pressure) is yet to be demonstrated. Results of coronary artery occlusion experiments in dogs, in which IABCP was combined with administration of a vasoconstrictor drug (thus elevating arterial blood pressure), suggest that increasing coronary perfusion is under these circumstances therapeutically a more important factor than decreasing LV afterload (Clayman et al., 1972).

Because the intra-aortic balloon, and similar counterpulsation devices, act in-series with the left ventricle, an increase in cardiac output can be

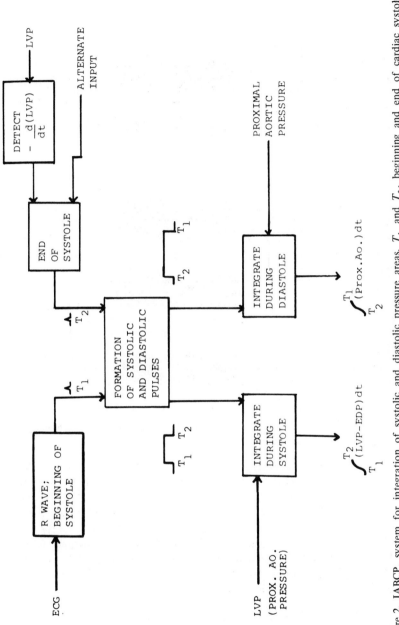

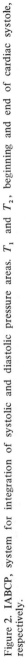

Figure 2. IABCP, system for integration of systolic and diastolic pressure areas. T_1 and T_2, beginning and end of cardiac systole, respectively.

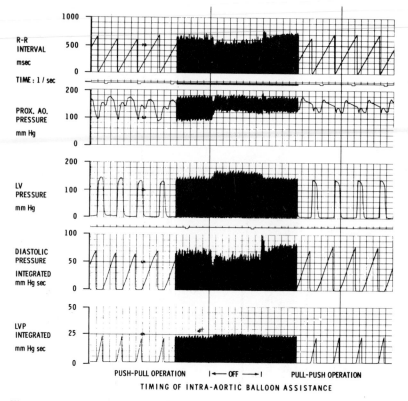

Figure 3. IABCP. *Left panel*, early balloon deflation; *right panel*, late balloon deflation.

attained only indirectly, by enhancing cardiac pump performance. This inherent limitation of the IABCP method manifests itself, unfortunately, under conditions when circulatory assistance is needed the most; on the basis of clinical experience, it is by now generally recognized that in low cardiac output states, accompanied by hypotension ($\overline{\text{BP}} < 60$ mm Hg), the balloon is likely to be ineffective (Noon, Normann, and DeBakey, 1975). Under these conditions, what is needed is an auxiliary power source in the form of a mechanical pump device.

PUMP ASSIST SYSTEMS

Experimentally and clinically, it has been demonstrated that an auxiliary circulatory pump can be therapeutically effective in reversing myocardial and secondary dysfunctions. By the employment of left ventricular bypass for left ventricular failure, e.g., in conjunction with cardiac surgery, recovery of cardiac function is favored by reductions of left ventricular preload, end-diastolic pressure (volume), and myocardial oxygen requirement, and, as a consequence of increased total left side output, by the interruption of a number of secondary, hemodynamic-metabolic vicious cycles.

Generally, cardiac assist pumps are either pulsatile or nonpulsatile and bypass either the total heart (veno-arterial) (Wakabayashi et al., 1974) or the left ventricle. In the various configurations, pump inflow connection is made either to systemic vein(s), to left atrium (DeBakey, Liotta, and Hall, 1966a), or to left ventricle (Bernhard et al., 1969; Pierce et al., 1974); pump outflow is connected to the aorta (Robinson et al., 1973) or a major peripheral artery.

Direct-Coupled Nonpulsatile Bypass

Nonpulsatile roller-pumps are employed both in circulatory and in pulmonary support systems. In the operating room, following cardiac surgery, the use of a roller-pump constitutes the most expedient method for bypass support. Unfortunately, because of the thrombogenicity of polyvinyl tubing, this approach requires continued heparinization (treatment with anticlotting drug) and is therefore limited to intraoperative applications. A scheme to circumvent this problem is the employment of indwelling, silicone elastomer cannulae, connected to left atrium and aorta during surgery. Postoperatively, through a small skin incision, precisely fitting cannulae obturators can be removed and roller-pump support instituted, in conjunction with partial heparinization (Litwak et al., 1973). Recently, however, relatively hemocompatible roller-pump tubing and cannulae have become available, making it possible to employ roller-pump support in the presence of normal hemostasis, i.e., without heparin (Wakabayashi et al., 1974).

Since left ventricular bypass is indicated most frequently, and, if in this configuration pump inflow tubing is connected to the left atrium—without any intervening reservoir—it follows that pump control is critical for achieving safe, optimal bypass support. We therefore designed and constructed the servo system presented schematically in Figure 4. Briefly, the processed left atrial pressure signal (voltage) is in an electronic control module compared to a reference voltage representing the desired left atrial pressure level. The difference between these voltages automatically determines the speed of the roller-pump. By the use of high system gain, left atrial pressure is safely and automatically locked to the set level. By contrast, attempts to manually control a roller-pump under conditions of high percentage bypass and a few mm Hg left atrial pressure, would be rather hazardous. For additional safety, the system (Figure 4) includes provision for automatic shutdown in 0.2 sec if line pressures exceed preset limits.

The servo locking of left atrial pressure is illustrated in the experi-

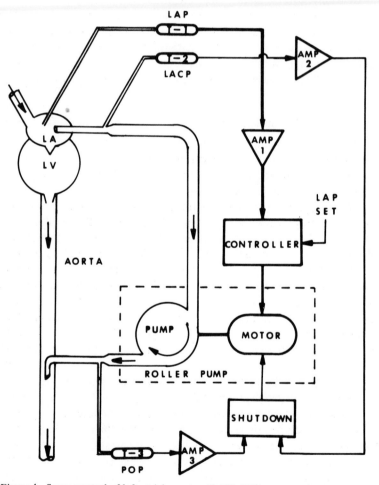

Figure 4. Servo control of left atrial pressure (LAP). POP, pump output pressure.

mental record reproduced in Figure 5. In a 28-kg dog, the ascending aorta was nearly occluded with a snare, and a roller-pump, automatically controlled, maintained circulation by pumping blood from left atrium to femoral arteries. Intravenous infusion of 150 ml blood over a 2-min period caused a near doubling of pump output, from 1.8 to 3.4 liters/min, while left atrial pressure increased by only 1 mm Hg, from 3 to 4 mm Hg. In clinical application, a critical factor in this system is the reliability of left atrial pressure measurement; stability and absence of position and other artifacts are prerequisites. An atrial cannula, incorporating a catheter-tip type transducer, is presently under development.

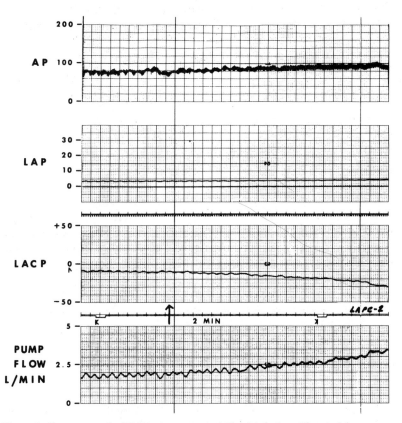

Figure 5. Servo control of LAP. *Arrow*, started blood infusion. AP, arterial pressure; LACP, left atrial cannula pressure. All pressures in mm Hg.

Reservoir-Coupled Nonpulsatile Bypass

Incorporation of a reservoir in the pump inflow line (Figure 6) serves three functions: (1) as a reservoir for blood drained by gravity; (2) as a trap for air or gas bubbles; and (3) as a capacitance element, constituting a decoupling between the blood drainage source and roller-pump. The reservoir is kept filled; thus it differs from reservoirs that contain both a fluid and a gas phase during use. A typical example of the latter is the bubble oxygenator commonly used in heart–lung machines. Currently, reservoir-coupled roller-pumps are used under conditions permitting the use of heparin (e.g., in pulmonary support with membrane oxygenator). Non-thrombogenic reservoirs and oxygenators (Hagler et al., 1975) are, however, under development and will provide important, therapeutic alternatives.

A reservoir used as indicated in Figure 6 typically consists of a 300-ml, flexible, plastic bag. Operationally, a pump operator adjusts the height of the reservoir and the speed of the roller-pump, usually keeping the reservoir completely filled in order to avoid the danger of pumping the reservoir empty. Consequently, because of human limitations, the system does not provide maximal system performance combined with a desirable margin of safety. We therefore designed and constructed the servo system presented schematically in Figure 7, depicting its use in atrio-aortic, left ventricular bypass. The essential feature is servo control of bag volume: voltage output from a volume sensor is electronically compared to a selectable reference voltage representing the desired reservoir volume (typically, half of full capacity); the difference between the two voltages determines the speed of the roller-pump (Normann et al., 1976). In this manner, for a given drainage pressure gradient, the pump output will automatically match the rate of blood drainage and, consequently, maximum flow can be obtained, safely, without exposing a human operator to stress and fatigue. The variation in reservoir volume (150 ml) is 0.8% of flow, i.e., increasing flow from 0 to 4 liters/min causes a volume change of 32 ml.

The primary safety requirement in the employment of these pump systems is the avoidance of embolism. In addition to the danger of clot formation, the pumping of air or gas constitutes a real threat. The servo control just described inherently reduces the possibility of pumping the reservoir empty because reduced inflow (e.g., by accidental clamping of inflow line) simply stops the pump when volume is down to the preset

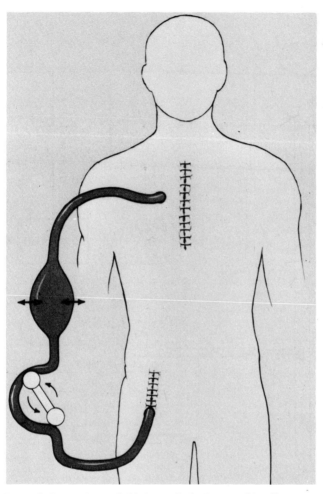

Figure 6. Reservoir-coupled left ventricular bypass with roller-pump.

control level. Additionally, an independent, volume-triggered shutdown circuit has been incorporated as a safety backup in the event of control module failure. Excessive pressure in pump outflow line also triggers a pump shutdown.

Performance of the servo control is illustrated in the experimental, representative record reproduced in Figure 8. In a left heart bypass configuration in dog, stepwise lowering of the bag from zero (equaling left

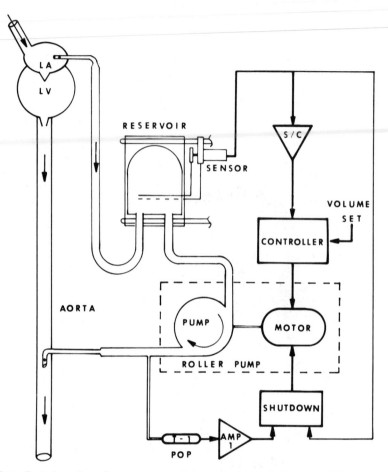

Figure 7. Automatic roller-pump control in reservoir-coupled bypass. POP, pump output pressure.

atrial level) to −53 cm caused, automatically, a stepwise increase in flow from 0.5 to 2.3 liters/min. The drop in left atrial pressure from 6.6 to 1.6 mm Hg and the gradual reduction in arterial pulse pressure reflect the increasing proportion of total output being bypassed by the roller-pump.

Pulsatile Bypass

The development of pulsatile blood pumps for clinical use goes back to the beginnings of the heart–lung machine; in one of the early models the

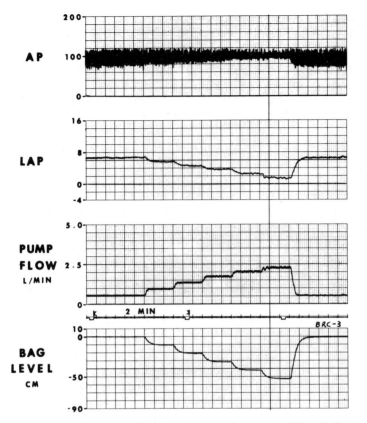

Figure 8. Experimental record obtained with control system in Figure 7. Reservoir level referenced to left atrium. Pressures in mm Hg.

pump was pulsatile (Dennis, 1956). Early clinical experiences with post-operative, paracorporeal, pulsatile left ventricular bypass of up to 10 days demonstrated reversal of severe left ventricular failure in some of the patients (DeBakey, 1971).

For short-term application, one approach to pulsatile bypass is to combine roller-pump support with IABCP, a combination that has been used in total cardiopulmonary bypass (Pappas et al., 1975). For longer-term support, days to weeks, a pulsatile assist pump is considered prefer-able.

Pulsatile bypass pumps are usually driven by a pneumatic power source; blood- and gas-containing compartments are separated either by a diaphragm or a bladder wall. Pump ejection is achieved by pulses of pressurized gas; filling is frequently assisted by the application of vacuum, particularly if blood is drained from the left atrium. Inlet and outlet valves are usually of a clinical, prosthetic type. Hookup of the pump varies with the institution—from placing it intra-abdominally, connected between apex of the left ventricle and abdominal aorta (Robinson et al., 1973) to placing it paracorporeally, connected between the left atrium and an auxiliary artery (Figure 9) (DeBakey, 1971). Filling of the pump from the left ventricle permits maximum unloading and therefore maximum reduction in myocardial oxygen requirement. On the other hand, the ventricular connection is more likely to involve complexities than is the atrial.

Operationally, pump performance is judged by visual observation of the pump (when possible) and by monitoring pneumatic line pressure, effects on physiologic parameters, and, in some instances, pump output by means of a flow probe incorporated in pump outflow tract. None of these

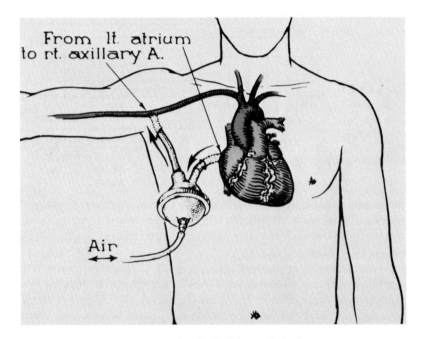

Figure 9. Hookup of paracorporeal, pulsatile left ventricular bypass pump.

methods provides precise information as to the beat-to-beat, operational behavior of the pump, and the standard method of control relies therefore on a human operator to select the timing (of ejection and filling) that appears appropriate. (If the pump is synchronized with the heart, then, naturally, ejection is triggered to occur in cardiac diastole.) Since pathophysiologic parameters, directly related to pump operation, can vary considerably from one pump beat to the next, it follows that optimized pump control needs to be based on precise, beat-to-beat measurement of pump dynamics. In choosing among possible measurement methods, important considerations are simplicity in application, long-term reliability, and, preferably, applicability to pumps implanted within the body.

The system we employ for *monitoring* pneumatic blood pumps is based on the measurement of electrical capacitance across the gas space within the pump (Normann et al., 1973, 1974a). Because the gas space varies reciprocally with pump blood volume, the latter can in this manner be measured. Depending on pump design, the magnitude of the capacitance can be from 0.5 to 50 pF. The only modification of the pump necessary for this measurement is the deposit of a thin, metallic film ("plate") on the inside of the gas-facing portion of pump housing (Figure 10). A thin cable, introduced via the pneumatic tubing, connects the plate with the signal processing unit, as indicated schematically in Figure 11. Output from the signal processor, representing the instantaneous position of the flexing member, provides on-line display and recording of stroke volume, flow into and out of the pump, plus pump output per minute (assuming intact valves). A special circuit design permits electronics to be located relatively remote from the pump, an important feature if the pump is employed intracorporeally (Normann et al., 1974b).

The availability of an electronic signal that directly and instantaneously reflects displacements within the pump, provides feedback information necessary for automatic, closed-loop *control* of pump events, as indicated in Figures 11 and 12. Trigger signals generated at preset levels of pump filling and emptying provide the control pulse for the pneumatic drive system. Consequently, each pump phase is initiated automatically, and stroke volume can be set at will. The various control options are illustrated in Figure 12; the two most commonly used are the free-running "volume-triggered" and the combined volume–ECG-triggered modes.

Satisfactory system performance has been demonstrated in numerous left ventricular bypass experiments in calves. The experimental record reproduced in Figure 13 illustrates some operational features: increasing

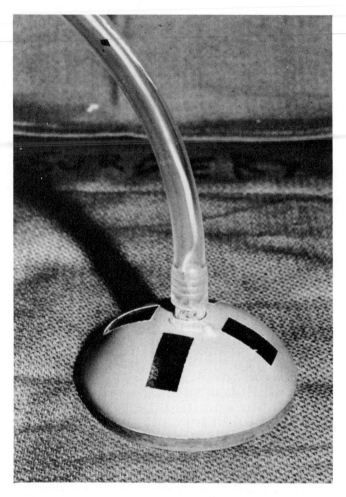

Figure 10. "Air-dome" of pneumatic bypass pump. Metallic coating, connected by intratubal cable, for pump capacitance measurement.

stroke volume, by changing the pump filling trigger point, was imme-diately accompanied by a reciprocal decrease in pump rate and by higher peak flows; continuity of operation is evident, i.e., at preset volume levels one pump phase is immediately followed by the next.

Summarized, the described monitor—control system provides the fol-lowing advantages: (1) automatic timing of pump events; (2) blood flow

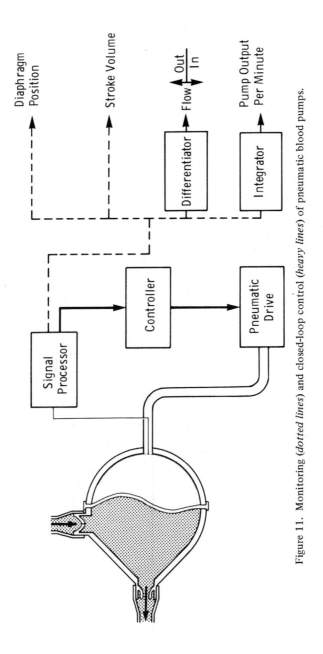

Figure 11. Monitoring (*dotted lines*) and closed-loop control (*heavy lines*) of pneumatic blood pumps.

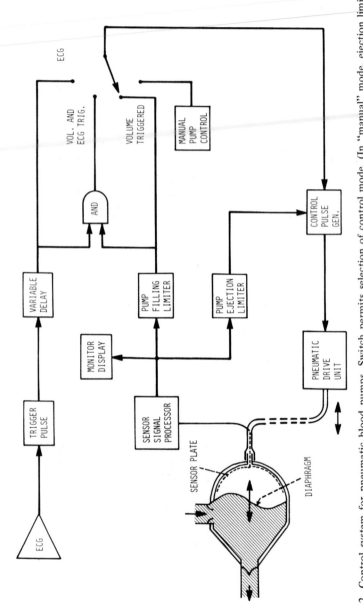

Figure 12. Control system for pneumatic blood pumps. Switch permits selection of control mode. (In "manual" mode, ejection limiter connection is interrupted.)

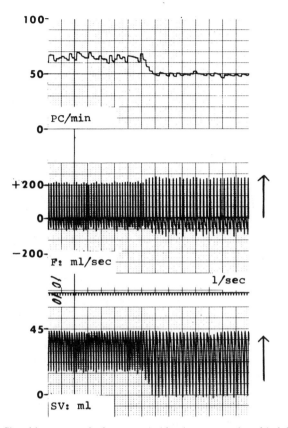

Figure 13. Closed-loop control of pneumatic blood pump employed in left ventricular bypass in calf. PC, pump cycles; F, flow; SV, stroke volume. Arrows indicate ejection, flow out of pump.

through the pump is continuous; (3) stroke volume and excursions of flexing member can be set at will; (4) it is applicable both to para- and to intracorporeal pneumatic blood pumps; (5) long-term reliability; (6) for the human operator, evaluation and control are greatly facilitated.

AUTONOMIC NERVOUS SYSTEM RESPONSES

It is well known that the cardiovascular system incorporates a great number of "biosensors," located in heart, lungs, large vessels, and carotid sinuses. Via nerves, the central nervous system (CNS) thus obtains feedback information necessary for carrying out cardiovascular control functions; outflows in autonomic nerves can profoundly affect cardiac function and peripheral circulation. Because mechanical circulatory assist is likely to alter hemodynamic inputs to biosensors, directly or indirectly, it is of more than academic interest to know the extent to which autonomic reflexes contribute to the total cardiovascular response. A typical example of the uncertainty in this general area is the still unresolved question concerning the relative merits of pulsatile versus nonpulsatile total cardiopulmonary bypass, a question which, at least partly, is related to the role of arterial baroreceptors: at the same mean arterial pressure, within the normal pressure range, baroreceptor output is significantly greater for pulsatile than for nonpulsatile pressures. One reflex effect of increased baroreceptor output is inhibition of sympathetic outflow to heart and peripheral vessels, tending to cause (among other things) slowing of heart rate, reduced cardiac contractility, and vasodilatation. Arterial baroreceptors are, of necessity, involved also in mechanical circulatory assist because the devices and systems used affect pressure and pressure waveforms in the systemic arterial tree.

The direct approach to a study of the effects on arterial baroreceptors is to record the activity in the nerves which connect baroreceptors with CNS. Having available to us special neurophysiologic instrumentation and techniques, we monitored, during IABCP in dogs, the output from baroreceptors (BRO) located in the aortic arch and the carotid sinuses. The tracings reproduced in Figure 14 illustrate the profound changes in the neurogram caused by intra-aortic balloon operation. The well-known sensitivity of these receptors to rate of pressure change (dP/dt) is evident, giving rise to characteristic diphasic bursts caused by cardiac and balloon pressure waves. The relative magnitude of these bursts and the increased total BRO per heart period varied in a sensitive manner with balloon timing and rate of inflation (Normann and Kennedy, 1971).

The next step in the analysis of reflex components concerns autonomic outflows from the CNS, particularly in sympathetic nerves to the heart and the peripheral vascular bed. The observed increase in BRO is consistent with the reported decrease in hind limb resistance during diastolic augmentation in unanesthetized dogs (Brown, Goldfarb, and Gott, 1966). Possibly of greater concern are the effects on sympathetic outflow to the heart itself—particularly if one considers the importance of adrenergic factors in cardiac pathophysiology. In preliminary experiments we monitored the outflow in cardiac sympathetic nerves and demonstrated

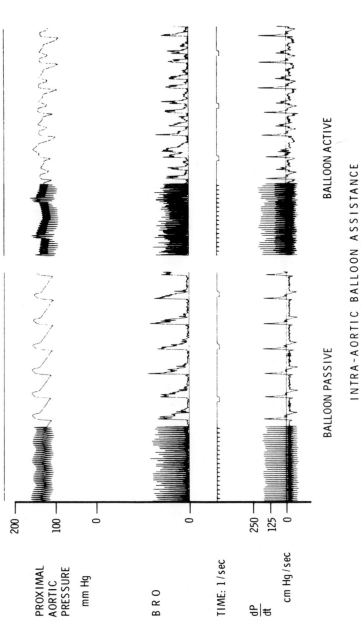

PROXIMAL AORTIC PRESSURE mm Hg

200

100

0

B R O

0

TIME: 1/sec

dP/dt cm Hg/sec

250

125

0

BALLOON PASSIVE

BALLOON ACTIVE

INTRA-AORTIC BALLOON ASSISTANCE

Figure 14. Monitoring of output from aortic baroreceptors (BRO) during IABCP (*right panel*). *Bottom trace*, derivative of proximal aortic pressure.

that in response to IABCP, the temporal pattern changed significantly, presumably caused by BRO alterations; unexpectedly, increased total BRO per cardiac cycle did *not* cause a reciprocal reduction in cardiac sympathetic outflow—although increased arterial pressure and BRO following injection of a vasoconstrictor did. If these preliminary results obtained in acute experiments can be extrapolated to the physiologically intact state, they bring into focus the very interesting and functionally important question of autonomic nervous system differentiation. Under a given set of circumstances, to what extent can responses in cardiac sympathetic outflow differ from those in sympathetic outflows to other organs? In the case of IABCP, it would be of considerable practical importance to substantiate the indication that the accompanying increase in total arterial baroreceptor output may not significantly reduce sympathetic outflow to the heart, although it may reduce the outflow to peripheral vessels, causing vasodilatation.

On general grounds and from an operational viewpoint, it seems prudent to further explore the possibility that employment of mechanical circulatory assist may induce neurohumoral responses that are likely to contribute significantly to the final therapeutic result.

SUMMARY COMMENTS

The primary obstacle to the development of circulatory assist systems has been the lack of blood-compatible materials and surfaces. Solutions to this primary problem, however, must be accompanied by flow dynamic and operational optimization if maximum safety and efficacy are to be achieved. Consequently, effective control of auxiliary, circulatory pump systems is of critical importance. At the basic level of control, the human operator is inadequate as the main feedback link. The employment of physical systems for sensing, signal processing, and control makes it possible to achieve high efficacy combined with enhanced safety. Additionally, the introduction of appropriate sensors and data processing provides on-line monitoring capability and thus the information necessary for evaluation of system performance. In further developments, the degree of therapeutic efficacy of mechanical circulatory assist will probably depend on the availability of a variety of blood pumps, used in various configurations, and on optimization of the functional interface between systems.

LITERATURE CITED

Bernhard, W. F., G. C. LaFarge, H. Jochin, S. Kitrilakis, and T. Robinson. 1969. Chronic left ventricular bypass with an implantable ventricular-aortic assist pump. Circulation 39, Suppl.: 99–103.

Brown, B. G., D. Goldfarb, and V. L. Gott. 1966. A vasomotor reflex contribution to systolic pressure reduction during diastolic augmentation. Trans. Amer. Soc. Artif. Int. Org. 12: 63–67.

Bruck, S. D. 1975. Biomedical applications of polymeric materials and their interactions with blood components: A critical review of current developments. Polymer 16: 409–417.

Clayman, R., K. H. Johansen, G. A. DeLaria, and E. F. Bernstein. 1974. The hypertensive balloon: A beneficial synergism for the salvage of ischemic myocardium. J. Thorac. Cardiovas. Surg. 68: 80–89.

DeBakey, M. E. 1971. Left ventricular bypass pumps for cardiac assistance. Amer. J. Cardiol. 27: 3–11.

DeBakey, M. E., D. Liotta, and C. W. Hall. 1966a. Left-heart bypass using an implantable blood pump. Mechanical Devices to Assist the Failing Heart, Chapter 18, pp. 223–239. National Academy of Sciences, National Research Council, Washington, D.C.

DeBakey, M. E., D. Liotta, and C. W. Hall. 1966b. Prospects for and implications of the artificial heart and assist devices. J. Rehab. 32: 106–107.

Dennis, C. 1956. Certain methods for artificial support of the circulation during open intracardiac surgery. Surg. Clin. N. Amer. 36: 423–436.

Hagler, H. K., W. M. Powell, J. W. Eberle, W. L. Sugg, M. R. Platt, and J. T. Watson. 1975. Five-day partial bypass using a membrane oxygenator without systemic heparinization. Trans. Amer. Soc. Artif. Int. Org. 21: 178–187.

Litwak, R. S., F. A. Lajam, R. M. Koffsky, G. Silvay, H. Shiang, S. A. Geller, and F. S. Pedersen. 1973. Obturated permanent left atrial and aortic cannulae for assisted circulation after cardiac surgery. Trans. Amer. Soc. Artif. Int. Organs 19: 243–250.

Moulopoulos, S. D., S. Topaz, and W. J. Kolff. 1962. Diastolic balloon pumping (with carbon dioxide) in the aorta—A mechanical assistance to the failing circulation. Amer. Heart J. 63: 669–675.

Noon, G. P., N. A. Normann, and M. E. DeBakey. 1975. Left ventricular bypass in treatment of pump failure. Transactions 2nd Henry Ford Hospital Internatl. Symp. on Card. Surg. In press.

Normann, N. A., M. E. DeBakey, G. P. Noon, and J. N. Ross. 1973. Monitoring and closed-loop control of pneumatic blood pumps. Cardiovasc. Res. Center Bull. 12: 3–12.

Normann, N. A., W. D. Johnson, D. H. Glaeser, and M. E. DeBakey. 1972. On-line data processing and experimental cardiac assistance. Proc. San Diego Biomed. Symp. 11: 59–61.

Normann, N. A., and J. H. Kennedy. 1971. Arterial baroreceptor responses to intraaortic balloon assistance. J. Surg. Res. 11: 396–400.

Normann, N. A., G. P. Noon, M. E. DeBakey, and J. N. Ross. 1974a. Automatic control of pneumatic blood pumps. Trans. Amer. Soc. Artif. Int. Organs 20: 685–690.

Normann, N. A., G. P. Noon, T. G. Cooper, and M. E. DeBakey. 1976. Automatic control of roller-pumps in cardio-pulmonary support systems. Proc. San Diego Biomed. Symp. 15: 119–124.

Normann, N. A., J. N. Ross, G. P. Noon, and M. E. DeBakey. 1974b. Instantaneous measurement of blood volume within implanted pneumatic blood pumps. Proc. 27th Am. Conf. Eng. Med. Biol. 15: 52.

Pappas, G., S. D. Winter, C. J. Kopriva, and P. P. Steele. 1975. Improvement of myocardial and other vital organ functions and metabolism with a simple method of pulsatile flow (IABP) during clinical cardiopulmonary bypass. Surgery 77: 34–44.

Pierce, W. S., W. O'Bannon, J. H. Donachy, J. L. Pennock, and J. A. Waldhausen. 1974. Preliminary Report. A new technique for insertion of a large-bore cannula into the left ventricule of the calf. J. Surg. Res. 17: 274–277.

Robinson, W. J., J. J. Migliore, J. Arthur, J. M. Fuqua, G. B. Dove, S. Coleman, F. N. Huffman, and J. C. Norman. 1973. An abdominal left ventricular assist device: experimental physiologic analyses II. Trans. Amer. Soc. Artif. Int. Organs 19: 229–234.

Wakabayashi, A., Y. Nakamura, K. J. Murphy, E. A. Stemmer, and J. E. Connolly. 1974. Heparinless venoarterial bypass. Its application in the treatment of experimental cardiogenic shock. Arch. Surg. 108: 497–501.

Cardiovascular Flow Dynamics and Measurements
Edited by N. H. C. Hwang and N. A. Normann
Copyright 1977   University Park Press   Baltimore

chapter 24

THE ARTIFICIAL HEART

The term "artificial heart" may represent any type of man-made blood pump, intracorporeal or extracorporeal ventricular assist device, or total heart replacement device. In this chapter, however, all papers except Chapter 24b deal with the total artificial heart (TAH). Since Chapter 24b describes power sources to drive the artificial heart, they may be applied to any type of blood pump.

In Chapter 24a Bücherl briefly covers every phase related to the entire project (design, material, material testing, turbulence, and stagnation in relation to thrombus formation, flow pattern—pulsatile or nonpulsatile, energy source, control and driving system, surgery, monitoring, and postoperative care). He describes major problems encountered in his laboratory: inflow occlusion of the right side of the heart, thrombus formation inside the artificial heart, pulmonary insufficiency, and infection. Finally, he points out that the problem of weight gain, when the calf survives for several months, requires a larger cardiac output than the maximum capacity of the TAH.

Chapter 24b, presented by Mohnhaupt and Unger, deals with various power sources, energy storage, and conversion systems that might be applicable to various blood pumps. Different approaches for producing hydraulic power, and limiting factors which determine the design of these components, are discussed. The authors enumerate five major design criteria in development of implantable energy systems: size, efficiency, service life, body interaction, and price. Finally, they describe three different power systems developed for their TAH.

In Chapter 24c, Lawson, who represents the Utah group, discusses postoperative pathophysiologic problems in calves with an implanted TAH. He mentions infection, hemolysis, and thrombus formation as three major problems in postoperative calves. He emphasizes that the eventual solution to the problem of infection will be the development of a completely implantable system. His group is trying to use the natural aortic and pulmonary valves of the experimental calf with the intention of reducing hemolysis, which they think is mainly caused by four prosthetic valves installed in the TAH. As for thrombus formation inside their TAH, Lawson mentions that one particularly troublesome area is usually around the atria and inflow valves.

In Chapter 24d Akutsu reports the results of 70 experiments performed between March 1971 and June 1975 using Silastic sac-type TAH in calves. He divided the calves into two groups according to their survival time: 43 calves that lived less than 100 hr and 27 calves that survived longer than 100 hr. The first group died mainly of technical and mechanical failures. Among 27 calves in the second group, 75% of the deaths occurred from causes related to pathophysiologic problems, thromboembolism, infection, low cardiac output, renal dysfunction, and pulmonary insufficiency. Akutsu shows the interrelationships between each step of the entire procedure and discusses the major problems encountered. He also discusses the mechanism of increase in right atrial pressure, frequently seen in long-term survivals, and its close relation to anemia.

The first TAH paper was presented by Akutsu and Kolff in 1958 in which one dog survived for 1.5 hr. Seventeen years later, the survival time of experimental animals has been prolonged to several months. Numerous problems still must be solved, however, and clinical application is some years away.

Cardiovascular Flow Dynamics and Measurements
Edited by N. H. C. Hwang and N. A. Normann
Copyright 1977   University Park Press   Baltimore

chapter 24a

TOTAL MECHANICAL HEART

E. S. Bücherl

In simple terms, we can say that the function of the heart is to transport blood according to the organism's actual needs. If we wish to replace this heart, we have to take over the transport by a pump that includes a driving system and an energy source. We have to realize that the transported fluid (blood) consists of water, proteins, electrolytes, and different kinds of living cells. To supply as much blood as an organism actually needs requires fast regulation of the pump. The basic parts of an artificial heart, then, include blood pump, driving system, energy source, and control system.

First of all, we need two blood pumps because we have two different circulatory systems: one with a high peripheral resistance and one with a low peripheral resistance. This looks quite simple but, as becomes clear later on, there are many problems in designing and fabricating an artificial heart.

To design an artificial heart replacing the natural heart we have to study carefully the volume and shape of the natural heart. A cast of the heart inside the chest shows us that there is actually very little space for the connections we must make between the artificial heart and the remnant of the natural heart (Figure 1).

Shortness of space and lack of flexibility in connecting sites are the first two difficult factors we have to confront and solve in the development of an intracorporeal (implantable) blood pump. This explains why blood pumps from different research groups look similar (Figures 2 and 3). In Figure 3 one can clearly distinguish four connectors. From the anatomic point of view this form cannot be changed for connections without drastically changing the direction of the blood flow. After the geometric design has been determined, the next important problem is the selection of materials from which the blood pump is fabricated.

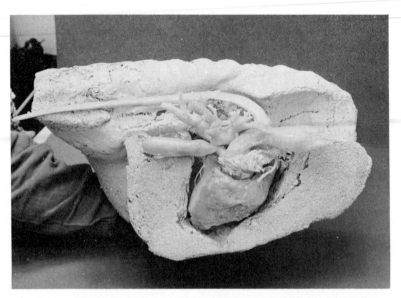

Figure 1. Cast of the thoracic cavity of a calf.

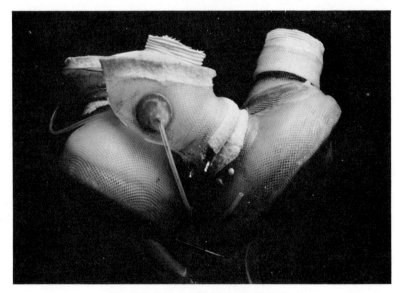

Figure 2. Total artificial heart (Berlin).

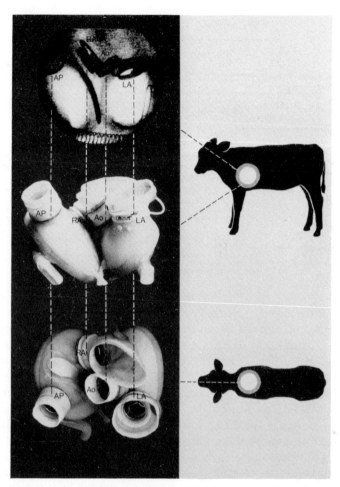

Figure 3. Position of total artificial heart in a calf.

We know that blood is a living fluid which coagulates rapidly when exposed to foreign material. Although the clotting mechanism is not yet completely understood, the following sequence of phenomena is speculated to occur: plasma proteins are irreversibly adsorbed and a few seconds later a macromolecular layer develops that allows (Figure 4) platelets to attach to this layer and thrombus formation starts, which may dislodge and cause embolism. One of the major factors effecting these

CONTACT BLOOD / ARTIFICIAL MATERIAL

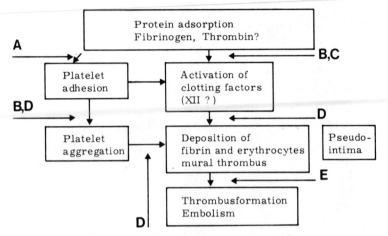

Figure 4. Anticoagulating precautions (*A–E*).

events is the electrical charge of the foreign material's surface. The initial adsorption of proteins to the surface influences this electrical charge, which is indicated by changes in the Zeta potential and the critical surface tension. Although this chapter does not present a detailed explanation, it might be helpful to discuss the possibilities of inhibiting these events. Possible means are (1) precoating the surface with proteins, (2) selecting materials with special surface properties, (3) incorporating anticoagulants on the surface, (4) utilizing low- or high-surface-energy materials, and (5) preclotting the plastic surface. We illustrate the most important problem at this time, namely, the contact of foreign material with blood.

In addition to biologic properties, we have to also look, from the mechanical point of view, for availability, workability, usability, and durability of the material.

Currently, we are investigating materials that can be divided into five groups: (1) specially prepared materials with heparin or albumin, (2) electrically loaded polymers, (3) neutral materials (polyurethane, hydrogels, pyrolytic carbons), (4) porous synthetics (nylon, dacron, Teflon, Ivalon), and (5) materials prepared with biologic cells.

Specially prepared materials usually mean those impregnated with heparin. According to our experience, vascular prostheses that were coated with albumin during the first implantation were found less thrombogenic during the second implantation.

The idea of an electrically loaded polymer comes from the physiologic fact that the normal vessel intima has a negatively charged surface. Therefore, Teflon, hydrogel, polyurethane, and other materials are prepared with small charcoal particles as conductive elements.

In the neutral group, urethane, hydrogel, and pyrolytic carbons are of special interest. Foreign material is more resistant to adsorption of blood elements if hydrated; the best known substance is Hydron, a three-dimensionally interlaced gel.

Currently, in our animal experiments, Silastic and polyurethane seem to be the best biocompatible materials. In contrast, porous synthetic materials such as nylon, dacron, and Teflon are known to have a very strong primary thrombogenicity. The purpose in using them is that, immediately after blood contact, a deposition of blood elements takes place and the foreign material is covered with a fine layer of host cells that finally grow into a new endothelial lining.

The last group, materials prepared with biologic cells, is very interesting because a lot of our problems would be solved if the blood were not in direct contact with the foreign material but with a preformed layer of cultured tissue. This means that we would have to cultivate fibroblasts on the surface of the foreign material several days before implantation in order to have a complete biologic lining.

How can we select the most suitable among these available materials? What are the proper materials to compare? We would be happy if there could be a screening test which would enable us to select the best material for more detailed investigation. Of course, there are many tests, e.g., measurement of coagulation time, erythrocyte traumatization, phagocytosis of leucocytes, platelet adherence, destruction, aggregation, Zeta potential, thrombus formation, thromboelastogramme, and critical surface tension. These are still very crude screening criteria, but at least it is possible to eliminate a large number of materials that are not suitable.

We have been quite successful with the technique involving thromboelastogrammes. If the material is thrombogenic, like Dacron flock, the coagulation is fast and the thrombus strong (Figure 5). If the material is antithrombogenic, the opposite is observed (Figure 6).

The drawback is that these in vitro tests do not always lead in the same direction as in vivo tests, but in vivo testing of biomaterial is still far more

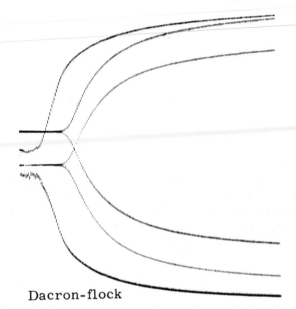

Dacron-flock

Figure 5. Thromboelastogram of Dacron-flocked silastic surface.

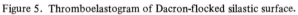

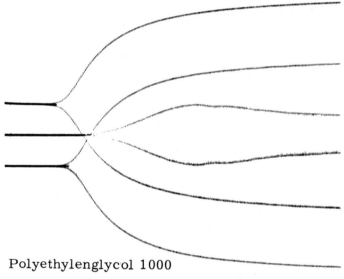

Polyethylenglycol 1000

Figure 6. Thromboelastogram with polyethylene glycol 1,000.

difficult and takes a lot of time (Figure 7). One approach is to implant the material into the wall of the right atrium or into the atrial cavity, thus bringing it in contact with the blood. Another possibility is to make a ring out of the material and implant it in a vein or an artery for observation. The most satisfying test is to put a tube of the material inside the aorta, thus creating a stenosis proximal to the renal arteries. Not only can the deposition of blood elements on this implanted tube be seen, but also whether thrombi were formed and embolism occurred. Because the blood goes straight to the kidneys, it is easy to detect infarcts there. Dr. Bert Kusserow, who introduced this test, has given this explanation: "If your gun-barrel is empty, you never know whether it has been fired or not." This means that the material, in place, can look satisfactory because any emboli that formed were dislodged. By this method, many materials were tested and compared. Visualization of the surface after contact with blood is done by using a scanning electron microscope at a magnification between 1,000 and 5,000 (Figure 8).

At present, we usually find various degrees of depositions in various locations after several days or weeks of contact with blood. We have to remember here that in cardiac patients with mitral valve disease and an abnormal blood flow in the left atrium, thrombus formation occurs also in a normal circulatory system. This, as well as our experiments with blood pumps, demonstrates that not only the antithrombogenicity of the material used is important, but also the blood flow pattern. It is important to

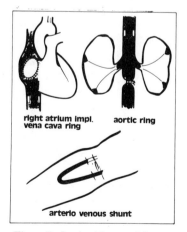

right atrium impl.   aortic ring
vena cava ring

arterio venous shunt

Figure 7. In vivo biomaterial test.

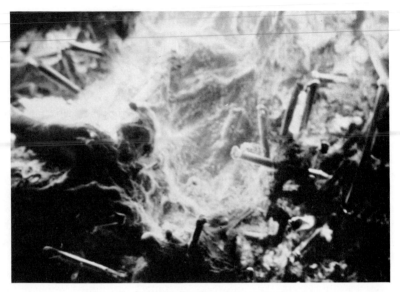

Figure 8. Scanning electron microscopic picture.

avoid, if possible, any areas of turbulent flow or of stasis; therefore, flow-dynamics tests of each pump are important.

Several different methods may be used for these tests; one of them is a flow visualization technique that uses suspended particles in the testing fluid. Another method is to dye the possible thrombogenetic area with a colored testing fluid (Figure 9).

Until now, we were not sure whether or not a pulsatile flow is necessary for the total artificial heart. Much physiologic data led to the conclusion that pulsatile flow is important for the regulation of the circulation. Therefore, our pump is designed to simulate this pulsatile flow. Because there is no material that can contract by itself, we use a flexible membrane that divides the pump into an air chamber and a blood chamber. In a pump with such a design, contact between the moving membrane and the housing is known to be a chief cause of thrombus formation (Figure 10).

To move this membrane requires energy. Because only the blood pump itself is inside the body, most groups use compressed air and special valves or magnetic pumps to move this membrane. In these systems it is possible to regulate many parameters, such as dp/dt and duration of systole and

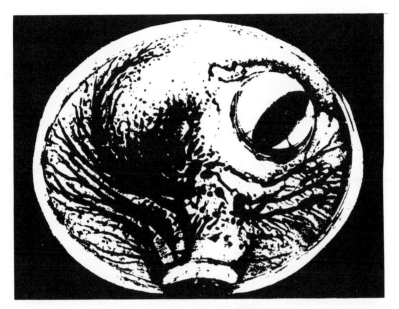

Figure 9. In vivo evaluation of possible thrombus formation (dye method).

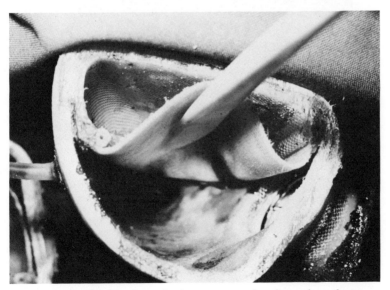

Figure 10. Thrombus formation between pump, housing, and membrane.

diastole, and thereby to achieve a desirable pulse wave. To have an outside control-driving unit requires a transcutaneous connection, which may cause a major problem of infection. The danger of infection is aggravated by the presence of foreign material in the wound. If this wound is protected very carefully, as is done in artificial-kidney patients with an extracorporeal shunt, one can maintain adequate asepsis. But unlike shunts to the kidney, in experimental animals the tube to the prosthetic heart has a diameter of about 2 cm and the tissue around the tube is permanently traumatized. Thus, infection is favored and often the animal dies from sepsis. Many attempts have been made to expect tissue ingrowth into the foreign material under the skin in order to create a barrier against infection (Figure 11). In a few animals, we demonstrated that these tubes healed in

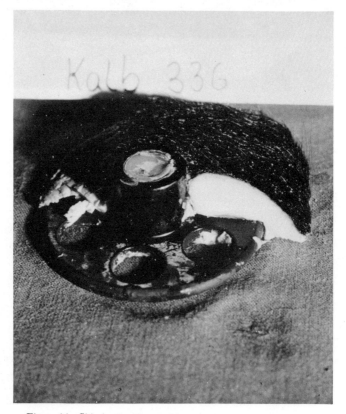

Figure 11. Skin button for extracorporeal energy transmission.

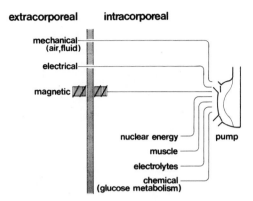

Figure 12. Energy source for incorporated blood pump.

quite nicely, but after several weeks abscesses did occur and the animals died of these infections.

The energy is also a problem especially if we want to bring it into the organism or to transmit energy into the body (Figure 12). Currently, the energy source is still outside the body and the pump is connected to it by a tube. Another possibility would be to use thin electrical wires. Many research groups, especially in Germany, are investigating the possibility of transmitting energy through the skin without a wound. The transmission of 1000 W/hr seems to be possible.

Of course, it would be most advantageous to use energy produced by the body itself, especially energy from chemical processes like glucose metabolism. This is indeed possible, but at the moment, the energy amount is so small that it is enough to drive a pacemaker but not an artificial heart. The greatest problem, without going into excessive detail, is that a few square meters of artificial material in contact with blood would be needed. The maximum energy needed is 5–6 W. However, if the efficiency of our driving system lies around 10–12%, the input must be around 50–60 W. The transmission of this energy by the drive system for our blood pump causes a certain amount of heat, and we have to consider whether the organism can dissipate it without a constant fever. From animal experiments we know that pigs are able to dissipate this heat without any difficulties.

Here, one returns to the problem mentioned earlier, the charging of an implanted battery from the outside. As mentioned, this would be fairly easy if one had a permanent connector on the surface of the body. The patient would then be able to move freely during the day and his battery could be charged during the night.

The preferred method, of course, would be to implant an energy source that would last a lifetime. At present, this is only conceivable with nuclear energy. From 50 to 60 g plutonium would drive an artificial heart for years, but the dangers of radiation are not satisfactorily under control. For research use, capsules with this amount of plutonium are being developed together with some kind of thermal engine, according to the principles of Rankine cycle engine and Sterling cycle engine. These machines, working with a temperature of over 1,000°C, can be insulated well enough for implantation. Experiments show that this approach could be realized, but, especially today, when nuclear radiation is regarded as being extremely dangerous, safety must come first, and this system cannot be applied. The radiation from 4 hr/wk contact with an animal carrying a nuclear capsule (at a distance of 45 cm) is less than the average environment radiation in the United States.

For the transmission of this energy, we need an actuator. This can be done mechanically by gas or fluid. To summarize, we have a blood pump, energy source, storage, and transmission; one hopes that one day everything can be implanted in the body. Last, but not least, we need a control system. The natural heart always works to supply as much blood as the organism actually needs. This need varies according to the various activities of the body. At rest, about 5 liters/min are enough; during periods of stress or hard work about 20 liters/min are necessary. It is quite easy to increase or decrease the perfusion volume of our blood pumps if the pump can be properly filled. The difficult problem is to determine how much the organism needs from moment to moment and how quickly any adjustment must be made by the mechanical heart.

Presently, regulation in our animal experiments is done by manually operated units according to Starling's law: cardiac output depends on atrial pressure. If atrial pressure increases, then, depending on the pressure-curve characteristics, cardiac output increases also. A careful look, however, tells us that the situation is not that simple (Figure 13). On a mock circulation loop, we see that the perfusion volume increases with increasing venous pressure, but the filling pressure is much higher than normal. Another important point is that the time available for filling is short. Therefore, a wider range of operating pressure is necessary (Figure 14). It is important to monitor the pressures, but presently we do not have an

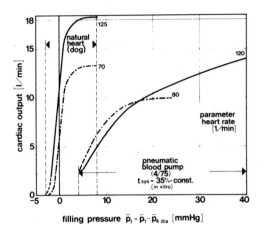

Figure 13. Starling's law of natural and artificial heart.

implantable pressure transducer that is stable enough to realize a fairly precise control.

A theorem of control theory states that the number of control variables must be smaller than or equal to the number of actuators of the system. In this case there are only *two* actuators: the cardiac output of the right ventricle and the cardiac output of the left ventricle. Out of the four pressures adjacent to the ventricles, two that can be controlled must be

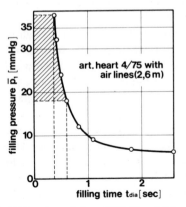

Figure 14. Filling time of the artificial heart (Type Berlin).

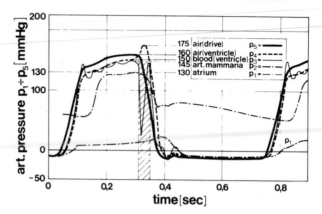

Figure 15. Comparison of driving pressure with the ventricular blood pressure.

selected. The best combination has to be selected on the basis of physiologic criteria.

We are currently investigating the possibility of regulating the driving system, which has no contact with blood. Actually, pressure in the driving system outside, in the air chamber, and in the blood chamber inside the chest, is all different (Figure 15). The important aspect of these curves is that at the end of systole there are a small peak in the air chamber curve and a straight fall in the blood chamber curve. This means that the membrane is distended to its endsystolic position, i.e., no more blood is ejected. If we could detect the beginning of this peak, we could regulate the ejection phase and also the filling phase.

This forward regulation perhaps is not enough because there are some other complications. For example, both pumps must provide, except for a few seconds, the same perfusion volume. If we watch only the right atrial and arterial pressure, the following could happen (Figure 16): The animal regulates itself very quickly by its peripheral resistance, which is increasing as seen in the figure. If the left pump does not respond immediately, or is not acting with a high reserve power, its perfusion volume decreases slightly. Otherwise, the right blood pump is working without any inhibition. The volume difference causes an increase of the left atrial pressure, which is followed by pulmonary edema. In this case it would be better to decrease the volume of the right pump. This is only one example, but it shows that we have to think both ways: first, in terms of normal perfusion pressures; second, in terms of protecting the organism from harm. After

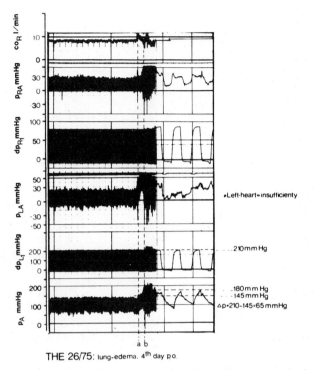

THE 26/75: lung-edema. 4th day p.o.

Figure 16. Driving and hemodynamic parameters during the occurrence of a hemorrhagic lung edema (animal experiment).

these general introductions we give a survey of our current status in animal experiments.

Although we are in a time of high standards within cardiac surgery, implant operation is major. A heart–lung machine takes over the blood transport and oxygenation for about 50–80 min, which results in some blood traumatization. The many tubes implanted interfere with other organ functions, especially the lung, and can, of course, cause dangerous thrombus formation in the circulatory system. Technical problems from surgery, especially bleeding, are rare. From our experiences with well over a hundred implantations on different animals, we feel that the most important point from the beginning is the position of the blood pumps (Figure 17). We test them very carefully by trying different positions, comparing rates of inflow of blood, and checking position by x-ray.

Special problems arise from the anatomy of the vena cava: the rigid

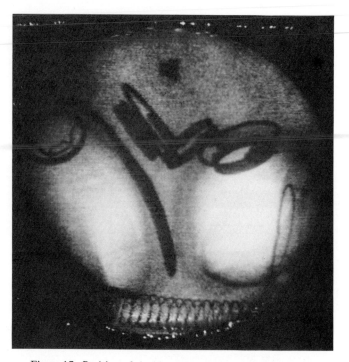

Figure 17. Position of the blood pump in the thoracic cavity.

housing of the pump can partly or completely occlude this thin-walled vein.

Most of our later problems are coming from the inflow. In many animals we see an increase of right atrial pressure without sufficient explanation. Valve insufficiency must also be discussed as a reason for higher blood volume, but in view of the curve from Starling's law, this higher pressure could be explained also by an increased perfusion volume (Figure 18). With all these measurements and with many implanted catheters, complications, especially thromboembolism and infection, can occur that can lead to termination of the experiment. Therefore, Dr. Kolff thinks that, first of all, surviving in good health is important and, therefore, measures only a few parameters in order not to endanger the animal. Perhaps because of his experience and including this precaution, he has the longest survival time of 95 days.

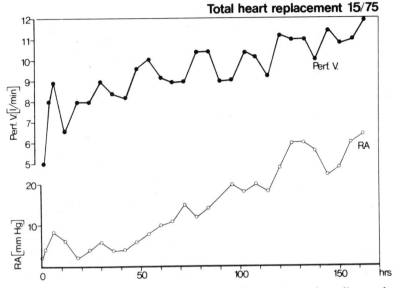

Figure 18. Increase of right atrial pressure and perfusion volume, depending on the surviving time.

We imagine that postoperative care is important. A weight gain in the experimental animal will be a serious problem in the future (Figure 19).

A few remarks on Dr. Atsumi's work in Japan should be included. The main difference is that their bilateral bypass-type, heart-assist pumps are fixed on the chest wall. The surprising thing is that their animals live for several weeks without infection.

If we draw a diagram of the survival times over the last 15 yr, we can be overoptimistic (Figure 20). First of all, we have to concede that these excellent results are rare. All over the world, I believe, out of roughly 600 experiments with total heart replacement, only three animals survived longer than 50 days and 50 more than 1 wk. We have to concede further that nearly all animals were connected with an energy source outside the body. This great progress is stimulating but, again, the deeper the investigation and the knowledge, the more problems become evident. At first, surgical and general technical difficulties were usually the main reasons for failure. In the second period, pathophysiology gave a broad spectrum of complications. We have seen pulmonary insufficiency, liver and kidney

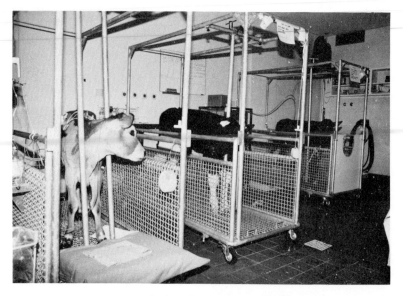

Figure 19. Intensive care unit in Berlin.

artifical heart - max. time of survival

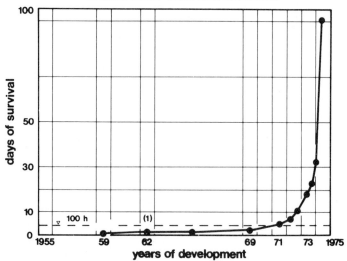

Figure 20. Statistics of the longest surviving time.

failure, gastrointestinal bleeding, electrolytes and metabolic changes, and many other signs of traumatization. Clotting problems with thrombus formation and embolism occurred in many animals. We have not yet overcome these complications; on the contrary, longer survival times will surely bring additional complications, especially from the artificial material.

All this could make us rather pessimistic; I am therefore happy to report that Dr. Kolff has successfully implanted an electrically driven prototype. This animal lived 21 days and was able to exercise on a treadmill. Measurements of the average power input correlated well with theoretical calculations.

Cardiovascular Flow Dynamics and Measurements
Edited by N. H. C. Hwang and N. A. Normann
Copyright 1977   University Park Press   Baltimore

chapter 24b

POWER SYSTEMS
FOR ARTIFICIAL HEARTS

Rainer Mohnhaupt and Volker Unger

Implantable circulatory assist devices and artificial heart (AH) systems for total replacement consist of five major components: energy source, energy storage, energy converters, transmission, and the blood pump. The different approaches for producing the hydraulic power and the limiting factors, which determine the design of these components, are discussed in this chapter. An implantable heart system is shown schematically and the interactions of a system like AH inside the body are demonstrated in Figure 1. These interactions are thermal load, radiation, tissue compatibility, infection, mechanical trauma of the blood, volume, noise, and vibration. Additionally, one has to design energy systems that are tolerated by the organism for long time. The major design criteria for the development of such systems are:

1. Size. A total volume of 1.5 liters and a weight of 1.5 kg can possibly be tolerated within the abdominal cavity and the chest.
2. Efficiency. Efficiency, the relation between useful hydraulic pump energy and useless energy, necessarily depends on the conversion process. Resultant energy in the form of heat and vibration needs to be minimized.
3. Service life. Because the replacement of defective mechanical components requires surgery, the desired durability should be at least 5, or better, 10 yr.
4. Body interaction. Thermal load, radiation, tissue compatibility, infection, mechanical damage of the blood, volume, noise, and vibration are the major factors (of Figure 1).
5. Price. This criterion can be discussed only on a relative basis. An estimated price of about $100,000 for a totally implantable nuclear power system constitutes probably the upper limit. Simpler systems can be designed, but one questions whether we can tolerate the greater restriction for the patient who has such a simpler system.

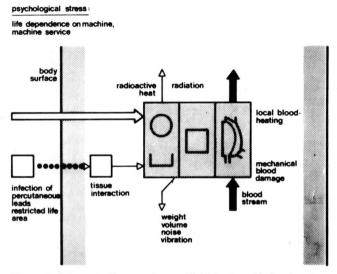

psychological stress:

life dependence on machine, machine service

body surface

radioactive heat   **radiation**

local blood-heating

mechanical blood damage

infection of percutaneous leads restricted life area

tissue interaction

blood stream

weight volume noise vibration

Figure 1. Schematic diagram of an artificial implantable heart system.

Figure 2 shows three different systems used today in animal experiments, the simplest at the top. Energy source, converters, and controls are located outside the body. The energy is transmitted to the blood pumps inside the chest by pneumatic gas tubes. The second system now in use for circulatory assist devices or total AH has thermal or electric energy storage, and the converter to hydraulic power is already inside the body. The electric energy is transmitted by a simple skin-transformer into the body. The system performance allows today an independence of 1–2 hr from external sources. The third system is the most advanced and all parts are implanted. From the view of energy it is totally independent for more than 10 yr. This ideal solution is today only possible with nuclear thermal energy sources. All technical problems for such a long time of service are not yet solved. Several thousand hours of continuous bench runs were performed, and a calf lived 1 wk with such a system.

Figure 3 shows an overview of all parts and technical approaches to perform the functions specified above: power source, storage, energy conversion, energy transmission, and consumption. Several technical solutions are already developed; others are in the stage of basic research. The different components and technical solutions of such power systems are discussed below.

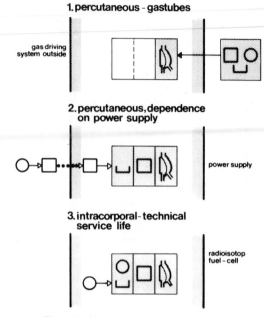

Figure 2. The three different AH systems.

RADIOISOTOPE
(Fowler, 1972; Mullins et al., 1972)

The criteria for radioisotope selection are:

1. Long half-life period.
2. High power density.
3. Radiation, which should be convertible almost totally into heat by a shielding of limited dimension and weight.
4. Decay products not harmful.
5. Moderate price.

The analysis of different radioisotopes as the thermal source for AH energy systems shows that today only ^{238}PU is suitable. ^{238}PU thermal sources are realized for artificial heart systems by several companies in the United States and used in several in vivo experiments. The half-life period is 87.5 yr. For 1 yr of service, about 80 g ^{238}PU are needed, which equals a power supply of about 50 W.

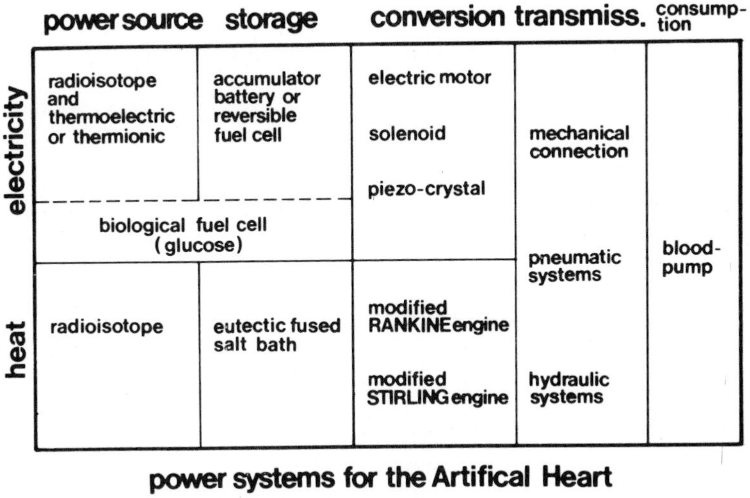

	power source	storage	conversion	transmiss.	consumption
electricity	radioisotope and thermoelectric or thermionic	accumulator battery or reversible fuel cell	electric motor		
			solenoid	mechanical connection	
			piezo-crystal		
	biological fuel cell (glucose)			pneumatic systems	blood-pump
heat	radioisotope	eutectic fused salt bath	modified RANKINE engine		
			modified STIRLING engine	hydraulic systems	

power systems for the Artifical Heart

Figure 3. Power systems for the AH.

THERMAL STORAGE
(Bleustein and Huffman, 1969; von Reth, 1974)

If energy is to be stored within the body, a low quotient of weight to stored energy has to be achieved. This storage is realized very effectively using the high melting heat of an eutectic mixture of salts. The parameters for such storage are:

1. Melting temperature.
2. Heat of fusion.
3. Weight.
4. Volume.
5. Chemical aggressivity.
6. Chemical stability.
7. By-products.

Three systems had been preferred until now:

1. NaF/LiF–Sodiumfluoride/Lithiumfluoride.
2. LiF/LiCL–Lithiumfluoride/Lithiumchloride.
3. LiH–Lithiumhydride.

The working temperature is about 650–800°C and the specific energy density ranges between 150 and 400 W-hr/liter. The storage capacity suitable for AH systems is about 30–100 W-hr. The heat loss through thermal isolation is about 4–6 W in realized systems.

RANKINE ENGINE AND STIRLING ENGINE
(Norman et al., 1968; Buck, 1969; Huffman, Robinson, and Kitrilakis, 1969; Martini, 1969; Peterson et al., 1969; Harmison, 1972; Harmison et al., 1972; Mott, 1972; Cole, Holman, and Mott, 1973; von Reth, 1974).

The thermodynamic conversion to hydraulic power to actuate the blood pump is possible using thermodynamic engines. Their working principles are based on two different thermodynamic processes:

1. Rankine-process with two phases: fluid and gas.
2. Stirling-process with only one phase: gas.

Both machines are manufactured for AH drive systems in the United States and Europe by different companies: Thermo Electron, Westinghouse Corp., Donald W. Douglas Labs, Aerojet-General Corp., Fluidonics Research Labs, and Messerschmitt-Bölkow-Blohm. Various bench models of both types are built. They differ in dimension, performance, and complexity.

Although lower in efficiency, the Stirling engine concept seems to be more promising for the future, because it needs fewer moving parts, which are the limiting factor for the machine's lifetime. Some machines are running only with frequencies of 1–2.5 Hz synchronized with the blood pump, reducing the hydraulic parts of the systems. But the efficiency is less than with engines running at 15–20 Hz as optimal frequency.

The aim of further development is to reduce the number of moving parts, to get high service life, and to improve the overall efficiency. An overall efficiency of 10% is achievable today. With heat sources (radioisotope or electric) of about 50 W, sufficient hydraulic power can be produced to pump the blood.

Depending on the engine type, different power transmission systems are used:

1. High hydraulic pressure of about 20 atm.
2. Low hydraulic pressure of about 1.3 atm. that is directly acting on a diaphragm type blood pump.
3. Mechanical transmission by a flexible shaft.

THERMOELECTRIC CONVERSION
(Allieri and Kudrick, 1971)

The thermal energy produced by a radioisotope or stored in thermal storage can be converted to electric energy by thermoelectric elements. Today, the efficiency of such elements is too small for AH driving systems. The Hittmann Corp. developed the most advanced thermoelectric power source with ^{238}PU, which produces 8 W with an efficiency of 12%. This was achieved by utilizing new materials arranged in a cascade system. After further development the converter may be suitable for AH systems. Today they are used as electric power sources for pacemakers. The power is about 9.7 W.

THERMIONIC CONVERSION
(Knapp, 1971)

The efficiency of thermionic converters is limited by the thermal conduction between the hot and cold plates of emitter and collector, but it can be improved by evacuating the converter. The decomposition of the emitter side of the element by the high temperature, 1500–2500°C, reduces the service life of the element. Some prototypes for pacemakers are already built. They are comparable in size and weight to chemical batteries, but they have longer service life.

ELECTRIC ENERGY STORAGE
(Hamlen et al., 1969)

The design criteria are:

1. High energy density.
2. No leakage.
3. Simple charge control.
4. High discharge rate.
5. Long service life.
6. Position independence.

The normal accumulator battery with different types of electrodes and electrolytes is not suitable for power consumption as high as the AH systems need. Different types are used as pacemaker batteries. They are used as short-time energy buffers in some circulatory assist devices.

REVERSIBLE FUEL CELL
(Miller and Glanfield, 1969)

The concept is based on the reversible fuel cell reaction. During charge mode the cell operates as an electrolysis cell and discharge is done by fuel cell reaction. In the charge mode water is electrolyzed to oxygen and hydrogen, which are stored in pressure-tight tanks. During discharge the two gases are combined and produce electrical power and water. General Electric developed a reversible fuel cell for the electrical energy storage for use with a circulatory assist device. The energy density of such a battery is about 40 W/kg with an overall efficiency of 28%. The high theoretic energy density of a fuel cell of about 3.6 kW/kg promises a much better performance for future developments. The problems today are caused by the decomposition of the electrolyte and the leakage of hydrogen.

BIOLOGIC FUEL CELL
(Batzold and Beltzer, 1969; Bocciarelli, 1969; Drake, 1969; Fishman and Henry, 1969; Giner and Malachesky, 1969; Kozawa et al., 1969)

The possibility of utilizing the dextrose and oxygen dissolved in blood for running a fuel cell to produce electric power for AH systems has been analyzed by several companies in the United States and Europe. Technically realized fuel cells are yet far from being sufficient for supplying power for AH systems. The problems on which the research is done are:

1. Oxygen reduction on different electrodes.
2. Active electrocatalysts for selective reduction.
3. Oxidation of glucose on different electrodes.
4. Fuel cell reaction in nearly neutral solution like blood.
5. Electrochemical kinetic problems at the surfaces.
6. Electrochemical reactions on other blood components.

Experimental fuel cells running with glucose and oxygen reach energy densities of about 1 mW/cm^2.

ELECTRODYNAMICAL CONVERSION

The energy conversion from electric power, which can come today only from outside the body, is widely used to run AH or circulatory assist devices in animal experiments. Electric motors, solenoids, and piezo-crystals are used for the conversion to mechanical or hydraulic power.

PIEZOELECTRIC CONVERTER
(Benson and Christie, 1969; Heimlich et al., 1969; Smiley et al., 1969; Smiley and O'Neill, 1972)

A piezoelectric driver consists of a number of thin piezoelectric ceramic disks. Applying a voltage, the thickness of the plates increases. This deflection is converted into hydraulic power to drive the blood pump. The piezoelectric converter has a good efficiency of 60–90% and the size is suitable. The problems are:

1. High voltage of up to 10 kV.
2. Low service life of the ceramic material.

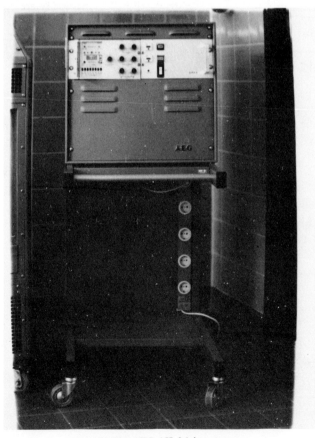

Figure 4. The AEG AH driving system.

3. Not implantable with today's electric energy storage.
4. Vibration.

SOLENOID CONVERTER
(Christie and Benson, 1969; Portner et al., 1973)

The solenoid energy converter is nearly the same in function, size, and technical feasibility as the piezo systems. The deflection of the solenoid is converted to hydraulic power. The overall efficiency of built systems can be as high as systems with good electric motors. The power density is about 50 W/kg and the efficiency is about 50%. Other problems arise with the complex electric control system.

ELECTRIC MOTOR
(Chambers, 1969; Griffith and Burns, 1969; Newgard, Woodbury, and Harmison, 1972)

The experimental systems with electric motors use piston pumps mechanically connected to the motor shaft, or rotational pumps, to produce the hydraulic power. Over a dozen different types of systems are built. They are also the oldest types of energy converters in the history of AH research.

The overall efficiency is about 40–50%, and, with a conventional battery pack as a storage system inside the body, could run 1.5 hr independently. The limiting factors are:

1. Mechanical wearing of the high-speed motors.
2. Efficiency of electric motors.

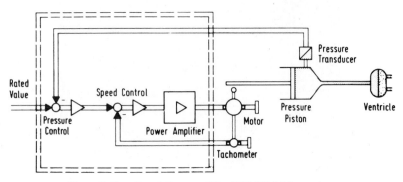

Figure 5. Functional diagram of the AEG AH driving system.

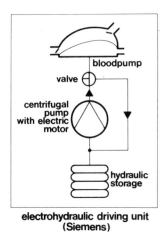

**electrohydraulic driving unit
(Siemens)**

Figure 6. Principle schematic of the Siemens left heart assist driving system.

TECHNICAL REALIZATION OF
THREE AH POWER SYSTEMS IN THE GERMAN AH PROJECT

In our current animal experiments for total artificial heart replacement, an extracorporeal driving unit is used, connected by two gas tubes with both

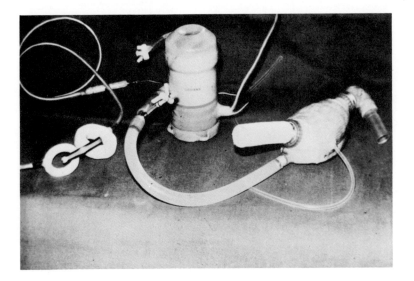

Figure 7. The Siemens–Westend Berlin implantable left heart assist system.

ventricles of the AH. With the last model (Figure 4), all driving parameters can be precisely maintained. The block diagram in Figure 5 shows the principle of operation of this unit built by AEG (Mohnhaupt and Mertig, 1974). The system consists of the pumping unit, the control unit, and the rated value generator. The main component is a low-inertia DC motor, which generates the pulsatile gas flow in the pneumatic cylinders by means of a rack-and-pinion mechanism. This concept ensures the required dynamics and decreased size. The driving unit is self-contained for 2 hr by means of high-performance batteries that are in the lower part of the housing. Further development is planned to control the driving parameters with a process control computer to avoid fatal incorrectness in handling the unit during animal experiments and to optimize the driving parameters automatically for different conditions at the AH.

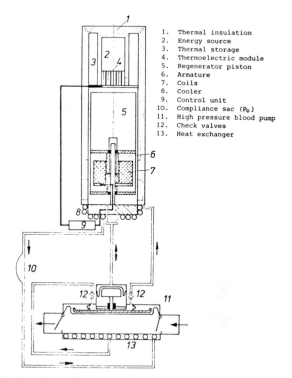

1. Thermal insulation
2. Energy source
3. Thermal storage
4. Thermoelectric module
5. Regenerator piston
6. Armature
7. Coils
8. Cooler
9. Control unit
10. Compliance sac (P_0)
11. High pressure blood pump
12. Check valves
13. Heat exchanger

Figure 8. Nuclear thermal energy converter for implantable AH systems build by MBB.

The Siemens Corp. (Haerten et al., 1974) developed, in cooperation with our group, several electrohydraulic driving systems for assist blood pumps. The unit consists of an implantable driving unit, a skin tunnel transformer for the transmission of electric power through the intact skin, and an extracorporeal power supply and control unit. Figure 6 shows the principle of the last design. It consists of a centrifugal pump combined with a brushless DC motor. The magnet rotor itself is the impeller of the pump. A valve is employed to reverse the flow during diastole and a hydraulic storage for a negative spring-loaded pressure during systole. The pump is activated only during the systolic cycle. The mean hydraulic power generated by this model is 2.7 W. This is sufficient to take over the whole work done by the left ventricle under normal physiologic conditions. The overall efficiency is about 5% (Figure 7).

The transcutaneous power transmission with the skin transformer is working well without biologic complications.

The MBB Corp. (von Reth, 1974) built several thermal converters on the basis of modified Stirling engine. The thermal energy can be supplied by a ^{238}PU capsule or a storage battery that is charged by electric power from outside the body. One of three models is shown in Figure 8. The

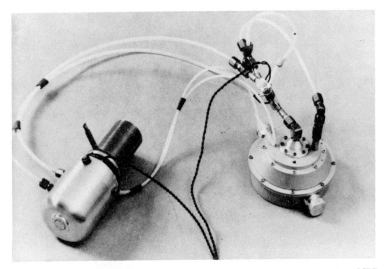

Figure 9. Working model of the thermal energy converter system for AH by MBB.

piston runs at frequencies synchronized with the pulsations of the blood pump, which must be connected to a pressure converter. The overall efficiency is now 3%. With a thermal power of about 55 W, sufficient hydraulic power for the AH system can be generated. With the thermal storage (100 W) the output of the blood pump can be maintained at 7 liters/min with a pressure at 120 mm Hg for 1 hr. Figure 9 shows a system with a high-pressure blood pump.

LITERATURE CITED

Allieri, F. D., and J. A. Kudrick. 1971. Implantable electrical power source for an AHS. Amer. Nucl. Soc. Trans. Washington, D.C.

Batzold, J. S., and M. Beltzer. 1969. Feasibility studies—Implantable biological fuel cell. Artif. Heart Progr. Conf. Proc., p. 817, Washington, D.C.

Benson, G. M., and J. W. Christie. 1969. Piezoelectric implantable energy converters. Artif. Heart Progr. Conf. Proc., p. 993, Washington, D.C.

Bleustein, M., and F. N. Huffman. 1969. Development of a heat source for an implantable circulatory support power supply. Artif. Heart Progr. Conf. Proc., Washington, D.C.

Bocciarelli, C. V. 1969. On the design of catalysts for biological fuel cells. Artif. Heart Progr. Conf. Proc., p. 861, Washington, D.C.

Buck, K. E. 1969. Development of a modified Stirling circle heart engine. Artif. Heart Progr. Conf. Proc., p. 1069, Washington, D.C.

Chambers, J. 1969. Implantable energy system for a cardiac assist device. Artif. Heart Progr. Conf. Proc., p. 945, Washington, D.C.

Christie, J. W., and G. M. Benson. 1969. Electromagnetic implantable energy conversion systems. Artif. Heart Progr. Conf. Proc., p. 969, Washington, D.C.

Cole, D. W., W. S. Holman, and W. E. Mott. 1973. Status of the USAEC nuclear-powered artificial heart. Amer. Soc. Artif. Int. Org. 19: 537.

Drake, R. F. 1969. Implantable fuel cell for an artificial heart. Artif. Heart Progr. Conf. Proc., p. 869, Washington, D.C.

Fishman, J. H., and J. F. Henry. 1969. Oxygen reduction on gold–palladium alloys in neutral media. Artif. Heart Progr. Conf. Proc., p. 825, Washington, D.C. 1969.

Fowler, E. E. 1972. Recent advances in applications of isotopes radiation in the United States—Artificial heart development. Isotop. Radiat. Tech. 9/3: 255.

Giner, J., and P. Malachesky. 1969. Anodic oxydation of glucose. Artif. Heart Progr. Conf. Proc., p. 839, Washington, D.C.

Griffith, Neil J., and Winton H. Burns. 1969. Development of an electro-hydraulic energy source to power and control circulatory assist devices. Artif. Heart Progr. Conf. Proc., p. 953, Washington, D.C.

Haerten, R., et al. 1974. In vitro and in vivo experiments with an implantable driving system for assist blood pumps. Europ. Soc. Artif. Organs I, Berlin.

Hamlen, R. P., E. G. Siwek, G. Rampel, and L. D. Wechsler. 1969. Internal energy storage for circulatory assist devices. Artif. Heart Progr. Conf. Proc., p. 1017, Washington D.C.

Harmison, L. T. 1972. Totally implantable nuclear heart assist and artificial heart. National Heart and Lung Institute, Washington, D.C.

Harmison, L. T., W. R. Martini, M. I. Rudnicki, and F. N. Huffman. 1972. Experience with implanted radioisotope-fuelled artificial hearts. Proc. 2nd Int. Symp. on Power from Radioisotopes, p. 731, Madrid.

Heimlich, L. A., P. D. Knerr, B. Hanson, R. Colville, and H. Chalifoux. 1969. High frequency piezoelectric motor pump for implanted energy conversion. Artif. Heart Progr. Conf. Proc., p. 1011, Washington, D.C.

Huffman, F. N., T. C. Robinson, and S. S. Kitrilakis. 1969. Development status of an implantable Rankine-cycle circulatory support system. Artif. Heart Progr. Conf. Proc., p. 1083, Washington, D.C.

Knapp, D. E. 1971. Thermionic and betavoltaic nuclear power sources for pacemaking. Amer. Nucl. Soc. Trans., Washington, D.C.

Kozawa, A., V. E. Zilionis, R. J. Brodd, and R. A. Powers. 1969. Search for a specific catalyst for electrochemical oxygen reduction in neutral NaCl solution. Artif. Heart Progr. Conf. Proc., p. 849, Washington, D.C.

Martini, W. R. 1969. Development of the thermocompressor as the power source for an artificial heart. Art. Heart Progr. Conf. Proc., Washington, D.C.

Miller, R. A., and E. J. Glanfield. 1969. Development of an electrical energy storage system for use with a circulatory assist device. Artif. Heart Progr. Conf. Proc., p. 1027, Washington, D.C.

Mohnhaupt, A., and L. Mertig. 1974. Pneumatic driving system for the artificial heart. Europ. Soc. Artif. Org. Vol. I, Berlin.

Mott, W. E. 1972. The USAEC nuclear-powered artificial heart program. Proc. 2nd Int. Symp. on Power from Radioisotopes, p. 713, Madrid.

Mullins, L. J., G. M. Matlack, J. Bubernak, and I. A. Leary. 1972. Characterisation and properties of biomedical 238 PU-fuels. Proc. 2nd Int. Symp. on Power from Radioisotopes, p. 49, Madrid.

Newgard, P. M., J. R. Woodbury, and L. T. Harmison. 1972. Implantable electrical power and control system for Artificial hearts. 7th IECEC Trans. 1972.

Norman, J. C., V. H. Covelli, W. F. Bernhard, and I. Spira. 1968. An implantable nuclear fuel console for an artificial heart. Trans. Amer. Soc. Artif. Int. Org. 14: 204.

Peterson, G. H., A. G. Kessler, G. H. Thorne, R. R. Clark, and O. L. Wood. 1969. All fluid control system to couple a Stirling engine gas compressor to left ventricular assist device. Artif. Heart Progr. Conf. Proc., p. 1093, Washington, D.C.

Portner, P. M., E. Dong, Jr., J. S. Jassawalla, and D. H. LaForge. 1973. Performance of an implantable controlled solenoid circulatory assist system. Amer. Soc. Artif. Int. Organs, 19.

Smiley, P. C., C. G. O'Neill, W. W. Olander, and J. C. Creighton. 1969. Development of a piezoelectric driver for an artificial left ventricle. Artif. Heart Progr. Conf. Proc., p. 981, Washington, D.C.

Smiley, P., and C. G. O'Neill. 1972. Development of an implantable, low-frequency piezoelectric driver for an artificial heart. 7th IECEC Trans.

von Reth, R. D. 1974. Development of an implantable thermal engine as power source for artificial blood pumps. Europ. Soc. Artif. Organs, Vol. I, Berlin.

Cardiovascular Flow Dynamics and Measurements
Edited by N. H. C. Hwang and Ñ. A. Normann
Copyright 1977   University Park Press   Baltimore

chapter 24c

PATHOPHYSIOLOGY OF CALVES WITH ARTIFICIAL HEARTS

John H. Lawson

An important series of problems associated with the artificial heart can be attributed to the body's justifiable suspicion of foreign objects. This suspicion is justifiable because foreign objects, including the artificial heart, can introduce infections. Artificial hearts—and particularly the artificial valves usually used with the artificial hearts—often cause hemolysis. In the face of infection, this hemolysis is accelerated.

The body reacts to the presence of foreign objects by trying to cover the objects. If, as in the case of the artificial heart, the object is in the blood stream, this attempt by the body to cover the object results in thrombus formation. Thrombus formation in turn leads to either reduced blood flow or thromboembolus, or both.

Infection caused by the artificial heart itself can be eliminated by standard techniques of sterilization. However, the most successful artificial hearts and ventricular assist devices (so far) are all pneumatically powered. Thus the power source is outside the body. Transferring the power to the artificial heart without introducing infection is difficult. Subcutaneous cuffs made from pyrolytic carbon or Dacron velour around the pneumatic drive lines, both of which promote tissue ingrowth, have been used with some degree of success (Fasching et al., 1975). Invasive monitoring is a less serious source of infection.

The eventual solution to the problem of infection lies in the development of implantable power sources. Two such power sources are being developed at this time. One is a plutonium power source with either a Stirling cycle or Rankine cycle engine (Smith et al., 1975). The other is an electric engine powered by rechargable batteries. The batteries could be recharged with a noninvasive high-frequency induction coil. Infection in calves is undoubtedly a greater problem than infection in humans would be.

Hemolysis leading to anemia, which may eventually lead to right heart failure, has been reported by several investigators (Honda et al., 1975). The principal cause of hemolysis appears to be the artificial valves used in the artificial heart. Early evidence indicates that the use of porcine xenografts, rather than valves made from Silastic or pyrolytic carbon, may reduce hemolysis. Saving the natural valves for use with the artificial heart is a surgically difficult but promising method of reducing hemolysis (Olsen et al., 1976).

The artificial heart itself is also responsible for some hemolysis. The amount of hemolysis can be greatly reduced if the heart is designed so that the moving portions of the heart do not touch (Kwan-Gett et al., 1970) and the optimal materials are used in the construction of the heart. Polyurethane hearts have kept calves alive for as long as 3 mo without transfusions and only slight anemia (Lawson et al., 1975). Reduction of infection also reduces the amount of hemolysis.

Thrombus formation may be encouraged in order to reduce thrombo-embolus through the promotion of a neo or pseudo intima. This is usually done by coating the interior of the artificial heart with Dacron fibrils. There is the possibility that the neo or pseudo intima may become thick enough to reduce the efficiency of the heart, thereby leading to rising venous pressures and eventual right heart failure (Lawson et al., 1975). There is evidence to indicate that the fibrils themselves often fail to adhere to the heart.

In artificial hearts with smooth intimas, thrombus formation is pathologic. It usually occurs in areas of low flow or in areas where there are sharp junctions (Lawson et al., 1975). One particularly troublesome area is usually around the atria and the inflow valves; in the artificial hearts we use at the University of Utah, in this area we have the junctions between the natural and the artificial atrium, and the artificial atrium and the artificial valve (Figure 1).

Thrombus buildup can lead to the reduced efficiency of the artificial heart. The reduced efficiency of the heart causes venous hypertension, which is quickly followed by the symptoms of right heart failure. These symptoms include increases in SGOT and indirect and total bilirubin, oliguria, and edema, particularly around the brisket of the calves. Less commonly, thrombus formation causes left heart failure with pulmonary edema followed by pulmonary failure. Even very brief periods of venous

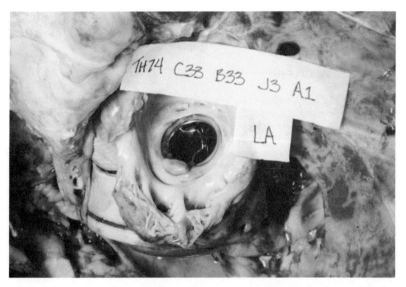

Figure 1. The left atrium and inflow valve of an artificial heart that kept a calf alive for 78 days. Note the large thrombus at the 7:00 o'clock position of the valve.

hypertension can be discerned in histopathologic examination of liver tissue and grossly by weighing the liver (Olsen et al., 1973). A normal calf's liver should weigh 1.65% of its total body weight. Calves that have had artificial hearts usually have livers that weigh 2–3% of their total body weight. This indicates that some degree of venous hypertension is common in calves with artificial hearts.

The occurrence of thromboembolus must be considered the greatest stumbling block in the path of the application of artificial hearts in humans. In our experience at the University of Utah, evidence of thromboembolic phenomena in the brain has been surprisingly rare, especially considering the frequent evidence of thromboemboli in the kidneys and the lungs of our calves (Olsen et al., 1975).

Improved methods of anticoagulation of our animals have reduced the occurrence of thromboemboli, but the ultimate elimination of the problem lies in improved heart designs and improved nonthrombogenic materials.

The development of nonthrombogenic materials with which to build a heart in which there are no areas of low flow or stagnation and no sharp junctures between materials, powered by an implantable power source, would eliminate the common pathology associated with the artificial heart, with which we are at this time familiar.

LITERATURE CITED

Fasching, W., M. Deutsch, U. Losert, et al. 1975. The "skin button:" A device for preventing infection along percutaneous lines. Amer. Soc. Artif. Int. Org. (ASAIO) Abstracts 4: 17.

Honda, T., Y. Kito, W. H. Gibson, J. V. Cockrell, and T. Akutsu. 1975. Circulatory pathophysiologic manifestations in two long-surviving calves with total artificial hearts. Cardiovasc. Dis. 2: 285.

Kwan-Gett, C. S., A. Kralios, T. Kessler, K. Backman, and W. J. Kolff. 1970. A prosthetic heart with hemispherical ventricles designed for lowered hemolytic action. Trans. Amer. Soc. Artif. Int. Org. 16: 409.

Lawson, J., E. Hershgold, D. B. Olsen, and W. J. Kolff. 1975. Comparison of polyurethane and silastic artificial hearts in 10 long survival experiments in calves. Trans. Amer. Soc. Artif. Int. Org. 21: 368.

Olsen, D., K. Van Kampen, J. Volder, and W. J. Kolff. 1973. Pulmonary, hepatic and renal pathology associated with the artificial heart. Trans. Amer. Soc. Artif. Int. Org. 19: 578.

Olsen, D., F. Unger, H. Oster, J. Lawson, T. Kessler, J. Kolff, and W. J. Kolff. 1975. Thrombus generation within the artificial heart. J. Thorac. Cardiovasc. Surg. 70: 248.

Olsen, D. B., J. Kolff, F. Stellwag, V. Ceccarelli, and H. Fukumasu. 1976. Saving the aortic and pulmonary artery valves with total heart replacement. Amer. Soc. Artif. Int. Org. Abstracts (in press).

Smith, L., D. Olsen, G. Sandquist, G. Arnett, S. Gentry, and W. J. Kolff. 1975. Power requirements for the A. E. C. artificial heart. Trans. Amer. Soc. Artif. Int. Org. 21: 540.

Cardiovascular Flow Dynamics and Measurements
Edited by N. H. C. Hwang and N. A. Normann
Copyright 1977   University Park Press   Baltimore

chapter 24d

RESULTS OF
70 EXPERIMENTS
IN CALVES WITH TOTAL
ARTIFICIAL HEARTS:
Causes of Death
and Problems

Tetsuzo Akutsu

INTRODUCTION

The first total artificial heart (TAH) implantation was performed in 1957 on a dog that survived 90 min (Akutsu and Kolff, 1958). Since that time extensive investigations have been performed all over the world. The initial goal of obtaining a 100-hour survivor, however, was not achieved until 1970. In 1971, the first 10-day survivor was reported by this laboratory (Akutsu et al., 1972). By 1973, other groups reported longer survivors (Nakasono et al., 1973; Kawai et al., 1974; Oster et al., 1976), and the first 25-day survivor was attained in this laboratory (Honda et al., 1975a). In 1974, one 94-day survivor was reported by Kolff's group (Lawson et al., 1975).

Recent progress in TAH experiments has resulted from the following factors. (1) Materials, design, and construction techniques have been improved, thus decreasing the incidence or grade of complications, such as hemolysis and breakage of the device, and leading to marked improvement in the function of the TAH. (2) An optimal control-driving condition has

Supported by the United States Public Health Service Contract No. NIH-NHLI-69-2185, Grant No. HL18084 and NSF No. GF34912.

been established with the aid of electronic and mechanical technology resulting in a more physiologic pumping pattern resembling the natural heart. (3) Long-term survivals have given us a chance to study the pathophysiology of the TAH implanted animal, and in turn, the understanding of the pathophysiology has led to further improvement of the experimental procedure.

This chapter describes causes of death of 70 calves implanted with the TAH between March 1971 and June 1975, and discusses major problems involved.

MATERIALS AND METHODS

Our air-driven TAH made of silicone rubber was designed to be implanted inside the pericardial sac of calves (Figure 1). Details of the device, the control and driving system, and the pumping procedure have already been reported (Akutsu, 1970; Akutsu, Takagi, and Takano, 1970; Akutsu et al., 1972).

Calves weighing 70–98 kg (average 82 kg) were used. They were checked particularly for upper respiratory infection and pneumonia; oral feeding was withheld for 24 hr prior to surgery. Anesthesia was induced by intravenous administration of sodium thiamylal 30 min after injection of 1 mg of Atropine, and was maintained with 0.5–1.0% Fluothane following intubation. Respiration was maintained by a mechanical respirator and was continued even during total heart–lung bypass. Every 15 min the lungs were manually inflated with an inspiratory pressure of approximately 20 cm H_2O. A muscle relaxant, succinylcholine chloride, was administered intravenously when the calf moved and spontaneous breathing appeared. The chest was opened through the left fifth intercostal space.

A bubble oxygenator was primed with 1 liter of heparinized fresh blood and 2 liters of lactated Ringer's solution. Sodium heparin (3 mg/kg) was injected prior to cannulation. After experiment no. 48, 30 mg/kg of methylprednisolone sodium succinate was administered before extracorporeal circulation (ECC) was started.

Following total excision of the natural heart, the device was connected in sequence to the right atrium, left atrium, aorta, and pulmonary artery. Residual air in the TAH was replaced with carbon dioxide first as a precaution against possible air embolism and then filled with heparinized saline. TAH pumping was begun at the time the ECC was stopped. All

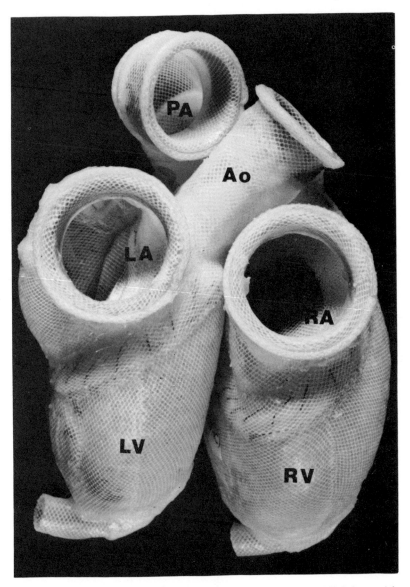

Figure 1. Akutsu total artificial heart. AO, aorta; LA, left atrium; LV, left ventricle; PA, pulmonary artery; RA, right atrium; RV, right ventricle.

residual fluid left in the oxygenator was gradually infused back to the calf while watching both atrial pressures and the arterial pressure.

All monitoring tubes and wires were exteriorized through the chest wall and the chest was closed in routine fashion. Continuous and simultaneous monitoring and recording of pressures were obtained in both atrial, aorta, and pulmonary artery. The cardiac output was also continuously recorded from the pulmonary artery by means of an electromagnetic flowmeter. Routine hematologic, biochemical, and bacteriologic examinations were carried out periodically. Fluid output and intake were calculated every 8 hr, and fluid balance was corrected every day. A broad spectrum antibiotic (4 g of sodium cephalothin/day) was administered to prevent infection, and sodium heparin (5 mg/kg/day) was given as an anticoagulant. At autopsy, the lungs, kidneys, liver, and spleen were examined for histopathologic alterations.

RESULTS

Figure 2 shows causes of death and the number of calves which died from each cause. The calves were divided into two groups according to their survival time; 43 calves that lived less than 100 hr and 27 calves which survived longer than 100 hr.

Group 1

Twenty-four calves out of 43 died from technical and mechanical failures (Figure 3). Breakage of the device caused seven deaths; surgical failure, seven; accident, seven; failure of the driving console, two; and failure of cardiopulmonary bypass, one.

Breakage of the device occurred only on the left side where the driving air pressure was 100 mm Hg higher than on the right side. When the pumping chamber broke, systemic air embolization occurred and the breakage of the outer housing resulted in pneumothorax. Various accidents involved the following: (1) massive bleeding caused by slippage of the left internal mammary artery catheter used for monitoring of the arterial pressure and (2) "cardiac arrest" caused by either slippage of the driving air tube or its accidental obstruction.

Failure of the unilateral driving system resulted in an insufficient air supply to the corresponding side and overpumping on the other side, eventually causing low cardiac output.

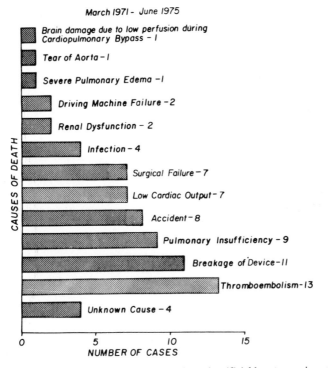

Figure 2. Causes and numbers of deaths in 70 total artificial heart experiments.

In one calf low perfusion pressure during cardiopulmonary bypass caused brain damage.

The causes of death of the remaining 19 calves were pulmonary insufficiency (eight deaths), low cardiac output (four deaths), thromboembolism (three deaths), and unknown causes (four deaths).

Pulmonary insufficiency was classified as either an acute type or a terminal type. The acute type was characterized by poor oxygenation when TAH pumping was begun. PaO_2 and arterial blood oxygen saturation (SaO_2) were 40 mm Hg and 70%, respectively; pH and $PaCO_2$ were usually within the normal range in these cases. Pulmonary artery pressure was 50 mm Hg, or even higher, immediately after the start of pumping, suggesting increased pulmonary artery resistance. The pulmonary histology in such a case is shown in Figure 4. There was a patchy distribution of pulmonary

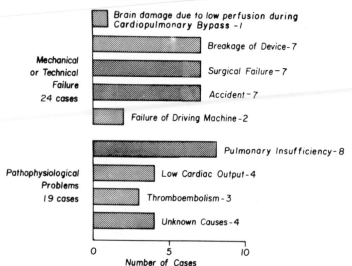

Figure 3. Group I. 43 calves that survived less than 100 hr.

edema characterized by alveolar spaces distended and filled with pink frothy material. The terminal type of pulmonary failure was usually accompanied by surgical complications such as traumatic damage of the left lung, atelectasis, hemothorax, etc. Death of these calves occurred within 3 days following gradual respiratory disorders.

Symptoms observed in four calves, whose causes of death were not determined, were rapid general deterioration within 50 hr after surgery accompanied by excessive bleeding, oliguria, or failure to recover from anesthesia.

Group 2

Among 27 calves that survived longer than 100 hr (Figure 5), five survived over 200 hr; the longest survival was 25 days. Average survival time was 177 hr. In this group, 74% of the deaths occurred from causes related to pathophysiologic problems: thromboembolism, ten deaths; infection, four; low cardiac output, three; renal dysfunction, two; and pulmonary insufficiency, one. The remaining seven calves died from mechanical or technical failures.

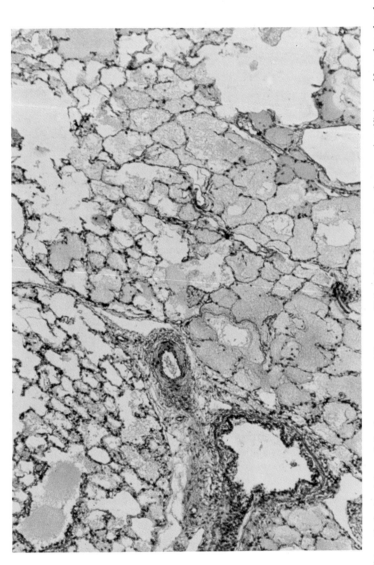

Figure 4. Histopathologic picture of the lung recovered from a calf that died from acute pulmonary insufficiency. Note that alveolar spaces are filled with frothy materials and distended. (Hematoxylin and eosin; original magnification × 63).

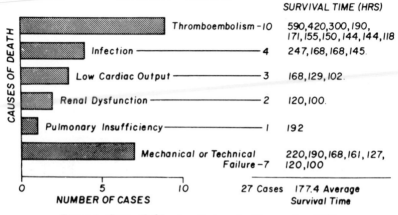

Figure 5. Group II. 27 calves that survived longer than 100 hr.

Frequency of thromboembolism was 37%. Typical clinical symptoms originating from affected organs such as the brain, lungs, and kidneys were convulsion, shortness of breath, and hematuria. At autopsy both lungs revealed multiple areas of hemorrhage in the peripheral portions probably caused by small infarctions; however, macroscopic infarcts, necrotic areas, and thromboemboli were found in only one calf. Histopathologic findings were interstitial edema, intraalveolar hemorrhage, focal collections of polymorphonuclear leukocytes, or multiple microthromboemboli. The kidney occasionally showed macroscopic multiple infarcts in the cortical area involving approximately 5–15% of both kidneys. Thromboemboli of renal arterioles and tubular necrosis were typical findings with renal infarction. Pathologic alterations of the stomach, gall bladder, small intestine, and mesentery were found in only two severe cases and were noted as several focal areas of hemorrhage, infarction, and necrosis. Thrombi formations inside the device were usually found in the transitional area from the atrium to the inlet valve and also at the bottom of both biscuspid-type outlet valves. Their size varied from 2X2X2 to 8X8X8 mm.

Insufficient cardiac output (absolute or relative) was seen in the following two occasions: (1) interference with the venous return when the metal ring embedded in the right atrial connector was pressing down on the inferior vena cava causing partial occlusion, and (2) development of excessive venous return to the TAH, which has a limited functional capacity. Symptoms resulting from the second situation became evident toward the terminal stage of experiments when the circulating blood volume increased in the presence of severe anemia or infection. The arterial pressure gradually decreased as deterioration proceeded. Although the total peripheral resistance decreased, the cardiac output did not increase after the maximum pumping capacity of the TAH had been reached. Consequently, the right atrial pressure rose to as high as 30 mm Hg in some calves. At autopsy, liver damage caused by long-lasting high atrial pressure was revealed. This was evidenced macroscopically by the swollen parenchyma, tense capsule, bluish-brown or purple surface, and yellow degeneration on cut section and, microscopically, by central necrosis with surrounding hemorrhage, hemorrhage around the central vein, fatty degeneration, and vacuole formation.

Four calves were terminated due to irreversible endotoxin shock by infection with *Escherichia coli* and *Pseudomonas aeruginosa.* In severe cases, the white blood cell count increased to over 30,000 and the body temperature rose to 42°C.

Two calves died from renal dysfunction; one calf had polyuria with a daily urine output of 23 liters and the other, on the contrary, went into anuria, probably due to renal shutdown caused by transfusion of mismatched donor blood.

Only one calf developed pulmonary insufficiency from pneumothorax; progressive deterioration of pulmonary function made us terminate the experiment after 192 hr of pumping.

Accidental death occurred in seven calves as follows: asphyxia, one; breakage of the device, four; rupture of the remnant aorta, one; pulmonary edema resulting from accidental hemo-pneumothorax, one. One calf, while standing, was strangulated by a canvas band that had been placed around her forelegs and neck to help her stand up. The accident occurred on the 10th postoperative day. Another calf died after 120 hr of pumping from massive bleeding caused by rupture of the remnant aorta. The aortic tissue, fixed by a single tie around the ring of the artificial aorta, developed ischemic necrosis resulting in sudden rupture.

DISCUSSION

The causes of death associated with the TAH can be classified into two categories: (1) technical and mechanical failures and (2) pathophysiologic problems. In the early stage deaths were mainly attributable to technical and mechanical problems and most of them occurred within 100 hr of pumping. As every phase of the entire procedure, from the design of the TAH through the postoperative care of the experimental animals, was improved and the survival time became longer, problems directly related to artificial heart pumping or relevant to pathophysiologic alterations came to the front.

Some of the innovations and procedures that contributed to the elimination of technical and mechanical failures are as follows. (1) Design of the outflow area of the left ventricle was changed so that the material in this area would not be subjected to excessive stress during ejection. (2) Fabrication techniques were changed, particularly in relation to the seam-lines in the layering of silicone rubber materials. (3) Two drive lines and all monitoring tubes were rearranged to prevent slippage, kinking, and snagging by the calf's leg. (4) In addition to the calf's body weight, the chest size was also considered for fitting of the device. (5) The control-driving console was put into operation and tested 24 hr before implantation surgery.

Figure 6 shows the interrelationships between each step of the entire procedure and the major problems encountered. Although some of these have been solved, those that have been particularly perplexing or cannot be solved at this time are discussed here. They include pulmonary insufficiency, infection, high right atrial pressure, and thromboembolism.

Acute pulmonary insufficiency, characterized by drastically poor oxygenation immediately after the beginning of TAH pumping, has been reported elsewhere (Akutsu et al., 1964; Honda et al., 1974). These calves showed PaO_2 as low as 40 mm Hg and never recovered. In general, mechanisms of pulmonary insufficiency can be divided into three major categories: (1) inadequate ventilation of the alveoli, (2) reduced gaseous diffusion through the respiratory membrane, and (3) decreased oxygen transport from the lungs to the tissues.

The cause of acute pulmonary insufficiency was thought to be related to the extracorporeal circulation (ECC), i.e., loss of surfactant, traumatic damage of blood cells in the pump oxygenator, hypoperfusion of the lung tissue, microthromboembolism in the pulmonary vessels, and opening of arteriovenous shunts in the pulmonary vascular bed. Wilson et al. (1970) have recently reported that ECC causes a hemodynamic condition similar to "controlled shock" and the pathologic picture of the pulmonary insufficiency found after the extracorporeal circulation was similar to that found in induced hemorrhagic shock. They stated that increased vascular perme-

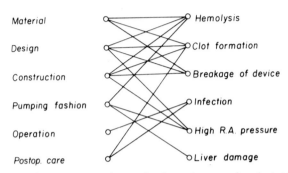

RELATIONSHIPS BETWEEN STEPWISE PROCEDURES OF TAH
AND MAJOR COMPLICATIONS

Material — Hemolysis

Design — Clot formation

Construction — Breakage of device

Pumping fashion — Infection

Operation — High R.A. pressure

Postop. care — Liver damage

Figure 6. Relationship between each step for the entire procedure in total artificial heart experiment and major complications.

ability and obstruction of pulmonary capillaries by leukocyte adherence, triggered by unknown mechanisms, might result in interstitial edema, hemorrhage into the alveoli, pulmonary edema, and shunting in the pulmonary vascular bed. Such pathologic alterations were successfully prevented when experimental animals were treated with an anti-inflammatory drug. We also thought that alveolocapillary block caused by inadequate perfusion and opening of arteriovenous shunts might have been responsible for pulmonary insufficiency in our experimental animals.

Keeping these facts in mind, management of the lung during implantation of the TAH was improved. The flow rate was maintained at approximately 70 ml/kg to keep the mean arterial pressure above 60 mm Hg, and moderate hypothermia was also applied when venous return was poor. In addition, two other steps were taken: (1) administration of 30 mg/kg of methylprednisolone sodium succinate before the ECC and (2) continuation of normal, intermittent, positive-pressure breathing through the entire course of surgery and periodic large inflations of the lung even during total perfusion. The second procedure prevented atelectasis or collapse of the alveoli more effectively than constant inflation (Edmunds and Austen, 1965). Thereafter, the frequency of acute pulmonary insufficiency in our laboratory has been markedly reduced. Terminal, pulmonary insufficiency is a secondarily induced phenomenon related to postoperative complications such as traumatic damage of the left upper lobe, pneumothorax, or hydro- or hemothorax.

Severe infection leading to septic shock was a major problem in the early stage. *Pseudomonas* and *E. coli* were always found as pathogenic microorganisms and experiments were terminated when septic shock developed. Specific situations in TAH experiments that readily lead to infection are as follows: (1) implantation of a large foreign body, (2) surgical wound not completely sealed because of external control-driving system and monitoring, and (3) frequent blood sampling and administration of drugs through monitoring lines. In addition to these factors related to the postoperative care, a preexistent factor, viz., that the calf is vulnerable to respiratory infection, must also be considered. Strict aseptic procedures and proper use of broad-spectrum antibiotics before, during, and after implantation surgery are of prime importance.

The incidence of high right atrial pressure (RAP) in long-term survivals has been previously described by our laboratory as well as by others (Akutsu et al., 1972; Moulopoulos, Jarvick, and Kolff, 1973; Honda et al., 1974; Urzua et al., 1974). The clinical and pathologic expressions are oliguria, ascites, hepatomomegaly, and central necrosis of the liver. The mechanism of its occurrence can be explained as follows. The TAH function curve in animal experiments is less steep than that of the natural heart (Figure 7). Because our TAH is driven by a manually regulated control-driving system, only one cardiac function curve is available under a certain set condition, which means that the cardiac output is completely controlled by venous return. Point A in Figure 7 shows the normal equilibrium point of the cardiac output and venous return of the natural heart. Point B is the initial equilibrium point of the TAH. The RAP stays within a reasonable range unless the venous return curve shifts. When the venous return curve shifts to the right, a new equilibrium point is established at point C because the cardiac function curve of the TAH is constant. Accordingly, a high RAP results. After the venous return has exceeded the pumping capacity of the TAH, RAP rises continuously unless the pathologic hemodynamic condition is corrected. The following factors cause a shift of the venous return curve to the right: (1) increase in the mean systemic pressure, (2) decrease in the peripheral vascular resistance, and (3) a combination of both (Guyton, Jones, and Coleman, 1973). They will possibly develop by numerous causes such as nervous stimulation, infection, hypervolemia, blood damage, respiratory insufficiency, drug effects, body movement, etc. Among these factors we have found that high RAP is closely related to anemia. Causes leading to anemia

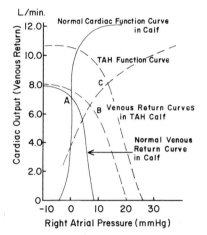

Figure 7. Graphical analysis of cardiac function curve and venous return curve in total artificial heart implanted calf.

can also be numerous and include blood damage induced during the heart–lung bypass as well as by the TAH pumping, blood loss, postoperative malnutrition, and infection. Anemia causes decrease in blood viscosity, decrease in oxygen transport, decrease in peripheral vascular resistance, increase in circulating blood volume, and, subsequently, increase in venous return. As long as the degree of increase in venous pressure does not exceed the pumping capacity of the TAH, RAP should remain normal. Since this mechanism was discovered, particular attention has been paid to maintaining hematocrit as close to the normal value as possible, and prevention of central necrosis of the liver has been successfully achieved (Honda et al., 1974). It is of prime importance to maintain the physiologic state of the experimental calves within a reasonable range so that the TAH with a limited capacity can fulfill the calves' metabolic demand, if possible, with normal cardiac output and RAP maintained reasonably low, thus eliminating the phenomenon of "right heart failure" (Honda et al., 1975*b*). It is necessary, however, for the device to be provided with low-resistance inflow valves, high compliance ventricular walls, and a sufficient cardiac reserve.

Thromboembolism, a major cause of death, killed 13 calves out of 70 (18.6%). It exhibited a mixture of clinical symptoms because the features of its onset and complications depended upon the damaged organs. The main manifestations were abnormal movement of the extremities, convulsion, hematuria, and dyspnea. In fact, thrombi formed inside the device may have scattered all over the body, but the main clinical symptoms were usually related to the brain and kidneys.

Three major factors are conceivably responsible for clot formation: (1) design and construction of the device, (2) physical and chemical properties of the materials, and (3) the blood coagulation status of the animal. Although approximately 40 different models of artificial hearts have been reported to date (Akutsu, 1975), none of these have been satisfactory in terms of nonthrombogenicity. It has been emphasized by every investigator that the design should eliminate any recess, groove, or pocket where blood might stagnate and result in clot formation. Definitive design criteria, however, have not yet been established. Materials presently in use for fabrication of the device were not originally developed for medical use. Although silicone rubber has been considered one of the best and most widely used materials, its surface property, as well as its physical property, in terms of durability, needs further improvement. In addition, it should be borne in mind that results are also related to the technique in handling of each material.

Imperfection of the material in antithrombogenicity can be compensated for to some extent by the use of anticoagulants. It is well known that whatever the surface, the initial common event in the interaction of blood with a foreign surface is rapid deposition of a strongly adherent proteinaceous film. Thereafter, according to a report by Mustard and Pakcham (1970), ADP-induced platelet aggregation plays a most important role in triggering clot formation. Mansfield, Sauvage, and Smith (1974) reported the important role of white blood cells and concluded that combined administration of Coumadin, Persantine, and aspirin was most effective. In four series of experiments such an anticoagulant regimen was used only in five recent calves; heparin was used in most of the calves. The results, however, did not show any significant difference.

SUMMARY

1. From March 1971 to June 1975, 70 artificial heart implantation experiments were carried out using calves weighing an average of 82 kg. The calves can be divided into two groups: 43 (61%) that survived less than 100 hr and 27 (39%) that survived longer than 100 hr. Five calves survived over 200 hr, and the longest survival was 25 days.

2. The calves in the first group (43 cases) died mainly from technical and

mechanical failures. Those early technical and mechanical failures were gradually eliminated with the improvements in every phase of the experiment. Consequently, in the second group 74% of the deaths were due to pathophysiologic problems.

3. Severe infection, which resulted in septic shock and killed four calves, was seen only in the early stage of the experiments. However, infection will be a serious problem when the survival time becomes longer.

4. Pulmonary insufficiency, which used to be one of the perplexing problems in TAH experiments, has been successfully eliminated by improving the respiratory management during ECC and postoperative care.

5. The mechanism of high right atrial pressure, which could not be controlled simply by readjusting the driving condition, has been elucidated. It is important to maintain physiologic parameters at a normal level to avoid an excessive increase in venous return. With this in mind, liver damage caused by high right atrial pressure has been remarkably reduced.

6. Regardless of postoperative anticoagulant therapy, clot formation inside the TAH and thromboembolism were revealed in most calves that survived longer than 100 hr.

ACKNOWLEDGMENTS

These 70 experiments were performed mainly at the University of Mississippi, Jackson, Mississippi, from 1971 to 1974. I would like to express my sincere appreciation to all the professional people and technicians who participated in this project during that time and who devoted their time, day and night, to this work.

LITERATURE CITED

Akutsu, T. 1970. Design criteria for artificial heart valves. J. Thor. Cardiovasc. Surg. 60: 34.

Akutsu, T. 1975. Artificial Heart; Partial Support and Total Replacement. Igakushoin Tokyo, Japan. pp. 92–353.

Akutsu, T., and W. J. Kolff. 1958. Permanent substitutes for valves and hearts. Trans. Amer. Soc. Artif. Intern. Org. 4: 230.

Akutsu, T., S. R. Topas, V. Mirkovitch, E. Panayotopoulos, and W. J. Kolff. 1964. Problems in calf lungs immediately after implantation of an artificial heart. Trans. Amer. Soc. Artif. Intern. Organs. 10: 162.

Akutsu, T., H. Takagi, and H. Takano. 1970. Total artificial hearts with built-in valves. Trans. Amer. Soc. Artif. Intern. Org. 16: 392.

Akutsu, T., H. Takano, H. Takagi, M. D. Turner, E. C. Henson, and J. W.

Crowell. 1972. Pathophysiology and new problems in total artificial heart. J. Thor. Cardiovasc. Surg. 64: 762.

Edmunds, L. H., and W. G. Austen. 1965. Effect of ventilation and pulmonary arterial occlusion during cardiopulmonary bypass on pulmonary function. Surg. Forum 16: 180.

Guyton, A. C., C. E. Jones, and T. G. Coleman. 1973. Circulatory Physiology: Cardiac Output and Its Regulation. W. B. Saunders, Philadelphia. pp. 137–492.

Honda, T., Y. Kito, W. H. Gibson, T. Nemoto, J. V. Cockrell, and T. Akutsu. 1974. Lung problems and liver damage in total artificial heart and their prevention. Trans. Amer. Soc. Artif. Intern. Org. 20: 27.

Honda, T., Y. Kito, W. H. Gibson, T. Nemoto, J. V. Cockrell, and T. Akutsu. 1975a. One 25-day survivor with total artificial heart. J. Thor. Cardiovasc. Surg. 69: 92.

Honda, T., I. Nagai, S. Nitta, S. R. Igo, C. H. Edmonds, C. W. Hibbs, Y. Kito, J. M. Fuqua, and T. Akutsu. 1975b. Evaluation of cardiac function and venous return curves in awake, unanesthetized calves with an implanted total artificial heart. Trans. Amer. Soc. Artif. Intern. Org. 21: 1975.

Kawai, J., J. Volder, F. M. Donovan, and W. J. Kolff. 1974. Long-term effects of the artificial heart. Ann. Surg. 179: 362.

Lawson, J., E. Hershgold, J. Kolff, D. B. Olsen, and W. J. Kolff. 1975. A comparison of polyurethane and silastic artificial hearts in ten long survival experiments in calves. Trans. Amer. Soc. Artif. Intern. Org. 21 (in press).

Mansfield, P. B., L. R. Sauvage, and J. C. Smith. 1974. Factors influencing thrombus generation in artificial hearts. Presented at the Symposium on Coronary Artery Medicine and Surgery. Texas Heart Institute, Houston, Texas, February.

Moulopoulos, S. D., R. Jarvick, and W. J. Kolff. 1973. State II problems in the project of the artificial heart. J. Thor. Cardiovasc. Surg. 66: 662.

Mustard, J. F., and M. A. Pakcham. 1970. Factors influencing platelet function: adhesion release and aggregation. Pharmacol. Rev. 22: 97.

Nakasono, M., T. Koami, K. Koiso, T. Agishi, and Y. Nose. 1973. One seventeen day survivor with intrathoracic artificial heart. Artif. Org. (Japan) 2 (Supplement): 117.

Oster, H., D. Olsen, T. H. Stanley, J. Volder, and W. J. Kolff. 1976. Artificial heart implantation with 19 days survival. Ann. Surg. (in press).

Urzua, J., R. J. Kiraly, J. I. Wright, R. Cloesmeyer, and Y. Nose. 1974. A rationally designed artificial heart for calves. Trans. Amer. Soc. Artif. Intern. Org. 20: 660.

Wilson, J. W., N. B. Ratlife, D. B. Hackel, E. Mikat, and T. Graham. 1970. Inflammatory response in reaction of lung to acute hemodynamic injury. Immunopathology of inflammation proceedings of a symposium of the International Inflammation Club, 1970.

Cardiovascular Flow Dynamics and Measurements
Edited by N. H. C. Hwang and N. A. Normann
Copyright 1977   University Park Press   Baltimore

Index

TCH CARDIOLOGY